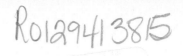

As a third-generation pediatric radiologist following in the footsteps of Drs. John Caffey and Frederic N. Silverman, I dedicate this book to the founding members of the Society for Pediatric Radiology (1958) and the European Society of Pediatric Radiology (1964).

Foreword

Ever since Dr. Hooshang Taybi began his career in radiology 43 years ago, his thirst for knowledge and his phenomenal memory have both amazed and benefited his colleagues from many fields of medicine. The first edition of his important work *Radiology of Syndromes* premiered in 1975. The most recent fourth edition—greatly expanded to cover the radiologic and clinical manifestations of over 1000 syndromes, metabolic disorders, and skeletal dysplasias, as well as a Gamuts chapter describing another 1250 entities—was published in 1996 under the title *Radiology of Syndromes, Metabolic Disorders, and Skeletal Dysplasias.*

In this *Handbook of Syndromes and Metabolic Disorders: Radiologic and Clinical Manifestations,* Dr. Taybi now makes available a concise version, almost in the form of a vade mecum, as a rapid recognition vehicle for the clinical and radiologic features of almost 700 conditions. Many bear descriptive, eponymic, mnemonic, or otherwise contrived names that may be unfamiliar to physicians who are not regularly engaged in recognizing syndromes but who do confront them in their professions. Frequently, a consultant in dysmorphology, genetics, or another clinical speciality may suggest a diagnosis that the attending physician, physician in training, or student cannot readily confirm. No comprehensive source of information to help verify or discard such suggested diagnoses has been available. In this newest publication, however, which lists conditions alphabetically and describes their clinical and radiologic manifestations thoroughly, Dr. Taybi now helps the reader to accept or discard a proffered diagnosis. The fourth edition of Dr. Taybi's standard reference book provides additional information and pertinent literature references.

The only similar compendium of syndromes of which I am aware is the *Encyclopedia of Medical Syndromes* by Robert H. Durham, published in 1960. In his foreword to that work, Dr. Tinsley Harrison states, "The syndromes...collected and clarified are so numerous that most of them cannot be mentioned in a textbook. Even in a dictionary, which must cover the whole range of medical words and phrases, these clinical patterns must either be omitted entirely or dismissed with a line or two." In the decades since Dr. Harrison's statement, the number of syndromes has increased exponentially. This *Handbook of Syndromes and Metabolic Disorders: Radiologic and Clinical Manifestations*, like Dr. Taybi's other contributions, will serve to remedy the difficulty in classifying them for some time to come.

Frederic N. Silverman, M.D.

Preface

The fourth edition of *Radiology of Syndromes, Metabolic Disorders, and Skeletal Dysplasias* was published in 1996. That book contains over 1000 entries—707 syndromes, 178 metabolic disorders, and 137 skeletal dysplasias. Another 1250 syndromes, metabolic disorders, skeletal dysplasias, and complex malformations are included in the Gamuts chapter. The comprehensive book is used as a reference source in hospital libraries and radiology and genetics departments, as well as in departments of pediatrics, orthopedics, and internal medicine.

Working from the bulk of information in my complete work, I have prepared this manageable and affordable *Handbook of Syndromes and Metabolic Disorders* for quick reference by radiologists and other physicians in their daily practices, as well as by medical students and physicians in training.

I have chosen not to include figures and references in this concise resource so that a maximum number of entities—691 total syndromes and metabolic disorders—can be included in this manual format.

I would like to acknowledge Dr. Ralph S. Lachman for contributing the excellent chapter on skeletal dysplasias to the third and fourth editions of my complete work, *Radiology of Syndromes, Metabolic Disorders, and Skeletal Dysplasias.* Since radiographs are absolutely essential in the study of skeletal dysplasias, I have decided not to include these disorders in this handbook.

The encouragement of my colleagues in radiology, in particular my mentor, Dr. Frederic N. Silverman, and the favorable response of readers have resulted in the extension of my original book on syndromes in 1975 to the fourth edition in 1996 covering syndromes, metabolic disorders, and skeletal dysplasias. I hope that this new practical handbook will make this information and subject matter available to a wider scope of readers.

The full support of Ms. Elizabeth Corra, the managing editor, and the cooperation and help of other members of the Mosby–Year Book staff, particularly Ms. Mia Cariño and Ms. Kathy Hillock, in preparing and publishing this book are most appreciated.

Hooshang Taybi

Notes on the Use of This Book

1. In the Alphabetic List of Syndromes and Metabolic Disorders, the syndromes and metabolic disorders discussed in the two chapters are combined. Synonyms, if any, of the syndromes and metabolic disorders are also listed so that the user can search for information about a given disease entity by more than one name.

2. The index is presented in the form of gamuts. This Index-Gamuts should be helpful to the user in the differential diagnosis of various clinical and radiologic manifestations of diseases described in the book.

3. The relatively more common clinical and radiologic manifestations of the syndromes and metabolic disorders appear in italics.

Contents

Alphabetic List of Syndromes and Metabolic Disorders, xiii

1   Syndromes, 1

2   Metabolic Disorders, 233

Index-Gamuts, 389

Alphabetic List of Syndromes and Metabolic Disorders

A

Aarskog syndrome, 2

Aarskog-Scott syndrome (AARSKOG SYNDROME), 2

Aase syndrome, 2

Aase-Smith syndrome II (AASE SYNDROME), 2

Abetalipoproteinemia, 234

Achalasia-adrenal-alacrima syndrome, 2

Acrocallosal syndrome, 3

Acrocephalopolysyndactyly, Carpenter type (CARPENTER SYNDROME), 29

Acrocephalopolysyndactyly, Goodman type (GOODMAN SYNDROME), 83

Acrocephalosyndactyly, Apert type (APERT SYNDROME), 11

Acrocephalosyndactyly, Pfeiffer type (PFEIFFER SYNDROME), 160

Acrodermatitis enteropathica, 234

Acrodystrophic neuropathy (THEVENARD SYNDROME), 208

Acrofacial dysostoses, 3

Acrofacial dysostosis (NAGER ACROFACIAL DYSOSTOSIS), 136

Acrofacial dysostosis (WEYERS ACRODENTAL DYSOSTOSIS), 226

Acrogeria, 4

Acromegaly and gigantism, 235

Acrorenal syndrome, 4

Adams-Oliver syndrome, 4

Addison disease, 237

Adducted thumbs syndrome (CHRISTIAN SYNDROME), 36

Adrenal cortical insufficiency (ADDISON DISEASE), 237

Adrenal hyperplasia (congenital), 238

Adrenogenital syndrome (ADRENAL HYPERPLASIA [CONGENITAL]), 238

Adrenoleukodystrophy and adrenomyeloneuropathy, 239

ADULT syndrome, 196

Afferent loop syndrome, 5

Afibrinogenemia (congenital), 241

Agammaglobulinemia, X-linked, 5

Aglossia-adactylia syndrome (HYPOGLOSSIA-HYPODACTYLIA SYNDROME), 98

Aicardi syndrome, 6

Ainhum, 6

Alagille syndrome, 6

Albright hereditary osteodystrophy (PSEUDOHYPOPARATHYROIDISM), 355

Albright syndrome (MCCUNE-ALBRIGHT SYNDROME), 125

Aldosteronism, 241

Aldrich syndrome (WISKOTT-ALDRICH SYNDROME), 228

Alexander disease, 242

Alien hand syndrome, 7

Alkaptonuria, 243

Allgrove syndrome (ACHALASIA-ADRENAL-ALACRIMA SYNDROME), 2

Alpers syndrome, 7

Alpers-Huttenlocher syndrome (ALPERS SYNDROME), 7

Alpha$_1$-antitrypsin deficiency, 243

Alpha-chain disease, 244

Alpha-thalassemia/mental retardation syndrome, 376

Alport syndrome, 8

Alport-leiomyomatosis syndrome, 8

Alström syndrome, 264

Aluminum intoxication, 245

Aluminum-related osteodystrophy (ALUMINUM INTOXICATION), 245

Aminopterin fetopathy, 8

Aminopterin fetopathy-like syndrome, 9

Amniotic band sequence, 9

Amyloidosis, 245

Amylopectinosis (GLYCOGEN STORAGE DISEASE TYPE IV), 277

Andermann syndrome, 9

Andersen disease (GLYCOGEN STORAGE DISEASE TYPE IV), 277

Anderson-Fabry syndrome (FABRY DISEASE), 266

Andre syndrome, 180

Androgen insensitivity syndrome (TESTICULAR FEMINIZATION), 373

Angelman syndrome, 10

Aniridia-Wilms tumor association, 10

Antecubital pterygium syndrome, 171

Anterior operculum syndrome (FOIX-CHAVANY-MARIE SYNDROME), 76

Antiphospholipid syndrome, 10

Antley-Bixler syndrome, 11

Apert syndrome, 11

Aplasia cutis congenita, 12

Aplasia cutis–limb defects (ADAMS-OLIVER SYNDROME), 4

AREDYLD syndrome, 264

Arens acrofacial dysostosis, 3

Arterial calcification of infancy, 12

Arteriohepatic syndrome (ALAGILLE SYNDROME), 6

Arteriomesenteric duodenal compression (SUPERIOR MESENTERIC ARTERY SYNDROME), 203

Arthro-dento-osteo-dysplasia (HAJDU-CHENEY SYNDROME), 87
Arthro-ophthalmopathy (STICKLER SYNDROME), 200
Arthropathy-camptodactyly syndrome, 13
Asherman syndrome, 13
Aspartylglucosaminuria, 247
Asplenia syndrome, 13
Ataxia-telangiectasia syndrome, 14
Austin disease (MULTIPLE SULFATASE DEFICIENCY), 334

B

Baller-Gerold syndrome, 14
Bamatter syndrome (GERODERMA OSTEODYSPLASTICA), 81
Bannayan-Riley-Ruvalcaba syndrome, 15
Banti syndrome, 15
Bardet-Biedl syndrome, 16
Barraquer-Simons syndrome, 311
Barry-Perkins-Young syndrome (YOUNG SYNDROME), 230
Bart hemoglobin hydrops fetalis syndrome, 375
Bartsocas-Papas syndrome, 172
Bartter syndrome, 16
Basal cell–nevus syndrome (GORLIN SYNDROME), 85
Bassen-Kornzweig syndrome (ABETALIPOPROTEINEMIA), 234
Batten disease (NEURONAL CEROID LIPOFUSCINOSIS), 336
BBB syndrome (OPITZ BBBG SYNDROME), 149
BBB/G syndrome (OPITZ BBBG SYNDROME), 149
Beals-Hecht syndrome (CONTRACTURAL ARACHNODACTYLY), 44
Bean syndrome, 17
Beare-Stevenson syndrome, 40, 50
Beckwith-Wiedemann syndrome, 17
Behçet syndrome, 18
Behr syndrome, 248
Berardinelli-Seip syndrome, 311
Berdon syndrome, 19
Beriberi (VITAMIN B_1 DEFICIENCY), 381
Bile plug syndrome, 19
Binder syndrome, 19
Biotinidase deficiency, 248
Bird-headed dwarfism (SECKEL SYNDROME), 188
Bixler syndrome (HYPERTELORISM–MICROTIA–FACIAL CLEFTING SYNDROME), 98
Blackfan-Diamond syndrome (DIAMOND-BLACKFAN SYNDROME), 54
Blind loop syndrome, 20
Blind pouch syndrome (BLIND LOOP SYNDROME), 20
Bloom syndrome, 20

Bloom-German syndrome (BLOOM SYNDROME), 20
Blue diaper syndrome, 249
Blue digit syndrome, 21
Blue rubber bleb nevus syndrome (BEAN SYNDROME), 17
Blue toe syndrome (BLUE DIGIT SYNDROME), 21
Bobble-head doll syndrome, 21
Boerhaave syndrome, 21
BOR syndrome (BRANCHIO-OTO-RENAL SYNDROME), 23
Börjeson-Forssman-Lehmann syndrome, 22
Bourneville-Pringle syndrome (TUBEROUS SCLEROSIS), 212
Brachmann–de Lange syndrome, 22
Brachymorphism-onychodysplasia-dysphalangism syndrome (SENIOR SYNDROME), 188
Brailsford-Morquio syndrome (MUCOPOLYSACCHARIDOSIS IVA), 331
Branchio-genito-skeletal syndrome, 23
Branchio-oculo-facial syndrome, 23
Branchio-oto-renal syndrome, 23
Branchio-skeleto-genital syndrome (BRANCHIO-GENITO-SKELETAL SYNDROME), 23
Bridges-Good syndrome (CHRONIC GRANULOMATOUS DISEASE OF CHILDHOOD), 256
Brown syndrome, 24
Brown-Séquard syndrome, 24
Bruns-Garland syndrome, 264
Bruton disease (AGAMMAGLOBULINEMIA, X-LINKED), 5
Buckley syndrome (HYPERIMMUNOGLOBULINEMIA E SYNDROME), 96
Budd-Chiari syndrome, 25
Buschke disease (MADELUNG DISEASE), 315

C
C syndrome (OPITZ TRIGONOCEPHALY SYNDROME), 149
Calcinosis universalis, 249
Calcium hydroxyapatite crystal deposition disease (HYDROXYAPATITE DEPOSITION
    DISEASE), 286
Calcium pyrophosphate dihydrate deposition disease, 249
Camptodactyly-arthropathy-pericarditis syndrome (ARTHROPATHY-CAMPTODACTYLY
    SYNDROME), 13
Canavan disease, 250
Canavan–van Bogaert–Bertrand disease (CANAVAN DISEASE), 250
Cantrell syndrome, 25
Caplan syndrome, 26
Carbohydrate-deficient glycoprotein syndrome, 251
Carbonic anhydrase II deficiency, 252
Carcinoid syndrome, 252
Cardiofacial syndrome, 26
Cardio-facio-cutaneous syndrome, 26

Cardiovocal syndrome, 27

Carey-Fineman-Ziter syndrome, 180

Carney complex, 27

Carney triad, 27

Carnitine deficiency syndromes, 253

Caroli syndrome, 28

Carotid sinus syndrome, 28

Carpal and tarsal osteolysis (OSTEOLYSIS WITHOUT NEPHROPATHY), 153

Carpal tunnel syndrome, 28

Carpenter syndrome, 29

Cast syndrome, 29

Cat-cry syndrome (CHROMOSOME 5: DEL (5P) SYNDROME), 37

Catel-Manzke syndrome, 30

Cat-eye syndrome, 30

Cauda equina syndrome, 30

Caudal dysplasia sequence, 31

Caudal regression syndrome (CAUDAL DYSPLASIA SEQUENCE), 31

Cayler syndrome (CARDIOFACIAL SYNDROME), 26

Celiac axis compression syndrome, 31

Celiac disease, 254

Central cord syndrome, 31

Central hypoventilation syndrome (congenital), 32

Cephaloskeletal dysplasia, 32

Cerebellar hypoplasia–endosteal sclerosis (STOLL-CHARROW-POZNANSKI SYNDROME), 201

Cerebro-costo-mandibular syndrome, 33

Cerebro-hepato-renal syndrome (ZELLWEGER SYNDROME), 386

Cerebro-oculo-facio-skeletal syndrome, 33

Cerebro-reno-digital syndromes, 34

Cerebroside lipidosis (GAUCHER DISEASE), 272

Cerebrotendinous xanthomatosis, 255

Cervical lipomatosis (MADELUNG DISEASE), 315

Cervico-oculo-acoustic syndrome (WILDERVANCK SYNDROME), 226

Charcot-Marie-Tooth disease, 34

CHARGE association, 34

Charlie M syndrome, 152

Chédiak-Higashi syndrome, 35

Cheiro-oral syndrome, 35

Chiari syndrome (BUDD-CHIARI SYNDROME), 25

Chilaiditi syndrome, 35

CHILD syndrome, 36

Childhood epileptic encephalopathy (LENNOX-GASTAUT SYNDROME), 113

Cholesterol embolization syndrome (BLUE DIGIT SYNDROME), 21

Cholesterol ester storage disease, 256

Christian syndrome, 36

Christ-Siemens-Touraine syndrome (ECTODERMAL DYSPLASIA [HYPOHIDROTIC]), 61

Chromosome 4: del (4p) syndrome, 36

Chromosome 5: del (5p) syndrome, 37

Chromosome 8 recombinant syndrome (RECOMBINANT (8) SYNDROME), 174

Chromosome 13 trisomy syndrome, 37

Chromosome 18 trisomy syndrome, 37

Chromosome 21 trisomy (DOWN SYNDROME), 57

Chromosome 22 trisomy/tetrasomy (CAT-EYE SYNDROME), 30

Chronic fatigue syndrome, 38

Chronic granulomatous disease of childhood, 256

Churg-Strauss syndrome, 38

Ciliary dyskinesia (IMMOTILE CILIA SYNDROME), 99

Claude syndrome, 39

Clouston syndrome, 39

Cloverleaf skull deformity, 39

Cockayne syndrome, 40

Coffin-Lowry syndrome, 42

Coffin-Siris syndrome, 42

Cogan syndrome, 43

COH syndrome, 40

Cohen syndrome, 43

Congenital chloride diarrhea, 257

Congenital indifference to pain (INSENSITIVITY TO PAIN [CONGENITAL]), 101

Congenital synspondylism (SPONDYLO-CARPO-TARSAL SYNOSTOSIS SYNDROME), 197

Conn syndrome (ALDOSTERONISM), 241

Contractural arachnodactyly, 44

Copper deficiency, 258

Cori disease (GLYCOGEN STORAGE DISEASE TYPE III), 276

Cornelia de Lange syndrome (BRACHMANN–DE LANGE SYNDROME), 22

Costello syndrome, 44

Cowden syndrome, 44

Cranio-carpo-tarsal dysplasia (FREEMAN-SHELDON SYNDROME), 78

Cranio-cerebello-cardiac dysplasia (RITSCHER-SCHINZEL SYNDROME), 179

Cranioectodermal dysplasia, 45

Craniofacial dysostosis (CROUZON SYNDROME), 47

Cranio-fronto-nasal dysplasia, 45

Craniosynostosis–radial aplasia syndrome (BALLER-GEROLD SYNDROME), 14

Craniotelencephalic dysplasia, 46

CREST syndrome, 46

Cri-du-chat syndrome (CHROMOSOME 5: DEL (5P) SYNDROME), 37

Cronkhite-Canada syndrome, 47

Cross syndrome, 47

Crouzon syndrome, 47
Crow-Fukase syndrome (POEMS SYNDROME), 161
CRST syndrome (CREST SYNDROME), 46
Cruveilhier-Baumgarten syndrome, 48
Cryptophthalmos-syndactyly syndrome (FRASER SYNDROME), 77
Currarino syndrome (OSTEOARTHROPATHY, FAMILIAL IDIOPATHIC), 152
Currarino triad, 49
Cushing syndrome, 258
Cutis laxa, 49
Cutis verticis gyrata, 50
Cystinosis, 259
Cystinuria, 260

D
Dandy-Walker malformation (DANDY-WALKER SYNDROME), 50
Dandy-Walker syndrome, 50
Darrow-Gamble disease (CONGENITAL CHLORIDE DIARRHEA), 257
Degos syndrome, 51
Déjérine-Sottas syndrome, 52
de Lange syndrome (BRACHMANN–DE LANGE SYNDROME), 22
Delleman syndrome, 52
Demons-Meigs syndrome (MEIGS SYNDROME), 126
de Morsier syndrome, 53
Denys-Drash syndrome, 53
Deprivation dwarfism, 260
Dermo-chondro-corneal dystrophy of François, 54
De Sanctis-Cacchione syndrome, 54
de Toni–Debré–Fanconi syndrome (FANCONI SYNDROME), 268
Diabetes insipidus, 261
Diabetes mellitus, 262
Diamond-Blackfan syndrome, 54
DIDMOAD syndrome (WOLFRAM SYNDROME), 229
Dieker-Opitz acrorenal syndrome (ACRORENAL SYNDROME), 4
Diencephalic syndrome, 55
Dietl syndrome, 55
DiGeorge syndrome, 55
Digito-reno-cerebral syndrome (ERONEN SYNDROME), 68
Digitotalar dysmorphism, 56
Distichiasis-lymphedema syndrome, 56
Donohue syndrome (LEPRECHAUNISM), 310
DOO syndrome, 56
DOOR syndrome, 56
Down syndrome, 57

Drash syndrome (DENYS-DRASH SYNDROME), 53

Dressler syndrome (POSTMYOCARDIAL INFARCTION SYNDROME), 166

Duane syndrome, 59

Dubin-Johnson syndrome, 265

Dubowitz syndrome, 59

Dumping syndrome, 60

Du Pan syndrome, 60

Dyke-Davidoff-Masson syndrome, 60

Dysendocrinism (LEPRECHAUNISM), 310

Dyskeratosis congenita, 60

E

Eagle syndrome, 61

Ectodermal dysplasia (hypohidrotic), 61

Ectrodactyly (SPLIT-HAND/SPLIT-FOOT DEFORMITIES), 196

Ectrodactyly–Ectodermal dysplasia–Clefting syndrome (EEC SYNDROME), 62

Edwards syndrome (CHROMOSOME 18 TRISOMY SYNDROME), 37

EEC syndrome, 62

Egger-Joubert syndrome, 151

Ehlers-Danlos syndrome, 63

Eisenmenger syndrome, 64

Elsahy-Waters syndrome (BRANCHIO-GENITO-SKELETAL SYNDROME), 23

Empty sella syndrome, 65

Encephalo-cranio-cutaneous lipomatosis, 66

Epidermal nevus syndrome, 66

Epidermolysis bullosa, 67

Erasmus syndrome, 26

Erdheim-Chester disease, 265

Eronen syndrome, 68

Escobar syndrome, 171

F

F syndrome, 68

Fabry disease, 266

Facio-audio-symphalangism syndrome (SYMPHALANGISM-SURDITY SYNDROME), 205

Facio-auriculo-radial dysplasia, 69

Facio-digito-genital syndrome (AARSKOG SYNDROME), 2

Facio-genito-popliteal syndrome, 171

Fahr disease, 267

Familial osteoectasia (HYPERPHOSPHATASIA), 293

Fanconi anemia, 69

Fanconi pancytopenia (FANCONI ANEMIA), 69

Fanconi syndrome, 268

Farber disease, 268

Fat embolism syndrome, 70

Felty syndrome, 70

Femoral hypoplasia–unusual facies syndrome, 70

Ferrocalcinosis (FAHR DISEASE), 267

Fetal akinesia sequence, 71

Fetal alcohol syndrome, 71

Fetal brain disruption sequence, 72

Fetal hydantoin syndrome, 72

Fetal hypokinesia sequence (FETAL AKINESIA SEQUENCE), 71

Fetal transfusion syndrome (TWIN-TO-TWIN TRANSFUSION SYNDROME), 216

Fetal trimethadione syndrome, 180

Fetal valproate syndrome, 73

Feuerstein-Mims syndrome (EPIDERMAL NEVUS SYNDROME), 66

FG syndrome, 73

Fibrodysplasia ossificans progressiva, 74

Fishman syndrome (ENCEPHALO-CRANIO-CUTANEOUS LIPOMATOSIS), 66

Fitch syndrome, 94

Fitz-Hugh–Curtis syndrome, 74

Fleischer syndrome, 299

Floating-Harbor syndrome, 75

Floppy valve syndrome, 75

Fluorosis, 269

Focal dermal hypoplasia (GOLTZ SYNDROME), 83

Focal scleroderma, 75

Foix-Chavany-Marie syndrome, 76

Forbes disease (GLYCOGEN STORAGE DISEASE TYPE III), 276

Foster Kennedy syndrome, 76

Fountain syndrome, 76

Fragile X syndrome, 77

François dyscephaly (HALLERMANN-STREIFF SYNDROME), 88

Fraser syndrome, 77

Freeman-Sheldon syndrome, 78

Frontodigital syndrome (GREIG CEPHALOPOLYSYNDACTYLY SYNDROME), 86

Fronto-facio-nasal dysplasia, 78

Frontonasal dysplasia, 78

Fryns syndrome, 79

Fucosidosis, 270

Fuhrmann syndrome, 79

G

G syndrome (OPITZ BBBG SYNDROME), 149

Galactosemia, 270

Galactosialidosis, 271

Galloway-Mowat syndrome, 80

Gangliosidosis GM_1 (GM$_1$ GANGLIOSIDOSIS), 278

GAPO syndrome, 80

Gardner syndrome, 80

Gardner-Silengo-Wachtel syndrome, 81

Gaucher disease, 272

Genito-palato-cardiac syndrome (GARDNER-SILENGO-WACHTEL SYNDROME), 81

Genoa syndrome, 94

Geophagia syndrome (PRASAD SYNDROME), 354

Geroderma osteodysplastica, 81

Gigantism, 236

Gilbert syndrome, 273

Gilles de la Tourette syndrome, 82

Gingival fibromatosis–abnormal fingers (ZIMMERMANN-LABAND SYNDROME), 231

Globoid cell leukodystrophy (KRABBE DISEASE), 307

Glossopalatine ankylosis syndrome, 152

Glucagonoma syndrome, 274

Glutaric aciduria type I, 274

Glycogen storage disease type I, 275

Glycogen storage disease type II, 276

Glycogen storage disease type III, 276

Glycogen storage disease type IV, 277

Glycogen storage disease type V, 277

GM_1 gangliosidosis, 278

GM_2 gangliosidosis, 279

Goldberg-Shprintzen syndrome, 82

Goldbloom syndrome, 82

Goldenhar syndrome (OCULO-AURICULO-VERTEBRAL SPECTRUM), 147

Goldenhar-Gorlin syndrome (OCULO-AURICULO-VERTEBRAL SPECTRUM), 147

Golden-Lakim syndrome, 82

Goldston syndrome, 51

Goltz syndrome, 83

Goltz-Gorlin syndrome (GOLTZ SYNDROME), 83

Goodman syndrome, 83

Goodpasture syndrome, 84

Gordon syndrome, 84

Gorham syndrome, 84

Gorlin syndrome, 85

Gottron Acrogeria (ACROGERIA), 4

Gougerot-Sjögren syndrome (SJÖGREN SYNDROME), 192

Gout, 280

Gradenigo syndrome, 85

Grant syndrome, 86
Graves disease (HYPERTHYROIDISM), 294
Greig cephalopolysyndactyly syndrome, 86
Griscelli syndrome, 86
Grisel syndrome, 87
Gruber syndrome (MECKEL SYNDROME), 125
Guillain-Barré syndrome, 87
Gunther disease, 353

H
Hajdu-Cheney syndrome, 87
Hallermann-Streiff syndrome, 88
Hallervorden-Spatz disease, 281
Hand-foot-genital syndrome, 89
Hand-foot-uterus syndrome (HAND-FOOT-GENITAL SYNDROME), 89
Hanhart syndrome, 152
"Happy puppet" syndrome (ANGELMAN SYNDROME), 10
HARD ±E syndrome (WALKER-WARBURG SYNDROME), 221
Head-bobbling "tic" (BOBBLE-HEAD DOLL SYNDROME), 21
Heart-hand syndrome II (TABATZNIK SYNDROME), 205
Hecht syndrome (TRISMUS-PSEUDOCAMPTODACTYLY SYNDROME), 212
HELLP syndrome, 89
Hemihypertrophy, 90
Hemochromatosis, 281
Hemolytic uremic syndrome, 90
Hemophilia, 282
Hemorrhagic shock–encephalopathy syndrome, 91
Hemosiderosis (idiopathic pulmonary), 284
Henoch-Schönlein syndrome, 91
Hepatic fibrosis–renal cystic disease, 92
Hepatolenticular degeneration (WILSON DISEASE), 383
Hepatopulmonary syndrome, 92
Hermansky-Pudlak syndrome, 284
Heyde syndrome, 93
Hinman syndrome, 93
Hippel-Lindau syndrome (VON HIPPEL–LINDAU SYNDROME), 220
Hirschsprung disease, 93
Hoffmann syndrome, 301
Holoprosencephaly, 94
Holoprosencephaly-polydactyly syndrome (PSEUDOTRISOMY 13 SYNDROME), 170
Holt-Oram syndrome, 94
Homocystinuria, 285
Horner syndrome, 95

Hughes-Stovin syndrome, 95

Hunter disease (MUCOPOLYSACCHARIDOSIS II), 329

Hurler syndrome (MUCOPOLYSACCHARIDOSIS I-H), 327

Hurler-Scheie compound (MUCOPOLYSACCHARIDOSIS I-H/S), 328

Hutchinson-Gilford syndrome (PROGERIA), 168

Hydrolethalus syndrome, 95

Hydroxyapatite deposition disease, 286

Hyperammonemic disorders, 286

Hypercholesterolemia, 288

Hypereosinophilic syndrome (idiopathic), 96

Hyperimmunoglobulinemia E syndrome, 96

Hyperinsulinism, 287

Hyperlipidemia (HYPERLIPOPROTEINEMIAS), 287

Hyperlipoproteinemias, 287

Hypermobility syndrome, 97

Hyperostosis frontalis interna (MORGAGNI-STEWART-MOREL SYNDROME), 132

Hyperostosis-hyperphosphatemia syndrome, 97

Hyperoxaluria (OXALOSIS), 343

Hyperparathyroidism, 290

Hyperperfusion syndrome, 97

Hyperphenylalaninemia (PHENYLKETONURIA), 350

Hyperphosphatasia, 293

Hyperprolactinemia, 293

Hypertelorism-hypospadias syndrome (OPITZ BBBG SYNDROME), 149

Hypertelorism–microtia–facial clefting syndrome, 98

Hyperthyroidism, 294

Hypertriglyceridemia, 289

Hypoglossia-hypodactylia syndrome, 98

Hypomelanosis of Ito, 98

Hypoparathyroidism, 296

Hypophosphatasia, 297

Hypopituitarism (anterior lobe), 298

Hypothenar hammer syndrome, 99

Hypothyroidism, 300

I

I-cell disease (MUCOLIPIDOSIS II), 323

Ichthyosis–limb reduction syndrome (CHILD SYNDROME), 36

Idiopathic periosteal hyperostosis with dysproteinemia (GOLDBLOOM SYNDROME), 82

Idiopathic pulmonary hemosiderosis (HEMOSIDEROSIS [IDIOPATHIC PULMONARY]), 284

Immotile cilia syndrome, 99

Immunoproliferative small intestinal disease (ALPHA-CHAIN DISEASE), 244

Inappropriate secretion of antidiuretic hormone syndrome (SYNDROME OF
INAPPROPRIATE SECRETION OF ANTIDIURETIC HORMONE), 373

Incontinentia pigmenti, 100
Incontinentia pigmenti achromians (HYPOMELANOSIS OF ITO), 98
Infantile multisystem inflammatory disease, 100
Insensitivity to pain (congenital), 101
Inspissated bile syndrome (BILE PLUG SYNDROME), 19
Iron deficiency anemia, 305
Irritable bowel syndrome, 102
Irritable colon syndrome (IRRITABLE BOWEL SYNDROME), 102
Iso-Kikuchi syndrome, 102
Ivemark syndrome (ASPLENIA SYNDROME), 13
Ivemark syndrome (RENAL-HEPATIC-PANCREATIC DYSPLASIA), 176

J
Jackson-Weiss syndrome, 102
Jadassohn-Lewandowsky syndrome, 103
Jaffe-Campanacci syndrome, 103
Jarcho-Levin syndrome, 197
Job's syndrome (HYPERIMMUNOGLOBULINEMIA E SYNDROME), 96
Johanson-Blizzard syndrome, 103
Joubert syndrome, 103
Juberg-Hayward syndrome, 104
Jugular foramen syndrome, 104
Juvenile Paget disease (HYPERPHOSPHATASIA), 293

K
Kabuki make-up syndrome, 104
Kallmann syndrome, 105
Karsch-Neugebauer syndrome, 196
Kartagener syndrome, 105
Kasabach-Merritt syndrome, 106
Kaufman-McKusick syndrome, 106
Kawasaki syndrome, 106
KBG syndrome, 107
Kearns-Sayre syndrome, 306
Kelly acrofacial dysostosis, 3
Keratoderma hereditaria mutilans (VOHWINKEL SYNDROME), 219
Keratosis palmaris et plantaris familiaris (tylosis), 107
Keutel syndrome, 108
Kinky-hair syndrome (MENKES SYNDROME), 319
Kleeblattschädel anomaly (CLOVERLEAF SKULL DEFORMITY), 39
Klein-Waardenburg syndrome, 108
Klinefelter syndrome, 108
Klippel-Feil syndrome, 109
Klippel-Trenaunay syndrome, 109

Klippel-Trenaunay-Weber syndrome (KLIPPEL-TRENAUNAY SYNDROME), 109
Klüver-Bucy syndrome, 110
Köbberling-Dunnigan syndrome, 311
Kocher-Debré-Sémélaigne syndrome, 307
Köhlmeier-Degos disease (DEGOS SYNDROME), 51
Krabbe disease, 307
Kugelberg-Welander syndrome, 110
Kuskokwim syndrome, 111
Kwashiorkor, 308

L
Lacrimo-auriculo-dento-digital syndrome, 111
Lactase deficiency, 308
Lactose intolerance (LACTASE DEFICIENCY), 308
LADD syndrome (LACRIMO-AURICULO-DENTO-DIGITAL SYNDROME), 111
Lambert-Eaton myasthenic syndrome, 112
Landau-Kleffner syndrome, 112
Laron syndrome, 309
Larsen syndrome, 112
Lateral medullary syndrome (WALLENBERG SYNDROME), 222
Launois-Bensaude disease (MADELUNG DISEASE), 315
Laurin-Sandrow syndrome, 113
Leigh disease, 309
Lennox-Gastaut syndrome, 113
Lenz microphthalmia syndrome, 113
LEOPARD syndrome, 113
Leprechaunism, 310
Léri syndrome, 114
Leriche syndrome, 114
Leroy I-cell disease (MUCOLIPIDOSIS II), 323
Lesch-Nyhan syndrome, 310
Lethal multiple pterygium syndrome, 171
Levine-Critchley syndrome (NEUROACANTHOCYTOSIS), 335
Levy-Hollister syndrome (LACRIMO-AURICULO-DENTO-DIGITAL SYNDROME), 111
Lhermitte-Duclos disease, 115
Lignac–de Toni–Fanconi syndrome (CYSTINOSIS), 259
Linear scleroderma "en coup de sabre" (FOCAL SCLERODERMA), 75
Linear sebaceous nevus sequence (EPIDERMAL NEVUS SYNDROME), 66
Lipoatrophy (LIPODYSTROPHIES), 311
Lipodystrophies, 311
Lipoglycoproteinosis (LIPOID PROTEINOSIS), 313
Lipogranulomatosis (FARBER DISEASE), 268
Lipoid dermatoarthritis, 115

Lipoid proteinosis, 313
Lissencephalies, 116
Lissencephaly, type I (MILLER-DIEKER SYNDROME), 130
Lobster-claw deformity (SPLIT-HAND/SPLIT-FOOT DEFORMITIES), 196
Locked-in syndrome, 117
Löffler syndrome, 118
Louis-Bar syndrome (ATAXIA-TELANGIECTASIA SYNDROME), 14
Lowe syndrome, 314
Lutembacher syndrome, 118
Lynch syndromes I and II, 118
Lysinuric protein intolerance, 314
Lysosomal acid lipase deficiency (WOLMAN DISEASE), 385

M

Macleod syndrome (SWYER-JAMES SYNDROME), 204
Macrodystrophia lipomatosa, 119
Madelung disease, 315
Maffucci syndrome, 119
Malabsorption syndrome, 119
Maladie de Basedow (HYPERTHYROIDISM), 294
Malignant atrophic papulosis (DEGOS SYNDROME), 51
Mallory-Weiss syndrome, 120
Mandibuloacral dysplasia, 120
Mandibulofacial dysostosis (TREACHER COLLINS SYNDROME), 211
Man-in-the-barrel syndrome, 120
Mannosidoses, 316
Maple syrup urine disease, 317
Marble brain disease (CARBONIC ANHYDRASE II DEFICIENCY), 252
Marden-Walker syndrome, 121
Marfan syndrome, 121
Marfanoid hypermobility syndrome, 122
Marinesco-Sjögren syndrome, 122
Maroteaux-Lamy syndrome (MUCOPOLYSACCHARIDOSIS VI), 333
Marshall syndrome, 123
Marshall-Smith syndrome, 123
Martin-Bell syndrome (FRAGILE X SYNDROME), 77
MASA syndrome, 124
Mauriac syndrome, 317
Mayer-Rokitansky-Küster syndrome, 124
Maxillonasal dysplasia (BINDER SYNDROME), 19
Mazabraud syndrome, 124
McArdle disease (GLYCOGEN STORAGE DISEASE TYPE V), 277
McCune-Albright syndrome, 125

McKusick-Kaufman syndrome (KAUFMAN-MCKUSICK SYNDROME), 106

Meckel syndrome, 125

Meconium plug syndrome, 126

Median cleft face syndrome (FRONTONASAL DYSPLASIA), 78

Megacystis-megaureter syndrome, 126

Megacystis–microcolon–intestinal hypoperistalsis syndrome (BERDON SYNDROME), 19

Meige-Nonne-Milroy disease, 126

Meigs syndrome, 126

MELAS syndrome, 318

Melnick-Fraser syndrome (BRANCHIO-OTO-RENAL SYNDROME), 23

Membranous lipodystrophy, 319

Mendelson syndrome, 127

Mendenhall syndrome, 264

Ménétrier syndrome, 127

Menkes disease, 319

Mermaid syndrome (SIRENOMELIA), 192

Metachromatic leukodystrophies, 321

Methylmalonic acidemia, 322

Mevalonic aciduria, 322

Michels syndrome, 127

Microcephalic osteodysplastic primordial dwarfism, 127

Microgeodic phalangeal syndrome (PHALANGEAL MICROGEODIC SYNDROME), 160

Mietens-Weber syndrome, 130

Mikulicz syndrome, 130

Milk-alkali syndrome, 323

Miller-Dieker syndrome, 130

Minkowski-Chauffard disease (SPHEROCYTOSIS), 372

Mirizzi syndrome, 131

Mitochondrial myopathy–encephalopathy–lactic acidosis–strokelike episodes (MELAS SYNDROME), 318

Mixed connective tissue disease, 131

Möbius syndrome, 132

Moersch-Woltmann syndrome (STIFF-MAN SYNDROME), 200

Mohr syndrome (ORO-FACIO-DIGITAL SYNDROME II), 150

Mohr-Majewski syndrome, 151

Molded baby syndrome, 132

Morgagni-Stewart-Morel syndrome, 132

Morning glory syndrome, 133

Morquio disease type A (MUCOPOLYSACCHARIDOSIS IVA), 331

Morquio disease type B (MUCOPOLYSACCHARIDOSIS IVB), 332

Mounier-Kuhn syndrome, 133

Mucolipidosis II, 323

Mucolipidosis III, 324

Mucolipidosis IV, 325

Mucopolysaccharidoses, 325

Mucopolysaccharidosis I-H, 327

Mucopolysaccharidosis I-H/S, 328

Mucopolysaccharidosis I-S, 329

Mucopolysaccharidosis II, 329

Mucopolysaccharidosis III, 330

Mucopolysaccharidosis IVA, 331

Mucopolysaccharidosis IVB, 332

Mucopolysaccharidosis VI, 333

Mucopolysaccharidosis VII, 334

Mucosal neuroma syndrome (MULTIPLE ENDOCRINE NEOPLASIA TYPE IIB), 135

Mucous colon syndrome (IRRITABLE BOWEL SYNDROME), 102

Muir-Torre syndrome, 134

Mulibrey nanism, 134

Multiple endocrine adenomatosis type I (MULTIPLE ENDOCRINE NEOPLASIA TYPE I), 134

Multiple endocrine adenomatosis type IIA (MULTIPLE ENDOCRINE NEOPLASIA TYPE IIA), 135

Multiple endocrine adenomatosis type IIB (MULTIPLE ENDOCRINE NEOPLASIA TYPE IIB), 135

Multiple endocrine neoplasia type I, 134

Multiple endocrine neoplasia type IIA, 135

Multiple endocrine neoplasia type IIB, 135

Multiple pterygium syndrome, 171

Multiple sulfatase deficiency, 334

Multiple synostosis syndrome, 136

Mutilating keratoderma (VOHWINKEL SYNDROME), 219

MURCS association, 136

Myositis ossificans progressiva (FIBRODYSPLASIA OSSIFICANS PROGRESSIVA), 74

Myxoma syndrome (CARNEY COMPLEX), 27

Myxoma–spotty pigmentation–endocrine overactivity (CARNEY COMPLEX), 27

N

Nager acrofacial dysostosis, 136

Nail-patella syndrome, 137

NAME syndrome (CARNEY COMPLEX), 27

Naso-maxillo-vertebral syndrome (BINDER SYNDROME), 19

Nasopalpebral lipoma-coloboma syndrome, 137

Nasu-Hakola disease (MEMBRANOUS LIPODYSTROPHY), 319

Navajo neuropathy, 335

Nelson syndrome, 335

Neonatal onset multisystem inflammatory disease (INFANTILE MULTISYSTEM INFLAMMATORY DISEASE), 100

Nephrogenic hepatic dysfunction syndrome, 138
Nephronophthisis, 138
Nephrotic syndrome, 138
Neu-Laxova syndrome, 139
Neuroacanthocytosis, 335
Neurocristopathy, 93
Neurocutaneous melanosis sequence, 139
Neurofibromatosis I, 140
Neurofibromatosis II, 144
Neuronal ceroid lipofuscinosis, 336
Neutrophil dysfunction syndrome (CHRONIC GRANULOMATOUS DISEASE OF
    CHILDHOOD), 256
NF-I (NEUROFIBROMATOSIS I), 140
NF-II (NEUROFIBROMATOSIS II), 144
Nielson syndrome, 171
Niemann-Pick disease, 336
Niikawa-Kuroki syndrome (KABUKI MAKE-UP SYNDROME), 104
NOMID (INFANTILE MULTISYSTEM INFLAMMATORY DISEASE), 100
Nonneurogenic neurogenic bladder (HINMAN SYNDROME), 93
Noonan syndrome, 145
Noonan-like/multiple giant cell lesion syndrome, 146
Norman-Landing disease (GM$_1$ GANGLIOSIDOSIS), 278

O
Occipital horn syndrome, 341
Ochoa syndrome (UROFACIAL SYNDROME), 217
Oculo-auriculo-vertebral spectrum, 147
Oculo-cerebro-cutaneous syndrome (DELLEMAN SYNDROME), 52
Oculo-cerebro-renal syndrome (LOWE SYNDROME), 314
Oculo-dento-digital dysplasia (OCULO-DENTO-OSSEOUS DYSPLASIA), 147
Oculo-dento-osseous dysplasia, 147
Oculo-mandibulo-facial syndrome (HALLERMANN-STREIFF SYNDROME), 88
Odonto-tricho-melic syndrome, 148
OFDS (ORO-FACIO-DIGITAL SYNDROMES), 150
Ogilvie syndrome, 148
Ondine's curse (CENTRAL HYPOVENTILATION SYNDROME [CONGENITAL]), 32
OPD-I syndrome (OTO-PALATO-DIGITAL SYNDROME TYPE I), 154
Ophthalmo-mandibulo-melic dysplasia, 148
Opitz BBBG syndrome, 149
Opitz trigonocephaly syndrome, 149
Opitz-Kaveggia syndrome (FG SYNDROME), 73
Opsoclonus-myoclonus syndrome, 150
Oral-facial-digital syndromes (ORO-FACIO-DIGITAL SYNDROMES), 150

Organoid nevus syndrome (EPIDERMAL NEVUS SYNDROME), 66

Ornithine transcarbamylase deficiency, 342

Oro-cranio-digital syndrome (JUBERG-HAYWARD SYNDROME), 104

Oro-facio-digital syndromes, 150

Oromandibular-limb hypogenesis, 152

Ortner syndrome (CARDIOVOCAL SYNDROME), 27

Osteitis fibrosa cystica, 292

Osteoarthropathy, familial idiopathic, 152

Osteolysis classification, 152

Osteolysis, familial expansile, 153

Osteolysis with nephropathy, 153

Osteolysis without nephropathy, 153

Osteoma cutis, familial, 154

Osteomalacia, 360

Osteopetrosis–renal tubular acidosis–cerebral calcification syndrome (CARBONIC
ANHYDRASE II DEFICIENCY), 252

Osteoporosis-pseudoglioma syndrome, 154

Oto-palato-digital syndrome type I, 154

Ovarian hyperstimulation syndrome, 342

Ovarian vein syndrome, 155

Oxalosis, 343

P

Pachydermoperiostosis, 155

Pachyonychia congenita (JADASSOHN-LEWANDOWSKY SYNDROME), 103

Paget-Schroetter syndrome, 156

Pallister-Hall syndrome, 156

Pallister-Killian syndrome, 156

Pancoast syndrome, 157

Papillon-Leage and Psaume syndrome, 150

Papillon-Lefèvre syndrome, 157

Paraneoplastic syndromes, 344

Paratrigeminal syndrome (RAEDER SYNDROME), 172

Parinaud syndrome, 158

Parry-Romberg syndrome (ROMBERG SYNDROME), 181

Patau syndrome (CHROMOSOME 13 TRISOMY SYNDROME), 37

Patterson syndrome, 347

Patterson-Stevenson-Fontaine acrofacial dysostosis, 3

Pearson syndrome, 348

Pegot-Cruveilhier-Baumgarten syndrome (CRUVEILHIER-BAUMGARTEN SYNDROME), 48

PEHO syndrome, 158

Pelizaeus-Merzbacher disease, 348

Pena-Shokeir syndrome type I (FETAL AKINESIA SEQUENCE), 71

Pena-Shokeir syndrome type II (CEREBRO-OCULO-FACIO-SKELETAL SYNDROME), 33

Pendred syndrome, 158

Pentalogy of Cantrell (CANTRELL SYNDROME), 25

Perisylvian syndrome (congenital bilateral), 158

Perlman syndrome, 159

Peroxisomal disorders, 349

Perrin syndrome, 94

Persistent müllerian duct syndrome, 159

Persisting mesonephric duct syndrome, 159

Peutz-Jeghers syndrome, 159

Pfeiffer syndrome, 160

Phalangeal microgeodic syndrome, 160

Phenylketonuria, 350

PHP (PSEUDOHYPOPARATHYROIDISM), 355

PIBI(D)S syndrome, 160

Pickwickian syndrome, 161

Pierre Robin syndrome (ROBIN SEQUENCE), 180

PKD (POLYCYSTIC KIDNEY DISEASE), 162

PKU (PHENYLKETONURIA), 350

Pleonosteosis (LÉRI SYNDROME), 114

Plummer-Vinson syndrome, 161

POEMS syndrome, 161

Poland sequence, 162

Pollitt syndrome (TRICHORRHEXIS NODOSA SYNDROME), 212

Polycystic kidney disease, 162

Polycystic ovary syndrome, 351

Polyglandular autoimmune disease, 352

Polyposis syndromes, 163

Polysplenia syndrome, 163

Pompe disease (GLYCOGEN STORAGE DISEASE TYPE II), 276

Popliteal artery entrapment syndrome, 163

Popliteal pterygium syndrome, 171

Porphyrias, 353

Postaxial acrofacial dysostosis, Miller type, 164

Postcardiotomy syndrome, 164

Postcholecystectomy syndrome, 165

Postcoarctectomy syndrome, 165

Postgastrectomy syndromes, 165

Postmyocardial infarction syndrome, 166

Postpericardiotomy syndrome (POSTCARDIOTOMY SYNDROME), 164

Postpneumonectomy syndrome, 166

Potter sequence, 166

PPHP (PSEUDOHYPOPARATHYROIDISM), 355

Prader-Willi syndrome, 166

Prasad syndrome, 354

Progeria, 168

Progressive encephalopathy–hypsarrhythmia–optic atrophy (PEHO SYNDROME), 158

Protein S deficiency, 354

Proteus syndrome, 169

Prune-belly syndrome, 170

Pseudoclaudication syndrome (CAUDA EQUINA SYNDROME), 30

Pseudo-Hurler polydystrophy (MUCOLIPIDOSIS III), 324

Pseudohypoaldosteronism type II, 84

Pseudohypoparathyroidism, 355

Pseudopseudohypoparathyroidism, 355

Pseudotrisomy 13 syndrome, 170

Pterygium syndromes, 171

Pyruvate dehydrogenase complex deficiency, 356

Pyruvate kinase deficiency anemia, 357

Q

Quadrilateral space syndrome, 172

R

Raeder syndrome, 172

Ramon syndrome, 172

Ramsay Hunt syndrome, 173

Rasmussen encephalitis (RASMUSSEN SYNDROME), 173

Rasmussen syndrome, 173

Rathbun disease (HYPOPHOSPHATASIA), 297

Raynaud syndrome, 173

Recombinant (8) syndrome, 174

Rectal ulcer syndrome (SOLITARY RECTAL ULCER SYNDROME), 195

Refsum disease, 357

Reifenstein syndrome, 174

Reiter syndrome, 174

Relapsing polychondritis, 175

Renal-genital-ear anomalies, 175

Renal-hepatic-pancreatic dysplasia, 176

Renal osteodystrophy, 292

Renal tubular acidosis, 358

Rendu-Osler-Weber syndrome, 176

Restrictive dermatopathy, 176

Rett syndrome, 177

Reye syndrome, 177

Reynolds acrofacial dysostosis, 3

Rheumatoid pneumoconiosis (CAPLAN SYNDROME), 26

Rib gap defect–micrognathia syndrome (CEREBRO-COSTO-MANDIBULAR SYNDROME), 33

Richieri-Costa acrofacial dysostosis, 3

Richter syndrome, 178

Rickets/osteomalacia, 359

Right middle lobe syndrome, 178

Rigid spine syndrome, 178

Riley-Day syndrome, 178

Riley-Smith syndrome, 15

Ritscher-Schinzel syndrome, 179

Roberts syndrome, 179

Robin sequence, 180

Robson-Mendenhall syndrome, 264

Rodríguez acrofacial dysostosis, 4

Rokitansky–van Bogaert syndrome (NEUROCUTANEOUS MELANOSIS SEQUENCE), 139

Romberg syndrome, 181

Rosenbloom syndrome, 264

Rotator cuff impingement syndrome (SHOULDER IMPINGEMENT SYNDROME), 189

Rothmund-Thomson syndrome, 181

Rotor syndrome, 361

Rubinstein-Taybi syndrome, 182

Rüdiger syndrome, 183

Russell syndrome (DIENCEPHALIC SYNDROME), 55

Ruvalcaba-Myhre-Smith syndrome, 15

RTA (RENAL TUBULAR ACIDOSIS), 358

S

Saethre-Chotzen syndrome, 183

Salla disease, 362

Sandhoff disease, 279

Sandifer syndrome, 184

Sanfilippo disease (MUCOPOLYSACCHARIDOSIS III), 330

Satoyoshi syndrome, 184

Say-Poznanski syndrome, 40

Scheie disease (MUCOPOLYSACCHARIDOSIS I-S), 329

Schimmelpenning-Feuerstein syndrome (EPIDERMAL NEVUS SYNDROME), 66

Schinzel syndrome (ULNAR-MAMMARY SYNDROME), 217

Schinzel-Giedion syndrome, 184

Schmidt syndrome, 352

Schwartz-Jampel syndrome, 185

Schwarz-Lélek syndrome, 185

Scimitar syndrome, 186

Scleroderma, 186

SC-phocomelia syndrome (ROBERTS SYNDROME), 179

Scurvy, 362

Sea-blue histiocyte syndrome, 188

Seckel syndrome, 188

Senior syndrome, 188

Sensenbrenner syndrome (CRANIOECTODERMAL DYSPLASIA), 45

Septo-optic dysplasia and pituitary dwarfism (DE MORSIER SYNDROME), 53

Shapiro syndrome, 188

Sharp syndrome (MIXED CONNECTIVE TISSUE DISEASE), 131

Sheehan syndrome, 363

Shone complex, 189

SHORT syndrome, 265

Short-bowel syndrome, 189

Shoulder impingement syndrome, 189

Shprintzen syndrome (VELO-CARDIO-FACIAL SYNDROME), 219

Shprintzen-Goldberg syndrome, 189

Shwachman syndrome, 363

Shwachman-Diamond syndrome (SHWACHMAN SYNDROME), 363

Shy-Drager syndrome, 190

Sialic acid storage disease, 364

Sialidosis, 364

Sialuria, Finnish type (SALLA DISEASE), 362

Sickle cell anemia, 365

Silver-Russell syndrome, 190

Simpson-Golabi-Behmel syndrome, 191

Singleton-Merten syndrome, 191

Sinusitis-infertility syndrome (YOUNG SYNDROME), 230

Sipple syndrome (MULTIPLE ENDOCRINE NEOPLASIA TYPE IIA), 135

Sirenomelia, 192

Sjögren syndrome, 192

Sjögren-Larsson syndrome, 369

Sleep apnea syndrome, 193

Slit ventricle syndrome, 193

Sly disease (MUCOPOLYSACCHARIDOSIS VII), 334

Small left colon syndrome, 193

Smith-Lemli-Opitz syndrome type I, 370

Smith-Lemli-Opitz syndrome type II, 371

Smith-Magenis syndrome, 193

Snapping hip syndrome, 194

Snapping tendon syndrome (SNAPPING HIP SYNDROME), 194

Sneddon syndrome, 194

Solitary rectal ulcer syndrome, 195

Solomon syndrome (EPIDERMAL NEVUS SYNDROME), 66

Somatostatinoma syndrome, 371

Sotos syndrome, 195

Spastic colon (IRRITABLE BOWEL SYNDROME), 102

Spherocytosis, 372

Spherophakia-brachymorphia syndrome (WEILL-MARCHESANI SYNDROME), 224

Sphingomyelin lipidoses (NIEMANN-PICK DISEASE), 336

Splenogonadal fusion/limb deformity, 196

Split notochord syndrome, 196

Split-hand/split-foot deformities, 196

Spondylo-carpo-tarsal synostosis syndrome, 197

Spondylocostal dysostoses, 197

Spondylothoracic dysostosis (SPONDYLOCOSTAL DYSOSTOSES), 197

Stagnant small-bowel syndrome, 198

Stauffer syndrome (NEPHROGENIC HEPATIC DYSFUNCTION SYNDROME), 138

Steele-Richardson-Olszewski syndrome, 198

Steinfeld syndrome, 94

Stein-Leventhal syndrome (POLYCYSTIC OVARY SYNDROME), 351

Sternal malformation–angiodysplasia association, 198

Sternal-cardiac malformations association, 198

Sterno-costo-clavicular hyperostosis, 199

Stevens-Johnson syndrome, 199

Stevenson syndrome, 181

Stewart-Treves syndrome, 199

Stickler syndrome, 200

Stiff-man syndrome, 200

Stokes-Adams syndrome, 201

Stoll-Charrow-Poznanski syndrome, 201

Straight back syndrome, 201

Streeter dysplasia (AMNIOTIC BAND SEQUENCE), 9

Sturge-Weber syndrome, 201

Sturge-Weber-Dimitri disease (STURGE-WEBER SYNDROME), 201

Subacute necrotizing encephalomyelopathy (LEIGH DISEASE), 309

Subclavian steal syndrome, 203

Sulfite oxidase deficiency, 372

Superior mesenteric artery syndrome, 203

Sweet syndrome, 204

Swyer-James syndrome, 204

Symphalangism-surdity syndrome, 205

Sympus apus (SIRENOMELIA), 192

Syndrome of inappropriate secretion of antidiuretic hormone, 373

Syndrome X, 205

Systemic sclerosis (SCLERODERMA), 186

T

Tabatznik syndrome, 205

Takatsuki syndrome (POEMS SYNDROME), 161

TAR syndrome, 206

Taybi syndrome (OTO-PALATO-DIGITAL SYNDROME TYPE I), 154

Taybi-Linder syndrome (CEPHALOSKELETAL DYSPLASIA), 32

Tay-Sachs disease, 279

Teebi hypertelorism syndrome, 206

Tel Hashomer camptodactyly syndrome, 207

Testicular feminization, 373

Tethered cord syndrome, 207

Tetrasomy 12p (PALLISTER-KILLIAN SYNDROME), 156

Thalassemia, 374

Thalidomide embryopathy, 207

Thevenard syndrome, 208

Thiamin deficiency (VITAMIN B_1 DEFICIENCY), 381

Thibierge-Weissenbach syndrome (CREST SYNDROME), 46

Third and fourth pharyngeal pouch syndrome (DIGEORGE SYNDROME), 55

Thoracic outlet syndrome, 208

Three M syndrome (THE 3-M SYNDROME), 208

3C syndrome (RITSCHER-SCHINZEL SYNDROME), 179

3-Hydroxy-3-methylglutaryl-coenzyme A lyase deficiency, 376

The 3-M syndrome, 208

Thrombocytopenia–absent radius syndrome (TAR SYNDROME), 206

Tietze syndrome, 209

Tolosa-Hunt syndrome, 209

Toriello-Carey syndrome, 210

Touraine-Solente-Golé syndrome (PACHYDERMOPERIOSTOSIS), 155

Tourette syndrome (GILLES DE LA TOURETTE SYNDROME), 82

Townes-Brocks syndrome, 210

Toxic shock syndrome, 210

Treacher Collins syndrome, 211

Tricho-dento-osseous syndrome, 211

Trichorrhexis nodosa syndrome, 212

Trismus-pseudocamptodactyly syndrome, 212

Trisomy/tetrasomy 22pter–q11 (CAT-EYE SYNDROME), 30

Troell-Junet syndrome, 212

Tuberous sclerosis, 212

Tumoral calcinosis, 377

Turcot syndrome, 214

Turner syndrome, 214

Twin-to-twin transfusion syndrome, 216

Tyrosinemia type I, 378

U

Ullrich-Turner syndrome (TURNER SYNDROME), 214

Ulnar drift (DIGITOTALAR DYSMORPHISM), 56

Ulnar-mammary syndrome, 217

Urbach-Wiethe disease (LIPOID PROTEINOSIS), 313

Urethral syndrome in women, 217

Urofacial syndrome, 217

Usher syndrome, 218

V

Váradi syndrome, 94

VACTEL (VATER ASSOCIATION), 218

VACTER (VATER ASSOCIATION), 218

VACTERL (VATER ASSOCIATION), 218

VATER association, 218

Velo-cardio-facial syndrome, 219

Verner-Morrison syndrome (VIPOMA SYNDROME), 379

VIPoma syndrome, 379

Vitamin A deficiency, 380

Vitamin A intoxication, 380

Vitamin B_1 deficiency, 381

Vitamin B_{12} deficiency, 381

Vitamin C deficiency (SCURVY), 362

Vitamin D intoxication, 382

Vohwinkel syndrome, 219

von Gierke disease (GLYCOGEN STORAGE DISEASE TYPE I), 275

von Hippel–Lindau syndrome, 220

von Recklighausen disease (NEUROFIBROMATOSIS I), 140

von Willebrand disease, 382

W

Waardenburg anophthalmia syndrome, 220

Waardenburg syndrome, 221

Wagner-Stickler syndrome (STICKLER SYNDROME), 200

Walker-Warburg syndrome, 221

Wallenberg syndrome, 222

Walt Disney Dwarfism (GERODERMA OSTEODYSPLASTICA), 81

Warfarin embryopathy, 222

Waterhouse-Friderichsen syndrome, 222

Watery diarrhea–hypokalemia–achlorhydria syndrome (VIPOMA SYNDROME), 379

Watson-Alagille syndrome (ALAGILLE SYNDROME), 6

WDHA syndrome (VIPOMA SYNDROME), 379

Weaver syndrome, 223

Weaver-Smith syndrome (WEAVER SYNDROME), 223

Weber-Christian syndrome, 223
Weil-Albright syndrome (McCune-Albright Syndrome), 125
Weill-Marchesani syndrome, 224
Weismann-Netter syndrome, 224
Wermer syndrome (Multiple Endocrine Neoplasia Type I), 134
Werner syndrome, 224
Wernicke-Korsakoff syndrome, 225
West syndrome, 225
Weyers acrodental dysostosis, 226
Weyers oligodactyly syndrome, 226
Whistling face syndrome (Freeman-Sheldon Syndrome), 78
Whitaker syndrome, 352
Wiedemann-Beckwith syndrome (Beckwith-Wiedemann Syndrome), 17
Wiedemann-Rautenstrauch syndrome, 226
Wildervanck syndrome, 226
Williams syndrome, 227
Williams-Beuren syndrome (Williams Syndrome), 227
Williams-Campbell syndrome, 228
Wilson disease, 383
Wilson-Mikity syndrome, 228
Winchester syndrome, 384
Wiskott-Aldrich syndrome, 228
WL syndrome (Symphalangism-Surdity Syndrome), 205
Wolcott-Rallison syndrome, 264
Wolff-Parkinson-White syndrome, 229
Wolf-Hirschhorn syndrome (Chromosome 4: del (4p) Syndrome), 36
Wolfram syndrome, 229, 264
Wolman disease, 385
Wrinkly skin syndrome, 230

X
Xanthine oxidase deficiency, 385
Xerodermic idiocy (De Sanctis-Cacchione Syndrome), 54
X-linked cutis laxa (Occipital Horn Syndrome), 341

Y
Yellow nail syndrome, 230
Young syndrome, 230
Youssef syndrome, 231

Z
Zellweger syndrome, 386
Zinsser-Engman-Cole syndrome (Dyskeratosis Congenita), 60
Zimmermann-Laband syndrome, 231
Zollinger-Ellison syndrome, 387

1

Syndromes

A

AARSKOG SYNDROME (AARSKOG-SCOTT SYNDROME; FACIO-DIGITO-GENITAL SYNDROME)

Clinical Manifestations: (a) *short stature;* (b) *facial features:* round face, hypertelorism, downward slanting of the palpebral fissures, blepharoptosis, maxillary hypoplasia, broad nasal bridge, short stubby nose, long and wide philtrum, linear dimple inferior to the lip, fleshy earlobes, abnormal placement and/or malrotation of the ears; widow's peak; (c) *saddle abnormality of the scrotum;* (d) *small hands; short fingers; small, broad, and flat feet; short thumbs with limited abduction; interdigital webbing;* (e) miscellaneous abnormalities: dental abnormalities; mild mental retardation; joint hypermobility; spastic hemiplegia due to cerebrovascular accidents; tortuousity of retinal vessels; (f) X-linked inheritance; autosomal dominant inheritance (sex-influenced); autosomal recessive inheritance.

Radiologic Manifestations: (a) *abnormalities of the hands and feet:* short and broad metacarpals and metatarsals; short fingers; clinodactyly of the fifth fingers; mild syndactyly; camptodactyly; hypoplasia of the terminal phalanges of the fingers; fusion of the middle and distal phalanges of the fifth toes; hypoplasia of the middle phalanges of the toes; (b) shortening of long tubular bones, with wide metaphyses; cervical spine anomalies (hypoplasia, fusion, and spina bifida occulta); mild laxity of the C1-C2 ligament; calcification of a thoracic intervertebral disc; 13 pairs of ribs; (c) miscellaneous abnormalities: maxillary hypoplasia; pelvic hypoplasia; asynchronic and delayed bone age.

AASE SYNDROME (AASE-SMITH SYNDROME II)

Clinical Manifestations: (a) *mild intrauterine growth retardation; congenital anemia* (hypoplastic, normocytic, and normochromic); *triphalangeal thumbs;* (b) X-linked recessive and autosomal recessive traits have been suggested.

Radiologic Manifestations: *Triphalangeal thumbs;* mild radial hypoplasia; absence of navicular bones; dysplastic middle phalanges of the fifth digits; long clavicles; "underdeveloped" ilia and sacrococcygeal vertebrae; skeletal maturation retardation.

ACHALASIA-ADRENAL-ALACRIMA SYNDROME (ALLGROVE SYNDROME)

Clinical Manifestations: (a) *lethargy; chronic vomiting; decreased tear production; acquired adrenocortical insufficiency; adrenocorticotropic hormone insensitivity; manometric evidence of achalasia of the* *gastroesophageal junction and dysmotility; progressive impairment of the nervous system:* motor and sensory neuropathy; ataxia; postural hypotension; episodically dilated and unequal pupils; parkinsonian features; optic atrophy; developmental delay; mild mental deterioration; (b) consistent with autosomal recessive inheritance.

Radiologic Manifestation: *Achalasia of the cardia;* velopharyngeal incompetence.

ACROCALLOSAL SYNDROME

Clinical Manifestations: (a) *craniofacial dysmorphism (macrocephaly; prominent forehead; hypertelorism); mental retardation; postnatal onset of growth retardation; foot anomalies (duplicated halluces; postaxial polydactyly of the toes); hand anomalies* (preaxial and/or postaxial polydactyly); seizures; hypotonia; strabismus; nystagmus; retinal pigmentation anomaly; optic atrophy; (b) probably autosomal recessive inheritance; most of the reported cases sporadic.

Radiologic Manifestations: (a) *agenesis or hypoplasia of the corpus callosum;* hydrocephalus; partial absence of the tentorium; cyst between the cerebrum and cerebellum; cerebral cortical atrophy; Dandy-Walker malformation; micropolygyria; large cisterna magna; arachnoidal cyst; (b) *preaxial or postaxial polydactyly of hands;* bifid terminal phalanges of thumbs; duplicated halluces; partial syndactyly of toes.

ACROFACIAL DYSOSTOSES

Classification of True Acrofacial Dysostoses
1. Arens acrofacial dysostosis: Presumed autosomal recessive; mandibulofacial dysostosis, postaxial oligodactyly, patent ductus arteriosus, talipes, feeding problems; death in early infancy.
2. Kelly acrofacial dysostosis: Autosomal recessive; growth and mental retardation; mild mandibulofacial dysostosis; hearing loss; symphalangism; radioulnar synostosis; hypospadias; cryptorchidism.
3. Postaxial acrofacial dysostosis, Miller type.
4. Nager acrofacial dysostosis.
5. Patterson-Stevenson-Fontaine acrofacial dysostosis: Autosomal dominant; mental retardation; cleft palate (submucous); abnormal auricles; oligosyndactyly of toes.
6. Reynolds acrofacial dysostosis: Autosomal dominant; mild mandibulofacial dysostosis; deafness; preaxial limb anomalies (duplication, hypoplasia); normal growth and IQ.
7. Richieri-Costa acrofacial dysostosis: Presumed autosomal recessive; mandibulofacial dysostosis; microtia; cleft lip/cleft palate; hypoplastic triphalangeal thumbs.

8. Rodríguez acrofacial dysostosis: Autosomal recessive or X-linked; severe mandibulofacial dysostosis; preaxial limb deficiencies; shoulder and pelvic girdle hypoplasia; central nervous system malformations; heart defects; lethal.

ACROGERIA (GOTTRON ACROGERIA)

Clinical Manifestations: (a) *thin and wrinkled skin; mottled skin pigmentation; prominent veins over the dorsa of the hands and feet and the upper part of the trunk; short stature; midfacial duskiness; pointed chin and nose;* thickened or dystrophic nails; skin biopsy (clumped and fragmented elastic fibers; atrophy of subcutaneous fat); (b) probably autosomal recessive inheritance; female preponderance.

Radiologic Manifestations: (a) *acro-osteolysis of distal phalanges;* (b) *micrognathia; antegonial notching of the mandible; delayed cranial suture closure; wormian bones;* (c) ankylosis of the interphalangeal joints of the hands; hourglass deformity of the distal phalanges of the hands and feet; hypoplasia of the terminal phalanges of the hands; absent distal phalanx of a toe; hallux valgus; mild osteopenia; cortical thickening; broad metaphyses; gracile bones, tubular lucencies in the long bones; congenital hip dislocation; slightly short forearm; short femoral neck; coxa valga deformity; aseptic necrosis of the femoral head; hypoplasia of the iliac wing; (d) craniostenosis (adult).

ACRORENAL SYNDROME (DIEKER-OPITZ ACRORENAL SYNDROME)

Clinical Manifestations: (a) *acral anomalies;* (b) *hypertension; proteinuria; hematuria; cylindruria; reduction of glomerular filtration; segmental glomerular sclerosis; renal interstitial fibrosis; oligomeganephronic renal hypoplasia;* (c) autosomal recessive inheritance.

Radiologic Manifestations: (a) *acral anomalies:* oligodactyly, ectrodactyly, brachydactyly, syndactyly, and polydactyly in varying combinations; various anomalies of the carpal and tarsal bones; split hands and feet; (b) *urinary system dysgenesis:* unilateral renal agenesis; duplication of the collecting system; renal hypoplasia leading to renal insufficiency; vesicoureteral reflux with hydronephrosis.

ADAMS-OLIVER SYNDROME (APLASIA CUTIS–LIMB DEFECTS)

Clinical Manifestations: (a) *scalp defect at the vertex* with or without skull defect; (b) *limb defects:* often asymmetric; usually limited to digits; (c) miscellaneous abnormalities: cutaneous syndactyly; hypoplastic nails; dilated and tortuous scalp veins; cutis marmorata; telangiectatica;

hemangioma; congenital cardiac malformations (13.4% occurrence); (d) consistent with autosomal dominant inheritance.

Radiologic Manifestations: (a) *skull defect at the vertex;* (b) *transverse limb reduction defects* (very minimal to absence of a limb); bone syndactyly; zygodactyly; ectrodactyly; polydactyly; brachydactyly; (c) direct association of the superior sagittal sinus with the base of the bony defect; communication of dilated scalp veins with the sagittal sinus.

AFFERENT LOOP SYNDROME

Clinical Manifestations: Symptoms appear following gastrectomy and gastrojejunostomy; altered afferent loop emptying with acute or chronic symptoms; in about 50% of the cases organic causes identified (perivisceritis; obstruction due to internal herniation or a kink; recurrent tumor; scarring of a stomal ulcer following a Billroth II gastrectomy; etc.): *epigastric distress; upper abdominal pain; abdominal distension; bilious vomiting; diarrhea; weight loss; anemia;* symptoms usually relieved by copious bilious vomiting; endoscopy (bile gastritis; bile esophagitis).

Radiologic Manifestations: (a) *prominent filling of the dilated proximal jejunal segment; marked active contractions of the distended proximal jejunal limb;* dilution of barium in the afferent loop by pancreatic and biliary juices; jejunogastric regurgitation; *retention of contrast medium in the proximal jejunal limb;* (b) ultrasound and computed tomography: *U-shaped cystic mass, with location of the distal portion posterior to the superior mesenteric artery and in front of aorta;* tracing of bile ducts into the cystic structure; gallbladder and biliary duct distension; hepatobiliary scanning (altered afferent loop emptying; atonic distension of the gallbladder).

AGAMMAGLOBULINEMIA, X-LINKED (BRUTON DISEASE)

Clinical Manifestations: Failure of pre-B cells to develop normally into mature B cells; onset of symptoms in infancy or early childhood: (a) *recurrent infections* (bacterial; viral); rheumatoid-like arthritis; dermatomyositis-like syndrome; growth hormone deficiency; delay of growth and puberty; *serum IgG equal to or less than 200 mg/dl with IgA and IgM markedly reduced for age; absence of functional serum antibody; normal cell-mediated immunity; deficiency of antibody-producing B-lymphocyte system; paucity of plasma cells and germinal centers in lymph nodes;* etc.; (b) fully penetrant X-linked inheritance; female carriers with normal immunologic parameters and clinically healthy; discordant phenotype in siblings reported; mapped to Xq22; Bruton tyrosine kinase gene mutations.

Radiologic Manifestations: (a) *recurrent pneumonias;* bronchial wall thickening; lobar or segmental atelectasis; bronchiectasis; tracheomegaly; *absence of lymphoid tissue in the nasopharynx;* absence of hilar adenopathy; (b) miscellaneous abnormalities: small-bowel pattern suggesting edema or malabsorption; synovial thickening without bone lesions; leptomeningeal inflammatory disease; meningeal enhancement following intravenous gadopentetate dimeglumine administration shown by magnetic resonance imaging; encephalopathy affecting white and gray matter; brain atrophy.

AICARDI SYNDROME

Clinical Manifestations: (a) *infantile spasm; subnormal intelligence; lacunar chorioretinopathy; hypsarrhythmia;* (b) miscellaneous abnormalities: multiple tumors; persistent hyperplastic primary vitreous; etc.; (c) probably X-linked dominant inheritance with male lethality.

Radiologic Manifestations: (a) *agenesis of the corpus callosum* (partial or total); (b) other central nervous system anomalies: gross asymmetry of the cerebral hemispheres; cerebellar hypoplasia; delayed myelination; asymmetric myelination; multiple intracerebral fluid collections with higher signal intensity than cerebrospinal fluid; etc.; (c) miscellaneous abnormalities: costovertebral malformations; microphthalmos; cystic intraorbital lesions.

AINHUM

Clinical Manifestations: Toes and fingers involved: *deep soft-tissue groove corresponding to a hyperkeratotic band partially or totally encircling the digit.*

Radiologic Manifestations: *Sharply demarcated thinning and narrowing of bone, then fracture and resorption;* autoamputation of the digit in some cases.

ALAGILLE SYNDROME (ARTERIOHEPATIC SYNDROME; WATSON-ALAGILLE SYNDROME)

Clinical Manifestations: (a) *dysmorphic facies:* small triangular face; broad forehead; pointed mandible; flattened cheeks; mild ocular hypertelorism; deep-set eyes; prominent or malformed ears; (b) *posterior embryotoxon; chorioretinal atrophy; pigment clumping;* Axenfeld anomaly; etc.; (c) *peripheral pulmonary stenosis or hypoplasia;* etc.; (d) *neonatal cholestasis; hypoplasia of the intralobular bile ducts;* cirrhosis; hepatic failure; hepatoma; hepatocarcinoma; focal liver hyperplasia; etc.; (e) *retarded growth;* (f) miscellaneous abnormalities: renal function abnormalities; cystic renal disease; endocrine and exocrine disorders; neuropsychiatric manifestations; cutaneous manifestations (keratoderma; cutaneous photosensitivity); (g) autosomal dominant transmission with very high penetrance and variable expressivity; various cytogenetic abnormalities involving 20p12; submicroscopic deletion within 20p12.

Radiologic Manifestations: (a) vertebral defects: *butterfly vertebrae;* small vertebral bodies; narrow interpedicular distances; irregular endplates; fused vertebral bodies; etc.; (b) limb deformities: short ulna; short distal phalanges; long and thin fingers; proximally placed thumbs; radioulnar synostosis; multiple lacunae, possibly representing intraosseous xanthomas; etc.; (c) diffuse hepatic increased echogenicity and loss of normal texture due to parenchymal disease; regenerative liver nodules; retention of Tc-99m IDA in the periphery of the liver; etc.; (d) hypoplastic kidneys; renal artery stenosis; unilateral absence of a kidney; medullary cystic disease with prominent renal echoes; duplicated ureters; renal stones; nephrocalcinosis; (e) miscellaneous abnormalities: hyperintensity of the globus pallidi and subthalamic nuclei on T_1-weighted magnetic resonance images; osteopenia.

Note: Presence of at least 3 of the 5 major manifestations (*peculiar facies; chronic intrahepatic cholestasis due to paucity of intralobular bile ducts; peripheral pulmonary artery hypoplasia or stenosis; posterior ocular embryotoxon; butterfly vertebral anomaly*) is required for the diagnosis of Alagille syndrome.

ALIEN HAND SYNDROME

Pathology: Two types: (a) frontal: damage to the supplementary motor area, anterior cingulate gyrus, and medial prefrontal cortex of the dominant hemisphere and anterior corpus callosum; (b) callosal: anterior callosal lesion.

Clinical and Radiologic Manifestations: *Involuntary movement of the extremity, contrary to the patient's intention;* restraining of the "alien hand" by the normal one; computed tomography and magnetic resonance imaging *(infarction; hemorrhage; tumor);* case reported with mirror movement.

ALPERS SYNDROME (ALPERS-HUTTENLOCHER SYNDROME)

Clinical Manifestations: Insidious onset of symptoms in infancy: (a) *developmental delay; failure to thrive; seizures;* (b) *liver disease:* liver failure, fatty change, loss of hepatocyte, bile duct proliferation, fibrosis, and cirrhosis; (c) central nervous system: gray matter disease with neuronal degeneration, gliosis and spongiosis of cerebral cortex, basal ganglia, brain stem, dentate nucleus, cerebellum, and lumbar spinal ganglia; presentation with seizures and multiple strokelike episodes; (d) autosomal recessive inheritance.

Radiologic Manifestations: *Low-density (computed tomography) regions, particularly in the occipital and posterior temporal lobes, involving both gray and white matter; progressive cerebral atrophy; occipital white matter softening.*

ALPORT SYNDROME

Clinical Manifestations: (a) *nephropathy: excretion of glomerular basement antigen, thickening and splitting of the glomerular basement membrane with electron-lucent areas containing small, dense granulations,* etc.; (b) *high-tone sensorineural deafness, usually progressive in childhood;* (c) *ocular abnormalities: anterior lenticonus and macular flecks,* etc.; (d) Alport-leiomyomatosis syndrome: leiomyomatosis (esophagus; tracheobronchial tree; vulva; clitoris) associated with hematuria, proteinuria, and glomerular lesions similar to those in Alport syndrome; (e) miscellaneous abnormalities: bilateral inguinal hernia; smooth muscle tumors with X-linked Alport syndrome (carrier detection in females); (f) dominant X-linked inheritance; mutations in Alport syndrome associated with diffuse esophageal leiomyomatosis.

Radiologic Manifestations: (a) *radiologic findings of renal failure;* (b) renal abnormalities: diffuse renal enlargement; minimal blunting of the calices; small and contracted kidney; renal cortical calcification; (c) congestive heart failure secondary to hypertension; (d) renal vascular changes: poor cortical opacification, severe tortuosity and crowded appearance at the corticomedullary junction, pruning of interlobar arteries, and indistinctness of the corticomedullary junction.

AMINOPTERIN FETOPATHY

Clinical Manifestations: Due to teratogenic effects of aminopterin and amethopterin used in the first trimester of pregnancy: *low birth weight; cranial dysplasia; abnormal facies: low-set ears; prominent eyes; hypertelorism; flat nasal bridge; micrognathia; cleft palate; upswept frontal hair pattern; shallow supraorbital ridges;* etc.

Radiologic Manifestations: *Cranial dysplasia (lack of normal ossification of the cranial vault at birth; poor ossification of the cranium and the development of multiple wormian bones in follow-up studies; cranium* *bifidum; aberrant longitudinal suture in the parietal bones; partial cranio-synostosis)*; etc.

AMINOPTERIN FETOPATHY-LIKE SYNDROME

Clinical Manifestations: Very similar to aminopterin syndrome, with no evidence of maternal exposure to the drug: (a) craniofacial dysmorphism: *temporal recession of the hairline with an upswept frontal hair pattern; ocular hypertelorism; prominent nasal root; low-set, posteriorly rotated earlobes; highly arched cleft palate;* (b) *dermatoglyphic anomalies*; (c) *short stature;* (d) *psychomotor retardation;* (e) reported in siblings; possibly autosomal recessive inheritance.

Radiologic Manifestations: *Parietal cranial bone defects;* small orbits; ossification defect of the orbital roof; facial asymmetry; micrognathia; hydrocephalus; mild scoliosis; spina bifida; small iliac wings; mildly hypoplastic thumb.

AMNIOTIC BAND SEQUENCE (Streeter Dysplasia)

Clinical Manifestations: (a) constrictive amniotic bands; amniotic adhesions; fetal malformations (limbs most commonly affected, followed by craniofacial defects): *single or multiple ring constrictions, most common distally;* facial clefts; calvarial defects; hydrocephalus; anencephaly; encephalocele; gastroschisis; omphalocele; Cantrell syndrome; etc.; (b) sporadic; familial amniotic bands and amniotic band disruption in twins have rarely been reported.

Radiologic Manifestations: (a) prenatal ultrasonography: *detection of limb, trunk, and craniofacial defects in association with the amniotic bands* (intrauterine bands without visualization of fetal defects is not diagnostic); (b) postnatal imaging: *limb, trunk, and craniofacial abnormalities.*

ANDERMANN SYNDROME

Clinical Manifestations: (a) *progressive motor-sensory neuronopathy*; facial dysmorphism (elongated face; hypertelorism; highly arched palate; hypoplastic maxilla; large angle of mandible; mild palpebral ptosis; mild facial diplegia); *mental retardation;* psychotic episodes; *electrophysiologic abnormalities* (absence of sensory action potentials; reduction of motor nerve conduction; signs of denervation and reinnervation); (b) autosomal recessive inheritance; majority of the reported cases originating in Quebec, Canada.

Radiologic Manifestations: *Agenesis of the corpus callosum* (partial or total).

ANGELMAN SYNDROME ("HAPPY PUPPET" SYNDROME)

Clinical Manifestations: (a) *dysmorphic craniofacial features: microcephaly; brachycephaly; pointed chin/prognathism; macrostomia*; midfacial hypoplasia; deep-set eyes; thin upper lip; widely spaced teeth; bowing of the upper teeth; (b) *feeding problems; delayed motor milestones; mental retardation; ataxic gait; stiff, jerky puppetlike movements and gait; truncal hypotonia; cortical myoclonus; limb hypertonia; paroxysmal laughter; seizures; inability to speak; persistent tongue thrusting; brisk reflexes;* autism; characteristic electroencephalographic abnormalities; (c) miscellaneous abnormalities: optic atrophy; hypopigmentation of skin, hair, and eyes, as compared with other family members (blue eyes; blond hair; oculocutaneous albinism); (d) sporadic; familial cases less common (autosomal dominant); maternally derived de novo deletion of chromosome 15q11–13 in most cases.

Radiologic Manifestations: *Microbrachycephaly;* vertical inclination of the base of the skull; horizontal occipital depression; prognathism; structural cerebral abnormalities (measuring the length of the banks of the sylvian fissure) shown by magnetic resonance imaging; brain atrophy; arachnoid cyst.

ANIRIDIA-WILMS TUMOR ASSOCIATION

Clinical and Radiologic Manifestations: (a) *Wilms tumor* (bilateral tumor in about one third of the cases); *congenital aniridia* (sporadic type); genitourinary abnormalities, including segmental cystic renal lesions histologically similar to autosomal dominant polycystic kidney disease; mental retardation; craniofacial dysmorphism; deformities of the pinna; cataracts; glaucoma; various skeletal defects; hamartomatous lesions; umbilical and inguinal hernias; hyperkinesis; (b) *deletion 11p13–14.1.*

ANTIPHOSPHOLIPID SYNDROME

Clinical and Radiologic Manifestations: (a) presence of *antiphospholipid antibodies:* lupus anticoagulant; anticardiolipin; (b) *venous and/or arterial thrombotic occlusion*; *livedo reticularis;* (c) central nervous system abnormalities: *cerebral ischemia;* multi-infarct dementia; migraine; epilepsy; chorea; transverse myelopathy; (d) miscellaneous abnormalities: myocardial infarction; intracardiac thrombosis; cardiac valve degeneration; pulmonary hypertension; renal vein thrombosis; intrarenal vascular lesions; malignant hypertension; renal insufficiency; recurrent abortion (placental vessel thrombosis; ischemia); Budd-Chiari syndrome; etc.

ANTLEY-BIXLER SYNDROME

Clinical Manifestations: (a) *trapezoidocephaly; midfacial hypoplasia;* low-set ears; choanal atresia; *joint contractures; fixed flexion at elbows;* clubfeet; narrow chest; renal and anal anomalies; esophageal atresia in a patient with trisomy 21 and Antley-Bixler syndrome; etc.; (b) autosomal recessive inheritance.

Radiologic Manifestations: *Craniosynostosis (coronals; lambdoids); humeroradial synostosis; bowed femurs;* antegonial notching of the mandible; high vertebral bodies; sclerosis at end-plates of vertebrae; carpal and tarsal fusion; bowed ulna; long bone fractures; gracile ribs; etc.

APERT SYNDROME (ACROCEPHALOSYNDACTYLY, APERT TYPE)

Clinical Manifestations: (a) *macrocrania; deformed head with high, broad, and flat forehead; brachycephaly; hypertelorism; depressed nasal bridge; down-slanting palpebral fissures; open mouth; trapezoid-shaped mouth with an associated highly arched palate and occasionally cleft palate; bifid uvula; relative prognathism*; (b) *"mitten hand" and "sock foot";* (c) dental anomalies: crowded teeth; malocclusion; anterior and posterior crossbites; delayed eruption; ectopic eruption; shovel-shaped incisors; (d) *proptosis;* strabismus; amblyopia; optic atrophy; papilledema; (e) *mental retardation;* (f) miscellaneous abnormalities: visceral abnormalities; musculoskeletal abnormalities; conductive hearing loss; acne vulgaris; cloverleaf skull deformity; etc.; (g) most cases sporadic; autosomal dominant inheritance in some cases.

Radiologic Manifestations: (a) *turribrachycephaly, macrocrania; premature closure of sutures (coronals in particular); shallow orbits; hypoplasia of the maxilla; prominent mandible; unilateral or bilateral canting of the temporal bone (upward tilting);* (b) central nervous system abnormalities: *megalencephaly*; frontal ventriculomegaly; partial or complete agenesis of the corpus callosum; absence of the septum pellucidum; cyst of the septum; malformations of the limbic structures; progressive hydrocephalus (uncommon); gyral abnormalities; encephalocele (frontal; occipital); pyramidal tract abnormalities; hypoplasia of cerebral white matter; heterotopic gray matter; convolutional atrophy; arrhinencephaly; hydromyelia; (c) *complete syndactyly involving the second to fifth digits (mitten hand and sock foot);* partial or complete duplication of the proximal phalanx of the great toes and first metatarsals; hallux varus; (d) miscellaneous abnormalities: skeletal abnormalities; upper airway obstruction; tracheal abnormalities (tracheal stenosis; cartilage sleeve abnormalities); prenatal ultrasonographic diagnosis (acrocephaly; cupped hands; fusion of the digits).

APLASIA CUTIS CONGENITA

Clinical Manifestations: (a) *aplasia cutis usually occurs in the midline of the scalp, less often on the trunk and limbs; often round or oval; sharply marginated; ulcerated or covered by thin membrane;* (b) *limb anomalies;* (c) superior sagittal sinus hemorrhage; (d) miscellaneous abnormalities: chromosomal abnormalities; seizures; central nervous system anomalies; cardiovascular anomalies; alimentary system anomalies; ocular abnormalities; skin lesions; ambiguous genitalia; cryptorchidism; acrania (absence of the flat bones of the cranial vault) associated with congenital scalp defect with or without distal limb anomalies; high myopia and cone-rod dysfunction in siblings; elevated α-fetoprotein; etc.; (e) autosomal dominant inheritance in some cases; variable intrafamilial expression; chromosome 12q abnormality.

Radiologic Manifestations: (a) *skull defect underlying the skin lesion* (in some); multiple wormian bones; enlarged parietal foramina; (b) anomalous scalp veins; drainage of scalp veins into intracranial venous sinuses; anomalous vessels of the face and eyes; hydrocephalus; (c) cerebral atrophy; meningocele; dural defects; etc.; (d) *limb anomalies:* acral reduction defects; absent lower limb below the midcalf; clubbing of the hands and feet; etc.; (e) miscellaneous abnormalities: intestinal lymphangiectasia; hemangiomas; vascular lesions of the face and eyes; hydrocephalus; cerebral malformations; dural defects; polycystic kidneys; meningocele; tracheoesophageal fistula; patent ductus arteriosus; occult spinal dysrhaphia underlying the cutaneous anomaly; etc.

ARTERIAL CALCIFICATION OF INFANCY

Clinical Manifestations: Onset of symptoms usually in the first few months of life: (a) respiratory distress; refusal to eat; vomiting; fever; *congestive heart failure;* periarticular swelling and joint stiffness; etc.; (b) occurrence in siblings; pattern of inheritance not definitely known.

Radiologic Manifestations: (a) *arterial wall calcification* shown by radiographic examination and sonography (very prominent echogenicity of the arterial wall and acoustic shadowing from the vessel walls); diffuse hyperechogenicity of the kidney; (b) *cardiomegaly; congestive heart failure;* pericardial effusion; thickened pulmonary and aortic valves; (c) miscellaneous abnormalities: periarticular calcification; epiphyseal calcification; earlobe calcification; cerebral arterial calcification and infarction; in utero diagnosis (hydramnios; fetal ascites; vascular calcification).

ARTHROPATHY-CAMPTODACTYLY SYNDROME (CAMPTO-DACTYLY-ARTHROPATHY-PERICARDITIS SYNDROME)

Clinical Manifestations: Onset of symptoms in childhood: (a) *arthropathy; camptodactyly;* pericarditis; (b) autosomal recessive inheritance.

Radiologic Manifestations: *Arthropathy* (primarily affecting the large joints; joint effusion; bone erosions); *camptodactyly* (bilateral and symmetric, secondary to flexion of the flexor tendons at the proximal interphalangeal joint level); pericarditis; coxa vara.

ASHERMAN SYNDROME

Pathology: Partial or complete uterine adhesions involving the endometrium and/or cervix as a result of trauma (curettage; manual removal of the placenta; enucleation of myoma) or inflammation (endometritis; septic abortion; schistosomiasis).

Clinical Manifestations: *Infertility; hypomenorrhea or amenorrhea; postpartum hemorrhage; placental retention; multiple pregnancy losses; hysteroscopic visualization of the adhesions.*

Radiologic Manifestations: Demonstration of the *adhesions* by hysterosalpingography, ultrasonography, or magnetic resonance imaging (*absence of normal endometrium and junctional zone signals on T_2-weighted images*).

ASPLENIA SYNDROME (IVEMARK SYNDROME)

Pathology: (a) *absent spleen;* rarely hypoplastic spleen; (b) *thoracic isomerism; right-sided appearance of left-sided organs* in the form of bilateral trilobed lungs; bilateral eparterial bronchi; extralobulation of the lungs; (c) isomerism of the atria; *complex cyanotic heart diseases* (bilateral superior venae cavae; a common hepatic vein; *anomalous pulmonary venous drainage; transposition of the great arteries; pulmonary stenosis or atresia; abdominal aorta and inferior vena cava on the same side);* (d) *alimentary system anomalies;* diaphragmatic hernia; *right and left lobes of the liver of almost equal size (symmetric liver);* (e) miscellaneous abnormalities: horseshoe adrenals; Jeune syndrome with situs inversus; etc.

Clinical Manifestations: *Cyanosis; congestive heart failure; polycythemia; Howell-Jolly bodies and Heinz bodies in the peripheral blood;* etc.

Radiologic Manifestations: (a) *horizontal liver; absent spleen* (computed tomography; dual radiopharmaceutical imaging with the use of ^{99m}Tc sulfur colloid and with the ^{99m}Tc PIPIDA [similarity of the images suggests asplenia, and a discrepancy in organ morphology between the two scans indicates the presence of a spleen]); (b) *vena cava and aorta on the same side of the spine in a "piggyback" fashion; absent splenic vein; midline portal vein;* (c) *bilateral pulmonary three lobes; bilateral eparterial bronchi; congenital heart anomalies;* etc.

ATAXIA-TELANGIECTASIA SYNDROME (LOUIS-BAR SYNDROME)

Clinical Manifestations: Onset of symptoms in childhood: (a) *oculocutaneous telangiectasia;* (b) *progressive cerebellar ataxia;* nystagmus; strabismus; failure of purposive eye movement; choreoathetosis; dysarthria; progressive mental deterioration; generalized muscle weakness; impassive face; progressive peripheral neuron degeneration; (c) recurrent sinopulmonary infections; (d) premature graying; (e) atrophic and sclerodermatous skin changes; follicular and solar keratoses; basal cell epithelioma; eczema; generalized skin pigmentation; cutaneous granulomatous lesions; (f) endocrinopathies; (g) *high sensitivity to ionizing radiation and various radiometric drugs; enhanced in vitro radiosensitivity of cultured skin cells; defect in deoxyribonucleic acid repair; predisposition to malignancies; abnormal humoral and cellular immunity; chromosomal instability;* (h) genetic heterogeneity; autosomal recessive inheritance.

Radiologic Manifestations: (a) *sinusitis; recurrent pulmonary infections; bronchiectasis; pulmonary fibrosis;* tracheomegaly; *lack of a thymic shadow in infancy; diminished or absent nasopharyngeal lymphoid tissues; absent nodal enlargement in pulmonary hili;* (b) miscellaneous abnormalities: diffuse cerebellar atrophy with marked involvement of the vermis, large cisterna magna; calcification in the lentiform nuclei; low density of white matter and cortical thickening consistent with pachygyria.

B

BALLER-GEROLD SYNDROME (CRANIOSYNOSTOSIS–RADIAL APLASIA SYNDROME)

Clinical Manifestations: (a) *skull deformity related to craniosynostosis;* facial dysmorphism (ocular hypertelorism; epicanthal folds; prominent nasal bridge; low-set dysplastic ears; cleft palate; bifid uvula; highly arched palate; micrognathia or prominent mandible); unusual hair pattern; (b) *preaxial limb anomaly;* (c) probably autosomal recessive inheritance; intrafamilial variability.

Radiologic Manifestations: (a) *craniosynostosis* (one or more sutures); (b) *radial hypoplasia or aplasia; hypoplastic or absent thumbs;* (c) miscellaneous skeletal anomalies: coxa valga; hypoplastic patella; slender fibula; foot deformities (tarsal coalition; metatarsus adductus; proximally placed halluces; brachyclinodactyly of individual toes; phalangeal aplasia/hypoplasia); shortening and curvature of the ulna; radial deviation of the hand; missing phalanges, metacarpals, and/or carpal bones; fused carpal bones; extensive agenesis of the frontal and parietal bones; vertebral anomalies; rib anomalies; (d) miscellaneous abnormalities: crossed renal ectopia; polyhydramnios; fetal hydrocephalus; osteosarcoma.

BANNAYAN-RILEY-RUVALCABA SYNDROME

Clinical Manifestations: (a) *macrocephaly; increased birth size; postnatal growth deceleration; tumors;* (b) miscellaneous abnormalities: macrodactyly; hypotonia; lipid myopathy; mild neurologic dysfunction; mild mental retardation; seizures; motor delay; speech delay; prolonged drooling; etc.; (c) autosomal dominant inheritance; sporadic.

Radiologic Manifestations: (a) *macrocephaly without ventricular enlargement;* (b) *tumors:* mesodermal hamartomas (subcutaneous; intracranial; visceral; intestinal; thoracic; skeletal); etc.; (c) miscellaneous abnormalities: hydrocephalus; diffusely thickened corpus callosum; increased T_2-weighted signals in deep white matter of the occipital and posterior parietal lobes (demyelination or dysmyelination).

Note: Considering Bannayan syndrome, Riley-Smith syndrome, and Ruvalcaba-Myhre-Smith syndrome as one etiologic entity, the name of Bannayan-Riley-Ruvalcaba syndrome has been proposed and used in this text. The originally described manifestations of each entity are as follows: (1) Bannayan: macrocephaly associated with multiple subcutaneous and visceral lipomas and hemangiomas; (2) Riley and Smith: macrocephaly associated with pseudopapilledema, and multiple hemangiomas; (3) Ruvalcaba, Myhre, and Smith: macrocephaly, intestinal polyposis, and pigmented spotting of the penis.

BANTI SYNDROME

Clinical Manifestations: *Splenomegaly; leukopenia; anemia; moderate thrombocytopenia;* upper alimentary tract hemorrhage; various manifestations of hepatic failure.

Radiologic Manifestations: *Esophageal and/or gastric varices; portal system obstruction* (intrahepatic: cirrhosis of the liver; extrahepatic); pancreatic fibrosis; tumor; etc.

BARDET-BIEDL SYNDROME

Clinical Manifestations: (a) *pigmentary retinal degeneration;* (b) *polydactyly;* (c) *obesity;* (d) *genital hypoplasia;* (e) *mental retardation;* (f) *nephropathy:* polydipso-polyuria; reduced concentrating ability; uremia; glomerular sclerosis; interstitial sclerosis; cystic renal dysplasia; (g) miscellaneous abnormalities: chorea; anomalies of the permanent dentition; (h) autosomal recessive inheritance; interfamilial and intrafamilial phenotypic variations.

Radiologic Manifestations: (a) *polydactyly;* syndactyly; clinodactyly of the fifth finger; (b) *urinary system anomalies:* cysts; calyceal diverticula; lobulated renal outlines of the fetal type; diffuse renal cortical loss; hypoplasia of the kidney; hydronephrosis; persistent urogenital sinus; vesicovaginal fistula; large echogenic kidneys mimicking infantile polycystic kidneys on prenatal and postnatal ultrasound examinations; (c) miscellaneous abnormalities: skull defects; hip dysplasia; atrophy of spinal cord associated with spinal stenosis; spina bifida; genu valgum; congenital cardiovascular defects; hypertrophy of interventricular septum; dilated cardiomyopathy; dilatation of intrahepatic bile ducts and common bile duct; enlargement of the lateral ventricles.

Note: Laurence-Moon syndrome: the cases reported by Laurence and Moon had mental retardation, hypogenitalism, pigmentary retinopathy, and spastic paraplegia. Bardet-Biedl and Laurence-Moon syndromes are considered different but interrelated autosomal recessive disorders.

BARTTER SYNDROME

Clinical Manifestations: (a) growth retardation; mental retardation; craniofacial dysmorphism; muscle weakness; tetany; vomiting; (b) *polydipsia; polyuria; normal blood pressure; hypokalemic alkalosis; hyperaldosteronism; normocalciuria or hypercalciuria; hyperplasia of the juxtaglomerular apparatus;* renal sodium wasting; plasma volume contraction; defect in platelet aggregation; inability to concentrate urine; elevated plasma renin and angiotensin levels; diminished pressor response to infused angiotensin; rise in aldosterone levels following the infusion of renin; hypophosphatemia due to hyperparathyroidism; retinopathy; (c) autosomal recessive inheritance most likely.

Radiologic Manifestations: (a) *nephromegaly;* marked renal medullary and minimal cortical hypertrophy; splayed minor calices; pyelectasis; hydroureters without obstruction; loss of cortical substance in the absence of vesicoureteral reflux; splaying of interlobar and arcuate arteries; *increased renal parenchymal echogenicity with a loss of corticomedullary differentiation;* hyperechoic pyramids; small cortical cysts;

nephrocalcinosis; (b) miscellaneous abnormalities: rickets; osteomalacia; chondrocalcinosis; transient gallbladder dilatation associated with hypokalemia; recurrent hydramnios.

Note: Hyperprostaglandin E syndrome is a neonatal variant of Bartter syndrome with enhanced renal and systemic formation of prostaglandin E_2: hypercalciuria, nephrocalcinosis, and osteopenia.

BEAN SYNDROME (BLUE RUBBER BLEB NEVUS SYNDROME)

Clinical Manifestations: (a) rubbery, raised bluish to black cutaneous *nevi* (cavernous hemangioma, 0.1 to 5 cm in diameter); gastrointestinal bleeding due to *mucosal hemangiomas;* other rare sites of hemangioma (lungs; liver; spleen; joint capsule; deep subcutaneous tissues; oral cavity; nasopharynx; pleura; peritoneal cavity; mesentery; conjunctiva; iris; retina; penis; uterus; urinary bladder; thyroid; heart; kidney; brain; spinal cord; meninges; cranial bones; muscles); (b) iron deficiency anemia; (c) most cases sporadic; autosomal dominant inheritance in a few families.

Radiologic Manifestations: *Single or multiple polypoid filling defects of the bowel of varying sizes;* phlebolith; *angiographic demonstration of visceral hemangiomas* (early opacification that then increases in the venous phase); magnetic resonance imaging: *bright signal on T_2-weighted images that probably is due to slow flow or thrombosis;* central nervous system involvement (hemangioma; intracranial calcification; venous thrombosis; brain atrophy; frontal sinus pericranii; venous angioma).

Note: Cellular blue nevus is a variant of blue nevus that arises in the dermis. It may be associated with local extension, including intracranial involvement.

BECKWITH-WIEDEMANN SYNDROME (WIEDEMANN-BECKWITH SYNDROME)

Clinical Manifestations: (a) *craniofacial dysmorphism*; *macroglossia*; *omphalocele, umbilical hernia, or diastasis recti*; *gigantism; visceromegaly;* (b) increased incidence of neoplasms (7.5%), especially if associated with asymmetry: nephroblastoma; adrenal cortical carcinoma; hepatoblastoma; hepatocellular carcinoma; etc.; (c) *hypoglycemia* (hyperinsulinism); (d) genetic heterogeneity; sporadic; familial (dominant inheritance; about 15% of the cases); male monozygotic twins discordant for Beckwith-Wiedemann syndrome.

Radiologic Manifestations: (a) *large tongue;* (b) *omphalocele or umbilical hernia;* (c) *nephromegaly;* diffuse increased echogenicity of the cortex; normal or proportionately enlarged nondilated calices; lobulated renal margin; corticomedullary cysts; nodules of mixed echogenicity;

medullary renal dysplasia mimicking renal tumor; pelvicalyceal distension; pelvicalyceal diverticula; duplex collecting system; medullary sponge kidney; (d) *hepatomegaly;* (e) prenatal ultrasonography: polyhydramnios; larger than expected fetus; enlarged fetal abdominal circumference; macroglossia; omphalocele; nephromegaly; cystic kidneys; accelerated growth profile; placentomegaly with or without associated cystic changes in the placenta; (f) miscellaneous abnormalities: advanced skeletal maturation (in some); neonatal cardiomegaly; widening of the metaphyses and cortical thickening of the long bones; hemihypertrophy (hemihyperplasia); posterior eventration of the diaphragm; microcephaly; adrenal calcification.

BEHÇET SYNDROME

Pathology: *Necrotizing arteritis*; aneurysmal dilatation of minor and major arteries; thrombotic occlusions of arteries; *thrombophlebitis.*

Clinical Manifestations: (a) *aphthous stomatitis;* absent or scanty lingual fungiform papillae; cutaneous and mucosal ulcerations; erythema nodosum; subungual infarction; (b) *genital ulcer;* ureteral obstruction with bladder involvement; epididymitis; (c) esophageal lesions; ulceration and perforation of the small bowel; colitis; diarrhea; pancreatitis; hepatomegaly; (d) *iridocyclitis with hypopyon;* (e) miscellaneous abnormalities: meningoencephalitis; oligoarthritis; polyarthritis; soft-tissue swelling; pericarditis; myocarditis; myocardial infarction; hypertension (renal artery stenosis); superior vena cava syndrome associated with chyloptysis and chylous ascites; association with Sweet syndrome; association with Budd-Chiari syndrome; association with relapsing polychondritis and human immunodeficiency virus infection; etc.

Radiologic Manifestations: (a) pulmonary parenchymal infiltrate; recurrent pneumonia, hilar adenopathy; pleural effusion; (b) *vasculopathies:* arterial aneurysm; venous thrombosis; pulmonary embolism; pseudoaneurysm; rupture of the coronary artery, with false aneurysm formation; arterial thrombosis; Budd-Chiari syndrome; prominent pulmonary arteries; perfusion defects on ventilation-perfusion scans; (c) esophageal ulceration; bowel stenosis, perforation, and functional disorder; enterocolitis; inflammatory polyposis of colon; (d) central nervous system involvement: infarction; edema; aneurysms; spontaneous arterial dissection; dural sinus thrombosis: (1) magnetic resonance imaging: acute phase (high signal intensity on T_2-weighted images within the brain stem, the basal ganglia, and the cerebral hemispheres; enhancement of the lesions using gadolinium-DTPA); chronic phase (atrophy of the posterior fossa structures; decreased signal intensity suggestive of hemosiderin deposition); (2) positron emission tomography or single photon emission computed tomography may detect abnormalities at an earlier stage, before their progression to a visible stage by computed tomography and magnetic resonance imaging: decreased regional cerebral blood flow and oxygen consumption; (e) miscellaneous abnormalities: osteoporosis; joint space narrowing; osseous erosions; spontaneous atlantoaxial subluxation; sacroiliitis; avascular necrosis of the femoral head; enthesopathy.

BERDON SYNDROME (MEGACYSTIS–MICROCOLON–INTESTINAL HYPOPERISTALSIS SYNDROME)

Clinical Manifestations: Onset of symptoms in the neonatal period: (a) *abdominal distension; decreased or absent bowel movements;* bilious vomiting; absent or decreased bowel sounds; manometric study of the stomach and duodenum (low frequency and low amplitude of the contractions); electrophysiologic study (decreased autonomic inhibitory input to the smooth muscle cells of the small intestine); (b) miscellaneous abnormalities: hydrometrocolpos and segmental colonic dilatation in a girl; (c) autosomal recessive inheritance.

Radiologic Manifestations: (a) *microcolon;* malrotation and malfixation of the bowel; *intestinal hypoperistalsis; dilated small bowel;* volvulus of the bowel; (b) *megalocystis;* hydronephrosis; hydroureter; absence of bladder outlet obstruction; vesicoureteral reflux; (c) miscellaneous abnormalities: dilated stomach; (d) antenatal ultrasound: polyhydramnios; rarely oligohydramnios (transient, followed by polyhydramnios); markedly enlarged bladder; hydroureter; hydronephrosis; dilated stomach; dilated bowel.

BILE PLUG SYNDROME (INSPISSATED BILE SYNDROME)

Clinical Manifestations: (a) association with: total parenteral nutrition; dehydration; massive hemolysis due to Rh or ABO incompatibility; cystic fibrosis; etc.; (b) *obstructive jaundice* in infancy due to impacted, thickened secretions and bile in the extrahepatic ducts; cholangitis in some cases; spontaneous resolution in many cases.

Radiologic Manifestations: (a) ultrasonographic demonstration of *dilated bile ducts and inspissated bile (low-level echoes);* (b) nuclear medicine hepatobiliary imaging: *lack of excretion of the radionuclide into the bowel indicates bile duct obstruction;* (c) *dilatation of the ducts and the intraluminal "mass" causing obstruction are demonstrated by an intraoperative cholangiogram.*

BINDER SYNDROME (MAXILLONASAL DYSPLASIA; NASO-MAXILLO-VERTEBRAL SYNDROME)

Clinical Manifestations: (a) *craniofacial dysmorphism:* nasal anomalies (obtuse or almost totally absent frontonasal angle; downward angling of the nasal pyramid; nasal kyphosis; hypoplasia of the alar cartilage; rounded appearance of the nares; hypoplastic and ptotic columella; "half-moon" appearance of the external nares; atrophy of the nasal mucosa); outward projection of the upper lip; projection of the chin; flatness of the mental area; aplasia of the maxilla and premaxilla around and under the nares and the columella; atrophy of the frenulum of the upper lip; dental occlusion problems; (b) cervical kyphosis and scoliosis; etc.

Radiologic Manifestations: (a) *craniofacial anomalies*: small glabella; flat nasofrontal angle; vertical position of the nasal bones; hypoplasia of the frontal process of the maxilla; thinness of the alveolar bone on the labial side of the upper incisors, vestibular version of the incisors; inversion of the incisors; pseudoprognathism or true mandibular prognathism; wide gonial angle; hypoplastic frontal sinuses; (b) cervical spine anomalies (in about one half of the cases): abnormality of the arch of C1; ossiculum terminale; separate odontoid process; spina bifida; block vertebrae; persistent chorda dorsalis (defective mineralization).

BLIND LOOP SYNDROME (BLIND POUCH SYNDROME)

Clinical Manifestations: *Intestinal stagnation resulting in bacterial overgrowth, bacterial breakdown of bile salts and deamination of protein leading to malabsorption, steatorrhea, and fat-soluble vitamin deficiencies:* abdominal cramps; feculent vomiting; melena; weight loss; malnutrition; growth retardation; macrocytic *anemia; hypoalbuminemia;* breath hydrogen test (high basal excretion of breath hydrogen after overnight fasting; an earlier and greater breath hydrogen value after oral lactose administration than is formed in lactose malabsorption alone; sustained hydrogen concentration rise over a period of several hours); etc.

Radiologic Manifestations: Usually a result of surgical side-to-side or end-to-side anastomosis after resection of a segment of bowel: spherical, tubular, or club-shaped gas-containing structure on a plain film of the abdomen; pseudotumor if filled with fluid or food debris; *demonstration of a pouch by contrast study of the bowel;* enterolith formation within the pouch.

BLOOM SYNDROME (BLOOM-GERMAN SYNDROME)

Clinical Manifestations: (a) *telangiectatic erythema of the face; dolichocephaly with malar hypoplasia; low birth weight and dwarfism; sensitivity to sunlight; hypersensitivity to chemotherapy and probably also to radiotherapy;* (b) unspecific and variable immunodeficiency (IgA; IgG; IgM); (c) increased susceptibility to infections; (d) high risk of malignancy; (e) *chromosomal breakage and rearrangement;* (f) autosomal recessive inheritance; predominance in males.

Radiologic Manifestations: Nonspecific: recurrent infections; digital anomalies (microdactyly; polydactyly; syndactyly; clinodactyly); hip dislocation; short lower limbs; pes equinus; absence of toes.

BLUE DIGIT SYNDROME (BLUE TOE SYNDROME; CHOLESTEROL EMBOLIZATION SYNDROME)

Etiology: Spontaneous microembolization to the peripheral small vessels from a proximal source (adherent fibrinoplatelet aggregates; thrombus; cholesterol-rich atheromatous plaque); cholesterol embolization after thrombolytic therapy.

Clinical Manifestations: *Digital ischemia with abrupt appearance of symptoms in the distal parts of extremities* (lower portion of the leg, toes, hands, fingers): *focal, painful, and cyanotic areas with sharp demarcation from the adjacent normally perfused skin; preservation of distal pulses;* peripheral gangrene.

Radiologic Manifestations: Angiography: *atheroma(s) in a major artery; small distal emboli;* transesophageal echocardiographic identification of thoracic aortic plaque-related thrombi; *audible pedal pulses* (Doppler ultrasonography).

BOBBLE-HEAD DOLL SYNDROME (HEAD-BOBBLING "TIC")

Pathology: (a) *suprasellar arachnoid cyst; third ventricle cyst; dilated lateral ventricles;* (b) miscellaneous abnormalities: aqueductal stenosis; large cavum velum interpositum; slow-growing mass in the anterior part of the third ventricle; cystic choroid plexus papilloma of the third ventricle; septum pellucidum cyst; ventriculoperitoneal shunt obstruction.

Clinical Manifestations: (a) *to-and-fro bobbing or nodding of the head and trunk;* (b) miscellaneous abnormalities: precocious puberty; memory loss; delayed developmental milestones; mild to moderate mental retardation; macrocephaly; hyperreflexia; truncal ataxia; optic pallor; optic atrophy; drop head attack.

Radiologic Manifestations: *Suprasellar arachnoid cyst; third ventricle cyst; aqueductal stenosis; hydrocephalus.*

BOERHAAVE SYNDROME

Clinical Manifestations: Rupture of all layers of the wall of the esophagus (posterolateral wall of the distal segment on the left side): (a) *vomiting; epigastric and chest pain; subcutaneous emphysema;* dyspnea;

cyanosis; painful swallowing; abdominal rigidity; positive cytologic study of pleural effusion in occult Boerhaave syndrome (detection of undigested food particles); (b) miscellaneous abnormalities: invasive candidiasis as a complication; duodenal gallstone ileus preceding the esophageal rupture.

Radiologic Manifestations: Early phase: *"V sign"* of Naclerio (localized mediastinal emphysema in the left retrocardiac region corresponding to the fascial planes of the mediastinal and diaphragmatic pleurae); late phase: *pleural effusion or hydropneumothorax; mediastinitis;* spontaneous formation of an esophageal-bronchial fistula; demonstration of the site of tear by contrast study of the esophagus; intramural hematoma.

BÖRJESON-FORSSMAN-LEHMANN SYNDROME

Clinical Manifestations: (a) *microcephaly; prominent supraorbital ridge; deep-set eyes; ptosis; nystagmus; large ears; "coarse" facial appearance*; *mental retardation; seizures; hypotonia; obesity; short stature; hypogonadism;* gynecomastia; ovarian dysfunction in female heterozygotes; *small hands with tapering, hyperextensible fingers;* (b) X-linked inheritance; the gene mapped to the q26–q27; variable expression in heterozygous females.

Radiologic Manifestations: Brain atrophy; thickened calvarium; skeletal abnormalities (steep radiocarpal angle; small femoral and/or humeral heads; short distal phalanges; narrow cervical spine canal; scoliosis; Scheuermann-like vertebral changes).

BRACHMANN–DE LANGE SYNDROME (DE LANGE SYNDROME; CORNELIA DE LANGE SYNDROME)

Clinical Manifestations: Marked clinical variability: (a) *low birth weight; growth failure;* (b) *low hairline; heavy confluent eyebrows; curly eyelashes; small, upturned nose; micrognathia; wide, thin, and downturned upper lip; microbrachycephaly;* (c) *hirsutism*; (d) *cryptorchidism;* (e) *marked mental, motor, and social retardation;* (f) *limb anomalies;* (g) miscellaneous abnormalities: initial hypertonicity; low-pitched, weak cry; various chromosomal abnormalities; tracheomegaly; etc.; (h) sporadic in most cases; autosomal dominant inheritance and presumed autosomal recessive cases.

Radiologic Manifestations: (a) *microbrachycephaly;* (b) *limb anomalies:* micromelia; phocomelia; hemimelia; oligodactyly; syndactyly; clinodactyly; proximally placed thumb; hypoplasia of the first metacarpal; abnormal pattern profiles of the hand; *dysplasia and dislocation of the radial head* with flexion and contracture of the elbow; *retarded skeletal maturation;* (c) rounded thoracic inlet; wide upper portion of the rib cage; short sternum; premature fusion of the ossification centers; 13 pairs of ribs;

thin rib cortices with undulating appearance; (d) prenatal ultrasonography: ulnar deficiency associated with congenital heart defect; small for gestational age; brachycephaly; short femoral length; diaphragmatic hernia.

BRANCHIO-GENITO-SKELETAL SYNDROME (BRANCHIO-SKELETO-GENITAL SYNDROME; ELSAHY-WATERS SYNDROME)

Clinical Manifestations: (a) mental retardation; seizures; craniofacial features (brachycephaly; ocular hypertelorism; midfacial hypoplasia; wide nasal tip; flared alae; nystagmus; strabismus; mild ptosis; submucous cleft palate; dysplastic dentin; unerupted teeth in adolescents); hypospadias; (b) probably autosomal recessive or X-linked inheritance.

Radiologic Manifestations: Dentigerous cyst; dysplastic dentine; partial obliteration of pulp chambers; excessive mastoid pneumatization; fusion of the second and third cervical vertebrae.

BRANCHIO-OCULO-FACIAL SYNDROME

Clinical Manifestations: (a) *branchial anomalies:* sinus/fistulous tract; atrophic skin lesions; aplasia cutis congenita; scarring; hemangiomatous branchial cysts; (b) *ocular anomalies:* lacrimal duct stenosis or atresia; dacryocystitis; microphthalmos; anophthalmos; etc.; (c) *auricular anomalies:* low-set, posteriorly rotated ears with thin helix and upturned lobules; conductive hearing deficit; etc.; (d) broad nose; short nasal septum; broad or divided nasal tip; depressed nasal bridge; (e) *oral anomalies:* abnormal upper lip (malformed; pseudocleft; partial cleft; complete cleft); cleft palate; alveolar ridge; cleft of the lower lip and chin; lip pits; dental abnormalities; highly arched palate; short upper lip/philtrum; etc.; (f) miscellaneous abnormalities: prenatal growth deficiency; developmental delay; mental retardation; seizures; neurogenic hearing loss; hypernasal speech; renal anomalies; thymic remnants in the branchial cleft; etc.; (g) autosomal dominant inheritance.

Radiologic Manifestations: Microcephaly; dolichocephaly; micrognathia; malar bone hypoplasia; premature closure of the metopic suture; hypoplasia of mastoids with absence of air cells; fusion and/or ankylosis of middle ear ossicles; hypoplastic thumbs; clinodactyly; preaxial polydactyly; kyphosis; lordosis.

BRANCHIO-OTO-RENAL SYNDROME (BOR SYNDROME; MELNICK-FRASER SYNDROME)

Clinical Manifestations: (a) asthenic appearance; long and narrow facies; *ear abnormalities (malformed pinnae; preauricular appendages;*

atretic ear canals; bilateral prehelical pits); deep overbite; constricted palate; bilateral branchial fistulae; *conductive, sensorineural, or mixed hearing deficit;* stapes fixation; myopia; aplasia or stenosis of the lacrimal ducts; (b) autosomal dominant inheritance; variable expressivity and penetrance.

Radiologic Manifestations: (a) *renal anomalies:* dysplasia; aplasia; polycystic kidney; etc.; (b) *ear malformations:* underdeveloped mastoid; abnormal internal auditory canal; malformations of the ossicles; smaller than normal cochlea with reduced number of turns; short upward-pointing lateral semicircular canal.

Note: (a) branchio-oto-renal syndrome and branchiooto syndrome (without renal abnormalities) may represent the same entity; (b) branchio-oto-ureteral syndrome (hearing loss, preauricular pit or tag, and duplication of the ureters or bifid renal pelvices) probably represents a variant of branchio-oto-renal syndrome; (c) an overlap between branchio-oto-renal syndrome and branchio-oculo-facial syndrome has been reported.

BROWN SYNDROME

Etiology: Caused by a mechanical obstacle to the passage of the superior oblique tendon through the trochlea: congenitally short or taut superior oblique tendon sheath complex; acquired (trauma; sinusitis; rheumatoid arthritis; lupus erythematosus; cardiopulmonary resuscitation; etc.).

Clinical Manifestations: *Diplopia during upward gaze, especially with the eye in adducted position; pseudopalsy (apparent inferior oblique "palsy"); "clicking" in the area of the trochlea; impaired ability to vertically elevate the eye in an adducted position;* cyclic characteristic (case report).

Radiologic Manifestations: Computed tomography and magnetic resonance imaging: thickening of the superior oblique tendon; *edema of the tendon* in acute inflammation and trauma; nodular superior oblique tendon sheath with low signal intensity on T_1-weighted images.

BROWN-SÉQUARD SYNDROME

Clinical Manifestations: Ipsilateral paresis or paralysis below the lesion; associated atrophy; loss of vibratory joint and tendon sensations; contralateral loss of pain and temperature sensibilities.

Radiologic Manifestations: Unilateral lesion of the spinal cord due to different etiologic factors: trauma; neoplasm; inflammation; cervical myelopathy in rheumatoid arthritis; degenerative disorders; delayed radiation myelopathy; acute herniated cervical disc; cervical spondylosis; ischemia; hemorrhage; cyst; congenital dysraphia; idiopathic spinal cord herniation; etc.

BUDD-CHIARI SYNDROME (CHIARI SYNDROME)

Pathology: Congenital obstruction of the hepatic venous outflow tract (web; diaphragm; interruption); acquired venous obstruction (thrombus; tumor; trauma; infections; etc.); liver pathology: fibrosis; hemorrhage; congestion; protein C deficiency; etc.

Clinical Manifestations: Abdominal pain; jaundice; hematemesis; ascites; hepatomegaly; laboratory manifestations of hepatocellular dysfunction; liver failure and shock.

Radiologic Manifestations: (a) ascites; (b) esophageal varices; (c) color Doppler: abnormal hepatic venous system (narrowing; flow reversal; tortuousity; absence of vessels; collaterals; compressed inferior vena cava; thickening and irregularity of hepatic vein walls; stenosis; proximal dilatation; venous thrombosis); cirrhosis; etc.; (d) computed tomography: hepatomegaly; hypodensity on a plain scan; absence of opacification of the hepatic veins on a postcontrast injection scan that is associated with a central "fan-shaped" patchy zone of increased attenuation followed by a decrease in attenuation; inhomogeneous liver density (slow blood flow and collateral venous opacification); (e) magnetic resonance imaging: reduction in the caliber or complete absence of the hepatic veins; "comma-shaped" intrahepatic collateral vessels; slow flow; thrombosis; laminar clot; tumor; hepatomegaly; inhomogeneity of the liver parenchyma; constriction of the vena cava; cirrhosis; varices; splenomegaly; adenomatous hyperplastic nodules of the liver in chronic Budd-Chiari syndrome; (f) venography: inferior vena constriction due to hepatomegaly; irregular filling defects in the inferior vena cava or the hepatic veins; web; clot; occlusion of the inferior vena cava with or without collateral vessels; "spider web" type of collateral intrahepatic veins shown by hepatic wedge venography; pressure measurement demonstrating a gradient at the site of obstruction; (g) arteriography: stretching, narrowing, and pruning of the hepatic arteries; hepatofugal flow; varices; (h) ^{99m}Tc sulfur colloid: normal or abnormal: decreased activity in the right and left lobes; caudate lobe appearing as a "hot spot," possibly because of a separate venous drainage into the inferior vena cava.

C

CANTRELL SYNDROME (PENTALOGY OF CANTRELL)

Pathology: *Combined anterior abdominal wall, diaphragmatic, sternal, pericardial, and intracardiac defects.*

Clinical Manifestations: *Diastasis, omphalocele or umbilical hernia; chest wall defect;* ectopia cordis through the defect in the distal portion of the sternum; *congenital heart disease;* association with amniotic band syndrome.

Radiologic Manifestations: S*ternal defect; dextroposition of the heart; intrapericardial herniation of abdominal organs; cardiac anomalies:* ventricular septal defect; atrial septal defect; pulmonary stenosis; tetralogy of Fallot; anomalous pulmonary venous drainage; ventricular diverticulum; etc.

CAPLAN SYNDROME (RHEUMATOID PNEUMOCONIOSIS)

Clinical Manifestations: *Occurrence in patients with rheumatoid arthritis in the setting of preexisting mild pneumoconiosis:* signs and symptoms of rheumatoid arthritis; cough, dyspnea; biopsy of lung nodules (dust particles; necrosis); energy-dispersive x-ray microanalysis of the dust particles that demonstrates silicon and other materials; occurrence in non–coal miners (foundry workers; roof tile makers; asbestos-related workers; a dolomite quarry worker).

Radiologic Manifestations: *Disseminated lung nodules,* some with cavitation; pleural thickening and calcification; calcification within some nodules; pulmonary fibrotic changes; roentgenologic findings of rheumatoid arthritis; the lung nodules may precede development of clinical arthritis.

Note: Erasmus syndrome consists of coal worker's pneumoconiosis in association with systemic sclerosis.

CARDIOFACIAL SYNDROME (CAYLER SYNDROME)

Clinical and Radiologic Manifestations: *Unilateral partial lower facial weakness in the neonate; congenital heart disease* (atrial septal defect; ventricular septal defect; patent ductus arteriosus; tetralogy of Fallot; right aortic arch; pulmonary stenosis; coarctation of the aorta; atrioventricular canal; etc.); genitourinary anomalies; musculoskeletal anomalies; etc.

CARDIO-FACIO-CUTANEOUS SYNDROME

Clinical Manifestations: Clinical variability: (a) *craniofacial dysmorphism:* relative macrocephaly; prominent forehead; shallow orbital ridges; bitemporal narrowing; posteriorly rotated ears; hypertelorism; prominent philtrum; down-slanting palpebral fissures; highly arched palate; (b) *congenital heart defects;* (c) *skin abnormalities:* atopic dermatitis; hyperkeratosis; ichthyosis-like lesions; multiple creases of palms and soles; (d) *hair abnormalities:* sparse, curly, and slow-growing; (e) *psy-*

chomotor retardation; (f) *postnatal short stature;* (g) ophthalmologic manifestations: poor vision; strabismus; nystagmus; exophthalmos; ptosis; retinal dystrophy; (h) neurologic manifestations: seizures; hydrocephalus; abnormal electroencephalogram; brain atrophy; (i) most reported cases sporadic; autosomal dominant inheritance.

Radiologic Manifestations: *Congenital heart defects* (atrial septal defect; pulmonary stenosis; etc.); dental abnormalities (amelogenesis imperfecta; pointed edges of teeth; decayed teeth); polyhydramnios; splenomegaly; delayed bone age; macrocephaly; microcephaly; cortical atrophy; hydrocephalus/ventriculomegaly.

CARDIOVOCAL SYNDROME (ORTNER SYNDROME)

Clinical and Radiologic Manifestations: *Hoarseness; unilateral (most common) or bilateral cord paralysis; cardiovascular pathology* (mitral valve stenosis; congenital heart defects; atherosclerotic heart disease; aortic aneurysm; ductus aneurysm; patent ductus arteriosus; Eisenmenger complex; primary pulmonary hypertension; recurrent pulmonary embolism; etc.); return to normal (laryngeal cords) after surgery for congenital cardiovascular defects.

CARNEY COMPLEX (NAME SYNDROME; MYXOMA SYNDROME; MYXOMA–SPOTTY PIGMENTATION–ENDOCRINE OVERACTIVITY)

Clinical and Radiologic Manifestations: (a) *cardiac myxoma,* single or multiple, located in atria and/or ventricles; (b) *pigmented skin lesions:* simple freckles; lentigines; multiple superficial nevi; cutaneous pigmented macules; blue nevi; (c) *endocrine overactivity:* Cushing syndrome; pheochromocytoma; testicular tumor; thyroid tumor; pituitary adenoma; etc.; (d) hyperpigmented macules of the mucous membranes; (e) ocular manifestations: eyelid lentigines; conjunctival and caruncle pigmentation; eyelid pigmentation; (f) peripheral tumors: myxoid tumors; neurofibromas; ductal adenoma of breast; testicular large-cell calcifying Sertoli cell tumor.

Note: (a) the origin of the acronym *NAME: N*evi, *A*trial myxoma, *M*yxoid neurofibromata, and *E*phelides; the alternative interpretation: *N*evi, *A*trial myxoma, *M*ucinosis of the skin, and *E*ndocrine overactivity; (b) LAMB syndrome (*L*entigines, *A*trial *M*yxoma, mucocutaneous *M*yxoma, *B*lue nevi) is considered to represent a variant of Carney complex.

CARNEY TRIAD

Clinical and Radiologic Manifestations: (a) *pulmonary chondroma* (smoothly lobulated nodules; computed tomographic demonstration of calcification in the periphery of the nodules); (b) *extraadrenal paraganglioma* (^{131}I scintigraphy to detect functioning tumor; magnetic resonance imaging as a screening tool); (c) *gastric epithelioid leiomyosarcoma or leiomyoblastoma.*

CAROLI SYNDROME

Clinical Manifestations: (a) *recurrent crampy upper abdominal pain; intermittent obstructive jaundice;* fever; (b) possibly autosomal recessive inheritance; reported in twin sisters.

Pathology: *Segmental saccular dilatation of intrahepatic bile ducts with extension to the liver periphery:* absence of liver cirrhosis or portal hypertension in the pure form of the disease; renal tubular ectasia or other renal cystic lesions; portal radicles partially or completely surrounded by dilated intrahepatic bile ducts; cholangitis; liver abscess; hepatic fibrosis; intrahepatic stones.

Radiologic Manifestations: (a) *saccular dilatation of bile ducts;* computed tomography before and after the infusion of cholangiographic contrast material: *a significant rise in computed tomography number of the cystic lesions; "the central dot sign": portal radicles partially or completely surrounded by dilated intrahepatic bile ducts;* (b) *color Doppler: signals of arterial wave pattern within the dilated bile ducts;* (c) Tc-99m DISIDA scintigraphy: areas of focally increased radiotracer accumulation persisting more than 2 hours; (d) miscellaneous abnormalities: intraductal biliary stones; renal tubular ectasia; recessive polycystic kidney disease; choledochal cyst; cholangiocarcinoma; fibroangioadenomatosis.

CAROTID SINUS SYNDROME

Clinical and Radiologic Manifestations: (a) attacks of syncope associated with bradycardia and/or hypotension; spontaneous occurrence or associated with known etiologic factors (benign or malignant mass lesions in the neck; inflammatory mass; radiation therapy; neck surgery; diagnostic angiography; embolization procedures; etc.); (b) diagnostic test: reproduction of symptoms by performing carotid massage for 10 to 15 seconds: development of symptoms, fall of blood pressure of more than 30 mm IIg, and bradycardia or asystole for more than 3 seconds.

CARPAL TUNNEL SYNDROME

Clinical Manifestations: Numbness, paresthesia, weakness, and burning pain on the anterior aspect of the wrist with extension to the fingers; abnormal clinical signs (wrist flexion, nerve percussion, carpal compression, and tourniquet tests), and abnormal electrophysiologic test results.

Radiologic Manifestations: (a) abnormal cross-sectional area of the carpal canal; swelling of the median nerve in the proximal part of the carpal tunnel; flattening of the median nerve in the distal part of the carpal tunnel; increased palmar bowing of the flexor retinaculum; thickening of synovial sheaths of flexor tendons; (b) abnormal dynamic gadolinium-enhanced magnetic resonance imaging: marked enhancement of the median nerve (nerve edema) or no enhancement of the nerve (ischemia).

CARPENTER SYNDROME (ACROCEPHALOPOLYSYNDACTYLY, CARPENTER TYPE)

Clinical Manifestations: (a) *acrocephaly;* (b) facial dysmorphism: broad cheeks and temples; depressed nasal bridge; lateral displacement of the medial canthi; epicanthal folds; downward thrust of the upper lids; (c) *obesity;* (d) *hypogenitalism;* (e) *brachysyndactyly of the hands; variable preaxial polysyndactyly of the feet; soft tissue syndactyly;* postaxial polydactyly in some cases; (f) *mental retardation;* (g) miscellaneous abnormalities: clinodactyly; camptodactyly; oligodontia; cloverleaf skull deformity; etc.; (h) autosomal recessive inheritance.

Radiologic Manifestations: (a) *premature closure of cranial sutures;* (b) *brachymesophalangia and soft-tissue syndactyly of the hands;* two ossification centers for the proximal phalanx of the thumb in childhood developing into duplication of the thumb in adulthood; (c) *preaxial polydactyly and syndactyly of the feet;* (d) prenatal diagnosis by ultrasonography; (e) miscellaneous abnormalities: coxa valga; genu valgum; pes varus; flared ilia; displaced patellae; congenital heart diseases; hernias; brain malformations.

CAST SYNDROME

Etiology: (a) obstruction of the third segment of the duodenum, probably caused by the superior mesenteric artery compression in patients who are undergoing treatment for scoliosis with or without the use of a body cast; (b) factors contributing to the development of obstruction: diminished compliance of the abdominal wall; lumbar hyperextension; primary lumbar hyperlordosis; traction on, or distraction of, the spine; asthenic body build; prolonged bed rest in the supine position; rapid weight loss; etc.

Clinical Manifestations: *Nausea; vomiting; abdominal distension.*

Radiologic Manifestations: *Gastroduodenal dilatation* extending to the third portion of duodenum.

CATEL-MANZKE SYNDROME

Clinical and Radiologic Manifestations: (a) *Robin anomaly:* mandibular hypoplasia; glossoptosis; U-shaped cleft palate; (b) *hyperphalangy (an accessory ossicle at the base of the index finger) and ulnar deviation;* (c) congenital heart disease; (d) miscellaneous abnormalities: ossicle between the base of the proximal phalanges of the third and fourth digits; clinodactyly; short fingers/toes; joint laxity/dislocation; dislocatable knees; talipes equinovarus; vertebral anomalies; rib anomalies; pectus excavatum; nuchal edema, costovertebral anomalies, and radial ray defect; etc.; (e) probably X-linked inheritance.

CAT-EYE SYNDROME (CHROMOSOME 22 TRISOMY/TETRASOMY; TRISOMY/TETRASOMY 22PTER–Q11)

Clinical Manifestations: Phenotypic and cytogenic variability: (a) *anorectal anomalies:* anal atresia; rectovestibular fistula; (b) *ocular hypertelorism with down-slanting palpebral fissures; lower, vertical iridal, and choroidal coloboma (cat eye);* (c) *auricular abnormalities:* preauricular tag and/or fistula; low-set ears; atretic auditory canal; (d) *genitourinary anomalies;* (e) chromosomal evaluation: *a small supernumerary chromosome shorter than a 22* (derived from duplicated regions of 22pter–22q11.2); parental origin of the extra chromosome; (f) miscellaneous abnormalities: cardiovascular anomalies; inguinal hernia; umbilical hernia; psychomotor retardation; physical retardation; oropalatal anomalies; unusual dermatoglyphics; Hirschsprung disease; renal dysfunction.
Radiologic Manifestations: *Anorectal anomalies; genitourinary anomalies;* skeletal abnormalities (scoliosis; rib anomalies; vertebral anomalies; hip dislocation; etc.).

CAUDA EQUINA SYNDROME (PSEUDOCLAUDICATION SYNDROME)

Clinical Manifestations: Narrowing of the sagittal diameter of the distal spinal canal secondary to various factors: intermittent "claudication" induced either by activity or by posture, lasting a few seconds to several minutes (numbness, coldness, or burning); muscle atrophy; minor degree of muscle weakness; reflex asymmetry; sensory abnormalities.
Radiologic Manifestations: (a) abnormalities of the vertebrae and spinal canal: ankylosing spondylitis; spondylolisthesis; herniated disc; narrow lumbar spinal canal; etc.; (b) neural elements compression; (c) gadolinium-enhanced magnetic resonance imaging: abnormal intrathecal enhancement at, and extending craniad (and in some also caudad) from the level(s) of severe spinal stenosis; (d) epidural venous stasis.

CAUDAL DYSPLASIA SEQUENCE (CAUDAL REGRESSION SYNDROME)

Clinical Manifestations: (a) *flat buttocks; short intergluteal cleft;* dimpling of the buttocks; "siren" or "mermaid" configuration in most severe cases; froglike deformity of the lower limbs in moderately severe cases; (b) neurologic deficits; (c) association with syndromes: Alagille syndrome; oculo-auriculo-vertebral spectrum; (d) miscellaneous associated anomalies: central nervous system; genitourinary; gastrointestinal, particularly anorectal; skeletal; cardiovascular; chromosomal; etc.

Radiologic Manifestations: (a) *vertebral agenesis that may vary from partial sacral agenesis to total agenesis below the first lumbar vertebra;* (b) *intraspinal anomalies:* tethered cord; dermoid cyst; lipoma; diastematomyelia; spinal cord syrinx; (c) limb anomalies of various type and severity, such as hip dislocation and equinovarus deformities of the feet; fused iliac bones in severe forms; (d) bowel dysfunction; neurogenic bladder; (e) intrauterine diagnosis by ultrasonography: normal or increased amniotic fluid; mild dilatation or normal urinary tract; nonfused extremities; sacral agenesis.

Note: The term *caudal regression syndrome* is usually used for the association of the anomalies of the entire caudal region: sacrum, anorectal, genitourinary, and lower limbs.

CELIAC AXIS COMPRESSION SYNDROME

Clinical Manifestations: *Periumbilical pain; epigastric discomfort;* nausea; vomiting; malabsorption (occasionally); weight loss; *systolic epigastric bruit;* carcinoma of the head of pancreas associated with the syndrome (case report).

Pathology: *Compression of the celiac artery against the aorta by the median arcuate ligament of the diaphragm.* This may cause a "stealing" of blood from the mesenteric artery via collaterals.

Radiologic Manifestations: *Narrowing of the celiac trunk with smooth eccentric compression of the anterior wall; dorsocaudal displacement of the celiac artery;* dilated peripancreatic collateral vessels; poststenotic dilatation of the distal celiac trunk; selective superior mesenteric arteriography (opacification of the celiac artery bed through collaterals, and delayed washout of contrast medium from the celiac artery territory).

CENTRAL CORD SYNDROME

Etiology: Cervical spondylosis; hyperextension injuries; fracture; fracture-dislocation; congenital abnormality; cervical disc protrusion.

Clinical and Radiologic Manifestations: Motor impairment, most pronounced in the upper limbs; variable degree of sensory loss below the level of the cord lesion; Lhermitte sign (sudden shooting paresthesia-like electric shocks spreading down the body or into the limbs on flexion of the neck); urodynamic abnormalities (detrusor hyperreflexia and external urethral sphincter dyssynergia).

CENTRAL HYPOVENTILATION SYNDROME (CONGENITAL) (ONDINE'S CURSE)

Clinical Manifestations: Diminished sensitivity of the respiratory center to reduced oxygen or increased carbon dioxide: (a) *persistent hypoventilation; recurrent apnea and cyanosis;* (b) difficulty in feeding and swallowing; (c) seizures related to hypoventilation; (d) *abnormal brain-stem auditory evoked responses during sleep:* delays in peak latencies pIII and interpeak latencies pI-III that imply a functional disturbance of brain-stem control of ventilation during sleep; (e) arterial blood gas analysis in sleep: *respiratory acidosis and hypercapnia;* (f) brain pathology: diffuse central nervous system astrocytosis, gliosis, and atrophy; *no primary brain-stem abnormality;* (g) association with Hirschsprung disease and neural crest tumors (neurocristopathy); (h) miscellaneous abnormalities: poor growth; below normal psychosocial performance; mental retardation in some; motor function deficiencies and eye-hand coordination deficits; gastroesophageal reflux.

Radiologic Manifestations: (a) mild brain atrophy in some cases; (b) miscellaneous abnormalities: neural crest tumors; Hirschsprung disease; association of Ondine's curse with Hirschsprung disease and cerebral arteriovenous malformation.

Note: *The triad of neurocristopathy includes Ondine's curse, congenital neuroblastoma, and Hirschsprung disease;* most of the reported cases with this association had total colonic aganglionosis.

CEPHALOSKELETAL DYSPLASIA (TAYBI-LINDER SYNDROME)

Clinical Manifestations: (a) *low birth weight; microcephaly;* (b) unusual facies, with bulging eyes, flat bridge of the nose, and highly arched palate; (c) spadelike hands and feet; (d) *mental and physical retardation;* (e) miscellaneous abnormalities: clubfoot deformity; cleft palate; absent hair; (f) probably autosomal recessive inheritance.

Radiologic Manifestations: (a) *severe microcephaly;* small fontanelles; ventricular dilatation; large subarachnoid space; (b) *deep intervertebral spaces* with a relative decrease in vertical diameter of the vertebral bodies; (c) *shortness of all long bones; splayed and irregular margins of the metaphyses of long bones and cup-shaped ends of the short tubular bones of the hands and feet; delayed ossification of tali, calcanei, and epiphyses at the knees; short iliac wings, near-zero acetabular angles, irregular ossification of acetabular roofs, and narrow sciatic notches;* (d) hydronephrosis.

Note: The types I and III of microcephalic osteodysplastic primordial dwarfism are considered to be a single entity. Some of the cases reported under this title have radiographic manifestations similar to cephaloskeletal dysplasia and probably represent the same entity.

CEREBRO-COSTO-MANDIBULAR SYNDROME (RIB GAP DEFECT– MICROGNATHIA SYNDROME)

Clinical Manifestations: (a) *micrognathia; respiratory distress due to flail chest; mental handicaps*; *palatal defect*; etc.; (b) most cases sporadic; genetic heterogeneity (autosomal dominant and autosomal recessive transmissions).

Pathology: Rib gaps consisting of fibrous, fibrovascular, or cartilaginous tissues; maxillomandibular abnormalities: multifocal growth retardation involving the septal cartilage, vomer, and mandibular condyle; abnormal genioglossus muscle and papillae of the tongue.

Radiologic Manifestations: (a) *micrognathia; gaps in the dorsal portion of the ribs, fragmented ossification of the ribs, and absence of normal costovertebral articulations;* (b) miscellaneous abnormalities: vertebral anomalies; subluxation of the elbows; hip dislocation; abnormal phalanges of the toes; multiple ossification centers of the calcaneus; vesicoureteral reflux; medullary renal cysts; renal ectopia; persistent urinary tract infection; dental defects; laryngeal and tracheal abnormalities; gastroesophageal reflux; aspiration pneumonia; polyhydramnios; etc.

CEREBRO-OCULO-FACIO-SKELETAL SYNDROME (PENA-SHOKEIR SYNDROME TYPE II)

Clinical Manifestations: Variability in clinical presentation and evolution: (a) *prenatal growth retardation; failure to thrive; mental retardation;* (b) *craniofacial dysmorphism:* microcephaly; sloping forehead; prominent bony ridge of the nose; high nose bridge; narrow palpebral fissures; upper lip overhanging the lower lip; large ears; long philtrum; micrognathia or retrognathia; (c) *microphthalmos; cataract;* blepharophimosis; cloudy corneas; nystagmus; (d) kyphosis; scoliosis; *contracture, mainly at the elbows and knees; permanently clenched fists;* camptodactyly, simian crease; longitudinal foot groove folding; *foot deformities; hypotonia;* etc.; (e) autosomal recessive inheritance.

Radiologic Manifestations: Acetabular dysplasia; hip dislocation; narrow pelvis; coxa valga; *foot deformities (vertical talus; rocker-bottom feet; calcaneovalgus;* hypoplasia of the second cuneiform, and proximal displacement of the second metatarsal); osteoporosis; renal anomalies; cerebral calcification (lenticular nucleus and hemispheric white matter).

CEREBRO-RENO-DIGITAL SYNDROMES

Clinical and Radiologic Manifestations: A community of syndromes with the following manifestations: (a) *brain dysgenesis:* microcephaly; agenesis of the corpus callosum; cerebellar vermis agenesis; micropolygyria; etc.; (b) *cystic renal dysplasia;* (c) *polydactyly.*

CHARCOT-MARIE-TOOTH DISEASE

Clinical Manifestations: The most common inherited peripheral neuropathy (anterior horn cells of the spinal cord and the peripheral nerves): (a) *chronic, slowly progressive demyelinating motor and sensory neuropathy; slow nerve conduction in type I; normal conduction in type II;* prenatal diagnosis of type Ia by multicolor in situ hybridization; etc.; (b) genetic heterogeneity (autosomal dominant inheritance most common).

Radiologic Manifestations: (a) *enlarged nerve roots, ganglia, and cauda equina;* (b) muscle atrophy; (c) miscellaneous abnormalities: posterior scalloping of the lumbar vertebrae; scoliosis; enlargement and erosion of intervertebral neural foramina; hip dysplasia in older children and adolescents; coxa valga; fatty infiltration and atrophy of calf muscles (magnetic resonance imaging evaluation).

CHARGE ASSOCIATION

Clinical Manifestations: (a) *coloboma of the eye* (C); *heart disease* (H); *atresia of the choana* (A) (posterior choanal abnormalities); *retarded growth and development* (R); *genital hypoplasia* (G); *ear anomalies and/or deafness* (E) (Mondini defect; hypoplastic incus; absent semicircular canal); (b) miscellaneous abnormalities: craniofacial dysmorphism; nervous system abnormalities; endocrine disorders; superior lacrimal canalicular atresia and nasolacrimal duct obstruction; (c) in association with other disorders: Joubert syndrome; DiGeorge sequence; VATER association; chromosomal abnormalities; etc.; (d) sporadic; dominant transmission in some families.

Radiologic Manifestations: (a) *choanal atresia;* (b) central nervous system anomalies: microcephaly; arrhinencephaly; holoprosencephaly; forebrain defects; hindbrain defects; (c) miscellaneous abnormalities: tracheoesophageal fistula; esophageal atresia; anal atresia; anal stenosis; renal anomalies.

CHÉDIAK-HIGASHI SYNDROME

Clinical Manifestations: (a) *partial albinism;* fragile appearance; predisposition to infections; development of lymphoma-like illness in the accelerated phase of the disease; (b) *massive lysosomal inclusions in the white blood cells;* neutropenia; anemia; thrombocytopenia; high zinc concentration in plasma, erythrocytes, lymphocytes, and granulocytes; defective neutrophil, monocyte, and lymphocyte locomotion; (c) *hepatosplenomegaly;* (d) prenatal diagnosis by examination of the hair shaft and polymorphonuclear cells; (e) autosomal recessive inheritance; mapped on chromosome 1q42–43.

Radiologic Manifestations: (a) hilar and mediastinal lymphadenopathy; hepatosplenomegaly; (b) lymphangiography: reticular pattern of enlarged inguinal and paraaortic lymph nodes; (c) central nervous system: diffuse brain atrophy; periventricular decreased density (computed tomography); increased signal intensity on the T_2-weighted images and lack of enhancement on the T_1-weighted images in periventricular and corona radiata regions; (d) hypoechoic periportal encasement.

CHEIRO-ORAL SYNDROME

Clinical Manifestations: Sensory disturbance around the corner of the mouth and the palm of the hand on the same side (cheiro-oral syndrome); sensory disturbance around the corner of the mouth, in the palm of the hand, and in the foot on the same side (cheiro-oral-pedal syndrome).

Radiologic Manifestations: Lesion in the central gyrus, in the thalamus, or in the brain stem (infarct; hematoma; etc.); bilateral subdural hematoma (case report).

CHILAIDITI SYNDROME

Clinical Manifestations: *Abdominal pain;* vomiting; anorexia; constipation; frequent passage of flatus; "tender hepatomegaly"; *marked diurnal abdominal distension;* absence of liver dullness; displaced liver edge.

Radiologic Manifestations: *Complete or incomplete interposition of the bowel between the liver and diaphragm;* abnormally long and mobile right colonic angle; strangulated volvulus of the sigmoid colon (case report).

CHILD SYNDROME (ICHTHYOSIS–LIMB REDUCTION SYNDROME)

Clinical Manifestations: Onset at birth or early childhood: (a) *ichthyosiform erythroderma*; (b) impaired hair growth and linear areas of alopecia on the affected side; (c) destruction of nails and replacement by keratotic clawlike material; onychorrhexis; (d) *limb deformity (ipsilateral):* varies from digital hypoplasia to complete absence of a limb; (e) *ipsilateral hypoplasia of other parts of the skeleton, brain, spinal cord, and viscera;* (f) miscellaneous abnormalities: endocrine defects; minor skin and visceral anomalies on the contralateral side; cleft lip; umbilical hernia; etc.; (g) probably X-linked dominant inheritance; majority female.

Radiologic Manifestations: (a) *unilateral hypoplasia or aplasia of a limb; unilateral hypoplasia of the calvaria, mandible, scapula, clavicle, pelvis, and ribs;* vertebral defects; (b) miscellaneous abnormalities: visceral anomalies (cardiovascular; renal; lung); punctate epiphyseal calcification.

Note: CHILD: *C*ongenital *H*emidysplasia with *I*chthyosiform erythroderma, and *L*imb *D*efects.

CHRISTIAN SYNDROME (ADDUCTED THUMBS SYNDROME)

Clinical and Radiologic Manifestations: (a) *microcephaly; craniosynostosis*; arthrogryposis; *myopathic face; ophthalmoplegia; downward slanting of the palpebral fissures; abnormal ear placement; bifid uvula; cleft palate; highly arched palate; adducted thumbs; talipes equinovarus or calcaneovalgus;* short first metacarpal; camptodactyly; limited extension of the elbows, wrists, and knees; muscular hypotonia; mental retardation; *dysphagia;* etc.; (b) autosomal recessive inheritance.

CHROMOSOME 4: DEL(4P) SYNDROME (WOLF-HIRSCHHORN SYNDROME)

Clinical Manifestations: *Mental and growth retardation;* craniofacial dysmorphism ("Greek warrior helmet" appearance; *microcephaly; prominent glabella; ocular hypertelorism;* broad-beaked nose; micrognathia; short philtrum with a down-turned mouth; *cleft lip and/or cleft palate*); deletion of 4p16; high perinatal mortality.

Radiologic Manifestations: *Microcephaly; hypertelorism; micrognathia;* retarded skeletal maturation; clubfoot; miscellaneous skeletal system abnormalities; hydrocephalus; cavum septum pellucidum; absent septum pellucidum; cerebellar anomalies; etc.

CHROMOSOME 5: DEL(5P) SYNDROME (Cri-du-Chat Syndrome; Cat-Cry Syndrome)

ClinicalManifestations: *Severe growth and mental retardation; catlike cry;* craniofacial dysmorphism (round-moon facies, micrognathia; retrognathia; *microcephaly;* low-set ears; downward slanting palpebral fissures; epicanthal folds; preauricular tags; posteriorly rotated pinnae; hypertelorism; strabismus); *muscular hypotonia;* congenital heart disease; etc.

Radiologic Manifestations: *Microcephaly and micrognathia;* abnormal development of the long bones related to muscular hypotonia; hands smaller than normal; disproportionate shortness of the third, fourth, and fifth metacarpals; elongation of the second, third, fourth, and fifth proximal phalanges; clinodactyly; scoliosis; small iliac wings; hip dislocation; talipes; malrotation of bowel; megacolon.

CHROMOSOME 13 TRISOMY SYNDROME (Patau Syndrome)

Clinical Manifestations: (a) *low birth weight;* (b) *craniofacial dysmorphism:* microcephaly; shallow supraorbital ridges; large, broad nose; cleft lip and palate; hypertelorism or hypotelorism; epicanthal folds; malformed and low-set ears; micrognathia; anophthalmia or microphthalmia; coloboma; retinal dysplasia; (c) *digital anomalies:* long, hyperconvex fingernails; camptodactyly; fifth finger overlapping the fourth; polydactyly; syndactyly; (d) *rocker-bottom feet;* (e) soft-tissue defects of the head and neck; (f) *severe mental defect;* (g) capillary hemangiomas; etc.

Radiologic Manifestations: (a) *microcephaly with a sloping forehead; hypotelorism or hypertelorism;* poor ossification of the calvaria; small orbits; spina bifida; *hand and foot deformities;* hypoplasia of the ribs; hypoplasia of the pelvis; low acetabular angles; (b) *arrhinencephaly/holoprosencephaly* (in about 80%); agenesis of the corpus callosum; cerebellar dysplasia; large cisterna magna; Dandy-Walker variant; hypoplasia of the inferior vermis; anencephaly; (c) miscellaneous abnormalities: various cardiovascular and renal anomalies; double vagina, bicornuate uterus; hydrops fetalis, fetal cystic hygroma.

CHROMOSOME 18 TRISOMY SYNDROME (Edwards Syndrome)

Clinical Manifestations: Great phenotypic variability: (a) *low birth weight; physical and mental retardation;* muscular hypotonia followed by hypertonia; (b) *craniofacial dysmorphism*: elongated skull with prominent occiput; micrognathia; small triangular mouth with short upper lip; low-set, malformed ears; highly arched palate; (c) short neck; shield deformity of the chest; (d) *flexion deformity of the fingers:* first digit adducted and second digit overlapping the third; (e) *foot deformities:* rocker-bottom; short first digit; dorsiposed hallux; (f) miscellaneous abnormalities: low-arched dermal ridge patterning on fingertips; neoplasms; etc.

Radiologic Manifestations: (a) thin calvaria with frontal bossing; *prominent occiput; J-shaped sella turcica; hypoplasia of the mandible and maxilla;* (b) *thin hypoplastic ribs; 11 pairs of ribs; short sternum;* (c) *hand deformities:* ulnar deviation of the digits; V-shaped deformity between the second and third digits; hypoplastic first metacarpal; flexion deformities; (d) *foot deformities:* rocker-bottom; short first digit; hammertoes; hypoplastic distal phalanges; (e) *small pelvis;* steep iliac angles; (f) central nervous system anomalies: small cerebellum; large cisterna magna; absence or hypoplasia of the corpus callosum; marked anteroposterior development of the temporooccipital lobes; a mild form of holoprosencephaly; absent septum pellucidum; heterotopias; (g) prenatal sonographic findings: intrauterine growth retardation; cardiac defects; clenched hands; cystic hygroma or nuchal thickening; omphalocele; large cisterna magna; brain dysgenesis; clubfeet or rocker-bottom feet; single umbilical artery; meningomyelocele; renal anomalies; (h) miscellaneous abnormalities: chondrodysplasia punctata; protrusio acetabuli; kyphoscoliosis.

CHRONIC FATIGUE SYNDROME

Clinical Manifestations: A multisystem disorder: disabling fatigue; myalgia; headache; sensory and motor dysfunction; low-grade fever; pharyngitis; adenopathy.

Radiologic Manifestations: (a) magnetic resonance imaging: foci of T_2-bright signal in the periventricular and subcortical white matter and in the centrum semiovale; (b) single photon emission computed tomography: multiple perfusion defects throughout the cerebral cortex (more extensive than that detected by magnetic resonance imaging); (c) radionuclide ventriculography: abnormal left ventricular myocardial dynamics: abnormal wall motion at rest and stress; dilatation of the left ventricle; segmental wall motion abnormalities.

CHURG-STRAUSS SYNDROME

Histology: *Necrotizing vasculitis; tissue infiltration by eosinophils; extravascular granulomas.*

Clinical Manifestations: (a) *asthma; systemic vasculitis;* (b) *eosinophilia;* (c) *allergic rhinitis;* nasal polyposis; sinusitis; (d) pericardial and myocardial disease; cardiac failure; mitral regurgitation; (e) miscellaneous abnormalities: abdominal pain; diarrhea; gastrointestinal bleeding; perforation; renal failure; skin lesions (purpura; nodules; erythema; urticaria); arthralgia; myalgia; arthritis; central or peripheral nervous system involvement (cerebral hemorrhage; brain infarct; cranial nerve palsies; ischemic optic neuritis; mononeuritis multiplex); exophthalmos and facial swelling (case report); detectable antimyeloperoxidase antibodies in patient's serum during active phase of the disease.

Radiologic Manifestations: Pulmonary infiltrates with variable features and distribution (transient; diffuse; peripheral; symmetric; patchy; nodular; cavitation); hilar adenopathy; pleural effusion; enlarged, irregular and stellate-shaped arteries on high resolution computed tomography (vascular wall eosinophilic infiltration); cerebral hemorrhage; brain infarct.

CLAUDE SYNDROME

Clinical and Radiologic Manifestations: *Ipsilateral fascicular third nerve palsy; contralateral ataxia;* computed tomography and magnetic resonance imaging: demonstration of the etiologic factor: neoplasm; vascular disease; mesencephalic paramedian infarct; hemorrhage.

Note: A fascicular nerve palsy in association with contralateral hemiplegia is called Weber syndrome.

CLOUSTON SYNDROME

Clinical Manifestations: (a) *ectodermal dysplasia:* rough, thick, and easily cracked *dyskeratotic skin on the palms and soles;* hyperpigmentation of the skin over the knuckles, elbows, knees, axillae, areolae, and pubic areas; thickening deformity; *hypoplasia and occasionally absent nails;* thin and *sparse hair* on the head, eyebrows, and body; normal teeth; (b) autosomal dominant inheritance.

Radiologic Manifestations: Thickening of the skull; tufting of the terminal phalanges.

CLOVERLEAF SKULL DEFORMITY (KLEEBLATTSCHÄDEL ANOMALY)

Classification
1. Isolated cloverleaf skull deformity.
2. Chromosomal abnormalities: dup(13q); dup(15q).
3. Craniosynostosis syndromes: Apert syndrome; Carpenter syndrome; Crouzon syndrome; Pfeiffer syndrome.
4. Skeletal dysplasias:
   - Osteoglophoinc dysplasia;
   - Micromelic bone dysplasia with cloverleaf skull and straight femora (as compared with typical thanatophoric dysplasia, which

has "telephone receiver" bowing of femora): narrow chest with small lungs; platyspondyly; cloverleaf skull deformity; narrow foramen magnum; hydrocephalus; hypoplastic cerebellum; etc;
- Camptomelic dysplasia (craniosynostotic type).
5. Syndromes:
   - Amniotic band syndrome;
   - Beare-Stevenson syndrome: cutis gyratum; acanthosis nigricans; hypertelorism; cleft palate; bifid scrotum; craniosynostosis with or without cloverleaf skull; etc.;
   - COH syndrome (Children's Orthopedic Hospital): cloverleaf skull; facial dysmorphism (proptosis; low nasal bridge; short, upturned nose; downturned mouth, narrow palate); thumb duplication; small fifth fingers; etc.;
   - Say-Poznanski syndrome: short-wide clavicles; winged scapulae; rib anomalies with prominent costovertebral junctions; wide ischial separation; angulated ulnae; polydactyly of the hands and feet; abnormal metacarpals and metatarsals;
   - Cloverleaf skull with elbow ankylosis only;
   - Shprintzen-Goldberg syndrome (marfanoid phenotype and craniosynostosis).
6. Iatrogenic: postbilateral subtemporal decompression for hydrocephalus.

Clinical Manifestations: *Trilobed skull; low-set ears; beaked nose; prognathism; recessed nasal root; severe exophthalmos;* limb anomalies; mental retardation.

Radiologic Manifestations: (a) *premature closure of cranial sutures (coronal, lambdoid, and squamous)* resulting in grotesque appearance; computed tomographic findings (near-complete absence of the lateral orbital wall; thin covering over the temporal lobe; enormous protrusion of the temporal fossa; hydrocephalus; shallow orbits; ocular hypertelorism; relative prognathism); (b) *limb anomalies:* subluxation of the radial heads; bony ankylosis of the elbows; shortness and bowing of the long bones; hip dislocation; webbed toes; webbed fingers; (c) prenatal ultrasonography: polyhydramnios; trilobed skull; increased biparietal diameter; hydrocephalus; intact temporal bone; absent corpus callosum; limb deformities.

COCKAYNE SYNDROME

Clinical Manifestations
(A) Classic Cockayne Syndrome (CS Type I): (a) normal or slightly low birth weight; *progressive growth failure;* (b) *developmental delay, progressive neurologic dysfunction:* motor weakness; muscle atrophy; myoclonus; decreased tone; increased tone; speech abnormalities; tremor; limb

ataxia; incoordination; gait abnormalities; seizures; etc.; (c) *cutaneous photosensitivity;* dry and sometimes scaly skin; (d) hair abnormalities: thin; dry; sparse; (e) *progressive pigmentary retinopathy;* enophthalmos; hyperopia; cataracts; optic disc atrophy; poor pupillary dilatation; decreased lacrimation; nystagmus; corneal opacities; etc.; (f) *sensorineural hearing loss;* (g) *dental caries;* (h) *characteristic physical appearance:* loss of adipose tissue; sunken eyes, slender nose, prominent superior maxillae, characteristic stance; etc.; (i) prenatal diagnosis with the use of cultured skin fibroblasts: demonstration of sensitivity to ultraviolet light in association with an anomalous response of nucleic acid synthesis in cultured fibroblasts after ultraviolet irradiation (lack of recovery); (j) autosomal recessive inheritance.

(B) SEVERE COCKAYNE SYNDROME (CS TYPE II): Earlier onset of symptoms as compared with CS type I: (a) *low birth weight; postnatal growth deficiency; microcephaly; poor or absent neurologic development;* (b) *rapid development of the characteristic facial and somatic abnormalities (within the first 2 years of life);* (c) eye abnormalities: *cataracts; microphthalmos; iris hypoplasia; microcornea;* (d) death usually within the first decade of life.

(C) MILD COCKAYNE SYNDROME: Minor symptoms with a delay in appearance of clinical manifestation; some with normal intelligence; normal growth and/or normal reproductive capacity.

Pathology: Reduced number of spinal motor neurons and nerve cells in the myenteric plexus of the colon; siderocalcific pericapillary deposits in the cerebellum, basal ganglia, and some parts of the cerebrum; increased sensitivity of cultured skin fibroblasts to ultraviolet light; hydrocephalus; segmental demyelination and granular lysosomal inclusion on ultrastructural examination.

Radiologic Manifestations: Abnormalities becoming noticeable after the first year of life: (a) *microcephaly; thick cranial vault; small sella turcica; intracranial calcifications (basal ganglia; subcortical white matter; cerebellum; pineal gland); brain atrophy; demyelination of the white matter (periventricular; subcortical); hydrocephalus;* (b) spinal abnormalities: ovoid vertebral bodies with anterior notching; biconcave vertebral bodies; increase in the anteroposterior diameter of vertebral bodies; scalloping and posterior wedging; thoracic kyphosis; intervertebral calcification; (c) various nonspecific skeletal abnormalities: slender long bones with narrow medullary canal, slightly bowed fibulae, and bulky metaphyses and epiphyses; large tarsal and carpal bones; large second metacarpal pseudoepiphyses; short and broad metacarpals, metatarsals, and phalanges; ivory epiphyses; cone-shaped epiphyses; asymmetric fingers; coxa valga; flexion deformities in the elbows and knees; short second toes; osteoporosis; thin, elongated ribs; (d) underdevelopment and sclerosis of the mastoids; underdevelopment of the paranasal sinuses; small mandible.

COFFIN-LOWRY SYNDROME

Clinical Manifestations: (a) *severe mental retardation* in males, less mental retardation in females; (b) *craniofacial dysmorphism:* square forehead with prominent outer lateral aspects; bitemporal narrowing; thickened supraorbital ridge and outer margins; thickened sagittal suture; thickened zygomatic arch; down-slanting, narrow palpebral fissures; heavy, arched eyebrows; ptotic upper lids; hypertelorism; broad nasal bridge; thick nasal septum; anteverted nostrils; thickened prominent lips with pouting lower lip; open-mouth facies; thick and prominent chin; prominent ears; (c) *large, flabby hands and tapering fingers;* (d) association with psychosis; etc. (e) X-linked semidominant inheritance; males more severely affected.

Radiologic Manifestations: (a) thickened facial bones; hyperostosis frontalis; large anterior fontanel; delay in the closure of the sutures; (b) pectus carinatum or excavatum; spinal deformities; drumstick-shaped terminal phalanx of the fingers and constriction of the adjacent shaft; coxa valga; lower-limb discrepancy; narrow iliac wings; short great toe; pseudoepiphysis of metacarpals; skeletal maturation retardation; (c) miscellaneous abnormalities: calcium phosphate crystal deposition in the ligamenta flava (spinal cord compression); sensorineural deafness associated with anomalous labyrinths; corpus callosum agenesis.

COFFIN-SIRIS SYNDROME

Clinical Manifestations: (a) *prenatal and postnatal growth deficiency; developmental delay; mental retardation;* (b) *craniofacial dysmorphism:* coarse face; microcephaly; prominent lips; wide mouth; low nasal bridge; wide nose; sparse scalp hair; bushy eyebrows; synophrys; (c) *nail hypoplasia or absence, with predominantly fifth finger and toe involvement; body hypertrichosis; lax joints; feeding difficulties in infancy;* hypoglycemia; (d) autosomal recessive inheritance.

Radiologic Manifestations: (a) *absent or hypoplastic terminal phalanges of the fifth fingers and toes;* absent or hypoplastic terminal phalanges of other fingers and toes; (b) other limb anomalies: clinodactyly; radial head dislocation; cone-shaped epiphyses; coxa valga; foot deformities (varus; valgus); absence of middle phalangeal ossification of the toes; small or absent patellae; (c) *retarded bone age;* (d) miscellaneous abnormalities: absent corpus callosum; pectus excavatum; hypoplastic clavicle; scoliosis; narrow intervertebral discs; eventration of the diaphragm; ureteropelvic junction obstruction; bladder diverticula; intestinal malrotation; Dandy-Walker malformation; vertebral fusion; supernumerary vertebrae and ribs; intussusception; gastric outlet obstruction.

COGAN SYNDROME

Clinical Manifestations: A form of *vasculitis* in young adults and older children, with equal sex distribution: (a) general symptoms: headaches; myalgia; arthralgia; abdominal pain; pleuritis; fever; (b) *ophthalmologic findings:* redness; photophobia; eye discomfort; disturbance of visual acuity; interstitial keratitis; conjunctivitis; excess lacrimation; ciliary flush; uveitis; episcleritis; scleritis; inflamed optic papilla; muscular involvement; papilledema; thinned sclera; cells in the anterior chamber; corneal ulceration; blindness; (c) *vestibuloauditory dysfunction,* mainly cochlear; sensorineural hearing defect; vertigo; tinnitus; nausea; intralabyrinthine osteogenesis; extensive endolymphatic hydrops in the cochlea (case report); (d) congestive heart failure; hypertension; vascular occlusion; aortic insufficiency; left ventricular hypertrophy; dysrhythmias; (e) cerebellar ataxia; (f) eosinophilia.

Radiologic Manifestations: (a) *congestive heart failure; aortic insufficiency* (aortitis; inflammatory or myxoid degeneration of valves); *vascular occlusion* (partial or complete); large-vessel vasculitis in about 10% of patients; pleural effusion; pericarditis; bowel ulcerations and other changes related to vasculitis; (b) computed tomography and magnetic resonance imaging of the inner ear: *calcific obliteration and soft-tissue obliteration of the intralabyrinthine fluid space.*

COHEN SYNDROME

Clinical Manifestations: (a) low birth weight for gestation; *short stature; obesity; mental retardation; hypotonia;* (b) *craniofacial dysmorphism:* microcephaly; high nasal bridge; hypotelorism; prominent ears; maxillary hypoplasia; malar hypoplasia; short philtrum; open mouth; micrognathia; down-slanted palpebral fissures; prominent upper incisors; narrow palate; gingival hyperplasia; (c) *hyperextensibility of the joints;* cubitus valgus; genu valgum; *narrow hands and feet;* finger syndactyly; hip dislocation; (d) delayed puberty; (e) *ophthalmologic abnormalities:* decreased visual acuity; hemeralopia; constricted visual fields; etc.; (f) probably autosomal recessive inheritance; reported in identical twins; intrafamilial variation.

Radiologic Manifestations: Mild shortening of the metacarpals and metatarsals; cubitus valgus; genu valgum; mild lumbar lordosis; mild thoracic scoliosis.

CONTRACTURAL ARACHNODACTYLY (Beals-Hecht Syndrome)

Clinical Manifestations: (a) craniofacial dysmorphism: oval-shaped head; somewhat deep-set eyes; small mouth; high palate; mild limitation in excursion of the jaw; *external ear deformity;* (b) *progressive kyphoscoliosis in childhood;* (c) *arachnodactyly; flexion contracture of the proximal interphalangeal joints of the fingers; flexion deformity of the elbows and knees;* adducted thumbs; ulnar deviation of the fingers; spontaneous improvement of the contracture with time; *dolichostenomelia; marfanoid habitus;* (d) keratoconus; ectopia lentis; ankyloblepharon; myopia; (e) mitral valve prolapse; mitral regurgitation; aortic root aneurysmal dilatation; (f) autosomal dominant inheritance with variable expressivity; sporadic.

Radiologic Manifestations: (a) slight osteopenia; *gracile bones;* mild bowing of the long bones; *elongation of the proximal phalanges of the fingers and toes;* (b) miscellaneous abnormalities: advanced bone age; vertebral malformations; restrictive lung disease resulting from kyphoscoliosis and thoracic constriction; esophageal atresia, duodenal atresia with an annular pancreas; mitral valve prolapse; cardiovascular anomalies; hypoplastic tibia and bowing of fibula.

COSTELLO SYNDROME

Clinical and Radiologic Manifestations: (a) *growth and developmental retardation;* (b) *"coarse" face;* large mouth; thick lips; macroglossia; thick earlobes; *loose, dark skin, particularly of hands and feet;* (c) miscellaneous abnormalities: acanthosis nigricans; dystrophic nails; curly hair; nasal papillomas; barrel chest; hyperextensible fingers; wide distal phalanges; restricted elbow motion; cubitus valgus; elbow dislocation; enamel hypoplasia; cerebral atrophy; short neck; relative macrocephaly.

COWDEN SYNDROME

Clinical Manifestations: (a) *macrocephaly; "birdlike" facies;* hypoplastic mandible and maxilla; microstomia; highly arched palate; (b) *breast lesions:* virginal hyperplasia; fibrocystic disease; neoplasm, benign gynecomastia in males; (c) *multiple facial papules; acral keratoses; palmoplantar keratoses;* acral verrucoid lesions; dermal fibromas; multiple skin tags; lipomas; cutaneous malignancies; (d) *multiple oral papillomas;* oral fibromas; scrotal tongue; oral malignancies; (e) *thyroid diseases:* goiter; adenoma; hyperthyroidism; hypothyroidism; thyroiditis; thyroglossal duct cyst; follicular adenocarcinoma; (f) menstrual irregularities; miscarriages; stillbirths; ovarian abnormalities; (g) leiomyomas in females; vaginal and vulvar cysts; adenocarcinoma of the uterus; carcinoma of the uterine cervix; carcinoma of the ovary, hydrocele; varicocele; transitional cell carcinoma of the renal pelvis; transitional cell carcinoma of the bladder; (h) polyps (juvenile, hamartomatous, hyperplastic, lymphomatous, inflammatory, or rarely adenomatous); diverticula of the colon; ganglioneuromas; neuromas; epithelioid leiomyoma of the rectosigmoid; adenocarcinoma of the colon; hepatic hamartoma; (i) dullness; seizures; intention tremors, neuroma of cutaneous nerves; neurofibroma; meningioma; hearing loss; (j) cataracts; angioid streaks; myopia; (k) autosomal dominant inheritance, with a high penetrance in males and females and interfamilial and intrafamilial differences in the expressivity of symptoms.

Radiologic Manifestations: Alimentary tract polyps; thyroid tumor; breast lesions; tumors at various sites.

Note: (a) *Cowden* is the family name of the first reported patient; (b) association with Lhermitte-Duclos disease (a possible component of Cowden phacomatosis).

CRANIOECTODERMAL DYSPLASIA (Sensenbrenner Syndrome)

Clinical Manifestations: (a) small stature; (b) *craniofacial dysmorphism:* large, dolichocephalic head; frontal bossing; anteverted nares; full cheeks; epicanthal folds; down-slanting of the eyes; posteriorly rotated ears; small helices; everted lower lips; highly arched palate; multiple oral frenula; capillary nevus on the forehead; (c) myopia; hyperopia; nystagmus; (d) *dental anomalies:* microdontia; hypodontia; fusion; widely spaced teeth; enamel dysplasia; (e) *fine, sparse, and slow-growing hair;* (f) short and narrow thorax; pectus excavatum; congenital heart disease; (g) limb anomalies: short limbs; hyperextensible joints; small hands; (h) renal dystrophy and tubulointerstitial nephropathy; etc.; (i) probably autosomal recessive inheritance.

Radiologic Manifestations: (a) osteoporosis; (b) limb anomalies: short tubular bones, especially in the hands and feet; thinness of the cortex of the tubular bones; slight widening of the metaphyses; flatness of the epiphyseal ossification center; delayed appearance of ossification of the femoral head; relative shortness of fibulae; (c) infantile type of vertebrae with biconvex upper and lower borders; narrow interpediculate distance in the lower lumbar region; (d) sagittal craniosynostosis (inconstant feature).

CRANIO-FRONTO-NASAL DYSPLASIA

Clinical Manifestations: (a) *craniofacial dysmorphism:* brachycephaly; plagiocephaly; acrocephaly; dolichocephaly; frontal bossing;

broad forehead; facial asymmetry; midface hypoplasia; ocular hypertelorism; broad nasal tip; bifid nose; strabismus; esotropia or exotropia; primary telecanthus; highly arched palate; cleft lip and/or cleft palate; bifid uvula; malocclusion; coronal synostosis; (b) *limb anomalies:* broad digits; long fingers; short fifth finger; digital hypoplasia; syndactyly; camptodactyly; polydactyly; clinodactyly; duplicated phalanx; hallux valgus; duplicated hallux; broad first toes; gap between the first and second toes; long toes; grooved nails; (c) increased incidence of miscarriage; (d) genetic heterogeneity (autosomal dominant; X-linked dominant with lethality in males); wide variation in the expression.

Radiologic Manifestations: *Coronal craniosynostosis; hypertelorism; midfacial hypoplasia;* pseudoarthrosis of the clavicle; Sprengel shoulder deformity.

CRANIOTELENCEPHALIC DYSPLASIA

Clinical Manifestations: (a) *frontal bone protrusion; neurologic abnormalities;* diminished brain growth; developmental delay; seizures; (b) probably autosomal recessive transmission.

Pathology: *Premature closure of cranial sutures; brain dysgenesis* (agyria; microgyria; heterotopic gray matter; partially fused frontal lobes; hydrocephalus; absent corpus callosum; etc.); optic nerve hypoplasia.

Radiologic Manifestations: *Premature closure of cranial sutures* (metopic; sagittal; coronal) with *prominent protrusion of the frontal bone;* short anterior fossa; vertical slope of the middle fossa, orbital hypotelorism; *brain dysgenesis.*

CREST SYNDROME (CRST SYNDROME; THIBIERGE-WEISSENBACH SYNDROME)

Clinical Manifestations: Onset of symptoms at the average age of 45 years: *sclerodactyly with ulcerations of the skin; scleroderma; limited to the fingers and face; Raynaud phenomenon; telangiectasia; dysphagia;* achalasia-like syndrome as the first manifestation; association with sick sinus syndrome; etc.

Radiologic Manifestations: *Soft-tissue calcification at various sites (fingers; shoulders; thoracic wall; cervical spine; etc.); osteopenia; bone erosions; intraarticular calcification; atlantoaxial joint destruction; subluxation of the upper cervical spine; abnormal motor function of the esophagus;* calcific constrictive pericarditis.

Note: *CREST:* Calcinosis, Raynaud phenomenon, Esophageal dysmotility, Sclerodactyly, Telangiectasia.

CRONKHITE-CANADA SYNDROME

Clinical Manifestations: Onset in middle or old age: (a) *gastrointestinal hamartomatous polyps of the juvenile type;* (b) *alopecia; (c) onychodystrophy;* (d) *skin hyperpigmentation;* abnormalities on light and electron microscopic studies (increased numbers of melanin granules in keratinocytes; increased numbers of melanosomes in melanocytes; areas with increased numbers of melanocytes; compact hyperkeratosis; perivascular inflammation and exocytosis).

Radiologic Manifestations: (a) *polyps of stomach, small bowel, and colon;* esophageal polyp very rare; patterns of involvement: (1) innumerable small polyps carpeting large areas; (2) scattered polyps of varying sizes; (3) sparse involvement with few small polyps; (b) coarsening of the mucosal folds of the small intestine with or without polypoid filling defects; segmentation of barium in the small bowel; intussusception (rare); carcinoma of the colon (rare); (c) erosive arthritis.

Note: Infantile form associated with the following: macrocephaly; clubbing of the fingers; alopecia; nail dystrophy; hypotonia; anemia; hepatosplenomegaly; protein-losing enteropathy.

CROSS SYNDROME

Clinical and Radiologic Manifestations: (a) *ocular and cutaneous hypopigmentation; mixed pattern of hair pigmentation; mental retardation; spasticity; microphthalmia; cloudy cornea;* (b) miscellaneous abnormalities: athetosis; gingival fibromatosis; cerebellar hypoplasia; Dandy-Walker malformation; osteoporosis; microdontia; (c) probably autosomal recessive inheritance.

CROUZON SYNDROME (CRANIOFACIAL DYSOSTOSIS)

Clinical Manifestations: (a) *brachycephaly or oxycephaly;* scaphocephaly and trigonocephaly less common; *parrot-beaked nose; bilateral exophthalmos; bilateral divergent pseudostrabismus; mandibular prognathism;* (b) mild to moderate mental retardation; (c) airway obstruction with cor pulmonale; sleep apnea; (d) exotropia; poor vision; blindness; optic atrophy; iris coloboma; keratoconjunctivitis; spontaneous luxation of the eyes; keratoconus; (e) atresia of the auditory meatus; hearing deficit; (f) autosomal dominant inheritance with complete penetrance and variable expressivity; sporadic in about one fourth of cases; mutations in the fibroblast growth factor receptor 2 gene; first trimester prenatal diagnosis by identification of the disease-causing mutation.

Radiologic Manifestations: (a) craniofacial deformities: *high vertex in the region of the anterior fontanelle, premature closure of any or all cranial sutures;* increased digital markings; basilar kyphosis with the plane of the clivus being more near vertical than normal; sphenoidal plane inclined downward and forward; downward displacement of the cribriform plate; medial and upward tilt of the petrous portion of the temporal bone; poor development or absence of development of the frontal sinus; shallow orbits; upward tilt of the roof of the orbit (frontal bone and lesser wing of the sphenoid); hypoplasia of the infraorbital rim; orbital hypertelorism resulting from enlarged ethmoidal air cells and lateral expansion and ballooning of the ethmoids; small and deformed optic foramina; exotropia; upward and medial tilt of the external auditory canal; poor pneumatization of the mastoids; deformity of the middle-ear ossicles in some cases; cloudy middle ears due to the presence of secretions (eustachian tube obstruction); stubby lateral and superior semicircular canals in some cases; elongated vertical portion of the carotid canal; more vertical direction of the groove of the sigmoid sinus; shallow sigmoid notch; hypoplasia of the maxillomalar facial mass; recession of the malar bone; short and distorted zygomatic arches; narrow pterygomaxillary fossa, marked thickening of the alveolar process of the maxilla; narrow V-shaped or semicircular deformity of the upper alveolar dental arch; crowding of the maxillary teeth; very short and high palate; lateral accumulation of soft tissue on the palatine processes; thick and long soft palate; relative mandibular prognathism; *nasopharyngeal airway constriction; narrow oropharynx;* (b) central nervous system: hydrocephalus; deformed ventricular system due to skull deformity; basilar impression; absent corpus callosum; chronic tonsillar herniation; (c) narrow trachea; (d) prenatal ultrasonography: abnormal cranial shape; proptosis; increased interorbital diameter; (e) miscellaneous abnormalities: anomalies of the craniocervical junction; cloverleaf skull deformity; sinus pericranii; calcification of the styloid ligament; calcaneocuboid coalition; subluxation of the radial heads; association with Pyle disease; hemangiomatous anomaly of bone.

CRUVEILHIER-BAUMGARTEN SYNDROME (PEGOT-CRUVEILHIER-BAUMGARTEN SYNDROME)

Clinical Manifestations: *Prominent umbilical or paraumbilical veins; venous hum; splenomegaly; portal hypertension with esophageal varices; liver disease (fibrosis; atrophy).*
Radiologic Manifestations: *Esophageal varices; splenomegaly; intrahepatic portal venous obstruction; patency of the umbilical vein in*

association with portal hypertension and abdominal collateral circulation demonstrable by various methods (ultrasound in combination with color-coded duplex sonography; computed tomography; percutaneous transhepatic portography; injection of superficial abdominal veins; superior mesenteric angiography).

CURRARINO TRIAD

The Triad: *Sacral defect; anorectal malformation; presacral mass.*

Clinical Manifestations: (a) *anorectal malformations (stenosis; anal ectopia; imperforate anus; rectovaginal fistula);* constipation; (b) miscellaneous abnormalities: progressive neurologic dysfunction; partial trisomy of chromosomes 13q and 20p; (c) autosomal dominant inheritance in about half of the cases; in the familial cases, one or two features may be missing.

Radiologic Manifestations: (a) *sacral bony abnormality* (scimitar sacrum; sacral hypoplasia; etc.); (b) *presacral mass* (anterior meningocele; teratoma; enteric cyst [isolated or in combination]); (c) miscellaneous abnormalities: hydrocephalus; lipomeningocele; tethered cord; low conus; dysplastic conus; dural sac ectasia; dural sac stenosis; neurogenic bladder; duplex ureter; hydronephrosis; vesicoureteral reflux; bicornuate uterus.

CUTIS LAXA

Clinical Manifestations: Variable clinical presentation and onset of symptoms: (a) *loose and pendulous skin, in particular, facial skin; growth retardation; looseness of the oropharyngeal mucosa;* airway obstruction due to lax and elongated vocal cords; deep voice; respiratory symptoms; *hernias; rectal and vaginal prolapse;* cor pulmonale; arrhythmia; degenerative changes in the cornea; mental retardation; etc.; (b) acquired cutis laxa: multiple myeloma; celiac disease; chronic urticaria; etc.; (c) autosomal dominant inheritance with variable penetrance (benign form); autosomal recessive; X-linked (occipital horn syndrome).

Pathology: Reduction in the amount and size of elastic fibers.

Radiologic Manifestations: (a) *pulmonary emphysema; cor pulmonale;* (b) *dilatation and tortuousity of blood vessels;* pulmonary artery stenosis; coarctation of the aorta; (c) diverticula of the gastrointestinal and urogenital tracts; gastric ulcer; esophageal dilatation; dilatation and tortuousity of the ureters; vesicoureteral reflux; hernias; diaphragmatic eventration; (d) miscellaneous abnormalities: radial head dislocation; pectus excavatum; osteoporosis with multiple fractures and flat vertebrae (compression fractures); punctate hip calcification.

CUTIS VERTICIS GYRATA

Classification
(A) PRIMARY: An isolated abnormality.
(B) SECONDARY: Endocrinopathies (acromegaly; myxedema; cretinism); skin lesions (cerebriform intradermal nevus; inflammatory dermatoses; leukemia; neurofibroma; dermatofibroma); central nervous system anomalies (fetal brain disruption sequence; hydranencephaly; polymicrogyria); rotational traction of scalp by long, matted hair.
(C) SYNDROMES: (1) Apert syndrome; (2) Beare-Stevenson cutis gyrata syndrome: acanthosis nigricans; cutis gyrata; furrowed palms and soles; scalp and neck skin folds; cutaneous/mucosal tags; small nails; craniofacial abnormalities (acrocephaly or cloverleaf deformity; craniosynostosis; ocular hypertelorism; choanal atresia; palatal anomalies; ear malformations); anogenital anomalies; prominent umbilical stump; etc.; (3) pachydermoperiostosis; (4) Turner syndrome.
Clinical Manifestations: (a) *corrugated or gyrate appearance of the scalp; sparse hair in the areas of the folds;* (b) mental retardation (frequent); (c) miscellaneous abnormalities: seizures; microcephaly; eye abnormalities (strabismus; cataract; blindness); cerebral palsy; hypotonia; developmental delay; presence of significant percentage of mitoses; etc.; (d) majority sporadic; autosomal recessive and dominant inheritance with varying expressivity in some.
Radiologic Manifestations: *Thick scalp folds;* microcephaly and skull asymmetry; small cerebellum; macroventriculy or microventriculy.

D

DANDY-WALKER SYNDROME (DANDY-WALKER MALFORMATION)

Etiology: Occurrence as an isolated malformation or in association with various chromosomal aberrations; single gene disorders, environmentally induced malformation syndromes, or other multifactorial abnormalities.
Association of Dandy-Walker Malformation with the Following
(A) SYNDROMES: (1) Aase-Smith syndrome; (2) Aicardi syndrome; (3) Coffin-Siris syndrome; (4) Brachmann–de Lange syndrome; (5) Ellis–van Creveld syndrome; (6) familial renal-hepatic-pancreatic dysplasia; (7) Fraser syndrome; (8) Joubert syndrome; (9) Klippel-Feil syndrome; (10) Meckel syndrome; (11) neurocutaneous melanosis sequence; (12) orofacio-digital syndrome type II; (13) Ruvalcaba syndrome; (14) Sjögren-

Larsson syndrome; (15) Walker-Warburg syndrome; (16) X-linked cerebellar hypoplasia; (17) X-linked mental retardation, seizures, basal ganglia disease, and Dandy-Walker malformation; (18) Goldston syndrome: renal cystic dysplasia and Dandy-Walker malformation (this may be a variant of Meckel syndrome); (19) sagittal craniosynostosis, Dandy-Walker malformation and hydrocephalus (Jones syndrome); (20) Dandy-Walker malformation with postaxial polydactyly; (21) facial dysmorphism, macrocephaly, myopia, and Dandy-Walker malformation (possibly an autosomal recessive syndrome); (22) Dandy-Walker malformation variant, cystic kidneys, and hepatic fibrosis (this may be a variant of Meckel syndrome); (23) Dandy-Walker malformation associated with Marden-Walker syndrome; (24) familial Dandy-Walker malformation, macrocephaly, facial anomalies, developmental delay, and brain stem dysgenesis.

(B) ENVIRONMENTALLY INDUCED MALFORMATION: Fetal alcohol syndrome; fetal cytomegalic infection; fetal isotretinoin syndrome; fetal rubella syndrome; maternal diabetes; warfarin embryopathy.

Clinical Manifestations: *Enlargement of the skull in the occipital region with prominent external convexity posterior to the foramen magnum; full fontanelles; wide sutures;* general symptoms: seizures; vomiting; irritability; opisthotonus; apnea; etc.

Radiologic Manifestations: (a) skull abnormalities: *enlarged dolichocephalic skull with a deep posterior fossa; thin occiput; high position of the tentorium cerebelli, torcular Herophili, and grooves for the lateral sinuses;* (b) brain abnormalities: *dilated fourth ventricle that extends to the inner table of the skull with a fingerlike extension into the upper cervical region;* torcular-lambdoid inversion; absent inferior vermis; dysplastic cerebellar hemispheres bounded posteromedially by the cyst; compression of basilar cisterns; bowing of the pericallosal artery; elevated branches of the middle cerebral artery; anterosuperior displacement of the proximal segment of the superior cerebellar artery; small or absent cerebellar blush; elongated great vein of Galen; elevated torcular Herophili; steep descent of the transverse sinuses.

Note: Owing to the association of large facial hemangiomas and Dandy-Walker malformation or similar posterior fossa abnormalities, imaging evaluation of the infants with these hemangiomas has been recommended.

DEGOS SYNDROME (KÖHLMEIER-DEGOS DISEASE; MALIGNANT ATROPHIC PAPULOSIS)

Clinical Manifestations: Often a male patient in the third decade; rare in children: *papular skin eruption progressing to ulceration;* involvement of the mucous membrane; *shallow ulcers of the mucosa of the stomach and* *bowel; bowel perforation; peritonitis;* malabsorption associated with intestinal ischemia; myocardial infarction; pericardial effusion; fibrous and fibrinous pericarditis; constrictive pericarditis; myocardial fibrosis; pulmonary infarct; renovascular hypertension; cerebral ischemia; ictus; deterioration of intellectual, social, and motor functions; prolonged purely cutaneous variant.

Pathology: Progressive cutaneovisceral *occlusive arteriopathy* (buccal mucosa; gastrointestinal tract; eyes; central nervous system; heart; kidneys; urinary tract; pleura; lungs; liver; pancreas): subendothelial fibromuscular proliferation; intimal deposits of lipid-laden cells (middle-sized and small arteries); often thrombus formation.

Radiologic Manifestations: Gastric perforation; bowel perforation; peritonitis; bowel infarction; pleural effusion; pericardial effusion; pleural and pericardial calcification; renal arteriopathy (occlusion of interlobular arteries; intrarenal collateral circulation; delayed nephrographic phase at the area of intrarenal collaterals); cerebral vasculopathy (multiple intracerebral arterial narrowing and ectasia ["beading"]; infarction; hemorrhage; necrosis; atrophy); visceral and peripheral arteriopathy (stenoses).

DÉJÉRINE-SOTTAS SYNDROME

Clinical Manifestations: Onset of disease usually in childhood, but often the disease is diagnosed in adult life: (a) symmetric diffuse or localized manifestations with a picture of *progressive motor and sensory neural involvement* and periodic phases of apparent remission: muscle weakness; pain; nystagmus; ataxia; areflexia; intention tremor; cranial nerve deficits; pupillary abnormalities; (b) enlarged and frequently palpable peripheral nerves; phrenic nerve involvement (case report); etc.; (c) autosomal dominant inheritance; a family with a gene mapped on chromosome 8 reported.

Pathology: *Thickening of affected nerves due to hyperplasia of the nerve sheath* (cranial nerves; spinal nerves; cauda equina; peripheral nerves).

Radiologic Manifestations: Vertebral abnormalities *(scalloping of the dorsal aspect of vertebral bodies; enlarged interpediculate distances; triangulation of the pedicle with flattening of the superior aspect of the pedicle; erosion of the pedicle);* rounded soft-tissue density masses at the apices of thorax; *thickening of nerve roots; enlarged sciatic trunks; blocked flow of contrast material within the spinal canal; distortion of contrast within the spinal canal.*

DELLEMAN SYNDROME (OCULO-CEREBRO-CUTANEOUS SYNDROME)

Clinical Manifestations: (a) *ocular anomalies: orbital cyst;* microphthalmos; eyelid coloboma; hamartoma; persistent hyaloid artery; (b) *psy-*

chomotor retardation; convulsions; (c) *skin anomalies:* appendages (peri-orbital; postauricular); aplasia; hypoplasia, punchlike defects; (d) miscellaneous abnormalities: generalized asymmetry; cleft lip; cleft palate; anophthalmia and congenital orbital hypoplasia; malformed ears; genital anomalies.

Radiologic Manifestations: (a) *orbital cyst;* microphthalmos; hamartoma; (b) *intracranial cysts; agenesis of corpus callosum; ectopic gray matter; brain hypoplasia; ventricular dilatation;* (c) miscellaneous abnormalities: skull defects; rib dysplasia; vertebral anomalies.

DE MORSIER SYNDROME (SEPTO-OPTIC DYSPLASIA AND PITUITARY DWARFISM)

Clinical Manifestations: (a) apnea, hypotonia, seizures, hypoglycemia, and prolonged jaundice in newborns; (b) *ocular abnormalities:* amblyopia; nystagmus; hemianopia; hypoplastic optic discs; irregular field defects; (c) normal or subnormal intelligence; (d) hormonal deficiencies (*growth hormone;* adrenocorticotropin hormone; thyroid-stimulating hormone; luteinizing hormone; follicular stimulating hormone; antidiuretic hormone with impaired osmotic regulation); excessive or deficient prolactin production; (e) miscellaneous abnormalities: short stature; various patterns of puberty (early, appropriately timed, or delayed); two siblings with septo-optic dysplasia from a consanguineous pedigree (case report); etc.

Pathology: *Agenesis of the septum pellucidum* (in the majority of the cases); *presence of a primitive optic ventricle; hypoplasia of the chiasm.*

Radiologic Manifestations: (a) *absence of the septum pellucidum; flattening of the roof and inferior pointing of the floor of the frontal horns of lateral ventricles; hypoplasia of the anterior optic pathways; prominent optic recess of the third ventricle;* dilatation of the suprasellar and chiasmatic cisterns; small optic nerves; (b) *retarded bone age;* (c) miscellaneous abnormalities: agenesis of the corpus callosum; enlargement of the pituitary stalk and infundibulum when septo-optic dysplasia is associated with diabetes insipidus; cortical atrophy with dilated sulci; sphenoidal encephalocele; association with schizencephaly (septo-optic dysplasia–schizencephaly complex); normal brain computed tomographic scan in the presence of typical endocrinologic and ophthalmologic manifestations of septo-optic dysplasia.

DENYS-DRASH SYNDROME (DRASH SYNDROME)

Clinical and Pathologic Manifestations: (a) *male pseudohermaphroditism; gonadal dysgenesis; progressive glomerular disease* (diffuse mesangial sclerosis; renal failure); (b) *nephroblastoma;* (c) chromosomal abnormalities: 46,XY in some of the phenotypic females; deletion of the region 11p13–p12 in 46,XX female; germline mutations in the Wilms tumor suppressor gene; exonic mutation of the WT1 gene; (d) miscellaneous abnormalities: gonadoblastoma; granulosa cell tumor; metanephric hamartoma; high incidence of intralobar nephrogenic rests in complete and partial Denys-Drash syndrome; diaphragmatic hernia.

Radiologic Manifestations: Increased echogenicity of the renal cortex; *Wilms tumor* (unilateral or bilateral).

DERMO-CHONDRO-CORNEAL DYSTROPHY OF FRANÇOIS

Clinical Manifestations: (a) *cutaneous xanthomatous nodules; corneal dystrophy: central and superficial, with whitish subepithelial opacities;* anterior cortical cataracts; acquired skeletal deformities with *contractures,* subluxations, and limitation of motion; (b) autosomal recessive inheritance.

Radiologic Manifestations: Osteochondral deformities detectable in the first decade of life: *defective endochondral ossification; defective and irregular ossification of some tarsal bones;* rarely extensive osteoarticular destruction involving the entire skeleton except the spine and skull.

DE SANCTIS–CACCHIONE SYNDROME (XERODERMIC IDIOCY)

Clinical Manifestations: Onset in infancy or early childhood: (a) *xeroderma pigmentosum; mental retardation; neurologic manifestations (speech disorders; convulsions; spasticity; choreoathetosis; cerebellar ataxia);* dwarfism; gonadal hypoplasia; etc.; (b) autosomal recessive inheritance.

Radiologic Manifestations: Microcephaly; diffuse leukodystrophy; olivo-ponto-cerebellar atrophy; cerebral cortical atrophy and ventricular dilatation; premature closure of cranial sutures; skeletal growth retardation.

DIAMOND-BLACKFAN SYNDROME (BLACKFAN-DIAMOND SYNDROME)

Clinical Manifestations: Insidious onset in infancy or childhood: (a) unusual facies in some cases (two-colored hair; wide-set eyes; snub nose; thick upper lip); (b) *macrocytic* (normocytic in some) *normochromic refractory anemia* with normal value of other formed elements; *complete or near complete absence of cells of the erythroid series in bone marrow;* (c) *triphalangeal thumb; thenar muscle hypoplasia;* (d) hydrops fetalis; (e) most cases sporadic; about 10% to 20% familial (autosomal recessive or autosomal dominant).

Radiologic Manifestations: (a) skeletal anomalies: *thumb malformations (triphalangeal; bifurcation; subluxation; hypoplasia; absence);* fusion of cervical vertebrae; Klippel-Feil syndrome; Sprengel deformity; hip dislocation; etc.; (b) renal anomalies: dysplasia; horseshoe deformity; ureteral duplication; etc.; (c) miscellaneous abnormalities: cardiac enlargement; refractory heart failure; altered fetal blood velocity pattern (increased intracardiac blood velocities with only moderate increase in cardiac output).

DIENCEPHALIC SYNDROME (Russell Syndrome)

Clinical Manifestations: *Emaciation;* hyperkinesia; normal or *increased appetite; euphoria; overalertness; initial growth acceleration.*

Pathology: Tumors in the region of the anterior hypothalamus (glioma most often); nondiencephalic tumors a less common cause of the syndrome.

Radiologic Manifestations: *Complete absence of subcutaneous fat;* sutural widening and other roentgenographic findings of increased intracranial pressure; hydrocephalus; *mass in the hypothalamic region* with indentation on the third ventricle; increased uptake of radionuclide (^{99m}Tc) in the vicinity of the sella turcica.

DIETL SYNDROME

Clinical Manifestations: Episodic symptoms associated with *ureteropelvic junction obstruction: acute dilatation of the renal collecting system due to complete or nearly complete obstruction at the ureteropelvic junction, causing crampy upper abdominal pain*, nausea, and vomiting; dehydration and resorption of urine from the collecting system may result in relief of symptoms; hematuria in some cases.

Radiologic Manifestations: *Demonstration of hydronephrosis by various imaging techniques, including diuretic augmented isotope renal scan.*

DiGEORGE SEQUENCE (Third and Fourth Pharyngeal Pouch Syndrome)

Clinical Manifestations: (a) *facial features:* broad nose; shortened philtrum; hypoplastic mandible; low-set ears; fused helix and anthelix; hypertelorism; (b) *hypocalcemic tetany in the newborn;* (c) *frequent infections;* wide immunologic spectrum (normal function to combined immunodeficiency); (d) *cardiovascular anomalies;* (e) chromosomal abnormalities: monosomy 10p13; duplication of the long arm of chromosome 9; interstitial deletion of 22q11; etc.; (f) most reported cases sporadic; autosomal dominant inheritance.

Radiologic Manifestations: (a) *absence of a thymic shadow in the first week of life on a chest roentgenogram;* (b) *cardiovascular anomalies*, especially aortic arch anomalies, including conotruncal anomaly, left common carotid artery arising from the pulmonary artery, and anomalous origin of left main pulmonary artery from the ascending aorta.

Note: (a) an overlap of the clinical manifestations of DiGeorge and velo-cardio-facial syndromes and microdeletions of chromosome 22q11 in both syndromes have been reported; (b) the acronym *CATCH 22* syndrome refers to the major manifestations of DiGeorge syndrome: *C*ardiac defects; *A*bnormal facies; *T*hymic hypoplasia; *C*left palate; *H*ypocalcemia; 22q11 deletions.

DIGITOTALAR DYSMORPHISM (ULNAR DRIFT)

Clinical and Radiologic Manifestations: (a) *flexion deformities; ulnar deviation and narrowing of the fingers; soft-tissue web causing abnormal position of the thumbs; vertical talus;* (b) autosomal dominant transmission has been suggested.

DISTICHIASIS-LYMPHEDEMA SYNDROME

Clinical Manifestations: (a) *extra rows of eyelashes;* partial ectropion of the lower lids (in some); *lymphedema of the lower limbs;* etc.; (b) autosomal dominant inheritance.

Radiologic Manifestations: (a) *hypoplastic lymph channels;* (b) miscellaneous abnormalities: kyphoscoliosis; spina bifida; spinal extradural cysts; mother with double uterus and son with Robin sequence.

DOOR SYNDROME

Clinical Manifestations: (a) *neurosensory deafness; onychodystrophy* (absent or small nails); *osteodystrophy of the terminal phalanges; mental retardation;* (b) miscellaneous abnormalities: congenital heart defects, hydronephrosis, hydroureter, dilatation of the bladder; (c) considerable heterogeneity; autosomal recessive inheritance (most cases); autosomal dominant inheritance.

Radiologic Manifestations: (a) *phalangeal anomalies:* hypoplasia; clinodactyly; cutaneous syndactyly; cone-shaped epiphyses; proximally placed thumbs; triphalangeal thumbs; etc.; (b) miscellaneous abnormalities: spinal anomalies; short femoral neck; metaphysial spur on the distal end of the femur; etc.

Note: It has been suggested that the acronym *DOO* be used for the autosomal dominant *D*eafness and *O*nycho-*O*steodystrophy and the acronym *DOOR* to be used for the autosomal recessive *D*eafness, *O*nycho-*O*steodystrophy, and *R*etardation.

DOWN SYNDROME (CHROMOSOME 21 TRISOMY)

Etiology: (a) chromosomal abnormality: nondisjunction in about 92%; translocation in about 5%; mosaicism in about 3%; (b) chance of recurrence in general about 1%.

Clinical Manifestations: (a) craniofacial dysmorphism: brachycephaly; flat occiput; short neck with a skin fold; straight hair; upward slanting of the palpebral fissures; epicanthal folds; small mouth; protruding tongue, narrow palate; fissured tongue; ear deformity (low-set, reduced ear length; small earlobes; angular, overlapping helix; prominent anthelix); dental abnormalities (delayed tooth eruption; small teeth; irregular tooth placement; abnormal sequence of tooth eruption; partial anodontia; low susceptibility to dental caries); (b) physical appearance: short stature; obesity; dry skin; alopecia; excess or loose skin of the hands; acromicria; brachydactyly; clinodactyly; small middle phalanx; second and fifth digits partial adactyly; wide space between the first and second toes; syndactyly of the second and third toes; simian creases; (c) ocular manifestations: Brushfield spots of the iris; strabismus; abnormalities of refraction; cataract; keratoconus; blepharoconjunctivitis; ectropion; iris hypoplasia; fundus changes; (d) neuropsychiatric manifestations: *mental and motor retardation; hypotonia;* Alzheimer disease in patients beyond the age of 30 or 40 years; (e) congenital heart disease; (f) respiratory system: obstructive sleep apnea; upper airway obstruction associated with midfacial hypoplasia (cor pulmonale and congestive heart failure); epiglottic enlargement (nonbacterial); etc.; (g) alimentary system anomalies; (h) genitourinary system: cryptorchidism; agonadism; renal hypoplasia; obstructive uropathy; cystic dysplastic kidney; Potter sequence; etc.; (i) endocrine disorders: thyroid dysfunction (hypothyroidism; hyperthyroidism); diabetes mellitus; precocious or delayed puberty; etc.; (j) immune disorders; (k) blood disorders: blood test abnormalities in newborns with benign natural history (increased hematocrit; decreased hematocrit; decreased platelet count; increased white cell count); transient neonatal leukemoid reactions; etc.; (l) neoplasias: leukemia (eighteenfold increased risk); testicular cancer; retinoblastoma; non-Hodgkin lymphoma; (m) α-fetoprotein: maternal and fetal low serum α-fetoprotein levels in midtrimester; (n) abnormally low unconjugated estriol; abnormally high chorionic gonadotropin.

Radiologic Manifestations: (a) alimentary system: esophageal dysfunction; congenital pyloric atresia; duodenal atresia; duodenal stenosis; annular pancreas; intraluminal duodenal diverticulum; Hirschsprung disease; anorectal anomalies (much higher prevalence than in general population); cholelithiasis; biliary sludge; (b) cardiovascular anomalies (cushion defects; ventricular septal defect; etc.); (c) central nervous system: round brain; smaller than normal whole brain volume (magnetic resonance quantitation); reduced anteroposterior diameter of the frontal lobes; narrow superior temporal gyrus; small posterior fossa; small cerebellum; small brain stem; large sylvian fissure in those under 1 year of age; high incidence of midline cava (cavum septi pellucidi; cavum vergae; cavum veli interpositi); posterior fossa ependymal cyst; spinal cord compression due to atlantoaxial dislocation (narrow canal); cervical cord myelopathy; delayed myelination; bilateral calcification of the basal ganglia; (d) respiratory system: epiglottic enlargement; tracheal stenosis (in particular mid-tracheal "hourglass" type); cystic lung disease; congenital pleural effusion; (e) skeletal system: brachycephalic microcephaly; hypoplasia of the facial bones and sinuses; short hard palate; high cribriform plate; thin calvaria with wide sutures and delay in closure; orbital hypotelorism, high orbital roofs; hypoplasia and sclerosis of mastoids (an indicator of undiagnosed otitis media in some cases); atlantooccipital instability and dislocation; atlantoaxial instability and dislocation (10% to 20% of individuals with Down syndrome have atlantoaxial instability); subluxation at cervical interspaces other than C1-C2; cervical spine anomalies (hypoplastic posterior arch of C1; persistent synchondrosis; ossiculum terminale; spina bifida; atlantoaxial fusion); congenital vertebral fusion; flattening of the cervical vertebrae; degenerative arthritis of the cervical vertebrae and intervertebral discs (patients usually over 20 years of age); upper cervical ossicles; increased height and decreased anteroposterior diameter of the lumbar vertebrae in newborns; scoliosis; extreme hyperextension of the fetal head with dorsiflexions of the cervicodorsal segment in the last trimester; 11 pairs of ribs; two ossification centers of the manubrium (in 85% to 90% of the cases); bell-shaped chest; gracile ribs; prominent conoid process of the clavicle; flared iliac wings with small acetabular angles and iliac index; distal tapering of the ischium in the first year of life; short hands with stubby digits; clinodactyly with dysplasia of the middle phalanges of the fifth fingers (shortened, disproportionately wide, and frequently wedge shaped); brachymesophalangia; severe joint laxity; hip dislocation; dislocation of radius at elbow; patellofemoral instability; pes planus; metatarsus varus; genu valgum; acetabular dysplasia with or without hip dislocation; slipped capital femoral epiphysis; tibiotalar slant; pseudoepiphyses of the hands; variable skeletal maturation; stippled epiphyses; (f) prenatal sonographic signs: thickened nuchal fold; fetal cystic hygroma; hypoplasia of the middle phalanx of the fifth digit; fetal hydrops; fetal cervical hyperextension in breech presentation; transient pleural effusion.

Note: Evaluation of the craniocervical junction: magnetic resonance imaging has shown the subarachnoid space width correlates with neural canal width on radiographs better than with either atlas-dens interval or clivus-posterior odontoid process distance.

DUANE SYNDROME

Clinical Manifestations: (a) *congenital strabismus with a deficiency of abduction and adduction; retraction of the globe; oblique movement of the globe and narrowing of the palpebral fissure during adduction; deficiency of convergence* (Duane retraction syndrome); (b) other syndromes or anomalies associated with Duane retraction syndrome: Rubinstein-Taybi syndrome; Goldenhar syndrome; Klippel-Feil syndrome; Wildervanck syndrome; Kallmann syndrome; Romberg syndrome; fetal alcohol syndrome; facial anomalies; cleft palate; external ear malformations; sensory neural hearing loss; facial palsy; syringomyelia; spastic diplegia; oculocutaneous albinism; short fingers and toes; Chiari I malformation; giant aneurysm of the vertebral-basilar arterial junction; chromosome 4q27–31 segment deletion; etc.; (c) most cases sporadic; familial cases in about 10%; autosomal dominant inheritance.

Radiologic Manifestations: (a) *various limb anomalies:* radial dysplasia; etc.; (b) magnetic resonance imaging of upshoot-downshoot phenomenon: vertical displacement of the lateral rectus muscle in relation to the orbit; (c) miscellaneous abnormalities: vertebral anomalies; spinal meningocele; rib anomalies; genitourinary anomalies.

Note: An association of radial ray defect and Duane syndrome has been reported to be transmitted as an autosomal dominant disorder and is called Duane/radial syndrome (DR syndrome; Okihiro syndrome).

DUBOWITZ SYNDROME

Clinical Manifestations: (a) *prenatal and postnatal growth failure; mild to severe mental retardation in about 60% of the cases;* (b) *craniofacial dysmorphism:* microcephaly; high and sloping forehead; flat supraorbital ridges; broad nasal bridge; dystopia canthorum or true ocular hypertelorism, blepharophimosis; highly arched palate; cleft palate; dysplastic ears; micrognathia; delayed dental eruption; severe dental caries; (c) *eczema on the face and limbs;* sparse hair; café au lait patches; (d) miscellaneous abnormalities: growth hormone deficiency; characteristic behavior pattern (shy, hyperactive, hates crowds, etc.); ichthyosiform eruption (case report); (e) probably autosomal recessive inheritance.

Radiologic Manifestations: Clinodactyly of the fifth fingers; preaxial polydactyly; cutaneous syndactyly of the second and third toes; pes planus; pes planovalgus; periosteal hyperostosis of the long bones; retarded bone age; progressive scoliosis.

DUMPING SYNDROME

Etiology: Ablation, alteration, or bypass of the pyloric sphincter; generalized autonomic dysfunction; total esophagogastrectomy.

Clinical Manifestations: Postprandial symptoms related to osmotic effect of foodstuff: *sense of fullness; cramps; diarrhea; nausea; vasomotor symptoms* (weakness; palpitation; sweating; flushing; dizziness); fluctuation in blood glucose levels (fainting; hypoglycemic seizures).

Radiologic Manifestations: Symptoms may be produced by a mixture of food and barium or 50% glucose mixed with barium; *rapid gastric emptying; dilution of a mixture within the small bowel due to a shift of fluid into the bowel;* radionuclide gastric emptying test.

Du PAN SYNDROME

Clinical and Radiologic Manifestations: (a) *complex type of brachydactyly:* buttonlike and radially deviated thumbs; short metacarpals; short phalanges; absent phalanges; hypoplasia of the carpal bones; etc.; (b) *fibular aplasia or hypoplasia;* knee dislocation in some; equinovalgus deformity of the feet; long or *hypoplastic metatarsal bones; ball-like hypoplastic toes; hypoplastic or absent phalanges; hypoplastic nails;* (c) sporadic and autosomal recessive inheritance.

DYKE-DAVIDOFF-MASSON SYNDROME

Clinical Manifestations: *Mental retardation; facial asymmetry; contralateral hemiplegia;* seizures.

Radiologic Manifestations: *Cerebral hemiatrophy with homolateral thickening and increased density of the calvaria; hypertrophy of the frontal sinuses and elevation of the sphenoid wing and petrous ridge;* asymmetry of the ventricles with a unilateral loss of brain substance; apparent shift of the ventricles, falx, and pineal to the atrophic side; crossed cerebellar atrophy.

DYSKERATOSIS CONGENITA (ZINSSER-ENGMAN-COLE SYNDROME)

Clinical Manifestations: Onset of the symptoms usually in the first decade of life: (a) *reticulated pigmentation;* skin atrophy; shiny fingertips; loss of dermatoglyphics; poikiloderma; generalized hyperpigmentation; telangiectasia; bullous lesions of the palms and soles induced by trauma; *leukoplakia of mucous membranes; nail dystrophy;* (b) *bone marrow dysplasia* (pancytopenia of Fanconi type); immune disorders; (c) blepharitis; conjunctivitis; ectropion; nasolacrimal duct obstruction; corneal cloudiness; cataracts; retinal atrophy; atherosclerotic changes of the retinal vessels; angioma of the retina; (d) enamel dystrophy; short, blunted roots; numerous dental caries; periodontitis; gingival recession; gingival bleeding; tooth mobility and severe alveolar bone loss; (e) predisposition to malignancy; marked sensitivity of the cultured skin fibroblasts to X-irradiation; chromosomal instability; (f) dysphagia; diarrhea; hemorrhage; nasopharyngeal atresia; etc.; (g) genetic heterogeneity; X-linked recessive inheritance (most likely location Xq22), with majority of the cases occurring in males; less commonly reported as autosomal dominant or autosomal recessive.

Radiologic Manifestations: (a) osteoporosis; increased bone fragility; radiolucent areas in diaphyses and coarse trabeculation in the metaphyses of the long bones; aseptic necrosis of the femoral head; (b) miscellaneous abnormalities: intracranial calcification; hepatosplenomegaly; liver cirrhosis; ascites; esophageal stricture; esophageal diverticula.

Note: The classic triad: *reticulated pigmentation, dystrophy of the nails, and leukoplakia of the mucous membranes.*

E

EAGLE SYNDROME

Clinical Manifestations: (a) the classic syndrome: *spastic and nagging pain in the pharynx with radiation into the mastoid region; dysphagia;* a feeling of a foreign body in the throat; *a palpable hard mass* in the tonsillar fossa (ossified stylohyoid ligament); a complete relief of the symptoms following surgical removal of the ossified stylohyoid ligament; (b) *carotodynia:* pain along the distribution of the carotid artery; subsidence of the symptoms following surgical resection of the stylohyoid process.

Radiologic Manifestations: *A smooth or bulky ossified stylohyoid process of varying length and degree of segmentation extending to the area of the lesser cornu of the hyoid bone;* external impression of the ossified ligament on the carotid artery.

ECTODERMAL DYSPLASIA (HYPOHIDROTIC) (CHRIST-SIEMENS-TOURAINE SYNDROME)

Clinical Manifestations: (a) *hypohidrosis; hypotrichosis;* (b) *oligodontia or anodontia;* abnormal crown form, with the contact point of the teeth being apically displaced (particularly the anterior teeth); (c) *unusual facies:* dish face; frontal bossing; saddle-shaped nose; prominent supraorbital ridges; protuberant lips; protruding ears; (d) *fever of unknown origin;* (e) miscellaneous abnormalities: mucus gland deficiencies; hearing problems; accumulation of wax in the auditory canals; persistent nasal crusting; dry and peeling skin at birth; eczema; deficiency of saliva; dental decay related to salivary gland dysfunction; lacrimation deficiency; (f) prenatal diagnosis: deoxyribonucleic acid–based linkage analysis during the first trimester of pregnancy; direct histologic analysis of fetal skin obtained by late second trimester fetoscopy; (g) X-linked recessive inheritance; fully expressed in males; partially expressed in heterozygous female carriers.

Radiologic Manifestations: *Deficient dentition;* apical displacement of the contact points of teeth; taurodontism; supernumerary lower incisor tooth; invagination of the tooth crown (talon cusps); "shovel-shaped" upper central incisors; upper and lower respiratory tract infections (sinusitis; pneumonia; etc.).

EEC SYNDROME (Ectrodactyly–Ectodermal Dysplasia–Clefting Syndrome)

Clinical Manifestations: (a) *ectodermal dysplasia; ectrodactyly* (clawhand and clawfoot; syndactyly; polydactyly); (b) facial dysmorphism: midfacial hypoplasia; *bilateral cleft lip/cleft palate;* prominent supraorbital ridges and nasal bridge; telecanthus; flat nasal tip; prominent ears; low position of the ears; hypoplasia of the earlobes; (c) xerostomia; absence of Stensen ducts; oral moniliasis; anodontia; oligodontia; enamel hypoplasia; dental caries; (d) eye abnormalities: anophthalmia or microphthalmia; absent lacrimal puncta; photophobia; chronic blepharitis; decreased tear formation; narrowing of the palpebral fissures; corneal vascularization; strabismus; astigmatism; ectropion; absent meibomian glands; (e) sporadic in most cases; autosomal dominant inheritance with great phenotypic variability; the penetrance of EEC mutation: 93% to 98%.

Radiologic Manifestations: (a) *clawhand; clawfoot;* various abnormalities of the carpals, tarsals, metacarpals, and metatarsals; (b) *genitourinary anomalies:* duplication of the collecting system; renal agenesis; hydronephrosis; hydroureter; bladder diverticulum; ureterocele; megaureter; vesicoureteral reflux; (c) prenatal detection of cleft lip/cleft palate and lobster-claw deformities by ultrasonography; (d) miscellaneous abnormalities: scoliosis; coxa vara; spina bifida; etc.

Note: (a) owing to the high occurrence of *U*rinary *T*ract abnormalities, *EECUT* has been suggested and included under "Synonyms"; (b) Czeizel-Losonci syndrome: split hand/split foot, syndactyly, urinary tract obstruction, radial, diaphragmatic, and neural tube defects (a possible new syndrome).

EHLERS-DANLOS SYNDROMES

Clinical Manifestations: Heterogeneous group of diseases of connective tissue with considerable overlap of the clinical manifestations: *joint hyperextensibility, abnormal stretchability of the skin, excessive bruisability, and fragility of blood vessels.*

- Type I (gravis type): autosomal dominant transmission with complete penetrance; new mutation common; *marked skin hyperextensibility and joint hypermobility; bruising tendency; "cigarette paper" scars*; fragility of fetal membranes; premature birth common.
- Type II (mitis type): autosomal dominant inheritance; *milder manifestations than the type I.*
- Type III (hypermobile type): autosomal dominant inheritance; *large and small joint hypermobility; mild skin hyperextensibility.*
- Type IV (vascular type): autosomal dominant and autosomal recessive; defect in type III collagen; diminished production and secretion of pro-α_2; *translucent skin; bruising tendency; mild skin hyperextensibility; laxity of the hand joints; ruptures* (artery; bowel; pregnant uterus); short life expectancy.
- Type V (X-linked type): X-linked recessive inheritance; *skin hyperextensibility;* bruising and joint hypermobility not constant features.
- Type VI (ocular-scoliotic type): autosomal recessive inheritance; lysyl hydroxylase deficiency in VI-A subtype; *microcornea; scleral perforation; retinal detachment; scoliosis;* soft, velvety, and hyperextensible skin.
- Type VII (arthrochalasis multiplex congenita): heterogeneous mode of inheritance (autosomal dominant; autosomal recessive); *marked articular hypermobility; soft skin and mild skin hyperextensibility;* short stature; micrognathia; structural defect of pro-α_1-collagen (VII-A) and pro-α_2-collagen (VII-B).
- Type VIII (periodontitis type): autosomal dominant inheritance; *fragile skin; bruising; abundant scarring; progressive periodontal disease; gingival recession; loss of teeth in the second and third decades.*
- Type IX: occipital horn syndrome: a disorder of copper metabolism; reclassified (removed from Ehlers-Danlos group).
- Type X: autosomal recessive; *petechiae, bruising; striae distensae; platelet aggregation defect; fibronectin abnormality.*
- Type XI: now classified as a joint instability disorder.

Radiologic Manifestations: (a) alimentary system: dilatation of the alimentary tract; spontaneous rupture; hemorrhage; mural hematoma; diverticula; malabsorption due to diverticula; constipation; rectal prolapse; diaphragmatic hernia; bile duct diverticula; (b) cardiovascular system: (1) heart: mitral valve prolapse; mitral insufficiency; aortic valve stenosis; aortic valve insufficiency; spontaneous left ventricular rupture; aneurysm of the sinus of Valsalva; papillary muscle dysfunction; tricuspid insufficiency; pulmonary valve stenosis; pulmonary valve insufficiency; pulmonary artery dilatation; myocardial infarction; congenital heart defects (septal defects; tetralogy of Fallot; dextrocardia; arch anomalies; bicuspid aortic valve; pulmonary artery anomalies; bicuspid tricuspid valve); (2) arterial: aneurysms; pseudo-aneurysm; aortic dissection; cystic medial necrosis; spontaneous rupture of the main arteries; elongated aortic arch; arterial stenosis; tortuous systemic or pulmonary arteries; arteriovenous fistulae; renovascular hypertension; intractable vasculitis and resorptive osteolysis; (3) venous: varicose veins; perforation of the superior vena cava (angiography complication), hepato-portal fistula; (c) craniofacial: (1) skull: delayed ossification of the vault; flat-tened orbits; micrognathia; hypertelorism; (2) temporomandibular joint dys-function; (3) teeth: malformed, stunted roots; pulp stones; etc.; (d) genitourinary system: hydronephrosis; infantile polycystic disease of the kid-neys; bladder diverticulum; bladder neck obstruction; medullary sponge kid-ney; adult polycystic kidney disease; pregnancy complications in type IV (rupture of the uterus, bowel, aorta, or vena cava; vaginal laceration; postpar-tum uterine hemorrhage); (e) nervous system: vascular malformations; dilata-tion of the fourth ventricle, lateral ventricles, and supracerebellar cistern; her-niated intervertebral disc; spontaneous carotid-cavernous fistulae; (f) respiratory system: mediastinal emphysema; spontaneous pneumothorax; subpleural blebs; transient, multiple, fluid-filled pulmonary cysts; hyperinfla-tion; tracheomegaly; bronchiectasis; severe irreversible obstructive pul-monary disease; pulmonary hypertension; (g) skeletal system and soft tissues: (1) spine: scoliosis; kyphosis; thoracic lordosis; lumbar platyspondyly; (2) chest wall: thoracic asymmetry; subluxation of the sternoclavicular joints; pectus recurvatum; pectus carinatum; elongated chest; costovertebral sublux-ations; (3) limbs: elongated ulnar styloid process; radioulnar synostosis; acro-osteolysis; flexion deformity of small hand joints; congenital hip dislocation; clawtoes and hammertoes; distraction of the pubic symphysis during deliv-ery; ectopic bone formation around hip joints; clubfoot; flatfoot; pes cavus; navicular-cuneiform synostosis; clinodactyly of the fifth finger; arachno-dactyly; syndactyly; carpal fusion; recurrent subluxation and dislocation; osteoarthritic changes; joint effusion; hemarthroses; secondary degenerative changes; (4) soft tissues: calcifications representing calcified subcutaneous lobules of fat; heterotopic ossification; (h) miscellaneous abnormalities: even-tration of diaphragm; external abdominal hernias; etc.

EISENMENGER SYNDROME

Clinical Manifestations: *Pulmonary hypertension with a bidirec-tional or reversed shunt at the atrial, ventricular, or aortopulmonary level;*

failure to thrive; cyanosis; exertional dyspnea; recurrent pulmonary infection; right ventricular hypertrophy; pulmonary ventilatory function abnormalities (raised residual volume and closing capacity and a reduction of other lung volumes and maximal expiratory flows); ocular manifestations (microaneurysms; hemorrhages; capillary dilatation; retinal collaterals; rubeosis iridis); congestive heart failure (uncommon); etc.

Radiologic Manifestations: (a) *heart size normal to moderately enlarged; mild to severely dilated pulmonary artery segment; dilatation of the central portion of the pulmonary arteries with abrupt tapering in the middle zone of the lung;* calcification in the wall of the pulmonary artery (in some); *reversed or bidirectional shunt;* (b) ultrasonography: (1) pulmonary valve: attenuation of the a wave; delayed opening; steep systolic opening slope and a complete midsystolic closure of the posterior leaflet, followed by a complete reopening of the valve in late systole; (2) aortic valve: sudden partial closure of the right coronary cusp in late systole.

EMPTY SELLA SYNDROME

Definitions: (a) empty sella: an extension of the subarachnoid space into the pituitary fossa with enlargement of the pituitary fossa, associated with compression and/or atrophy of the pituitary gland; (b) empty sella syndrome: association of empty sella and symptoms such as headaches, visual disorders, and endocrinopathies.

Etiology: (a) idiopathic empty sella; (b) empty sella in association with endocrine disorders; (c) secondary empty sella (Sheehan syndrome; perinatal trauma; etc.)

Clinical Manifestations: (a) *headaches; difficulty in walking; lightheadedness; weakness; numbness;* (b) *visual disorders:* blurred vision; diminished acuity; diplopia; optic atrophy; visual field constriction; (c) *endocrinopathies;* (d) miscellaneous abnormalities: 18 monosomy with growth hormone deficiency and empty sella; growth hormone deficiency and empty sella in DIDMOAD syndrome; etc.

Radiologic Manifestations: (a) *normal or enlarged sella with various configurations* (normal; cuplike; quadrangular; omega-shaped; balloonlike deep sella); erosion of the cortical margin of the sella; thin cranial vault; increased digital marking of the calvaria; (b) normal course of the pituitary stalk traversing the cistern to the pituitary gland and inserting in the midline of a flattened pituitary gland located posteroinferiorly; (c) miscellaneous abnormalities: coexistence of an empty sella and a pituitary adenoma; normal-sized sella in most cases of Sheehan syndrome, rarely enlarged sella in this syndrome; intrasellar herniation of suprasellar visual system, and anteroinferior third ventricle.

ENCEPHALO-CRANIO-CUTANEOUS LIPOMATOSIS (FISHMAN SYNDROME)

Clinical Manifestations: *Seizures; spasticity; mental retardation; large, hairless soft-tissue masses; eyelid excrescences; scleral lipodermoid cysts; cloudy cornea; iris dysplasia;* etc.

Pathology: *Unilateral temporofrontal lipomatosis of the scalp and neck; homolateral multiple intracranial lipomas and cervical spinal cord lipoma;* leptomeningeal lipogranulomatosis; porencephalic cyst; cortical atrophy; hydrocephalus; micropolygyria; defective lamination of the cerebrum; cortical calcifications in the homolateral cerebral hemisphere; lipomatosis of the skull, eye, and heart.

Radiologic Manifestations: *Ipsilateral cerebral atrophy and ventricular dilatation; defective opercularization of the insula; large porencephalic cyst in the posterior part of the brain; superficial and deep brain calcification;* arachnoid cyst; absent corpus callosum; localized area of widening of the diploic space; vascular malformations.

EPIDERMAL NEVUS SYNDROME (SOLOMON SYNDROME; FEUERSTEIN-MIMS SYNDROME; SCHIMMELPENNING-FEUERSTEIN SYNDROME; LINEAR SEBACEOUS NEVUS SEQUENCE; ORGANOID NEVUS SYNDROME)

Clinical Manifestations: (a) three types of nevi: *sebaceous nevi, keratocystic nevi, and follicular nevi* (least common type); (b) *adnexal tumors:* syringocystadenoma papilliferum; nevus sebaceus of Jadassohn; mammary gland adenocarcinoma; (c) pigmentary skin changes: *hypopigmentation; café au lait spots; junction nevi; intradermal nevi;* (d) *vascular lesions:* extranuchal nevus flammeus; cavernous hemangiomas; sclerosing hemangiomas; (e) *cutaneous malignancies:* keratoacanthoma; basal cell carcinoma; squamous cell carcinoma; (f) *neurologic manifestations:* seizures; infantile spasms; mental retardation; hyperkinesia; cerebrovascular accidents; hemiparesis; quadriplegia; cranial nerve and cranial nuclei abnormalities; cortical blindness; neoplasms; unilateral hypsarrhythmia; Lennox-Gastaut electroencephalographic pattern; microcephaly; macrocephaly; hemimegalencephaly; hypertonia; hypotonia; (g) *ocular abnormalities:* epidermal nevus extension to the eyelid conjunctiva; lipodermoid tumors of the subconjunctiva; ectopic lacrimal glands; coloboma of the lid, iris, choroid, and retina; corneal opacity and pannus formation; oculomotor dysfunction; nystagmus; ptosis; macrophthalmia; conjunctival growth; retinal changes; exotropia, esotropia; (h) *predilection for hamartomas and systemic malignancies;* (i) rarely familial (possibly autosomal dominant inheritance with decreased penetrance).

Radiologic Manifestations: (a) skull abnormalities: focal cranial thickening; asymmetry of the facial bones and orbits; ipsilateral facial hemihypertrophy; premature closure of the sphenofrontal suture; sphenoid bone malformations; abnormalities of the sella turcica; giant cell granuloma of the maxilla; (b) limb abnormalities (hypoplasia; localized gigantism; duplication; etc.); bone cyst; joint ankylosis; scoliosis; kyphosis; lordosis; pelvic deformities; lytic bone defects; bowing of the tubular bones; bone sclerosis; monostotic fibrous dysplasia; finger and toe deformities; (c) central nervous system abnormalities: (1) *cerebral atrophy;* neuronal migration abnormalities; porencephaly; unilateral megalencephaly; isolated enlargement of one temporal lobe; hemiacrocephaly; hydrocephalus; widening of the subarachnoid space; widened insula; low computed tomographic density of the white matter; brain calcification; coarctation of the lateral ventricle; focal thickening of the calvarium associated with hypoplasia of the white matter; cortical calcification, and leptomeningeal drape that is enhanced after contrast injection (magnetic resonance imaging) in the parietooccipital region ipsilateral to a facial sebaceous nevus in a patient with epidermal nevus syndrome; spinal cord compression; (2) vascular dysplasia; aneurysm; myelomeningocele and spinal arteriovenous malformation; ischemia; hemorrhage; (d) miscellaneous abnormalities: cardiac malformations; renal malformations; hypophosphatemic rickets or osteomalacia; intrascleral bone formation; odontodysplasia; soft-tissue thickening and calcification.

EPIDERMOLYSIS BULLOSA

Clinical Manifestations: (a) minimal trauma causing disruption of cohesion between the dermis and epidermis and the formation of *ulcers, vesicles, and bullae; deformed or absent nails; mucosal involvement;* (b) enamel hypoplasia; dental caries; (c) fetal and infantile manifestations: elevated maternal serum α-fetoprotein levels associated with fetal epidermolysis bullosa lethalis with pyloric atresia; prenatal diagnosis by fetal skin biopsy and ultrasonography; oral lesions in newborn due to negative pressure of sucking in utero; pyloric, esophageal, and anal atresia (a case report); etc.

Radiologic Manifestations: (a) *osteoporosis of hand and feet; deformed hands and feet with flexion contracture and webbing of the fingers and toes; wedge-shaped or hooklike appearance of the terminal phalanges;* subluxations in severely involved extremities; soft-tissue calcification adjacent to the terminal phalangeal tufts; superficial fascial calcification; acro-osteolysis; resorption of the metacarpal and metatarsal heads; shortened metatarsal bones; metacarpal and metatarsal subluxation; bony ankylosis of the proximal interphalangeal joints; distal trophic changes; carpal and tarsal fusion and destruction; cystic changes of the distal radius and ulna; encasement of the whole extremity in a pouch of skin; (b) hypoplastic upper maxilla; increased mandibular angle and prognathism; loss of teeth; dental caries; periapical abscesses; jagged contours of the crowns; retained roots; stenosis of the pharynx; (c) digestive system: esophageal abnormalities (diffuse inflammatory changes; nodular filling defects due to blisters of bullae; motility disorders; ulcers; scars; webs; pseudodiverticula; shortening of the esophagus; esophageal rupture; hiatal hernia; gastroesophageal reflux; stricture; complete obstruction of the lumen; membranous congenital esophageal atresia); congenital pyloric atresia; acquired pyloric obstruction; fecal impaction; prenatal detection of gastric dilatation due to pyloric atresia and echogenic particles in the amniotic fluid; (d) genitourinary system abnormalities: mucosal pseudopolyp of the bladder; ulceration of the glans tip with scarring producing obstruction and secondary ureterectasia and hydronephrosis; vaginal stenosis; chronic vaginal urinary reflux; urinary retention; (e) miscellaneous abnormalities: skeletal maturation retardation; slender long bones; hip dysplasia with premature osteoarthritis; knee joint bony ankylosis; scoliosis; diaphragmatic hernia in sibs; squamous cell carcinoma of the maxillary sinus and palate; localized epidermolysis bullosa acquisita of esophagus in a patient with Crohn disease.

ERONEN SYNDROME (Digito-Reno-Cerebral Syndrome)

Clinical and Radiologic Manifestations: (a) digital anomalies (absence or hypoplasia of the distal phalanges of fingers and toes; hypoplastic nails); renal anomalies (cystic disease; duplication; unilateral agenesis); seizures; brain dysgenesis; facial dysmorphism (full tip of the nose; high and sloping forehead; wide nasal bridge); etc.; (b) autosomal recessive inheritance.

F

F SYNDROME

Clinical Manifestations: (a) syndactyly, polydactyly; prominence of the sternum with or without pectus excavatum; (b) autosomal dominant inheritance.

Radiologic Manifestations: *Carpal and tarsal synostoses;* deformity of the first and second fingers with frequent *syndactyly* between these digits; *hypoplasia, deformity, and proximal synostosis of the metatarsals;*

proximal polydactyly of the toes and extensive webbing of adjacent toes; pectus excavatum; spina bifida occulta.

FACIO-AURICULO-RADIAL DYSPLASIA

Clinical and Radiologic Manifestations: (a) *dysmorphic facies; conductive deafness; deformity of the pinna* (primitively formed); *asymmetric radial dysplasia;* etc.; (b) autosomal dominant inheritance; variable expression.

FANCONI ANEMIA (Fanconi Pancytopenia)

Clinical Manifestations: Extreme clinical heterogeneity: (a) hematologic disorders usually appearing between 5 and 10 years of age: bleeding tendency; *pancytopenia;* increased levels of fetal hemoglobin; hypocellular bone marrow; (b) *brown pigmentation of the skin;* (c) *radial ray deformity;* radial ray reduction deformities; supernumerary thumbs; (d) *small stature;* microcephaly; (e) chromosomal abnormalities: spontaneous chromosomal instability; *chromosomal breakage in lymphocytes in response to treatment with deoxyribonucleic acid cross-linking agents;* (f) postnatal and prenatal diagnosis and carrier detection by exposure of blood lymphocytes or amniotic fluid cells to diepoxybutane; (g) malignancies: leukemia; squamous cell carcinomas; hepatic tumor; brain tumor; (h) endocrine disorders: growth hormone deficiency, isolated or combined with other hypothalamopituitary defects; primary testicular failure associated with cryptorchidism; (i) anomalies of the genitourinary system, heart, central nervous system, ears, and eyes; (j) autosomal recessive inheritance; genetic heterogeneity; clinical and cytogenetic diversity; equal male/female sex ratio; a locus for Fanconi anemia on 16q determined by homozygosity mapping.

Radiologic Manifestations: (a) *absent, hypoplastic, or supernumerary thumb; hypoplasia or absence of the first metacarpal, greater multangular, and navicular bones;* hypoplasia or absence of the radius; digitalized thumb; bifid thumb; (b) retarded skeletal maturation; (c) *renal anomalies;* (d) miscellaneous abnormalities: microcephaly; thickened calvaria; vertebral anomalies; Klippel-Feil deformity; scoliosis; kyphosis; spina bifida; sacral agenesis; Sprengel deformity; epiphyseal hypertrophy of the first metacarpal; leg length discrepancy; congenital hip dysplasia; genu valgum; clubfoot deformity; navicular aplasia; arachnodactyly; brachydactyly; short toes; nonossifying fibroma-related osteomalacia; alimentary system anomalies; biliary atresia; hydrocephaly; absent septum pellucidum; absent corpus callosum; neural tube defect; migration defects; Arnold-Chiari malformation; moyamoya; etc.

FAT EMBOLISM SYNDROME

Clinical Manifestations: *Acute respiratory failure due to deposition of marrow fat within pulmonary capillaries , which results in a capillary leak within the lung, pulmonary edema, hemorrhage, and microatelectasis;* signs and symptoms evident within 12 to 72 hours after injury: *fever; tachypnea; hyperpnea; dyspnea; tachycardia; cyanosis;* hemoptysis; altered sensorium; petechiae; fat in the retinal vessels; lipuria; fat in a cryostat-frozen section of clotted blood; increase in platelet adhesiveness; decrease in platelets, hemoglobin, and hematocrit; normal or reduced fibrinogen levels in initial phase, followed in some cases by a delayed rise above normal levels; hypercalcemia; can lead to adult respiratory distress syndrome.

Radiologic Manifestations: (a) *widespread increase in lung density (alveolar and interstitial),* more marked in the perihilar region initially, followed by extension to the periphery and generalized pulmonary involvement; (b) normal heart and pulmonary vasculature; (c) perfusion imaging: diffuse, subsegmental mottled appearance of the lungs; normal ventilation images; (d) brain magnetic resonance imaging: multiple high signal abnormalities on both T_1- and T_2-weighted images; (e) hypoperfusion on HMPAO–single photon emission computed tomography study.

FELTY SYNDROME

Clinical Manifestations: (a) triad: *rheumatoid arthritis; splenomegaly; hypersplenism* (anemia; leukopenia; granulocytopenia); (b) miscellaneous abnormalities: generalized lymphadenopathy; hepatomegaly; nodular regenerative hyperplasia; portal fibrosis; abnormal lobular arrangement; portal hypertension; esophageal varices; T cell lymphoma; IgG antibodies against white blood cells; impaired granulocytopoietic activity; skin pigmentation; eye manifestations (episcleritis; nodular scleritis; corneal ulcer; sicca syndrome; iridocyclitis; retinal vasculitis); etc.

Radiologic Manifestations: *Rheumatoid arthritis; splenomegaly;* scintigraphy (^{99m}Tc sulfur colloid): a reversal of the liver-to-spleen uptake ratio despite normal liver function test results; virtually no visualization of the bone marrow of the sternum, vertebrae, and ribs.

FEMORAL HYPOPLASIA–UNUSUAL FACIES SYNDROME

Clinical Manifestations: (a) *facial dysmorphism:* short nose with broadened tip; elongated philtrum; thin upper lip; micrognathia; up-slanting palpebral fissure; cleft palate; ear deformities (overfolded helices; posterior rotation; cupped; microtic; hypoplastic cartilage); (b) *short thighs;*

(c) miscellaneous abnormalities: clubfoot deformity; preaxial polydactyly; limited motion of the shoulder or elbow; infant of the diabetic mother; etc.

Radiologic Manifestations: (a) *short or absent femurs;* short or absent fibulae; (b) miscellaneous abnormalities: mild shortness of the humeri; constricted ilial base; vertical ischial axis; acetabular hypoplasia; large obturator foramina; Sprengel deformity; radiohumeral synostosis; radioulnar synostosis; rib anomalies; vertebral anomalies; foot deformities; genitourinary anomalies; cardiovascular anomalies; alimentary tract anomalies; etc.

FETAL AKINESIA SEQUENCE (PENA-SHOKEIR SYNDROME TYPE I; FETAL HYPOKINESIA SEQUENCE)

Clinical Manifestations and Pathology: (a) *intrauterine growth retardation;* (b) *facial dysmorphism:* low-set and malformed ears; hypertelorism; epicanthal folds; small mandible; depressed nasal tip; (c) *limb anomalies:* small or prominent joints; fixed joints in flexion or extension position; lack of normal growth; clubfoot; camptodactyly; (d) miscellaneous abnormalities: short umbilical cord; polyhydramnios; lethal familial fetal akinesia syndrome and type III lissencephaly; etc.; (e) sporadic; autosomal recessive inheritance; genetic heterogeneity; intrafamilial heterogeneity.

Radiologic Manifestations: (a) prenatal ultrasonographic abnormalities: hydramnios; hydrops/edema; scalp edema; micrognathia/retrognathia; restricted limb movement; decreased or absent fetal breathing; small narrow chest; absent stomach echo; arthrogryposis; rocker-bottom foot deformity; clubfoot; fixed flexion of the knees; fixed extension of the knees; fixed flexion of the elbows; flexion deformities of the wrists and ankles; shortness of the long bones; camptodactyly; depressed nasal tip; cryptorchidism; kyphosis of the thoracic spine; reduced muscle bulk; (b) limb abnormalities: *thin, gracile, sticklike, or cylindric long bones; talipes equinovarus; camptodactyly; subluxation at the interphalangeal joints of the fingers; dislocations; fractures;* (c) *thin ribs; small thorax; pulmonary hypoplasia;* (d) miscellaneous abnormalities: scoliosis; vertebral segmentation anomalies; extra ribs; various urinary system anomalies; renal hamartomas; renal cysts; intestinal malrotation; etc.

FETAL ALCOHOL SYNDROME

Clinical Manifestations: (a) *prenatal and postnatal growth retardation;* decreased adipose tissue; *mental retardation; poor coordination; hypotonia; irritability in infancy; hyperactivity in childhood;* (b) *craniofacial dysmorphism:* microcephaly; midfacial hypoplasia; retrognathia in infancy; micrognathia or relative prognathism in adolescence; posterior rotation of the ears; poorly formed concha; hypoplastic philtrum; small vermilion border of the lips; cleft lip/palate; highly arched palate; short palpebral fissures; etc.; (c) cutaneous abnormalities: hemangiomas; hirsutism in infancy; absence or dysplasia of the nails; (d) cardiovascular and urinary system abnormalities; (e) association with neoplasm: neuroblastoma; adrenal carcinoma; hepatoblastoma; ganglioneuroblastoma; sacrococcygeal teratoma; rhabdomyosarcoma; nephroblastoma; endodermal sinus tumor; medulloblastoma; Hodgkin disease; acute lymphocytic leukemia; (f) miscellaneous abnormalities: hepatobiliary abnormalities; cutaneous tuberous angioma; Gilles de la Tourette syndrome (a case report); etc.

Radiologic Manifestations: (a) *skeletal anomalies:* scoliosis; hemivertebrae; Klippel-Feil syndrome; pectus excavatum; pectus carinatum; clubfoot; flexion contracture; radioulnar synostosis; camptodactyly; clinodactyly; tetradactyly; short metatarsals; punctate epiphyseal calcification; congenital hip dislocation; a distinctive hand pattern profile (shortness of the metacarpals and phalanges of about 2 SD below the mean, in particular, at the fifth terminal phalanx; narrowness of the terminal phalanges); bilateral tibial exostoses; (b) *nervous system anomalies: microcephaly;* malformation of neuronal and glial migration; hydrocephaly; anencephaly; porencephaly; agenesis of the corpus callosum; meningomyelocele; lumbosacral lipoma; Dandy-Walker deformity; holoprosencephaly; reduction in the size of the basal ganglia and thalamic structures; (c) *urogenital anomalies:* renal anomalies (hypoplasia; aplasia; hydronephrosis; hamartoma; caliceal cyst; fused kidneys; duplication; cystic kidneys); bladder diverticula; vesicovaginal fistula; urogenital sinus; hypospadias; labial hypoplasia.

FETAL BRAIN DISRUPTION SEQUENCE

Etiology: Fetal brain disruption sequence is considered to be secondary to vascular disruption or infection (parasitic; viral) in the second or third trimester of pregnancy, resulting in decreased intracranial hydrostatic pressure and fetal skull collapse.

Clinical and Radiologic Manifestations: *Microcephaly; cutis verticis gyrata; overlapping sutures; prominent occipital bone; mental retardation; neurologic deficits; various degrees of cerebral hemisphere destruction;* ventriculomegaly; widening of the extraaxial fluid spaces; cortical brain calcification; reported in two female siblings.

FETAL HYDANTOIN SYNDROME

Clinical Manifestations: (a) *prenatal and postnatal growth deficiency; psychomotor development retardation;* (b) *microcephaly; ridging* *of metopic suture; large anterior and posterior fontanelles; short and broad nose; depressed nasal bridge; mild hypertelorism; inner epicanthal folds; strabismus; ptosis of the eyelids; low-set ears; wide mouth; relative prognathism; prominent lips; cleft lip and/or cleft palate;* low posterior hairline; short neck; (c) limb anomalies: *hypoplasia of the nails; fingerlike thumb; hypoplasia of the distal phalanges of the hands and feet; anonychia/hyponychia;* nail pigmentation; single palmar crease; adactyly; acheiria; pes cavus; clubfoot; polydactyly; (d) cardiovascular anomalies: atrial septal defect; ventricular septal defect; pulmonary stenosis; coarctation of the aorta.

Radiologic Manifestations: (a) *skeletal abnormalities:* apparent distal hyperphalangia due to the division of an otherwise normal phalanx; extra phalanx located between the metacarpal and proximal phalanx; poor skeletal mineralization; slenderness of the diaphyses of long bones; transverse radiolucent metaphyseal band; clinodactyly; distal digital hypoplasia; adactyly; digital hypoplasia; triphalangeal thumbs; syndactyly; polydactyly; clubfeet; congenital scoliosis; various anomalies of the ribs, sternum, and spine; (b) miscellaneous abnormalities: cerebral and cerebellar underdevelopment; medullary sponge kidneys; diaphragmatic hernia.

FETAL VALPROATE SYNDROME

Clinical and Radiologic Manifestations: (a) *craniofacial dysmorphism:* midface hypoplasia; short nose with a broad and/or flat bridge; anteverted nostrils; shallow philtrum; thin upper lip; thick lower lip; epicanthal folds; minor abnormalities of the ear; micrognathia; ridging of the metopic suture; outer orbital ridge deficiency; bifrontal narrowing; (b) *developmental delay, neurologic abnormalities; neural tube defects;* segmentation anomalies of vertebrae; etc.

FG SYNDROME (OPITZ-KAVEGGIA SYNDROME)

Clinical Manifestations: (a) *craniofacial dysmorphism:* high and broad forehead; prominent nose; hypertelorism; frontal hair upsweep; medial eyebrow flare; small ears with a simple structure; micrognathia; inverted V-shaped upper lip; large mouth; protruding tongue; gingival hyperplasia; malocclusion; (b) *psychomotor retardation; hypotonia and hyperextensible joints at birth; constipation;* joint contractures, apparent spasticity, and unsteady gait later; friendly, sociable, and overly talkative; (c) *short stature;* (d) keloids; (e) X-linked inheritance, incompletely recessive.

Radiologic Manifestations: Spinal anomalies; lumbar hyperlordosis; clubfoot; broad thumbs and big toes; minimal cutaneous syndactyly; anal anomaly (stenosis; imperforate anus); pyloric stenosis; megalencephaly;

agenesis of the corpus callosum; heterotopia of neuroglial tissue; pachygyria; cortical dysgenesis; "cystic" cavum septi pellucidi.

Note: *F* and *G* represent the initials of the families.

FIBRODYSPLASIA OSSIFICANS PROGRESSIVA (MYOSITIS OSSIFICANS PROGRESSIVA)

Clinical Manifestations: (a) *heat; muscle pain; inflammatory swelling; induration; torticollis;* (b) *microdactyly* (thumbs; hallux); webbed toes; (c) exacerbation related to various factors: trauma; operation to excise ectopic bone; biopsy of the lumps; intramuscular injections and venipuncture; dental treatment; (d) miscellaneous abnormalities: reduction defects of all digits; restrictive movement of the spine and shoulder; submandibular swelling (heterotopic calcification); ankylosis of temporomandibular joints; etc.; (e) most cases sporadic; autosomal dominant inheritance with complete penetrance and variable expressivity.

Pathology: *A mesodermal disorder; progressive swelling and ossification of the fascia, aponeuroses, ligaments, tendons, and connective tissue of skeletal muscle; the biopsied specimen containing normal endochondral osteogenesis at heterotopic sites.*

Radiologic Manifestations: (a) *progressive ossification in muscles and subcutaneous tissues in an apicocaudal direction, with the neck involved in an early stage; swelling of the muscular fascial planes before the development of ectopic ossification;* ossification with a multifocal site pattern adjacent to and extending around muscles (neck, spine, and shoulder girdle most common sites); (b) *high signal intensity of the soft tissues; especially with* T_2 *weighting;* (c) soft tissue mass lesions within muscles and connective tissue containing *echogenic material;* (d) *ankylosis of interphalangeal, carpometacarpal, and metatarsophalangeal joints; microdactyly (great toes and thumbs)* caused by shortness of the metatarsals and metacarpals, monophalangic great toe resulting from synostosis; (e) miscellaneous abnormalities: ossification of ligamentous insertions producing pseudoexostoses; association with synovial chondromatosis; etc.

FITZ-HUGH–CURTIS SYNDROME

Etiology and Pathology: (a) genitourinary infection *(Neisseria gonorrhoeae; Chlamydia trachomatis);* intrauterine device; (b) anterior perihepatitis ("violin string" adhesions between the anterior surface of the liver and the anterior abdominal wall).

Clinical Manifestations: *Acute right upper quadrant abdominal pain* that may be referred to the right shoulder and back; guarding; positive

Murphy sign; laparoscopy: *perihepatitis; adhesions between the liver sur-face and the abdominal wall;* salpingitis (not in all cases).

Radiologic Manifestations: *Prehepatic peritoneal fluid collection;* thickening of the Glisson capsule; violin-string adhesions between the liver surface and the abdominal wall; focal hepatic lesion; peritoneal fluid around the spleen; *salpingitis;* absence of right renal, hepatic, or biliary system abnormalities.

FLOATING-HARBOR SYNDROME

Clinical Manifestations: (a) *intrauterine growth retardation, short stature; triangular face; bulbous nose; long eyelashes; deep-set eyes; short philtrum; thin lips; posteriorly located ears; malocclusion*; *expressive language delay;* usually normal motor development; (b) miscellaneous abnormalities: somatic asymmetry (a case report); celiac disease (a case report); etc.; (c) autosomal recessive and autosomal dominant modes of inheritance have been suggested.

Radiologic Manifestations: (a) *skeletal maturation retardation;* (b) miscellaneous abnormalities: cone-shaped epiphyses (hands); pseudoarthrosis of clavicle; Legg-Perthes disease.

Note: The name of the syndrome originates from Boston Floating Hospital and Harbor General Hospital (Torrance, California), where the original cases were reported.

FLOPPY VALVE SYNDROME

Pathology: Disruption and loss of normal valvular architecture and an increase in ground substance (aortic and mitral valves primarily involved).

Clinical Manifestations: Dyspnea; chest pain; cardiomegaly; cardiac murmur; congestive heart failure (in some); left ventricular hypertrophy; arrhythmias; echocardiography (fluttering and large excursion of valves; cardiac chamber enlargement); etc.

Radiologic Manifestations: Cardiomegaly; cardioangiographic demonstration of cardiac chamber enlargement; left ventricular hypertrophy; valvular insufficiency; prolapsing valvular cusps.

FOCAL SCLERODERMA (Linear Scleroderma "en Coup de Sabre")

Clinical Manifestations: (a) skin lesions on the face, trunk, and limbs of different size and shape, often unilateral; scalp and facial lesions having a "coup de sabre" appearance; *erythema and edema in the early phase, followed by a waxy color and finally skin atrophy and hypopigmentation;* (b) immune disorders (present in about one half of the cases): hypergammaglobulinemia, antinuclear antibodies, and antibodies to single-stranded deoxyribonucleic acid.

Radiologic Manifestations: (a) *demineralization and muscular atrophy underlying the skin lesions;* (b) soft-tissue calcification; (c) ipsilateral white matter abnormalities in patients with progressive facial hemiatrophy (increased signals on T_2-weighted images); intracranial calcification.

Note: Some consider focal scleroderma and Romberg syndrome part of the same disease spectrum.

FOIX-CHAVANY-MARIE SYNDROME (ANTERIOR OPERCULUM SYNDROME)

Pathology: *Bilateral anterior perisylvian lesions:* cerebrovascular disease; infections; developmental defect; reversible form in children with epilepsy; neurodegenerative disorders.

Clinical Manifestations: Usually a sudden *loss of speech and bilateral loss of voluntary control of muscles supplied by cranial nerves V, VII, IX, X, and XII: loss of voluntary control of facial, masticatory, lingual, pharyngeal, and in some cases ocular muscles.*

Radiologic Manifestations: Demonstration of the cerebral lesion: *vascular occlusion; encephalitis; infarction; developmental defects* (bilateral central macrogyria); etc.

FOSTER KENNEDY SYNDROME

Etiology: Intracranial basofrontal lesion.

Clinical and Radiologic Manifestations: *Ipsilateral optic atrophy and central scotoma; contralateral papilledema;* ipsilateral proptosis (in some); *depression or a loss of the sense of smell; tumor* located in frontal lobe, olfactory groove, sphenoidal wing (medial third), pituitary fossa, or nasopharynx (carcinoma).

FOUNTAIN SYNDROME

Clinical Manifestations: (a) mental retardation; deaf mutism; "coarse" facial features; full lips; swelling of the face with "edematous" infiltration of the subcutaneous tissue; short, stubby hand; (b) autosomal recessive inheritance most likely.

Radiologic Manifestations: Anomalies of the turns of the cochlea; marked thickness of the calvarium; short metacarpals and phalanges with a thick cortex.

FRAGILE X SYNDROME (Martin-Bell Syndrome)

Clinical Manifestations: Caused by a mutation in the FMR-1 gene: (a) *craniofacial dysmorphism:* head circumference over the 50th percentile; prognathism; narrow, long face; flattened nasal bridge; hypertelorism; epicanthal folds; large, cupped, or protruding ears; highly arched palate; strabismus; (b) *language difficulties; learning disability; mild to marked mental retardation; short attention span; behavior disorders of various types and severity;* (c) mild increase in birth weight; reduced adult height in males; (d) *macro-orchidism;* (e) prenatal diagnosis and carrier detection: amniotic fluid; chorionic villus specimen; fetal blood sampling and molecular methods; (f) X-linked inheritance; the fragile site at Xq27.3.

Radiologic Manifestations: (a) decreased size of the posterior cerebellar vermis and increased size of the fourth ventricle; age-related increase in the hippocampus and age-related decrease in the volume of the superior temporal gyrus; (b) mitral valve prolapse; mitral regurgitation; aortic root dilatation; aortic and tricuspid valve abnormalities; mild aortic coarctation associated with hypoplasia of the descending aorta; (c) miscellaneous abnormalities: flexible flatfeet; clubfoot deformity; scoliosis; pectus excavatum.

FRASER SYNDROME (Cryptophthalmos-Syndactyly Syndrome)

Clinical Manifestations: (a) *unilateral or bilateral cryptophthalmos;* extended hair growth on the forehead; ear abnormalities; hypertelorism; nose abnormalities; midline fissure; dental abnormalities; lacrimal duct defects; coloboma of the upper eyelid; cleft lip/palate; (b) *syndactyly of the fingers;* (c) miscellaneous abnormalities: urinary system abnormalities; genital anomalies; etc.; (d) autosomal recessive inheritance; wide range of phenotypic expression; sporadic.

Radiologic Manifestations: (a) *ocular abnormalities: calcified lens; absence of the lens; abnormal size and contour of the globe; thin rectus muscles; cystic structure within the orbit; absence of lacrimal glands;* (b) parietal lacunae; flattening of the frontal eminence or temple; microcephaly; meningoencephalocele; (c) *urogenital anomalies;* (d) *syndactyly;* (e) prenatal ultrasonography: oligohydramnios; uropathy; microphthalmia; hypertelorism; syndactyly; markedly enlarged lungs; (f) miscellaneous abnormalities: wide separation of the pubic symphysis; bowel malrotation; central nervous system anomalies; calcification of falx cerebri.

FREEMAN-SHELDON SYNDROME (WHISTLING FACE SYNDROME; CRANIO-CARPO-TARSAL DYSPLASIA)

Clinical Manifestations: (a) *characteristic facies:* microstomia; lip protrusion held as in whistling, H-shaped groove of the chin; flatness of the midface; small nose; sunken eyes; highly arched palate; small tongue; ocular hypertelorism; long philtrum; epicanthus; (b) short and broad neck; mild pterygium colli; (c) *ulnar deviation of the hands; finger contractures;* nonopposable thumbs; camptodactyly; *clubfoot deformity;* (d) miscellaneous abnormalities: small stature; epilepsy; etc.; (e) genetic heterogeneity: sporadic most common; autosomal dominant inheritance with variable expressivity; autosomal recessive.

Radiologic Manifestations: (a) *craniofacial disproportion;* dolichocephaly; steep anterior fossa; small malar bones; small mandible; (b) *ulnar deviation of the hands; flexed thumbs; contracture of the fingers and toes; equinovarus feet;* retarded skeletal maturation; disharmonious maturation with retarded development of the carpal centers when compared with those in the phalanges; (c) prenatal diagnosis: abnormal extremities and mouth on ultrasonography (positive family history); (d) miscellaneous abnormalities: tall vertebrae with a narrow anteroposterior diameter; flattened vertebrae; kyphosis or kyphoscoliosis; spina bifida occulta; spatulate ribs; increase in the width of the long bones, radial head dislocation; hip contracture; hip dislocation; long and vertically oriented ischia; genu valgum deformity; vertical talus deformity; renal anomalies; hiatal hernia.

FRONTO-FACIO-NASAL DYSPLASIA

Clinical and Radiologic Manifestations: (a) craniofacial dysmorphism (facial hypoplasia; cranium bifidum occultum defect; widow's peak; frontal lipoma; nasal hypoplasia; bifid nose; deformed nostrils; clefts [lip; premaxilla; palate; uvula]); blepharophimosis; lower lid lagophthalmos; primary telecanthus; S-shaped palpebral fissures; eyelid coloboma; microphthalmos; etc.; (b) autosomal recessive inheritance.

FRONTONASAL DYSPLASIA (MEDIAN CLEFT FACE SYNDROME)

Clinical Manifestations: (a) *unilateral or bilateral notching of the nose or the alae nasi; ocular hypertelorism; broad nasal bridge; absence of the tip of the nose; anterior cranium bifidum;* widow's peak scalp hair anomaly; primary telecanthus; median cleft upper lip; median cleft palate;

(b) ocular abnormalities: epicanthal folds; eyelid ptosis; accessory nasal eyelid tissue with secondary displacement of the inferior puncti laterally; colobomas; microphthalmos; congenital cataracts; refractory errors; strabismus; nystagmus; vitreoretinal degeneration with retinal detachment; inflammatory retinopathy; epibulbar dermoid tumors; corneal dermoid; optic nerve hypoplasia; optic nerve coloboma; (c) miscellaneous abnormalities: micropenis; choanal atresia; etc.; (d) sporadic; very few familial cases reported.

Radiologic Manifestations: (a) *cranium bifidum frontalis; orbital hypertelorism; midline cleft involving various bony structures; maxillary hypoplasia; hypoplastic frontal sinuses;* deformed anterior portion of the lateral ventricles and anterior cerebral arteries; agenesis or hypogenesis of the corpus callosum; lipoma of the corpus callosum; vertical bony bar in the intracranial midline; (b) miscellaneous abnormalities: macrocephaly; hydrocephalus; holoprosencephaly; basal encephalocele.

FRYNS SYNDROME

Clinical and Pathologic Manifestations: (a) *diaphragmatic defects (not in all cases);* (b) *lung hypoplasia;* (c) *cleft palate;* (d) *cardiovascular anomalies:* septal defects, aortic arch anomalies; (e) *urinary system anomalies:* renal cysts, renal agenesis; hydronephrosis; etc.; (f) *digestive system anomalies:* duodenal atresia; esophageal atresia; bowel malrotation; etc.; (g) *short limbs; distal limb hypoplasia (brachytelephalangy); hypoplastic nails;* (h) *"coarse" facial features;* macrostomia; broad, flat nasal bridge; anteverted nares; abnormal helices/lobules; narrow palpebral fissures; micrognathia; facial hirsutism; (i) miscellaneous abnormalities: Fryns syndrome phenotype and trisomy 22; etc.; (j) autosomal recessive inheritance.

Radiologic Manifestations: (a) delayed ossification of the basiociput and cervical vertebral bodies; broad medial ends of the clavicles; broad ribs, thin ribs, and abnormal rib-vertebral junctions; globularly formed ilium; shortness of long bones; (b) prenatal ultrasonography: *polyhydramnios; diaphragmatic hernia;* cystic hygroma.

FUHRMANN SYNDROME

Clinical and Radiologic Manifestations: (a) *right-angle bowing of femora and absent fibulae; absent nails;* polydactyly; foot deformity; (b) autosomal recessive inheritance.

G

GALLOWAY-MOWAT SYNDROME

Clinical and Radiologic Manifestations: (a) *microcephaly;* large, floppy ears; receding forehead; micrognathia; optic atrophy; *seizures; developmental delay; hypotonia; nephrotic syndrome; glomerulopathy; cerebral dysgenesis* (gyral abnormalities; migrational anomalies; hydrocephalus); etc.; (b) autosomal recessive inheritance.

GAPO SYNDROME

Clinical Manifestations: (a) *shortness that simulates a rhizomelic type of dwarfism;* normal mental development; *alopecia; pseudoanodontia* (failure of tooth eruption); *optic atrophy; craniofacial dysmorphism* (high and bossing forehead; wide anterior fontanelle; midface hypoplasia; thick lips; protruding eyes; micrognathia); (b) miscellaneous abnormalities: dermal deposit of PAS-positive, diastase-resistant amorphous hyaline substance and collagen fibers; widespread interstitial fibrosis; audible intracranial bruit with narrowing of the sigmoid sinuses; etc.; (c) autosomal recessive inheritance.

Radiologic Manifestations: *Unerupted teeth (pseudoanodontia); skeletal maturation retardation;* mandibular hypoplasia; shallow orbits; protruding eyes; thickening of the lateral orbital walls; hypertelorism; thick ribs; dilatation of the intracranial and scalp veins (venous obstruction).

Note: *GAPO:* **G**rowth retardation, **A**lopecia, **P**seudoanodontia, and **O**ptic atrophy.

GARDNER SYNDROME

Clinical Manifestations: (a) *soft-tissue tumors:* epidermoid inclusion cysts of the skin; dermoid tumors; fibroma; lipoma; lipofibroma; leiomyoma; intraabdominal tumors (desmoids and peritoneal fibromas); (b) *osteomatosis;* (c) *gastrointestinal polyposis;* (d) abnormal dentition; (e) malignancies; cancer development in the rectal remnant (post–colon resection); (f) miscellaneous abnormalities: increased skin pigmentation; multiple familial pilomatricoma-like changes in epidermal cysts (a cutaneous marker for Gardner syndrome); keloids; mammary fibrosis; hypertrophy of the retinal pigment epithelium; thyroid carcinoma preceding diagnosis of hereditary polyposis; (g) autosomal dominant inheritance, complete penetrance, and variable expressivity; both sexes equally affected.

Radiologic Manifestations: (a) *benign osteomatosis:* skull, trunk, and limbs, in particular, lobulated osteomas of the mandibular angle most characteristic; (b) dental abnormalities: supernumerary teeth; unerupted teeth; numerous dental caries; odontomas; (c) *gastrointestinal polyposis; desmoid tumor* with involvement of the mesenteric root, causing vascular obstruction; spiculation of the small-bowel pattern and mural changes; small-bowel obstruction; (d) miscellaneous abnormalities: diffuse uptake of Tc-99m HDP after colectomy (due to mesenteric fibromatosis); hydronephrosis and hydroureter due to obstruction by desmoid tumor; intense uptake of radiotracer within maxilla and mandible; polypoid lymphoid hyperplasia of the small bowel; leontiasis ossea.

Note: (a) approximately 50% of patients with the familial adenomatous polyposis syndromes have osseous lesions; (b) occult bone lesions of the jaw and ocular fundus lesions may be detectable before the appearance of colonic polyps in affected and at-risk relatives.

GARDNER-SILENGO-WACHTEL SYNDROME (GENITO-PALATO-CARDIAC SYNDROME)

Clinical and Radiologic Manifestations: (a) craniofacial dysmorphism (micrognathia; low-set ears; cleft palate; cleft alveolar ridge; prominent occiput; depressed nasal bridge; anteverted nares; "carp" mouth); congenital heart disease; limb anomalies (clubfeet; prominent heels; flexion deformity of the thumbs); 46,XY, female internal genitalia; hypospadias; gonadal dysgenesis; (b) either autosomal recessive or X-linked recessive inheritance.

GERODERMA OSTEODYSPLASTICA (WALT DISNEY DWARFISM; BAMATTER SYNDROME)

Clinical Manifestations: Symptoms with onset in infancy: (a) *short stature; senile facial features;* sagging cheeks; sunken eyes; tendency to microcornea; *thin skin with poor turgor and elasticity; easily wrinkled; prominent veins;* defects in dental implantation; muscular hypotonia; *hyperlaxity of joints;* severe flatfoot deformity; etc.; (b) autosomal recessive inheritance.

Radiologic Manifestations: *Generalized osteoporosis; predisposition to fractures; platyspondyly;* biconcave vertebral bodies; bone-within-bone appearance; multiple parallel lines in the vertebral bodies; scoliosis; *dislocated hips;* knee subluxation; flatfoot; posterior displacement of the maxilla with relative mandibular prognathism; extension of the mandibular premolar and molar roots below the inferior dental canal, and of the second molars into the lower border of the mandibular cortex; hypercementosis of the maxillary incisors and mandibular molars surrounded by a radiolucent halo; etc.

GILLES DE LA TOURETTE SYNDROME (TOURETTE SYNDROME)

Clinical Manifestations: (a) *behavioral disorders:* obsessive-compulsive behavior; manic depressive symptoms; learning disorders; attention deficit; hyperactivity; sleep disorders; *motor and vocal tics;* (b) miscellaneous abnormalities: association with fetal alcohol syndrome (a case report); (c) autosomal dominant inheritance.

Radiologic Manifestations: Reduced basal ganglia volumes; difference for measures of symmetry in the putamen and lenticular region as compared with the control group; Tc-99m HMPAO–single photon emission computed tomography brain imaging: hypoperfusion with no characteristic pattern.

GOLDBERG-SHPRINTZEN SYNDROME

Clinical and Radiologic Manifestations: (a) short stature; (b) psychomotor retardation; (c) microcephaly; sloping forehead; highly arched eyebrows; hypertelorism; bulbous nose; pointed chin; large ears; submucous cleft palate; coloboma iridis; (d) Hirschsprung disease; (e) miscellaneous abnormalities: tapering fingers; computed tomography findings suggesting "defective neuronal migration and/or brain dysgenesis"; (f) autosomal recessive inheritance.

GOLDBLOOM SYNDROME (IDIOPATHIC PERIOSTEAL HYPEROSTOSIS WITH DYSPROTEINEMIA)

Clinical Manifestations: (a) nonspecific upper respiratory infection; fever; (b) *limb pain; warm, deep induration of the involved region;* (c) *elevated serum proteins; marked elevation of γ-globulin; hypoalbuminemia;* variable values of α_1-, α_2-, and β-globulins; (d) elevated sedimentation rate; anemia (normocytic and normochromic); normal or elevated white blood cell count; normal platelet count; (e) recovery in several weeks or months.

Pathology: Periosteal new bone formation with mucinous edema, and increased plasma cells with variable degrees of fibrosis in the bone marrow adjacent to the periosteal changes.

Radiologic Manifestations: (a) *lamellar new bone formation:* long bones most common sites; facial bones, metatarsals, and metacarpals less common sites; (b) radionuclide bone scan (increased uptake).

GOLDEN-LAKIM SYNDROME

Clinical and Radiologic Manifestations: Dolichocephaly; pointed facies; small mandible; bifid uvula; pterygium colli; limb deformities (flexion deformity of the knees without popliteal webs; pes cavus; club-foot; atrophy of the calf muscles; camptodactyly of the fifth digits); kyphoscoliosis; defective ossification of the lamina of some vertebrae; pectus excavatum.

GOLTZ SYNDROME (GOLTZ-GORLIN SYNDROME; FOCAL DERMAL HYPOPLASIA)

Clinical Manifestations: (a) *poikiloderma with focal dermal hypoplasia* (skin atrophy, linear pigmentations, and fat deposit in the superficial layers of the skin); *papillomas of the mucous membranes;* sparse scalp hair; nail dystrophy (grooves; spooned); dermatoglyphic abnormalities; (b) *limb anomalies;* (c) *eye abnormalities:* hypertelorism; anophthalmia; aniridia; heterochromia; colobomas; hypopigmented or hyperpigmented retina; cloudy vitreous; subluxation of the lens; strabismus; nystagmus; discrete vascularized peripheral subepithelial corneal opacifications; obstructed tear ducts; (d) craniofacial abnormalities: facial asymmetry; absent uvula; split soft palate; hypoplasia of the external ear; fragile enamel; dental caries; conductive deafness; (e) about 95% of all reported cases sporadic; 90% female; X-linked dominant inheritance with lethality in hemizygous males.

Radiologic Manifestations: (a) *syndactyly;* (b) *dental anomalies:* microdontia; oligodontia; deformed teeth; retarded eruption; etc.; (c) renal anomalies; (d) hypoplasia of the craniofacial skeleton; steep clivus; (e) scoliosis; segmentation errors of the vertebrae; rudimentary tail; hypoplasia of the ribs; bifurcation of the ribs; oligodactyly; polydactyly; adactyly; foot deformities; hypoplasia of the pelvic bones; (f) miscellaneous abnormalities: association with osteopathia striata; generalized osteopenia; pelvic hemangioma; microcephaly; diaphragmatic hernia; midclavicular aplasia or hypoplasia.

GOODMAN SYNDROME (ACROCEPHALOPOLYSYNDACTYLY, GOODMAN TYPE)

Clinical and Radiologic Manifestations: (a) craniofacial dysmorphism: acrocephaly; highly arched eyebrows; downward slant of the palpebral fissures; epicanthal folds; prominent nose; flared nares; highly arched palate; crowding of teeth; micrognathia; facial hirsutism; protruding, deformed ears; (b) upper limbs: polydactyly; syndactyly; brachydactyly; clinodactyly; camptodactyly; ulnar deviation of the fingers; angulation of the elbow; (c) lower limbs: muscle hypoplasia; genu valgum; pes cavus; pes equinovarus; syndactyly; (d) three siblings from a consanguineous family.

GOODPASTURE SYNDROME

Clinical Manifestations: Weakness; cough; pallor; low-grade fever; tachycardia; *pulmonary hemorrhage; hemoptysis*; *renal disease (hematuria; albuminuria; uremia); high titers of circulating antibodies to glomerular basement membrane radioimmunoassay and enzyme-linked immunosorbent assay* (most sensitive and specific diagnostic test); microcytic anemia.

Pathology: Proliferative glomerulonephritis with or without crescents; linear immunofluorescence for IgG and C3 along the glomerular basement membrane; diffuse pulmonary hemorrhage with linear immunofluorescence for IgG and C3 along the alveolar basement membrane.

Radiologic Manifestations: *Pulmonary infiltration of various types:* patchy, fine, powdery, stippled, linear, nodular, mottled, and massive consolidation; perihilar pattern with apices and bases relatively clear; pleural effusion; cardiomegaly.

GORDON SYNDROME

Clinical Manifestations: (a) *camptodactyly; clubfoot;* distal arthrogryposis; *cleft palate;* etc.; (b) autosomal dominant inheritance, reduced penetrance in females, variable expressivity.

Radiologic Manifestations: *Camptodactyly;* pseudoepiphysis of the second metacarpal; atypical carpal ossification sequence; *clubfoot deformities;* stenosis of the spinal canal; narrow intervertebral discs.

Note: The term *Gordon syndrome* is also used for pseudohypoaldosteronism type II (association of hypertension, hyperkalemia, and normal glomerular filtration rate).

GORHAM SYNDROME

Clinical Manifestations: Onset usually in childhood or young adult life: (a) *progressive deformity without systemic findings, with or without overlying skin or soft-tissue angiomas; pain; increased focal skin temperature (thermography);* (b) chylous or serosanguineous pleural effusion; (c) miscellaneous abnormalities: respiratory distress due to massive osteolysis of chest; spinal cord transection; paraplegia; partial remission; association with colonic carcinoma.

Radiologic Manifestations: (a) *patchy osteoporosis in the early stage; progressive, extensive, partial, or total unicentric bone resorption* (one or more bones may be involved); tapering of the end of the bone involved; may cross the joint; no evidence of reossification; pathologic fracture; (b) ^{99m}Tc pyrophosphate scan: decreased isotope uptake in affected areas; rarely increased uptake; (c) magnetic resonance imaging: high signal replacing bone on both T_1- and T_2-weighted images; heterogeneous appearance in the presence of both fibrosis (low signal intensity) and osteolysis (high signal intensity); (d) arteriography: abnormal vascular blush in the affected area; angiomatous bone lesion demonstration by computed tomography–guided intraosseous angiography.

GORLIN SYNDROME (BASAL CELL–NEVUS SYNDROME)

Clinical Manifestations: (a) *characteristic craniofacial features:* large calvaria with frontal and biparietal bulging; low position of the occiput; prominent supraorbital ridges; heavy eyebrows; wide nasal root, mild hypertelorism; exotropia; pouting lower lips; exaggerated mandibular length; (b) skin abnormalities: *multiple nevoid basal cell carcinomas;* milia and cysts; *palmar and/or plantar pits;* comedones; café au lait pigmentations; (c) oral lesions: *odontogenic keratocysts;* defective dentition; prognathism; fibrosarcoma of the jaws; ameloblastoma; cleft lip; cleft palate; (d) ocular abnormalities: hypertelorism; congenital blindness; dystopia canthorum; cataracts; coloboma of the choroid and optic nerve; etc.; (e) central nervous system abnormalities: mental retardation; facial nerve palsy; nerve deafness; congenital hemiparesis; seizures; (f) genital abnormalities; (g) miscellaneous abnormalities: benign and malignant tumors; microphthalmia; etc.; (h) autosomal dominant inheritance.

Radiologic Manifestations: (a) *odontogenic cysts of the maxilla and mandible;* hypoplastic mandible; (b) *rib anomalies; vertebral anomalies;* (c) frontal and temporoparietal bossing; *lamellar calcification of the falx;* bridging of the sella; other calcified structures (diaphragma sellae; tentorium cerebelli; petroclinoid ligaments; dura; pia; choroid plexus); cerebellar atrophy; absent corpus callosum; cyst of the septum pellucidum; hydrocephalus; hyperpneumatized sinuses; small sella turcica; (d) skeletal abnormalities: supracondylar humeral spurs; widening of the distal segments of the radii; spotty osteoblastic deposits in the phalanges; syndactyly; oligodactyly; brachymetacarpal; tarsal and carpal fusions; extrametatarsal bone; cysts in the bones and the hands and feet; defective medial segment of the clavicle; widespread cystlike osteolytic bone lesions; osteoblastic spotty "osteopoikilotic" lesions; (e) miscellaneous abnormalities: calcification within ovaries; ovarian fibroma and other tumors; soft-tissue calcification; renal anomalies.

GRADENIGO SYNDROME

Clinical Manifestations: (a) the triad: (1) otitis media; (2) mastoiditis; (3) pain in the region innervated by the first and second divisions of the trigeminal nerve and ipsilateral abducens nerve paralysis; (b) miscellaneous abnormalities: hearing loss; meningitis; facial paralysis; nerves VIII, IX, and X involvement.

Radiologic Manifestations: *Mastoiditis; petrositis* with osteoporosis in the early phase and bone destruction at the apex in the late phase of the disease; dural involvement; cerebritis; phlebitis; thrombosis.

GRANT SYNDROME

Clinical Manifestations: (a) camptomelia; blue sclerae; mandibular hypoplasia; short stature; no tendency to fracture; no dentinogenesis imperfecta; (b) consistent with autosomal dominant inheritance.

Radiologic Manifestations: Wormian bones persistent beyond childhood; brachycephaly; osteopenia in infancy; bowing of the long bones of the lower limb with improvement after infancy; shallow glenoid fossae; tendency to shoulder dislocation.

Note: The eponym *Grant* originates from the affected family's surname.

GREIG CEPHALOPOLYSYNDACTYLY SYNDROME
(FRONTODIGITAL SYNDROME)

Clinical and Radiologic Manifestations: (a) *craniofacial dysmorphism:* macrocephaly; broad nasal root; frontal bossing; scaphocephaly; brachycephaly; large fontanelle; hypertelorism; ear anomaly; (b) hand anomalies: *postaxial* (occasionally preaxial) *polydactyly;* broad thumbs; syndactyly; (c) foot anomalies: *preaxial* (rarely postaxial) *polydactyly;* syndactyly; broad hallux; (d) miscellaneous abnormalities: advanced bone age in newborn; camptodactyly of the fingers and toes; inguinal hernia; mental retardation; macrosomia; association with sinus node disease; cystic hygroma, omphalocele, hydrocephaly, and cardiac malformations; craniosynostosis; (e) autosomal dominant inheritance with complete penetrance and variable expressivity.

GRISCELLI SYNDROME

Clinical Manifestations: (a) *partial albinism; frequent pyogenic infections;* recurrent episodes of fever; hypotonia; *multiple immunodeficiencies;* neutropenia; thrombocytopenia; anemia; visceral lymphohistiocytic infiltration with erythrophagocytosis; central nervous system, cranial nerves, and spinal cord involvement; etc.; (b) probably autosomal recessive inheritance.

Radiologic Manifestations: Progressive demyelination and eventual loss of brain tissue.

GRISEL SYNDROME

Etiology: Spontaneous subluxation of C1 on C2, associated with inflammatory conditions of the head and neck (pharyngitis; abscess; tonsillitis; ear infection; pharyngeal surgery; etc.), causing ligamentous laxity.

Clinical and Radiologic Manifestations: *Torticollis; unilateral or bilateral anterior subluxation of C1 on C2;* permanent spinal deformity, if the disease not recognized and treated early; spinal cord compression.

GUILLAIN-BARRÉ SYNDROME

Clinical Manifestations: Acute inflammatory demyelinating polyradiculoneuropathy: *paresthesias; weakness (arms; legs; face; oropharynx); areflexia; sensory loss; typical electrophysiologic features; elevated cerebrospinal fluid protein;* ophthalmoparesis; sphincter dysfunction; ataxia; pain; respiratory failure; autonomic dysfunction; severe hypertension; etc.

Radiologic Manifestations: (a) *widening of the nerve roots and obliteration of the root sleeves (edema of the nerves and roots in the acute phase; fibrous thickening and inflammatory exudates in the chronic phase);* (b) magnetic resonance imaging: *markedly abnormal enhancement of the thickened nerve roots and cauda equina;* (c) complications: recurrent atelectasis; pneumonia; pneumothorax; aspiration; peptic ulcer; urinary tract infection; (d) sequelae: scoliosis; deformities of the extremities.

H

HAJDU-CHENEY SYNDROME (ARTHRO-DENTO-OSTEO-DYSPLASIA)

Clinical Manifestations

(A) INFANCY AND CHILDHOOD: (a) *craniofacial dysmorphism:* prominent occiput, low hairline, synophrys, long lashes, thick eyebrows, low-set ears, highly arched palate, dental maleruption and malocclusion; structural changes in the dentine and cementum of the teeth; (b) *short stature;* failure to thrive; retarded puberty; (c) miscellaneous abnormalities: short neck; hernia; hirsutism; (d) autosomal dominant inheritance; sporadic.

(B) ADULTS: (a) *short stature;* (b) *craniofacial dysmorphism:* prominent occiput; highly arched palate; epicanthal folds; telecanthus; downslanting palpebral fissures; early loss of teeth; stenotic ear canal; conductive hearing loss; myopia; loss of vision; disc pallor; constriction of the visual field; nystagmus; abducens palsy; ptosis; exotropia; optic atrophy; (c) miscellaneous abnormalities: low-pitched voice; compression-related neurologic symptoms (cerebellum; lower cranial nerves; etc.); painful paresthesia of the fingers; pseudoclubbing of the fingers; short nails; curved nails; joint laxity; normal or near-normal intelligence; etc.

Radiologic Manifestations: (a) *craniofacial abnormalities:* bathrocephaly; flat cranial base; basilar invagination; multiple wormian bones; persistence of cranial sutures in late adult life; deep sella turcica; hypoplastic facial bones; underdevelopment of sinuses; horizontal clivus; craniofacial osteoporosis; anterior nasal spine resorption; alveolar resorption of the mandible and maxilla; micrognathia, obtuse mandibular angle; edentulism in young adults; (b) *osteolysis of the terminal phalanges of the hands and feet; generalized osteoporosis* (high turnover); miscellaneous skeletal abnormalities (fractures; vertebral abnormalities; modeling defects in tubular bones; bowing of the paired long bones; mesomelic shortening of the arms; hypoplastic radial head; displacement of radial head; hip dislocation; genu valgum; metatarsophalangeal subluxation); (c) central nervous system abnormalities: *upwardly shifted brain stem caused by the tip of the odontoid process associated with basilar invagination;* hydrocephalus; Arnold-Chiari malformation; atrophic pituitary gland; empty sella; expanded pituitary fossa; symmetric fluid collection along the optic nerve sheath; distortion of the optic nerves and infundibular stalk; enlarged internal auditory canals; syringohydromyelia; (d) miscellaneous abnormalities: progressive cardiac valvular dysfunction and conduction disease; calcified aneurysm of ductus arteriosus; hypothyroidism; cervical osteolysis and instability.

HALLERMANN-STREIFF SYNDROME (Oculo-Mandibulo-Facial Syndrome; François Dyscephaly)

Clinical Manifestations: (a) *brachycephaly; small face; small and pinched nose; microstomia; thin lips; micrognathia; low-set ears; highly arched palate;* ocular abnormalities (*congenital cataracts; microphthalmia;* nystagmus; strabismus; blue sclerae; etc.); *dental defects;* (b) miscellaneous abnormalities: *proportionate dwarfism; hypotrichosis; skin atrophy; hyperextensible joints; mental, motor, and speech retardation;* etc.; (c) sporadic; reported in one of dizygotic twins.

Radiologic Manifestations: (a) *craniofacial abnormalities:* brachycephaly; often delayed closure of the fontanelles and persistent wide sutures; frontal and parietal bossing; thin calvaria; small face and orbits; hypoplasia of the mandibular rami with anterior displacement of temporomandibular joints; abnormally obtuse gonial angle; shallow sella turcica; wormian bones; platybasia; elevated anterior cranial fossa; prominent nasal bones; hypotelorism; poor pneumatization of paranasal sinuses;

narrow upper airway due to abnormal craniofacial configuration; (b) tracheomalacia; (c) *dental abnormalities;* (d) skeletal abnormalities: *gracile tubular bones;* poor demarcation of the cortex from medullary portion of the long bones in infancy; vertebral abnormalities (platyspondyly; lordosis; scoliosis; cervical vertebral anomalies; spina bifida); decreased number of sternal ossification centers; (e) miscellaneous abnormalities: osteoporosis; elevated scapulae; hip dislocation, coxa valga; anomalies of radius and ulna; syndactyly; scaphocephaly; calcification of the falx.

HAND-FOOT-GENITAL SYNDROME (HAND-FOOT-UTERUS SYNDROME)

Clinical Manifestations: (a) *small feet; short great toes;* hallux varus; *abnormal thumbs; thenar eminence hypoplasia;* clinodactyly of the fifth fingers; (b) *genital anomalies in females; various degrees of hypospadias in males;* (c) autosomal dominant inheritance with full penetrance and variable expression (male and female).

Radiologic Manifestations: (a) *hand anomalies:* short first metacarpals; short middle phalanx of the fifth fingers; pseudoepiphyses; pointed distal phalanx of the thumbs; fusion of the trapezium and scaphoid; os centrale; long ulnar styloid; split ulnar epiphysis; a typical "pattern profile" of the metacarpals and phalanges; (b) *feet anomalies*: short first metatarsals; pointed distal phalanx of the great toe; tarsal and phalangeal coalition; absence of most secondary ossification centers of the middle and distal phalanges; short proximal phalanx; abnormal navicular bone; short calcaneus; fusion of the cuneiform to other bones; delay in appearance or maturation of medial and intermediate cuneiforms; (c) *genitourinary anomalies in females:* bifid uterus; double uterus; septated vagina, opening of the urethral meatus into the vaginal vault; subsymphyseal epispadias; patulous urethra; urinary incontinence; vesicoureteral reflux; (d) *genitourinary anomalies in males: hypospadias;* vesicoureteral reflux; ureteropelvic junction obstruction.

HELLP SYNDROME

Clinical and Radiologic Manifestations: (a) *H*emolysis; *E*levated *L*iver enzymes; *L*ow *P*latelet count; *toxemia of pregnancy;* right upper quadrant or epigastric pain; shoulder pain; (b) hepatic imaging: "geographic" areas of increased liver echogenicity; hepatic necrosis (computed tomography: low attenuation); hemorrhage, subcapsular hematoma; spontaneous liver rupture; (c) miscellaneous abnormalities: ascites; pleural effusion; disseminated intravascular coagulation.

HEMIHYPERTROPHY

Clinical Manifestations: *Range of asymmetry from enlargement of one digit to hypertrophy of the entire one half of the body:* (a) associated reported conditions: mental deficiency; skin lesions (hemangiomas; nevi; telangiectasia; café au lait spots; unilateral folliculitis; acne); unilateral hypertrichosis; precocious development of genital hair; Beckwith-Wiedemann syndrome; Silver-Russell syndrome; hypospadias; Sotos syndrome; phakomatoses; hamartomatous lesions; testicular hypertrophy; cryptorchidism; Möbius syndrome and crossed total hemihypertrophy; (b) oncogenic potential: hepatoblastoma; hepatic hemangioendothelioma; Wilms tumor; nephroblastomatosis; adrenocortical tumors; adrenal hyperplasia; gonadoblastoma; carcinoma of an undescended testicle; clear-cell adenocarcinoma of the uterine cervix; pheochromocytoma; retroperitoneal sarcoma; cerebellar hemangioblastoma; etc.

Radiologic Manifestations: (a) asymmetry, with the difference usually greatest in the limbs (longer and thicker bones on the large side); difference in bone maturation and unequal paired internal organs in some cases; (b) genitourinary abnormalities: bilateral or unilateral nephromegaly; medullary sponge kidney; renal ectopia; cysts; calyceal diverticulum; ovarian cysts; (c) miscellaneous abnormalities: liver cyst; focal nodular hyperplasia of the liver; cerebral vascular abnormalities; intestinal lymphangiectasia; crossed hemihypertrophy with Wilms tumor.

Note: The HEMI 3 syndrome refers to a developmental syndrome of: *H*emihypertrophy, *H*emihypesthesia, and *H*emiareflexia.

HEMOLYTIC-UREMIC SYNDROME

Clinical Manifestations: (a) upper respiratory tract infection or "flu-like" illness as prodromal symptoms; *vomiting; diarrhea, often bloody;* abdominal symptoms that may simulate an acute surgical condition in the abdomen or ulcerative colitis; (b) *hematuria; proteinuria;* renal failure; (c) purpura; petechiae; (d) hypertension; congestive heart failure; dilated cardiomyopathy; (e) *central nervous system manifestations;* (f) *hemolytic anemia; thrombocytopenia; azotemia;* hyponatremia; hyperuricemia; hyperphosphatemia; hyperkalemia; hyperlipidemia; abnormally shaped red blood cells; elevated white blood cell count with a shift to the left; elevated total bilirubin level; (g) miscellaneous abnormalities: intravascular coagulation; hypoproteinemia; association with *Escherichia coli* 0157:H7 infection; post–solid organ transplant development of hemolytic-uremic syndrome; etc.

Radiologic Manifestations: (a) cardiomegaly; congestive heart failure; pulmonary edema; (b) *colon changes simulating ulcerative colitis;*

prominent filling defects; mucosal edema; marginal serrations; focal or total colonic infarction; gangrene; perforation; stricture; gangrenous appendicitis; intussusception; small bowel wall thickening; (c) acute renal cortical necrosis (hyperechogenicity of the renal cortex; sonolucent renal pyramids); poor renal function by radionuclide renal scan; renal atrophy; cortical calcification; abnormal intrarenal arterial Doppler patterns during oliguria or anuria; (d) cerebral infarction: cerebral microthrombi, in particular, in the basal ganglia; large-vessel thrombotic strokes less common; (e) miscellaneous abnormalities: bone marrow necrosis in the adult; pancreatic calcification; hemoperitoneum; ascites associated with mesenteric inflammatory changes; pituitary hemorrhage.

HEMORRHAGIC SHOCK–ENCEPHALOPATHY SYNDROME

Pathology: Hemorrhagic foci in the brain and some other organs; cerebral edema; cerebral infarction; fatty liver.

Clinical Manifestations: An acute and life-threatening (mortality of about 60%) disease of childhood with rapid onset of multisystem failure (central nervous system; kidneys; cardiovascular system; liver): *seizures; shock; coma; increased intracranial pressure; hyperthermia; coagulopathy; renal and hepatic dysfunction;* gastrointestinal bleeding; diarrhea; electroencephalogram: diffuse slowing.

Radiologic Manifestations: *Cerebral edema; cerebral infarction; decreased cerebral perfusion in the areas of infarction* (single photon emission computed tomography); non-hem iron deposition in the thalami and basal ganglia.

HENOCH-SCHÖNLEIN SYNDROME

Clinical Manifestations: (a) *insidious or sudden onset of pain in the abdomen;* vomiting; (b) *painful joints;* (c) *cutaneous purpura;* maculopapular or urticarial rash in some (in addition to the purpura); painful scalp and facial edema; (d) gastrointestinal hemorrhage; superficial ulcer; erosive gastritis; hemorrhagic-erosive duodenitis; purpuric lesions; ulcers of the rectosigmoid colon; (e) *nephritis;* (f) miscellaneous abnormalities: edema; headaches; behavioral changes during acute phase; seizures; testicular and scrotal swelling; arrhythmias; cardiac failure; elevated erythrocyte sedimentation rate; leukocytosis; polynucleosis; hypoproteinemia; thrombocytosis; decrease in factor XIII levels during acute phase; etc.

Pathology: Allergic necrotizing arteritis with submucosal hemorrhage and mucosal ulceration of the bowel.

Radiologic Manifestations: (a) intestinal lesions: *spiking or cobble-stone appearance of the bowel wall resulting from mucosal edema; thumbprints resulting from submucosal intestinal hemorrhage; colonic wall edema;* intussusception; spontaneous bowel perforation; mucosal erosion; intestinal stricture as a late complication; mural thickening; luminal narrowing; intramural hemorrhage; edema; functional intestinal obstruction; (b) urinary system abnormalities: hemorrhagic ureteritis; ureteral obstruction at different levels with variable degree of upper urinary tract dilatation; hemorrhagic cystitis; irregular mural filling defect in the urinary bladder; swelling of the bladder wall; scrotum and contents abnormalities (edema of the scrotal skin and contents, intact vascular flow; hemorrhage; normal or increased perfusion); (c) miscellaneous abnormalities: pulmonary hemorrhage; pulmonary infiltrates; pleural effusion; free peritoneal fluid; intracranial hemorrhage; hydrops of the gallbladder; skeletal muscle involvement.

HEPATIC FIBROSIS–RENAL CYSTIC DISEASE

Clinical Manifestations: (a) *portal hypertension* manifested by hematemesis or melena; *hepatosplenomegaly; renal failure;* etc.; (b) autosomal dominant and autosomal recessive modes of inheritance have been suggested; various combinations of hepatic and renal fibrocystic lesions in the same family.

Radiologic Manifestations: (a) *renal tubular dilatation* similar to that described in medullary sponge kidney with or without calcification; renal cystic disease; nephromegaly; distorted renal echo pattern; (b) high level of echoes in the liver; *dilatation of intrahepatic biliary ducts;* duplication of intrahepatic venous channels; (c) miscellaneous abnormalities: esophageal varices; giant intrahepatic biliary cyst; ascites; cerebellar hemangioma; cerebral aneurysm; etc.

HEPATOPULMONARY SYNDROME

Clinical Manifestations: Shortness of breath; *chronic liver disease; absence of intrinsic heart or lung disease; abnormal arterial oxygenation;* etc.

Radiologic Manifestations: Bi-basilar, medium-sized (1.5 to 3 mm) nodular or reticular lung opacities; *extrapulmonary appearance on intravenous radiolabeled microspheres* (intrapulmonary shunting); *positive contrast enhanced echocardiogram* (intrapulmonary shunting); *pulmonary vascular dilatation; anastomosis between large arteries and veins near hilum, and in the lung periphery; angiographic and computed tomographic demonstration of vascular dilatation.*

HEYDE SYNDROME

Clinical and Radiologic Manifestations: *Aortic stenosis; gastrointestinal bleeding; angiodysplasia of the gastrointestinal tract,* in particular, the ascending colon; demonstrable by endoscopy (usually multiple lesions: red, flat, or slightly elevated) and by angiography (early venous filling, vascular tufting, and slow venous emptying); subsidence of intestinal bleeding following aortic valve replacement.

HINMAN SYNDROME (NONNEUROGENIC NEUROGENIC BLADDER)

Clinical Manifestations: Day and night wetting; infected urine; fecal retention; normal neurologic evaluation; usually normal vesicoureteral anatomy.

Radiologic Manifestations: Large bladder capacity; "neurogenic type" bladder configuration; significant postvoid residual; secondary upper urinary tract disease in some (hydroureter/hydronephrosis; vesicoureteral reflux); normal urethral configuration in the early phase of urination, followed by distension of the urethra due to contraction of the external sphincter in the later phase of urination (carrot-shaped proximal urethra).

HIRSCHSPRUNG DISEASE

Syndromes Associated with Hirschsprung Disease: (1) chromosomal abnormalities (Down syndrome; chromosome 13 microdeletion; deletion of chromosome 10; etc.); (2) Shah-Waardenburg syndrome: autosomal recessive inheritance; white forelock; isochromia iridis; long segment Hirschsprung disease; (3) Bardet-Biedl syndrome; (4) metaphyseal chondrodysplasia, McKusick type; (5) Goldberg-Shprintzen syndrome; (6) Aarskog syndrome; (7) the syndrome of congenital heart malformation, broad big toes, and ulnar polydactyly in siblings; (8) cat-eye syndrome; (9) familial neuroblastoma, neurofibromatosis, aganglionosis, and jaw-winking syndrome; (10) Hirschsprung disease associated with polydactyly, unilateral kidney agenesis, hypertelorism, and congenital deafness; autosomal recessive inheritance; (11) Ondine's curse; (12) syndrome of infantile osteopetrosis and Hirschsprung disease; consanguineous union.

Association of Hirschsprung Disease with Other Abnormalities: (1) colonic atresia; (2) congenital muscular dystrophy; (3) neurocristopathy: Hirschsprung disease, ganglioneuroblastoma, and autonomic nervous system dysfunction; (4) neurointestinal dysplasia; (5) rubella embryopathy; (6) fetal cytomegalovirus infection; (7) type D brachydactyly; (8) hyperthermia during pregnancy; (9) deafness; (10) tumors: neuroblastoma; multifocal ganglioneuroblastoma; pheochromocytoma; (11) macrocephaly; (12) familial midline field defects: hypoplasia of the corpus callosum and/or cerebellar hypoplasia; Robin sequence; pharyngeal and laryngeal hypoplasia; cardiac defect; etc.

HOLOPROSENCEPHALY

Syndromes Associated with Holoprosencephaly or Arrhinencephaly (Hypoplasia or Absence of the Olfactory Bulbs and Tracts)
1. Agnathia-holoprosencephaly-situs inversus triad
2. Anosmia-radiohumeral synostosis syndrome
3. Aprosencephaly syndrome: aprosencephaly, radial aplasia, and genital anomalies
4. Camptomelic dysplasia
5. COH syndrome (*C*hildren's *O*rthopedic *H*ospital): cloverleaf skull, facial dysmorphism (proptosis; low nasal bridge; short upturned nose; downturned mouth; narrow palate), thumb duplication, and small fifth fingers
6. DiGeorge syndrome
7. Fitch syndrome: arrhinencephaly, absent corpus callosum, hydrocephaly, absent left leaf of the diaphragm, ventricular septal defect, and absent fifth fingernails
8. Genoa syndrome: holoprosencephaly and craniosynostosis (possibly autosomal recessive inheritance)
9. Goldenhar spectrum–arrhinencephaly
10. Kallmann syndrome
11. Meckel syndrome
12. Pallister-Hall syndrome
13. Perrin syndrome: anosmia, mental deficiency, hypogonadism, and congenital ichthyosis
14. Pseudotrisomy 13 syndrome
15. Steinfeld syndrome: holoprosencephaly, bilateral hypoplasia of radius and ulna, absent thumbs, midline cleft lip and palate with absent philtrum, congenital heart defect, renal dysplasia, and absent gallbladder
16. Váradi syndrome: cleft lip/palate, growth deficiency, mental retardation, duplicated halluces, supernumerary fingers, and lingual nodule

HOLT-ORAM SYNDROME

Clinical Manifestations: (a) *congenital cardiovascular diseases;* (b) *fingerlike* or *absent thumb;* etc.; (c) autosomal dominant inheritance with variable expressivity; penetrance of 100%; gene localization: 12q12.

Radiologic Manifestations: Hand anomalies: *thumb anomalies* (digitalized; absent; hypoplastic; triphalangeal; bifid); first metacarpal anomalies (absent; hypoplastic; abnormal plane; etc.); *finger anomalies* (clinodactyly; syndactyly; absent; hypoplastic); second to fifth metacarpal anomalies; *carpal anomalies* (delayed or absent ossification; hypoplastic; fused, irregular; extracarpal/os centrale; enlarged; etc.); anomalies of the forearm; anomalies of the humerus; shoulder anomalies; chest wall anomalies; rib anomalies; vertebral anomalies.

Note: The classic syndrome is that of *combination of triphalangeal thumb with a secundum type of atrial septal defect,* but various combinations of cardiac defects and skeletal manifestations ranging from phocomelia to minor abnormalities have been reported.

HORNER SYNDROME

Clinical Manifestations: *Homolateral miosis; ptosis of the upper lid, narrowing of the interpalpebral fissure; minimal enophthalmos; facial flushing and anhidrosis.*

Radiologic Manifestations: Radiologic demonstration of the etiologic factors: trauma; neoplasm; thrombosis and infarction; aneurysm of innominate artery; goiter; etc.

HUGHES-STOVIN SYNDROME

Clinical Manifestations: *Headaches, fever, cough, dyspnea, hemoptysis, and papilledema;* clinical manifestation of peripheral *phlebothrombosis.*

Pathology: *Thromboses* occurring in the legs, vena cava, superior sagittal sinus, jugular vein, or right side of the heart in association with *pulmonary artery aneurysms.*

Radiologic Manifestations: *Round densities on a chest radiograph, representing aneurysms; diminished vascularity in different section of the lung; aneurysms of segmental branches of pulmonary arteries.*

HYDROLETHALUS SYNDROME

Clinical Manifestations: (a) *hydrocephalus,* occipitoschisis extending from the foramen magnum; (b) *facial anomalies: micrognathia; deformed ears;* hypoplastic eyes; cleft lip and/or palate; poorly formed nose; tongue anomalies; (c) *polyhydramnios;* (d) limb anomalies: *polydactyly;* hallux duplex; clubfeet; short limbs; (e) miscellaneous abnormalities: airway obstruction; stillborn (majority); (f) autosomal recessive inheritance.

Radiologic Manifestations: (a) macrocrania; *dorsal midline defect of the skull;* keyhole-shaped deformity of the base of the skull with a dorsal midline defect of the occipital bone posterior to the foramen magnum; *hydrocephalus; marked brain dysgenesis; severe micrognathia;* (b) limb anomalies: *crossed polydactyly in the hands and feet* (hand: postaxial; feet: preaxial); proximal hypoplasia of tibiae; short upper limbs; short first metatarsal bone; double hallux varus and short hallux varus; cutaneous syndactyly between the double halluces; (c) fetal ultrasonography: atypical hydrocephalus, absent midline structures, and clubfoot deformity (a case report).

HYPEREOSINOPHILIC SYNDROME (IDIOPATHIC)

Criteria for Diagnosis: *Eosinophilia of 1500 cells/mm³ or higher; persistence of eosinophilia for at least 6 months or fatal in a short time; eosinophilia-related organ system dysfunction; absence of a recognized cause for the eosinophilia.*

Clinical Manifestations: (a) *pulmonary symptoms and angioedema*; (b) cardiomyopathy; endomyocardial fibrosis; organic heart murmur; congestive heart failure; (c) behavioral disturbances; upper neuron signs; peripheral neuropathy; central nervous system abnormalities related to embolic disorders; (d) immune disorders: combined immunodeficiency; hypergammaglobulinemia; elevated levels of serum IgE and circulating immune complexes; clonal proliferation of type 2 helper T cells; (e) miscellaneous abnormalities: transition to eosinophilic gastroenteritis; presentation with central nervous system dysfunction; chromosome 20: del(20q); etc.

Radiologic Manifestations: (a) myocardial disease with both left-sided and right-sided heart failure; mitral regurgitation; cardiac dilatation; mitral regurgitation with echographic demonstration of localized thickening of the posterobasal left ventricular wall behind the posterior mitral leaflet and absent or diminished motion of the posterior mitral leaflet; apical obliteration of one or both ventricles by echogenic material suggestive of fibrosis or thrombosis; computed imaging demonstrating mural thrombosis; (b) patchy parenchymal pulmonary infiltrate; pleural effusion; (c) alimentary system eosinophilic infiltration, in particular gastric outlet obstruction; (d) hepatomegaly; multiple hepatic focal lesions (sharply or poorly defined nodules with varied echogenicity; hypodense on computed tomographic studies; decreased radionuclide uptake on scintigrams).

HYPERIMMUNOGLOBULINEMIA E SYNDROME (JOB'S SYNDROME; BUCKLEY SYNDROME)

Clinical Manifestations: (a) *eczematoid dermatitis; recurrent "cold" suppurative skin infections, usually by pyogenic staphylococci;* (b) *chronic purulent sinusitis and otitis media; chronic pulmonary infections;* (c) *impaired neutrophil chemotaxis; high levels of serum IgE* (at least 10 times normal: 2000 IU/ml); depressed specific cell-mediated immune responses; deficient antibody-forming capacity; (d) miscellaneous abnormalities: colon perforation; associated severe diarrhea, diabetes mellitus, and absence of islets of Langerhans in a neonate; necrotizing fasciitis; ventricular aneurysm and myocarditis in a child; etc.; (e) autosomal recessive inheritance.

Radiologic Manifestations: *Sinusitis; mastoiditis; recurrent pneumonia; pneumatocele formation* with variable persistence and expansion; spontaneous pneumothorax; osteoporosis; recurrent fractures; craniosynostosis.

HYPERMOBILITY SYNDROME

Criteria for Diagnosis: The ability of the patients to perform at least three of the following five maneuvers: (a) *extension of the wrists and metacarpal phalanges so that the fingers are parallel to the dorsum of the forearm;* (b) *passive apposition of thumbs to the flexor aspect of the forearm;* (c) *hyperextension of the elbows (10 degrees or more);* (d) *hyperextension of the knees (10 degrees or more);* (e) *flexion of the trunk with the knees extended so that the palms rest on the floor.*

Clinical and Radiologic Manifestations: (a) pain, most common in the knees, hands, and fingers; (b) miscellaneous abnormalities: joint dislocation; ligamentous injury; premature osteoarthritis; joint effusion; temporomandibular joint dysfunction; poor proprioceptive feedback.

HYPEROSTOSIS-HYPERPHOSPHATEMIA SYNDROME

Clinical Manifestations: Onset of symptoms in childhood: *swelling, pain, tenderness, and heat in the involved limbs; fever;* long periods of well-being between the symptomatic episodes; laboratory findings (not constant in all reported cases): *elevated sedimentation rate; hyperphosphatemia; hyperglobulinemia;* anemia; elevated alkaline phosphatase level.

Pathology: Periosteal fibrous thickening and subperiosteal bone formation; nonspecific inflammation.

Radiologic Manifestations: *Minimal to extensive subperiosteal bone formation along the shaft of tubular bones of the limbs; healing with slight osteosclerosis of the affected remaining bone;* increased uptake on skeletal scintigraphic examination.

HYPERPERFUSION SYNDROME

Clinical and Radiologic Manifestations: A complication of revascularization procedures for severe cerebrovascular occlusive disease (carotid endarterectomy; balloon angioplasty; aortocarotid bypass surgery): (a) ipsilateral headaches; migraine variants; confusion; lateralized focal seizures; hemiparesis; (b) increase in cerebral perfusion (nuclear studies); (c) computed tomography: low cerebral density, sulcal effacement, and cerebral hemorrhage; (d) transcranial Doppler evaluation of changes in cerebral perfusion.

HYPERTELORISM–MICROTIA–FACIAL CLEFTING SYNDROME (BIXLER SYNDROME)

Clinical and Radiologic Manifestations: (a) *hypertelorism; clefting (lip, palate, and nose); broad nasal tip; bifid nose; microstomia;* mandibular arch hypoplasia; flattened angle of the mandible; conductive deafness; *microtia; meatal atresia;* hypoplasia of the auditory ossicles; psychomotor retardation; microcephaly; etc.; (b) probably autosomal recessive inheritance.

HYPOGLOSSIA-HYPODACTYLIA SYNDROME (AGLOSSIA-ADACTYLIA SYNDROME)

Clinical Manifestations: (a) *microstomia; micrognathia; syngnathia; hypoglossia of variable degrees; absence of development of the distal segments of the limbs* (digits in particular); (b) miscellaneous abnormalities: Goldenhar and Möbius syndromes associated with hypoglossia-hypodactylia syndrome (a case report).

Radiologic Manifestations: (a) *micrognathia;* (b) *hypoplasia of the extremities:* peromelia to absence of the distal segments of the digits; (c) dental anomalies: absence of mandibular incisors; natal teeth; (d) miscellaneous associated anomalies: dextrocardia; transposition of abdominal organs; bony fusion of the jaws; jejunal atresia; short bowel; "apple peel" bowel.

HYPOMELANOSIS OF ITO (INCONTINENTIA PIGMENTI ACHROMIANS)

Clinical Manifestations: (a) skin manifestations: *irregular hypopigmented whorls, patches, streaks, or zig-zag pattern, often bilateral and asymmetric;* (b) *central nervous system manifestations:* seizures; psychomotor delay; hypotonicity; hypertonicity; hemiparesis; speech delay; ataxia; asymmetric reflexes; sensory deficits; macrocephaly; microcephaly; focal electroencephalographic abnormalities; mental retardation; sensorineural deafness; hyperkinesia; hydrocephaly; etc.; (c) *ocular abnormalities;* (d) miscellaneous abnormalities: coarse facial features; dental abnormalities; chromosomal abnormalities; neuroblastoma; (e) majority of the cases sporadic; autosomal recessive, autosomal dominant, and X-linked dominant transmission have been suggested but not confirmed.

Radiologic Manifestations: (a) *hemimegalencephaly; gray matter heterotopias; white matter lesions similar to leukodystrophies; small periventricular cysts; cerebral lesion in centrum semiovale suggestive of massive demyelination;* absence of normal demarcation between gray and white matter; asymmetry of the cerebral hemispheres; atrophy of the cerebellar vermis; (b) pectus carinatum; pectus excavatum; clinodactyly; syndactyly; polydactyly; ectrodactyly; short fingers; genu valgum; pes valgus; pes varus; short limb; lordosis; scoliosis; spinal fusion; congenital hip dislocation; skeletal maturation retardation.

HYPOTHENAR HAMMER SYNDROME

Clinical Manifestations: Occlusion of the distal ulnar artery or superficial volar arch of the hand subjected to repetitive blunt trauma (hammer, push, or pound; tennis playing): *cold sensation; painful digits; paresthesias; cyanosis, pallor or mottling;* aggravation of symptoms with exposure to cold; Raynaud phenomenon; positive Allen test (with clenched fist blood is pressed out from the palm, the radial artery is pressed tightly, and the fist is opened: delay in disappearance of the palmar pallor due to the ulnar artery obstruction); digital coldness; hypothenar callus or mass; atrophy and softening of finger pads; tender hypothenar eminence; ischemic ulcer; subungual hemorrhage; gangrene.

Radiologic Manifestations: Angiography: *occlusion of the distal ulnar artery, a superficial volar arch, or a digital artery;* corkscrewlike configuration of the ulnar artery in Guyon canal (intramural necrosis and fibrosis and nonocclusive intraluminal thrombosis); aneurysm with or without occlusion of the palmar arterial system; embolism to the digital arteries from thrombi formed on damaged intima of the distal ulnar artery.

I

IMMOTILE CILIA SYNDROME (CILIARY DYSKINESIA)

Clinical Manifestations: (a) *rhinorrhea; chronic productive cough; recurrent pneumonia; recurrent bronchitis; recurrent otitis; recurrent sinusitis;* nasal polyp; episodic and/or persistent wheezes; abnormal pulmonary function tests; abnormal mucociliary clearance test result; (b) digital clubbing; (c) *oligospermia, absent or marked decrease in sperm motility;* (d) autosomal recessive inheritance.

Radiologic Manifestations: Pulmonary consolidations; peribronchial thickening; atelectasis; bronchiectasis; obstructive lung disease with hyperinflation; *sinusitis, mucosal thickening.*

Note: About one half of the cases of primary ciliary dyskinesia are associated with Kartagener syndrome.

INCONTINENTIA PIGMENTI

Clinical Manifestations: A multisystem, ectodermal disorder: (a) skin lesions *(erythema, vesicles, and pustules; papules, verrucous lesions, and hyperkeratosis; hyperpigmentation; pallor, atrophy, and scarring);* nail dystrophy; hair abnormalities (lusterless, wiry, and coarse hair; alopecia, especially at the vertex); (b) eye abnormalities: retinal ischemia; bleeding; fibrosis; retrolental "mass"; hyperpigmentation of the conjunctiva, iris, and retina; microphthalmos; cataract; optic atrophy; (c) teeth abnormalities: *hypodontia; delayed eruption; impaction; crown malformation;* (d) breast abnormalities: hypoplasia or aplasia; supernumerary nipples; nipple hypoplasia; abnormalities in nipple pigmentation; (e) neurologic abnormalities: seizures; spastic paralysis; motor retardation; mental retardation; microcephaly; abnormal electroencephalogram; (f) X-linked dominant with lethality in the male hemizygotes; very high penetrance (near 100%); variable expression.

Radiologic Manifestations: (a) microcephaly; brain edema; brain atrophy; hydrocephalus; porencephalic cyst; gyral dysplasia; hypoplasia of the corpus callosum; neuronal heterotopias; periventricular white matter damage; destructive encephalopathy; magnetic resonance imaging findings compatible with small vessel occlusion; acute hemorrhagic necrosis; optic atrophy; (b) skull deformities; (c) skeletal abnormalities: vertebral anomalies; syndactyly; supernumerary ribs; hemiatrophy; shortening of the legs and arms; (d) dental abnormalities: partial anodontia; malformed teeth; impactions; pegged teeth; cysts; (e) miscellaneous abnormalities: internal carotid artery aneurysm with reduced middle cerebral flow; skeletal maturation retardation; subungual dysplastic nodules associated with dorsal scalloped erosion of the terminal tuft of the phalanx.

INFANTILE MULTISYSTEM INFLAMMATORY DISEASE
(NEONATAL ONSET MULTISYSTEM INFLAMMATORY DISEASE; NOMID)

Clinical Manifestations: Symptoms usually present at birth or during early infancy: *evanescent rash; relapsing arthropathy,* mostly involving the knee and elbow joints; *fever; lymphadenopathy; persistent open fontanelle; cerebrospinal fluid pleocytosis; anemia; leukocytosis; elevated sedimentation rate; IgG elevation*; etc.

Radiologic Manifestations: (a) *osteoporosis*, vertebral compression fractures; *swelling at the end of the long bones (bony and cartilaginous overgrowth); minimal joint effusion; joint contracture; muscle and soft-tissue wasting; shortening of the long bones of the limb in association with bowing (varus deformities of the proximal portions of the femora and tibiae); widening of the shaft of the long bones in association with a periosteal reaction that cloaks the ends of the long bones* (the ulnae and fibulae relatively unaffected); *irregularity and cupping of the metaphyses; large, irregular, and fragmented epiphyses; premature fusion of the physes; cone-shaped epiphysis and notching of the corresponding metaphysis of the distal segment of the femur;* relatively tall vertebrae and a short anteroposterior diameter; gibbous deformity at the thoracolumbar junction; (b) macrocrania; frontal bossing; wormian bones; thickened and dense base of the skull; slightly peaked orbits; widened mandibular angle; slight antegonial notching; adequate tooth mineralization; (c) hepatosplenomegaly; (d) miscellaneous abnormalities: mild cardiomegaly; ventriculomegaly; wide extraaxial fluid spaces.

INSENSITIVITY TO PAIN (CONGENITAL) (CONGENITAL INDIFFERENCE TO PAIN)

Clinical Manifestations: (a) *absence or marked diminution of the sense of pain; touch perception not affected; ulcers of the lips and tongue due to biting;* early loss of teeth; corneal opacity; infection of fingers, toes, and the mandible; neglected fractures; (b) miscellaneous abnormalities: multiple bruises; high plasma α-endorphin levels associated with a reduction in the expression of natural killer cells; (c) autosomal recessive inheritance.

Radiologic Manifestations: *Microfractures and macrofractures; epiphyseal separation; osteomyelitis* (mandible, fingers, and toes in particular); aseptic necrosis in the juxtaarticular regions of weight-bearing long bones; subperiosteal hemorrhage in infancy; degenerative changes and loose bodies in the joints in older cases; neuropathic joints; recurrent dislocation of the hip.

Differential Diagnosis: Congenital insensitivity to pain with anhidrosis (autosomal recessive inheritance); hereditary sensory radicular neuropathy (autosomal dominant inheritance); congenital sensory neuropathy (sporadic); familial dysautonomia (autosomal recessive inheritance); Lesch-Nyhan syndrome (X-linked inheritance); autosomal dominant insensitivity to pain; child abuse.

IRRITABLE BOWEL SYNDROME (IRRITABLE COLON SYNDROME; SPASTIC COLON; MUCOUS COLON SYNDROME)

Clinical Manifestations: Criteria for Diagnosis (Thompson: *Lancet* 341:1569, 1993): *Continuous or recurrent symptoms enumerated under* (A) *(at least 3 months duration), plus two or more of the criteria enumerated under* (B) *(at least a quarter of occasions or days).*

(A) Abdominal pain or discomfort that is relieved by defecation; and/or associated with a change in frequency of stool; and/or associated with changes in consistency of stool.

(B) (a) altered stool frequency; (b) altered stool form (lumpy/hard or loose/watery); (c) altered stool passage (straining, urgency, or feeling of incomplete evacuation); (d) passage of mucus; (e) bloating or feeling of abdominal distension.

Radiologic Manifestations: (a) *excessive colonic motility; reduced width of the lumen; increased number of haustral markings; segmental spasm;* (b) dynamic ^{99m}Tc bran scan: significantly slow ileocecal clearance; (c) ultrasonography: small percentage of the studied cases have shown abnormalities in other intraabdominal organs (not recommended as a routine procedure; not significant in management).

ISO-KIKUCHI SYNDROME

Clinical and Radiologic Manifestations: (a) *congenital nail dysplasia (micronychia; anonychia; etc.) involving the index fingers and sometimes their neighbors; dorsal spurlike protrusion of the distal phalanx of the involved digit;* (b) autosomal dominant inheritance with variable expression most likely.

J

JACKSON-WEISS SYNDROME

Clinical and Radiologic Manifestations: (a) *craniosynostosis,* midfacial hypoplasia; (b) *foot abnormalities:* medially deviated toe; tarsal bone fusion; phalangeal, tarsonavicular, and calcaneonavicular fusions; short and broad metatarsals; short and broad phalanx of the toes; coned epiphyses; hallux valgus; (c) hand abnormalities: coned epiphyses; distal and middle phalangeal hypoplasia; carpal bone malsegmentation; (d) autosomal dominant inheritance.

JADASSOHN-LEWANDOWSKY SYNDROME (PACHYONYCHIA CONGENITA)

Clinical Manifestations: (a) *palmoplantar keratosis and hyperhidrosis; follicular keratosis; epidermal cysts; pachyonychia congenita:* hypertrophy and subungual hyperkeratosis of all nails; (b) *mucous membrane lesions:* oral leukokeratosis; hoarseness due to laryngeal involvement; (c) complications of pachyonychia; (d) autosomal dominant inheritance.

Radiologic Manifestations: Narrowing of the esophagus; intestinal diverticula; osteomas.

JAFFE-CAMPANACCI SYNDROME

Clinical Manifestations: (a) pain; swelling; *café au lait spots;* (b) miscellaneous abnormalities: mental retardation; hypogonadism; cryptorchidism; gonadotropin deficiency; eye anomalies; congenital heart disease; alopecia; precocious puberty.

Radiologic Manifestations: *Disseminated "nonossifying fibromas"* of the long bone and pelvis (spindle and giant cells; hemorrhagic foci; hemosiderin pigment); pathologic fracture(s); kyphoscoliosis; scoliosis associated with stenosis of the aortic isthmus, chylothorax, and chylopericardium (a case report).

JOHANSON-BLIZZARD SYNDROME

Clinical Manifestations: Phenotypic variability: (a) *low birth weight; motor, somatic, and mental retardation; hypotonia;* (b) *hyperextensibility of joints;* (c) *craniofacial anomalies:* microcephaly; aplastic alae nasi; skin dimples and defects over the fontanelles; (d) *severe oligodontia; small teeth;* micrognathia; maxillary hypoplasia; (e) *sensorineural deafness;* (f) *exocrine pancreatic insufficiency;* hypothyroidism; hypopituitarism; (g) *recto-urogenital anomalies;* (h) miscellaneous abnormalities: malabsorption; hair anomalies; eyelid ptosis; strabismus; cutaneolacrimal fistula; (i) probably autosomal recessive inheritance.

Radiologic Manifestations: Cystic dilatation of the cochlea and the vestibulum; hydronephrosis; caliectasis; skeletal maturation retardation; pancreatic lipomatosis.

JOUBERT SYNDROME

Clinical Manifestations: (a) facial dysmorphism: low-set ears; highly arched palate; epicanthus; upward slanting of the eyes; short neck; (b) *neonatal tachypnea or apneic spells; mental retardation; ataxia; episodic hyperpnea; rhythmic protrusion of the tongue;* (c) *ocular motor abnormalities;* congenital retinal dysplasia; *bilateral chorioretinal coloboma;* (d) miscellaneous abnormalities: hepatic fibrosis; unilateral facial paralysis; cystic kidneys; (e) autosomal recessive inheritance; male preponderance.

Radiologic Manifestations: *Partial or complete absence of the cerebellar vermis;* absent corpus callosum; enlarged cisterna magna with abnormally shaped anterior and upper borders; cisterna magna connected with a malformed fourth ventricle via an anomalous channel; dilatation of the fourth ventricle with convexity of the upper part of the roof posteriorly and of the floor toward the brain stem; hypoplasia of the medulla and upper cervical spinal cord.

JUBERG-HAYWARD SYNDROME (Oro-Cranio-Digital Syndrome)

Clinical and Radiologic Manifestations: (a) *growth retardation;* (b) craniofacial dysmorphism: *microcephaly; cleft lip and/or cleft palate; broad and flat nasal bridge; bowed and upward-slanting eyebrows;* cupped ears; preauricular tags; (c) skeletal abnormalities: *hypoplasia or aplasia of thumbs; proximal or distal displacement of thumbs;* interphalangeal inflexibility of the thumbs; short metacarpals and phalanges; anomalous carpal bones; *limitation of extension of elbows;* radial head luxation; radial hypoplasia; minor anomalies of toes; minor vertebral and rib anomalies; (d) autosomal recessive inheritance with variable expression most likely.

JUGULAR FORAMEN SYNDROME

Clinical and Radiologic Manifestations: *Unilateral palsy of the ninth, tenth, and eleventh cranial nerves as a result of the following etiologic factors at the base of the skull and retroparotid space:* tumor; trauma; vascular occlusion; infection; etc.

K

KABUKI MAKE-UP SYNDROME (Niikawa-Kuroki Syndrome)

Clinical Manifestations: (a) *facial features reminiscent of the Kabuki actors' make-up:* arching eyebrows, sparse in the lateral half; long eyelashes; long palpebral fissures; ectropion of the lower eyelids; broad and depressed nasal tip; prominent ears; short nasal septum; (b) missing and widely spaced teeth; (c) *mental retardation* (slight to moderate); (d) *growth deficiency;* (e) *stubby fingers; finger pads; abnormal dermatoglyphic pattern;* (f) miscellaneous abnormalities: congenital heart defect; acquired hypogammaglobulinemia and anti-IgA antibodies; congenital velopharyngeal incompetence; growth hormone deficiency and premature thelarche; chronic idiopathic thrombocytopenic purpura; etc.

Radiologic Manifestations: Nonspecific: brachydactyly, particularly of fingers three through five; brachymesophalangy V; pseudoepiphyses; vertebral abnormalities (scoliosis; butterfly deformity; sagittal cleft; narrow intervertebral disc spaces; etc.); rib anomalies; hip dislocation; coxa valga; dislocated hypoplastic patella; ventriculomegaly; etc.

KALLMANN SYNDROME

Clinical Manifestations: (a) *hypogonadotropic hypogonadism;* (b) *anosmia or hyposmia;* (c) neurologic deficits outside the olfactory and hypothalamic regions: congenital mirror movements; spastic paraplegia; cerebellar dysfunction; gazed-evoked horizontal nystagmus; spatial attentional abnormalities; color vision disturbance; neurosensory deafness; (d) miscellaneous abnormalities: mental retardation; arachnoid cyst of the middle fossa; chromosomal abnormalities; etc.; (e) the X-linked Kallmann syndrome gene assigned to Xp22.3; autosomal recessive inheritance; autosomal dominant inheritance.

Radiologic Manifestations: (a) *abnormalities of the olfactory system (hypoplasia of the olfactory sulci; aplasia or hypoplasia of olfactory bulb and tracts);* (b) miscellaneous abnormalities: small anterior pituitary gland; extensive brain calcification; suprasellar cyst; enlarged paranasal sinuses; choanal atresia; renal abnormalities; malrotation of the bowel; hand anomalies; hypogonadism with delayed closure of epiphyseal growth zone resulting in epiphysiolysis of proximal femoral epiphysis after trauma.

KARTAGENER SYNDROME

Clinical Manifestations: (a) *situs inversus;* (b) *sinusitis with mucopurulent nasal discharge from infancy;* (c) *ciliary dyskinesia (about 50% of the patients with ciliary dyskinesia have Kartagener syndrome);* (d) spermatozoa variations: normal spermatozoa and fertility; motile cilia with immotile spermatozoa; motile cilia with abnormal waveforms and structurally defective axonemes; (e) miscellaneous abnormalities: hemangiomatous proliferation of lung capillaries; presenting as neonatal respiratory distress; etc.; (f) autosomal recessive inheritance.

Radiologic Manifestations: *Situs inversus* or *isolated dextrocardia;* absent or underdeveloped paranasal sinuses; *sinusitis; bronchiectasis.*

Variants: (a) complete situs inversus and congenital heart disease without sinusitis; (b) dextrocardia, congenital heart disease, sinusitis, and bronchiectasis; (c) sinusitis and bronchiectasis without situs inversus.

KASABACH-MERRITT SYNDROME

Clinical Manifestations: (a) *systemic hemangioma* or hemangioendothelioma of different sizes and locations; (b) *thrombocytopenia;* decreased platelet survival time; *prolonged clotting time; bleeding;* (c) miscellaneous abnormalities: Kaposiform hemangioendothelioma; malignant vascular tumors in adults; multifocal congenital hemangiopericytoma.

Radiologic Manifestations: Findings depend on the involved organs: osteolytic lesions; visceromegaly; hydronephrosis; hydrocephalus; lung involvement with pneumothorax; progressive increase in the uptake of ^{111}In-labeled platelets within the lesion; imaging of liver with Tc-99m–labeled erythrocytes (hypertrophy of the artery; greatly hypervascular mass; pooling of blood within the lesion).

KAUFMAN-McKUSICK SYNDROME (McKUSICK-KAUFMAN SYNDROME)

Clinical Manifestations: (a) *postaxial polydactyly* (unilateral or bilateral; hands and/or feet); (b) *abdominal "mass"; external genital anomalies in females; urinary retention;* (c) miscellaneous abnormalities: hypospadias; undescended testes in males; supernumerary nipple; (d) autosomal recessive inheritance; phenotypic variability.

Radiologic Manifestations: (a) *hydrometrocolpos; hydronephrosis and hydroureter;* (b) *postaxial polydactyly;* (c) miscellaneous abnormalities: hip dislocation; knee dislocation; vertebral anomalies; oligohydramnios; syndactyly; peritoneal cyst (refluxing vaginal secretion).

KAWASAKI SYNDROME

Clinical Manifestations: Acute multisystem vasculitis; most patients (80%) under 5 years of age: *Fever persisting at least 5 days; changes in peripheral extremities: erythema and edema of hands and feet (acute phase); membranous desquamation of fingertips (convalescent phase); polymorphous exanthem; bilateral, painless bulbar conjunctival injection without exudate; changes in lips and oral cavity: erythema and cracking of lips, strawberry tongue, and diffuse injection of oral and pharyngeal mucosae; nonpurulent cervical lymphadenopathy (1.5 cm or larger in diameter), usually unilateral.*

Fever and at least four of the aforementioned features are required to be present to establish the diagnosis. However, in the presence of fever and coronary artery disease, fewer than four of the principal symptoms can be used for diagnosis of the syndrome.

Radiologic Manifestations: (a) coronary, peripheral, cerebral, and visceral arterial abnormalities (*thrombosis, stenosis, and aneurysm* [spherical; fusiform]; rupture of an aneurysm; arterial wall calcification); (b) *cardiomegaly;* myocardial damage (scintigraphy); ventricular aneurysm; pericardial effusion; valvular regurgitation (mitral; tricuspid; aortic); left ventricular wall motion abnormalities; myocarditis; myocardial infarction; (c) pneumonia, reticulogranular pattern of the lungs; peribronchial cuffing; atelectasis; air trapping; pleural effusion; (d) hydrops of the gallbladder; gallbladder necrosis; gallbladder perforation; marked impairment of meal-stimulated gallbladder emptying; intestinal pseudoobstruction; bowel necrosis; ischemic colitis; bowel obstruction (stricture as a complication of the disease); (e) avascular necrosis of the femoral head; aseptic necrosis of the calcaneus; presentation as pyarthrosis of the hip; (f) miscellaneous abnormalities: parapharyngeal adenopathy; necrotic pharyngitis; peritonsillar abscess; renal involvement: increased cortical echogenicity; enhanced corticomedullary differentiation; renomegaly; cerebral vascular disease; aneurysm; cerebral infarction.

KBG SYNDROME

Clinical Manifestations: (a) *craniofacial dysmorphism:* round face, brachycephaly, biparietal prominence, a distinctive nose, broad eyebrows, and telecanthus; (b) dental anomalies: short alveolar ridges; *macrodontia;* oligodontia; malposition; enamel hypoplasia; (c) *short stature;* (d) *mild to moderate mental retardation;* (e) probably autosomal dominant inheritance with significant variability of expression.

Radiologic Manifestations: (a) *skeletal maturation retardation;* (b) skeletal abnormalities: anomalies of vertebrae; pectus excavatum; cervical ribs; shortness of the tubular bones of the hands; hexadactyly; clinodactyly of fifth fingers; syndactyly of toes 2 and 3.

Note: *KBG*: the patients' initials.

KERATOSIS PALMARIS ET PLANTARIS FAMILIARIS (TYLOSIS)

Clinical Manifestations: Onset of symptoms between the ages of 3 and 12 months: (a) *diffuse extensive symmetric cornification of the skin beginning on the palms and soles with extension of the process dorsally in some cases; keratoma; hyperhidrosis;* maceration; autoamputation in severe cases; (b) autosomal dominant inheritance; gene mapped to 17q12–24.

Radiologic Manifestations: Thickening and disorganization of normal soft-tissue planes; *osteoporosis; tapering of the distal phalanges; progressive amputation of the phalanges, metacarpals, and metatarsals;* luxation of joints; fusion of carpal bones.

KEUTEL SYNDROME

Clinical Manifestations: (a) *brachytelephalangia;* (b) *hearing loss* (external; mixed; conductive); (c) characteristic facies *(midfacial hypoplasia, depressed nasal bridge, and small alae nasi);* (d) autosomal recessive inheritance.

Radiologic Manifestations: (a) *widespread cartilage calcification/ ossification:* external ears; nose; larynx; tracheobronchial tree; ribs; (b) miscellaneous abnormalities: stippled epiphyses; peripheral pulmonary stenosis; ventricular septal defect.

KLEIN-WAARDENBURG SYNDROME

Clinical Manifestations: (a) *facial dysmorphism:* lateral displacement of the medial canthi, heterochromia of the iris, blepharophimosis, heavy eyebrows, large root of the nose, hypoplastic alae, "cupid bow"–shaped upper lip, prognathism, and white forelock; (b) deafness, unilateral or bilateral; (c) albinotic skin patches; (d) *thin upper limbs with hypoplasia of musculoskeletal structures; flexion deformity* (elbow; wrist; fingers); (e) autosomal dominant inheritance.

Radiologic Manifestations: Syndactyly of the hands; *carpal bone fusion.*

KLINEFELTER SYNDROME

Clinical Manifestations: (a) tall/thinly built male; *eunuchoid appearance;* (b) normal or slightly underdeveloped penis; *testicular atrophy; azoospermia;* seminiferous tubule dysgenesis; *gynecomastia; elevated gonadotropin excretion in the urine; low normal, or decreased 17-ketosteroid excretion in the urine;* (c) mild mental retardation; (d) cardiovascular manifestations: subarachnoid hemorrhage due to aneurysm; mitral valve prolapse; varicose veins; hypostatic leg ulcers; subacute ischemia of the lower limbs; Takayasu arteritis; venous thromboemboli; (e) miscellaneous abnormalities: association with neoplastic lesions; bilateral aplasia of mandibular ramus and condyle; ischemic priapism; etc.; (f) *chromosomal abnormalities:* 47,XXY in about 80% to 85%, variants and mosaics in about 15% to 20%.

Radiologic Manifestations: Nonspecific and nonconstant: (a) radioulnar synostosis; positive metacarpal sign; phalangeal preponderance (normally the length of the fourth metacarpal is equal to length of distal plus proximal phalanges); pointed appearance or squared ends of fingers; brachymesophalangia with or without clinodactyly of fifth finger; high metacarpal index (length/width); (b) skull dysmorphism: temporal flattening; decreased width of vault; short anteroposterior diameter of skull; shortening of anterior fossa; decrease in length of base; thinning of vault at major fontanelle; premature and excessive calcification of coronal suture; deepening of posterior fossa, shortening of mandibular rami; increase in size of pituitary fossa associated with thinning of posterior clinoid and dorsum sella and a double floor; (c) dental anomalies: short roots; elongated body; enlarged pulp chamber.

KLIPPEL-FEIL SYNDROME

Clinical Manifestations: (a) *"absent" neck, decreased mobility of the head; low occipital hairline;* (b) deafness (in about 30%); (c) miscellaneous abnormalities: thenar hypoplasia due to aberrant radial artery; hypoparathyroidism; familial Klippel-Feil syndrome and paracentric inversion inv(8)(q22.2–q23.3); reciprocal translocation between 5q11.2 and 17q23; (d) autosomal recessive and autosomal dominant modes of inheritance have been suggested; sporadic.

Radiologic Manifestations: (a) *fused cervical or cervicothoracic vertebrae; hemivertebrae deformities;* cervical spondylosis; (b) ear anomalies: absent auditory canal; microtia; deformed ossicles; underdevelopment of the bony labyrinth; Mondini defect; small or absent internal auditory canal; etc.; (c) genitourinary anomalies; (d) central nervous system abnormalities: Chiari I malformation; hydromyelia; syringomyelia; disc herniations; diastematomyelia; spinal cord compression; atlantoaxial instability; recurrent vertebrobasilar embolism; (e) miscellaneous abnormalities: atlantooccipital fusion; spinal canal stenosis; spina bifida; Sprengel deformity; micrognathia; rib fusion; intraspinal tumor; frontonasal dysplasia and postaxial polydactyly; isolation of the right subclavian artery with subclavian steal; congenital duplication of mandibular rami; abnormal masses in the mandibular ramus region.

Note: The classical *triad of low posterior hairline, short neck, and limitation of head and neck motion* is not present in all cases.

KLIPPEL-TRENAUNAY SYNDROME (KLIPPEL-TRENAUNAY-WEBER SYNDROME)

Clinical Manifestations: Usually monomelic (lower limb in about three fourths of the cases): (a) *superficial varices; port-wine telangiectatic nevi; soft-tissue and bone hypertrophy;* internal organ involvement; craniofacial involvement; (b) miscellaneous abnormalities: erectile dysfunction; abdominal hamartoma with undescended testis; a 5:11 balanced translocation; splenic lymphangioma; etc.

Radiologic Manifestations: Various imaging modalities including angiography, computed tomography, ultrasonography, and scintigraphy: (a) *elongation and widening of the bones of a limb (hypertrophy) and cortical thickening;* (b) *hypoplasia or atresia of some major deep veins; abnormal venous channels connecting deep veins to dilated superficial veins;* nonvisualization of valves in some veins; decompensation of superficial veins; (c) *other associated vascular abnormalities:* abdominal hemangiomas; varicose pulmonary veins; cutaneous lymphangiomas; Sturge-Weber syndrome; aplasia of the cervical internal carotid artery and malformation of the circle of Willis; duplication of the inferior vena cava; absent inferior vena cava; (d) scintigraphic abnormalities: venous occlusion; collateral venous channels; extensive radionuclide uptake in the enlarged limb; pulmonary emboli; (e) lymphatic hyperplasia, aplasia, or hypoplasia in the limbs; abnormal dermal lymphatic flow; (f) central nervous system abnormalities: cerebral and cerebellar hemihypertrophy; cerebral atrophy; cerebral calcifications; angiomatous leptomeningeal enhancement; markedly enhancing choroid plexus; aplasia of the cervical internal carotid artery and malformation of the circle of Willis; aneurysm of transverse cervical artery; cerebral arteriovenous fistula; spinal cord arteriovenous malformation; (g) miscellaneous abnormalities: macrodactyly; dental abnormalities; atrophy of involved areas; nephroblastomatosis; hemihypertrophy of the face; syndactyly; polydactyly; dislocation of the hip; scoliosis; kyphosis; phleboliths.

Note: The diagnostic triad: *vascular nevus, congenital varicose veins, and bone and soft-tissue hypertrophy.*

KLÜVER-BUCY SYNDROME

Clinical Manifestations: *Severe behavioral problems; hyperactivity; rage reaction; marked emotional liability; urge to place all objects into the mouth;* visual agnosia; hypersexuality; alteration in dietary habits; problems in intermediate memory; partial expression in some cases.

Radiologic Manifestations: *Hydrocephalus ex vacuo in the temporal lobe region (temporal hydrocephalus); central nervous system changes related to the etiologic factors.*

KUGELBERG-WELANDER SYNDROME

Clinical Manifestations: A degenerating disease of the anterior horn cells of the spinal cord; onset usually between 3 and 18 years of age: (a) *atrophy and weakness of proximal limb muscles followed by involvement of the distal muscles;* (b) *electromyographic and muscle biopsy findings of a lower motor neuron lesion;* (c) cardiomyopathy associated with arrhythmias; (d) autosomal recessive inheritance; autosomal dominant in some families has been suggested.

Radiologic Manifestations: (a) computed tomography: *development of patches of low-density tissue in the muscles; progressive spread and enlargement of the low-density areas all over the surface of the muscles, with the muscles developing a ragged outline; progressive submergence of muscles into the adipose tissue;* (b) *cardiomegaly* and echocardiographic manifestations of cardiac chamber enlargement; (c) esophageal dilatation with absence of peristalsis; small-bowel dilatation; loss of colonic haustrations.

KUSKOKWIM SYNDROME

Clinical Manifestations: (a) *multiple congenital joint contractures;* kyphosis in infants; atrophy or compensatory hypertrophy of associated muscle groups; normal intelligence; etc.; (b) autosomal recessive inheritance.

Radiologic Manifestations: *Hypoplasia of the first or second vertebral body;* progressive elongation of the pedicles of the fifth lumbar vertebra with *spondylolisthesis; osteolytic areas in the outer one third of the clavicles in childhood; osteolytic lesions of the proximal humeral metaphysis* in infancy and childhood; *hypoplasia of patellae;* etc.

L

LACRIMO-AURICULO-DENTO-DIGITAL SYNDROME (LADD SYNDROME; LEVY-HOLLISTER SYNDROME)

Clinical and Radiologic Manifestations: (a) *lacrimal anomalies:* absent or hypoplastic lacrimal gland or puncta and/or nasolacrimal ducts and/or tear sac; diminished or absent tears or recurrent or chronic tearing; (b) *dental anomalies:* delayed tooth eruption; peg-shaped teeth; enamel dysplasia; anodontia; dental hypoplasia; (c) *digital anomalies:* thumb anomalies; finger anomalies; polydactyly; abnormal metacarpophalangeal profile pattern; (d) miscellaneous abnormalities: salivary gland abnormalities (absent gland; salivary gland hyposecretion); malformed ear(s); hearing disorder; etc.; (e) autosomal dominant inheritance.

LAMBERT-EATON MYASTHENIC SYNDROME

Clinical and Radiologic Manifestations: Association with bronchial carcinoma (often small-cell carcinoma) in about two thirds of cases: *weakness, easy fatigability of the legs secondary to proximal muscle weakness, especially the pelvic girdle and proximal limb muscles, usually sparing cranial muscles; paradoxical potentiation in electromyographic studies;* the autoantibodies directed against the voltage-gated calcium channels of motor nerve terminals; *respiratory muscle weakness.*

LANDAU-KLEFFNER SYNDROME

Clinical and Radiologic Manifestations: Onset in childhood: (a) *regression of receptive and/or expressive language abilities; convulsive disorders;* (b) electroencephalography: *bilateral spike- and slow-waves arising from variable foci;* (c) single photon emission computed tomography: decreased regional perfusion; perfusion asymmetry; (d) positron emission tomography: hypometabolism, in particular over the temporal lobes.

LARSEN SYNDROME

Clinical Manifestations: (a) *distinctive facies:* flat face; hypertelorism; depressed nasal bridge; prominent forehead; cleft palate; cleft uvula; periodontitis; (b) *laxity of the joints; dislocated elbows, hips, and knees;* cylindric fingers; spatulalike thumbs; short and broad fingertips; resistant clubfoot deformity; (c) sensorineural or mixed hearing loss; abnormal ear anatomy; (d) most cases autosomal dominant inheritance or sporadic; autosomal recessive inheritance; a gene of autosomal dominant Larsen syndrome mapped to chromosome region 3p21.1–14.1.

Radiologic Manifestations: (a) *joint dislocations* (usually the large joints); abnormal skeletal mineralization; accessory ossicles of the hands, wrists, knees, elbows, and feet; double or triple calcaneal ossification center; *short metacarpals, metatarsals, and distal phalanges; spatulate thumbs;* (b) *flattened frontal bone; small base of the skull and facial bones; shallow orbits; hypertelorism; micrognathia;* (c) abnormal segmentation of the vertebrae; flat vertebrae; cervical kyphosis; scoliosis; cervicothoracic lordosis; hypoplasia of the cervical vertebrae; dislocation of the upper cervical vertebrae in association with congenital defects; (d) miscellaneous abnormalities: short humerus with hypoplasia of the distal end; short fibulae; increased anterior bowing of tibiae; foot deformities; toe deformities; "square" tubular bones; skeletal maturation retardation; finger clubbing; thin ribs; long clavicles; deficiency of pubic bone ossification; laxity of the trachea, larynx, and costochondral cartilages; aortic root dilatation; cervical cord compression; congenital heart disease; (e) early prenatal diagnosis by transvaginal ultrasonography.

LAURIN-SANDROW SYNDROME

Clinical and Radiologic Manifestations: (a) polysyndactyly of the hands; hands held in a "semicupped position"; mirror polysyndactyly of the feet; duplication of the ulna and fibula; absence of the radius and tibia; (b) miscellaneous abnormalities: hypoplasia of the nasal alae with coloboma and short columella; tarsal bone anomalies; (c) autosomal dominant inheritance in one family.

LENNOX-GASTAUT SYNDROME (CHILDHOOD EPILEPTIC ENCEPHALOPATHY)

Clinical Manifestations: Onset of symptoms usually before the age of 5 years: *mixed seizure disorder:* minor motor; tonic-clonic; atypical absence; partial seizures; disordered sleep; electroencephalography *(generalized 1.5 to 2.5 per second spike-wave discharges; etc.); intellectual impairment.*

Radiologic Manifestations: Ventricular dilatation; cerebral atrophy; double cortex (subcortical neuronal tissue separated from the cortex by a layer of white matter); positron emission tomographic scan *(hypometabolism:* unilateral focal; unilateral diffuse; bilateral diffuse).

LENZ MICROPHTHALMIA SYNDROME

Clinical Manifestations: (a) *microphthalmia or anophthalmia; mental retardation; microcephaly; malformations of the pinnae* (tags; pits); *dental anomalies:* peglike teeth; diastemas; irregular tooth eruption; etc.; (b) X-linked recessive inheritance.

Radiologic Manifestations: Renal anomalies (horseshoe kidneys; ectopic kidney; duplication); kyphoscoliosis; lordosis; thin clavicles; clinodactyly; camptodactyly; syndactyly; webbed toes; intestinal anomalies.

LEOPARD SYNDROME

Clinical Manifestations: (a) *lentigines;* (b) cardiac conduction defect; hypertrophic obstructive cardiomyopathy-lentiginosis (Moynahan syndrome); pulmonary valvular stenosis; (c) genital anomalies: hypospadias; cryptorchidism; gonadal hypoplasia; late puberty; (d) retardation of growth; (e) sensorineural deafness; (f) miscellaneous abnormalities: association with steatocystoma multiplex and hyperelastic skin; Chiari I malformation; etc.; (g) autosomal dominant inheritance.

Radiologic Manifestations: (a) *cardiovascular abnormalities:* pulmonary valvular stenosis; hypertrophic cardiomyopathy; infundibular or supravalvular pulmonic stenosis; subaortic stenosis; (b) skeletal abnormalities: skeletal maturation retardation; pectus carinatum or excavatum; kyphoscoliosis; winging scapulae; hypermobile joints; cubitus valgus; rib anomalies; hypoplastic fifth digit; syndactyly, zygodactyly; cervical spine fusion; spina bifida occulta; Madelung deformity of the wrist; delayed healing of fractures; severe scoliosis with posterior spinal fusion.

Note: *LEOPARD* is an acronym: *L*entigines; *E*lectrocardiographic conduction abnormalities; *O*cular hypertelorism; *P*ulmonary stenosis; *A*bnormal genitalia; *R*etardation of growth; *D*eafness.

LÉRI SYNDROME (PLEONOSTEOSIS)

Clinical Manifestations: (a) *shortness of stature; mongoloid facies;* (b) *limb abnormalities:* short and spadelike hands; flexion contractures of the digits of the hands and feet, broad thumbs in the valgus position; cubitus valgus; limitation of motion of the joints; carpal tunnel syndrome; genu recurvatum; Morton metatarsalgia; (c) autosomal dominant inheritance with good penetrance and variable expression.

Radiologic Manifestations: (a) *increase in width of the bones, in particular those of the hands, feet, and vertebrae;* bizarre enlargement of the posterior neural arches of the cervical vertebrae; a relative decrease in the anteroposterior diameter of the vertebral bodies of L2 and L3; *flexion contractures of the digits of the hands and feet;* (b) miscellaneous abnormalities: skeletal maturation retardation; ischemic necrosis of the femoral heads; spinal cord compression.

LERICHE SYNDROME

Clinical Manifestations: *Intermittent claudication;* weakness of lower limbs; soft-tissue atrophy of both lower limbs; pallor of the legs and feet on standing; absence of trophic changes of the skin or nails; slow wound healing; *inability to maintain erection;* absent or very poor pulse over the aorta and iliac arteries and in the periphery.

Radiologic Manifestations: Calcification at the aortic bifurcation; *aortic occlusion at the bifurcation; collateral circulation;* contrast computed tomography with bolus injection demonstrating a sclerotic, normal-caliber aorta with a hypodense center below the level of the renal arteries.

LHERMITTE-DUCLOS DISEASE

Clinical Manifestations: (a) *symptoms related to the mass effect: intracranial hypertension; cerebellovestibular signs;* visual disturbances; respiratory arrest; (b) miscellaneous abnormalities: megalencephaly in about 50% of the cases; polydactyly; association with Cowden syndrome; cutaneous hemangiomas; parotid carcinoma; local gigantism; neurofibromatosis; malignant occipital astrocytoma.

Pathology: Marked enlargement of cerebellar folia (focal or diffuse); hypertrophied granular-cell neurons and hypermyelinization of their axons (dysplastic gangliocytoma).

Radiologic Manifestations: (a) *cerebellar enlargement, prominent cerebellar folia; deformed fourth ventricle; hypodense nonenhancing mass in the posterior fossa (computed tomography);* obstructive hydrocephalus; focal calcification associated with the lesion; *inhomogeneous signal on short TR/short TE MR, increased signal intensity on TR/long TE, no enhancement of the lesions with gadolinium administration* (exception: a case with enhancement reported); heterotopia; (b) miscellaneous abnormalities: leontiasis ossea; thinning of the occipital squamosa adjacent to the cerebellar lesion; vascular contrast enhancement.

Note: Owing to the association of Lhermitte-Duclos disease and Cowden syndrome, the possibility of these two conditions representing a single "phacomatosis" has been suggested.

LIPOID DERMATOARTHRITIS

Clinical Manifestations: Onset of symptoms between adolescence and senescence: (a) *cutaneous papules; cutaneous and subcutaneous nodular lesions* (ears, bridge of the nose, scalp, dorsum of the hands, and nail beds the most common sites); (b) polyarthritis usually preceding the cutaneous eruptions by an average of 3 years; progressive crippling deformities of the hands; (c) leonine facies in advanced stage of disease.

Pathology: Lipid-laden giant histiocytes in the skin and synovial lesions.

Radiologic Manifestations: (a) *juxtaarticular erosions at insertion of synovia;* (b) *destruction of articular cartilage and subchondral bones of the phalanges,* which may in progressive cases result in telescoping of soft tissues; destruction of odontoid process and atlas; atlantoaxial subluxation; (c) thinning of distal phalanges; (d) miscellaneous abnormalities: marginal erosion (feet; shoulders; wrists; hips; knees; sternomanubrial joints); sacroiliac joint ankylosis; nonclassified soft-tissue masses.

LISSENCEPHALIES

A group of migrational disorders of brain, classified into three types:
Tables SY-L-1, SY-L-2, and SY-L-3.

Table SY-L-1   Characteristics of Patients with Type I Lissencephaly

	Miller-Dieker Syndrome	Norman-Roberts Syndrome	Neu-Laxova Syndrome
Brain	Lissencephaly	Lissencephaly	Lissencephaly
Head and face	Microcephaly, bitemporal hollowing, prominent occiput, *high forehead with vertical midline wrinkling, anteverted nares, low-set ears with anomalies* and micrognathia	Microcephaly, bitemporal hollowing, slightly prominent occiput, sloping forehead. *Nares are not upturned, normal ears,* eyes widely set with prominent nasal bridge, micrognathia	Microcephaly, *malformed low-set ears,* receding forehead, grotesque facial appearance with bulging eyes
Neurologic	Early hypotonia with subsequent hypertonia with opisthotonic posturing, seizures, severe mental retardation, decreased spontaneous movement and poor feeding	Profound mental retardation, decreased spontaneous activity, poor feeding, seizures	
Growth	Low birth weight with severe postnatal growth deficiency	Poor (delayed)	
Others	Congenital heart defects, polydactyly and other visceral anomalies	Clinodactyly, chordee	Atrophic muscles, camptodactyly, syndactyly of toes and fingers, hypoplastic genitalia
Etiology	Deficiency (partial deletion) in the 17th chromosome	Autosomal recessive or sporadic	Autosomal recessive or sporadic
Survival	3 to 18 months	2 to 12 months	Death in utero

From Byrd SE, Osborn RE, Bohan TP et al: The CT and MR evaluation of migrational disorders of the brain. Part I. Lissencephaly and pachygyria, *Pediatr Radiol* 19:151, 1989. Used by permission.

Table SY-L-2   Characteristics of Patients with Type II Lissencephaly—Walker-Warburg and Cerebro-Oculo-Muscular Syndrome

Brain	Lissencephaly, hydrocephalus, Dandy-Walker cyst or cerebellar atrophy or posterior cephaloceles
Head and face	Macrocephaly; no typical facial characteristics, but the ears may be low-set and malformed; micrognathia
Neurologic	Profound mental retardation, decreased spontaneous activity, severe hypotonia, seizures
Growth	Normal at birth, subsequently growth deficiency
Eyes	Retinal dysplasia, microphthalmia, colobomas, leukomas, optic nerve hypoplasia and/or gliosis
Muscles	Congenital muscular dystrophy in all patients with cerebro-oculo-muscular syndrome
Other	Cryptorchism
Etiology	Autosomal recessive or sporadic
Survival	Birth to 5 months

From Byrd SE, Osborn RE, Bohan TP et al: The CT and MR evaluation of migrational disorders of the brain. Part I. Lissencephaly and pachygyria, *Pediatr Radiol* 19:151, 1989. Used by permission.

Table SY-L-3   Characteristics of Patients with Type III Lissencephaly

	Isolated Lissencephaly Syndrome	Cerebro-Cerebellar Lissencephaly Syndrome
Brain	Lissencephaly	Lissencephaly, severe cerebellar and brain-stem atrophy
Head and face	Microcephaly, no typical facial features, bitemporal hollowing, prominent occiput, micrognathia	Microcephaly, no typical facial features, mild bitemporal hollowing, sloping forehead, micrognathia
Neurologic	Profound mental retardation, decreased spontaneous activity, early hypotonia, poor feeding, seizures	Severe hypotonia and seizures with no spontaneous movements
Growth	Markedly delayed	
Etiology	Autosomal recessive or sporadic	Autosomal recessive or sporadic
Survival	1 to 6 years	Birth to 1 month

From Byrd SE, Osborn RE, Bohan TP et al: The CT and MR evaluation of migrational disorders of the brain. Part I. Lissencephaly and pachygyria, *Pediatr Radiol* 19:151, 1989. Used by permission.

LOCKED-IN SYNDROME

Clinical and Radiologic Manifestations: *Paralysis (loss of all voluntary movements) except for eye and eyelid movements; usually normal* *mental state and consciousness; lesion in the ventral pontine* (infarct; tumor; hemorrhage; trauma; inflammatory diseases).

LÖFFLER SYNDROME

Clinical Manifestations: *Chest pain; dyspnea; slight fever; cough; wheezing; peripheral eosinophilia;* bronchoalveolar lavage: eosinophilia.

Radiologic Manifestations: *Transient and migratory patchy pulmonary infiltrations:* single or multiple peripheral areas of consolidation, often homogeneous, ill-defined, and nonsegmental; changing pattern (chest radiographs and computed tomography).

Note: The original description of the disease by Löffler included the following manifestations: *fleeting and transient pulmonary infiltrates with peripheral blood eosinophilia in mildly infected or asymptomatic patients.*

LUTEMBACHER SYNDROME

Clinical and Radiologic Manifestations: (a) *atrial septal defect associated with mitral valve stenosis;* continuous murmur originating from the accelerated blood flow passing through the small atrial septal defect (Doppler echography); varying degrees of *cardiomegaly; marked right atrial enlargement;* normal or slightly enlarged left atrial and ventricular chambers; *dilated pulmonary artery and branches; diminished rate of mitral valve closure; thickened mitral leaflet; abnormal diastolic anterior motion of the posterior mitral valve leaflet; paradoxical motion of the interventricular septum;* (b) miscellaneous abnormalities: cyanosis and digital clubbing in a patient with iatrogenic atrial septal defect (balloon dilatation of the mitral valve).

LYNCH SYNDROMES I AND II

(A) LYNCH SYNDROME I (SITE-SPECIFIC FAMILIAL COLONIC CANCER): Colonic mucinous or colloid-type malignancies (without polyposis) occurring usually at early ages and often located in the proximal segment of the colon; multiple primary carcinomas may be present at the time of initial investigation; high likelihood of cancer recurrence if part of the colon is not removed; autosomal dominant inheritance.

(B) LYNCH SYNDROME II (CANCER FAMILY SYNDROME): Features of Lynch syndrome I associated with cancer in the female genital tract and other sites, in particular carcinoma of the endometrium and ovary; also reported are transitional cell carcinoma, carcinoma of the pancreas, gastric carcinoma, complete intestinal metaplasia, chronic atrophic gastritis restricted to the antrum, carcinoma of the ureter, and laryngeal carcinoma.

M

MACRODYSTROPHIA LIPOMATOSA

Clinical Manifestations: A form of localized gigantism due to progressive hypertrophy of all the mesenchymal elements (fibroadipose, vessels, nerves, tendons, and bones) with a disproportionate increase in the fibroadipose tissue: *slowly progressive unilateral focal gigantism;* progressive arthropathy; psoriasiform rash.

Radiologic Manifestations: (a) *marked proliferation of subcutaneous fat; enlargement of bones; marginal erosions; exostoses; joint destruction; irregular periosteal reaction; ankylosis by bands of dense bone*; absence of angioma or arteriovenous fistula; (b) miscellaneous abnormalities: early maturation of epiphyseal ossification centers in the involved area; thinning of metacarpals; thinning of metatarsals; syndactyly; polydactyly; brachydactyly; symphalangism; exostosis-like bony overgrowth along interphalangeal joints.

MAFFUCCI SYNDROME

Clinical Manifestations: *Hemangiomatosis of skin,* often cavernous, often of limbs and other soft tissues; arteriovenous shunts; *dwarfism with deformity of affected extremities; huge and hard nodules and masses (enchondromas);* associated with malignant tumors; platelet trapping.

Radiologic Manifestations: (a) large expansile *enchondromas* of long bones and bones of hands and feet; soft-tissue masses and *phleboliths; hemangiomas of soft tissues and bones; phlebectasia;* (b) miscellaneous abnormalities: malignant degeneration of bone lesions; cervical spine involvement; chondrosarcoma of the nasal septum; adrenal Cushing syndrome; multiple enchondromas associated with spindle cell hemangioendotheliomas (a variant of Maffucci syndrome); pathologic fractures; etc.

MALABSORPTION SYNDROME

Classification: (a) primary: celiac disease; nontropical sprue; tropical sprue; (b) constitutional diseases; small-bowel diseases; postsurgical; etc.

Clinical Manifestations: *Bulky, fatty, and foul-smelling stools;* weight loss; growth retardation; abdominal distension; skin pigmentation; atrophy of intestinal villi; development of intestinal lymphoma or carcinoma in long-standing sprue; etc.

Radiologic Manifestations: (a) *dilatation of the small bowel with abnormal contractility; segmentation; hypersecretion; decrease in promi-*

nence of mucosal folds; prolonged transit time; moulage sign; duodenal changes (dilatation; decrease in the number of mucosal folds; thickening and asymmetry of the mucosal folds); nonhomogeneous appearance of barium granules throughout colon (less common with modern barium suspension); adaptation of the ileum in nontropical sprue (increase in the ileal fold pattern and a decrease in the jejunal fold pattern; reversed pattern representing chronic inflammation and atrophy of the jejunum and compensatory hypertrophy of the ileum); floating feces (horizontal beam, double-contrast enema); (b) miscellaneous abnormalities: small-bowel ulcer; intramural hematoma; thick mesentery in sprue; mixed connective tissue disease complicated by pneumatosis cystoides intestinalis and malabsorption syndrome.

MALLORY-WEISS SYNDROME

Clinical Manifestations: (a) *painless hematemesis (*usually following straining or vomiting); *pallor and tachycardia;* endoscopic visualization of the *laceration* site; (b) miscellaneous abnormalities: Mallory-Weiss syndrome complicating pregnancy in a patient with scleroderma; association with hemophilia A and chronic liver disease.

Radiologic Manifestations: Barium outlining the laceration in the form of a *streaky collection of media in the wall* (roentgenographic detection uncommon); *arteriographic demonstration of the site of laceration in patients with active bleeding* (distal esophagus: gastroesophageal junction).

MANDIBULOACRAL DYSPLASIA

Clinical Manifestations: Very variable phenotype: (a) *atrophic skin; poikiloderma; nail dysplasia; alopecia; broad short phalanges; facial hypoplasia; mandibular hypoplasia; pseudoexophthalmos; beaked nose; short stature; stiff joint;* (b) autosomal recessive inheritance.

Radiologic Manifestations: *Delayed cranial suture closure; wormian bones; mandibular hypoplasia; acro-osteolysis;* clavicular hypoplasia; rib hypoplasia; soft-tissue calcification.

MAN-IN-THE-BARREL SYNDROME

Clinical Manifestations: *Acute cerebral hypoperfusion* associated with severe hypotension; brachial diplegia without motor disturbance of the legs; facial grimacing; coma.

Radiologic Manifestations: *Bilateral watershed infarction in the temporooccipital area and in the frontal white matter between the supply territories of the anterior and middle cerebral arteries.*

MARDEN-WALKER SYNDROME

Clinical Manifestations: (a) *psychomotor retardation;* (b) *growth retardation;* (c) *fixed facial expression; blepharophimosis; low-set ears; micrognathia; hypertelorism; epicanthal folds; strabismus; cleft palate; small mouth; everted lower lips; long philtrum; upturned nose tip;* (d) *congenital joint contractures; reduced muscle mass; hypotonia; kyphoscoliosis;* (e) neurologic abnormalities; (f) probably autosomal recessive inheritance.

Radiologic Manifestations: (a) microcephaly; cortical atrophy; ventriculomegaly, agenesis of the corpus callosum; hypoplastic brain stem; hypoplasia of the inferior vermis and of the cerebellar hemispheres; enlarged cisterna magna and fourth ventricle; colpocephaly; (b) miscellaneous abnormalities: hypoplastic kidney; microcystic renal disease; congenital heart disease; dextrocardia; pyloric stenosis; Dandy-Walker malformation.

MARFAN SYNDROME

Clinical Manifestations: A disorder of connective tissue with multisystem manifestations.

(A) GENERAL MANIFESTATIONS: (a) *tall stature; long limbs; arachnodactyly; ectopia lentis;* cardiovascular abnormalities; dolichocephaly; narrow and highly arched palate; dental crowding; (b) miscellaneous abnormalities: learning disability; endocrine and growth disorders; microhematuria and proteinuria.

(B) INFANTILE MARFAN SYNDROME: (a) dolichocephaly; a characteristic facies (broad nasal bridge, down-slanting palpebral fissures, and low-set ears); crumbled ears; highly arched palate; cleft palate; micrognathia; blue sclerae; retinal detachment; iridodonesis; megalocornea; *dislocated lenses;* (b) *serious cardiovascular pathology (mitral valve prolapse; valvular regurgitation; aortic root dilatation);* (c) *respiratory problems* (pneumonia; emphysema; atelectasis); anterior chest deformity; (d) *hyperextensible joints; flexion contracture; arachnodactyly;* (e) miscellaneous abnormalities: hip dislocation; foot deformities; femoral fracture.

(C) Autosomal dominant inheritance with variable expressivity and high degree of penetrance; prenatal diagnosis by identification of a fibrillin-1 mutation in chorionic villus sample.

Radiologic Manifestations

(A) SKELETAL SYSTEM: (a) long, tall, and thick skull; long face with retrognathia (associated with pulmonary dysfunction in some cases); enlarged paranasal sinuses; (b) atlantoaxial instability; kyphoscoliosis; laxity of lumbar vertebral joints; spondylolisthesis; increased interpediculate space and wide spinal canal; thoracic meningocele; sacral abnormalities (expansion of the central sacral spinal canal; enlargement of sacral foramina in association with extensive bony erosion; sacral meningocele); straight back; Schmorl nodes; dislocation of the sternoclavicular joint; (c) elongated fingers; abnormal metacarpophalangeal pattern profile (a relatively long metacarpal 1 and short distal phalanx 1); hip dislocation; perilunate dislocation unrelated to trauma; patella alta, genu recurvatum; protrusio acetabuli; flexion deformities; clinodactyly; foot deformities (pronation; pes planus; calcaneoplanovalgus; clubfoot; vertical talus; calcaneal spur; hallux valgus; hammer toe; long first digit); slipped capital femoral epiphysis; (d) osteoporosis, in particular in women; (e) bone maturity in childhood between chronologic and statural age.

(B) CHEST: Pectus carinatum or pectus excavatum; rib notching; congenital malformations of the bronchi; bronchiectasis; *pulmonary dysaeration* (pulmonary emphysema; bullae); spontaneous pneumothorax; cystic disease; diffuse reticular interstitial densities; lung perfusion abnormalities.

(C) CARDIOVASCULAR SYSTEM: *Mitral abnormalities* with insufficiency; *aortic sinus dilatation; aortic insufficiency;* aortic and pulmonary arterial aneurysm; aneurysm of the ductus arteriosus; isolated aneurysm of the abdominal aorta; *cystic medial necrosis of the aorta* and occasionally of peripheral vessels; aortic dissection; multiple small intimal flaps; coarctation of the aorta; dissecting aneurysm of the ductus arteriosus; echocardiography (aortic enlargement; abnormal compliance of the aortic wall; prolapse of the posterior leaflet of the mitral valve; appearance of shaggy echoes on the anterior mitral leaflet); calcification of an incompetent foramen ovale; atrial septal aneurysm; massive calcification of the mitral valve annulus in young adults.

(D) CENTRAL NERVOUS SYSTEM: *Dural ectasia;* thoracic meningocele; pelvic meningoceles; meningeal cysts.

(E) DIGESTIVE SYSTEM: Gastrointestinal diverticulosis; achalasia of the esophagus.

MARFANOID HYPERMOBILITY SYNDROME

Clinical and Radiologic Manifestations: *Marfanoid habitus; generalized hypermobility of the joints; hyperextensibility of the skin;* cardiovascular abnormalities (floppy mitral valve; aortic aneurysm; aortic regurgitation; dissecting aortic aneurysm; coarctation of the aorta); pectus excavatum; genu recurvatum; scoliosis.

MARINESCO-SJÖGREN SYNDROME

Clinical Manifestations: A degenerative disease: (a) *cerebellar ataxia; spasticity; mental deficiency; cataracts; myopathy;* neurogenic muscular atrophy; progressive ophthalmoplegia; reduced cytochrome c oxidase in muscle; etc.; (b) autosomal recessive inheritance.

Radiologic Manifestations: (a) diffuse brain atrophy of mild to moderate degree involving primarily the white matter of the cerebrum, cerebellum, brain stem, and cervical spinal cord; small cerebellar vermis and absence of the posterior pituitary gland (case report); (b) positron emission tomography: decreased metabolic rate in the thalamus; (c) miscellaneous abnormalities: microcrania; skeletal abnormalities (talipes equinovarus; pes planus; short digits; kyphosis; skeletal maturation retardation); irregular teeth.

MARSHALL SYNDROME

Clinical Manifestations: (a) *short nose; anteverted nostrils; flat malar bones; myopia with vitreoretinal degeneration;* congenital cataract; prominent upper incisors; mental retardation; retinal tear and detachment; cleft palate; hypohidrotic ectodermal dysplasia; short stature; Robin sequence; deafness; (b) autosomal dominant inheritance.

Radiologic Manifestations: Thickened calvaria; beaked or bullet-shaped vertebra in the younger patient; platyspondyly with irregular ossification of end-plates; small iliac bones with irregular lateral border; mild bowing of the radius and ulna; coxa valga; poorly formed and irregular epiphyses; dural calcification.

MARSHALL-SMITH SYNDROME

Clinical Manifestations: (a) *craniofacial dysmorphism:* long cranium; prominent forehead; micrognathia; prominent eyes associated with shallow orbits; underdeveloped and upturned nose; blue sclerae; coarse eyebrows; (b) *relative failure to thrive (underweight for length; accelerated linear growth);* (c) *motor and mental retardation;* (d) *widening of proximal and middle phalanges of hands;* (e) *respiratory difficulties:* apneic spells; pneumonia; stridor; laryngomalacia; pulmonary hypertension.

Radiologic Manifestations: (a) *premature appearance of secondary ossification centers (prenatal);* (b) *prominent forehead; shallow orbits; hypoplastic mandibular rami;* (c) *wide proximal and middle phalanges of hands with pointed distal ends (bullet-shaped); narrowness of the distal phalanges;* (d) pneumonia; atelectasis; (e) miscellaneous abnormalities: unusual protrusion of the supraoccipital bone behind the foramen magnum and the posterior arch of C1; hypoplasia of the odontoid; instability at craniocervical junction; atlantoaxial subluxation; compression and kinking of medulla and cord; decreased anteroposterior diameter of vertebral bodies; mild anterior wedging of vertebrae.

MASA SYNDROME

Clinical and Radiologic Manifestations: Clinical variability: (a) *M*ental retardation; *A*phasia; *S*huffling gait, *S*pasticity; *A*dducted thumbs; (b) miscellaneous abnormalities: hydrocephalus, agenesis of the corpus callosum; (c) X-linked inheritance; linkage to Xq28; occurrence of MASA syndrome and X-linked hydrocephalus in one family.

MAYER-ROKITANSKY-KÜSTER SYNDROME

Classification: (a) type A (typical form): normal appearing external genitalia; *absent vagina* (only a shallow vaginal pouch present); *absent uterus* (only symmetric uterine remnants present); normal fallopian tubes; normal ovaries; normal ovarian function; no renal anomalies; (b) type B (atypical form): *asymmetric uterine muscular buds* (aplasia of one or both buds, or asymmetry of the buds, if both present); *abnormally developed fallopian tubes* (hypoplasia or aplasia of one or both tubes); *ovarian anomalies* (inguinal hernia containing an ovary; no descent of ovary; absent ovary; streak ovaries); *renal anomalies* (unilateral agenesis, pelvic kidney).
Clinical Manifestations: (a) *primary amenorrhea; sterility; dyspareunia; absent vagina; normal genotype, phenotype, and endocrine status;* (b) miscellaneous abnormalities: stapedial ankylosis; pseudohematuria caused by uterourethral fistula; ovarian cancer; ovarian teratoma; pseudocyst of the thyroglossal duct; etc.
Radiologic Manifestations: (a) *genitourinary anomalies*: absence of vagina; thin uncanalized vaginal plate; uterus anomalies; renal anomalies; (b) skeletal anomalies: brachymesophalangia of digits 2 to 5; long proximal phalanx of digits 3 and 4; long metacarpals of digits 1 to 4; radial dysplasia; carpal abnormalities; phocomelia; vertebral anomalies.

MAZABRAUD SYNDROME

Pathology: *Intramuscular myxoma; fibrous dysplasia.*
Clinical Manifestations: (a) *skeletal deformity and fracture associated with fibrous dysplasia;* (b) *intramuscular mass;* (c) oncogenic osteomalacia.
Radiologic Manifestations: (a) *skeletal fibrous dysplasia;* (b) soft-tissue tumor(s): hyperechoic intramuscular tumor(s); magnetic resonance imaging: hypointense to muscle on T_1-weighted images and hyperintense on T_2-weighted and STIR images; angiography: avascular soft-tissue mass.

McCUNE-ALBRIGHT SYNDROME (Albright Syndrome; Weil-Albright Syndrome)

The Triad: (a) *patchy cutaneous pigmentation;* (b) *sexual precocity;* (c) *polyostotic fibrous dysplasia.*

Clinical Manifestations: Onset of symptoms in childhood: (a) *precocious puberty;* (b) *café au lait spots,* often unilateral on the same side as the bone manifestation; (c) *various endocrinopathies;* (d) miscellaneous abnormalities: height and weight greater than 95th percentile for age; high-output cardiac failure; (e) sporadic; female preponderance; reported familial cases questionable; mutations in the gene for the alpha subgroup of the G1 protein in a patchy mosaic pattern.

Radiologic Manifestations: (a) *advanced skeletal maturation;* premature closure of growth plates resulting in short stature; (b) *polyostotic fibrous dysplasia;* (c) pathologic fractures; (d) upward convexity of the intrasellar contents, focal area of abnormal attenuation of the pituitary; increase in the height (greater than 7 mm) of the pituitary; pituitary adenoma; (e) miscellaneous abnormalities: ovarian cysts in childhood; nephrocalcinosis in an infant with the clinical diagnosis of McCune-Albright syndrome associated with Cushing syndrome; kyphoscoliosis; soft-tissue myxoma and hypophosphatemic rickets; heteromultinodular thyroid gland in euthyroid girls with McCune-Albright syndrome.

Note: (a) sexual precocity may be gonadotropin dependent (true precocious puberty), or gonadotropin independent (precocious pseudopuberty) due to autonomous ovarian hyperactivity; (b) autonomous multiendocrine hyperfunction in some cases (at least four primary endocrinopathies in one case: precocious puberty, hyperthyroidism, primary hyperparathyroidism, and hyperprolactinemia).

MECKEL SYNDROME (Gruber Syndrome)

Clinical Manifestations: Phenotypic variability: (a) *microcephaly; occipital encephalocele; cleft lip; cleft palate;* (b) *polydactyly* (hands; feet); (c) miscellaneous abnormalities: clubfeet; microphthalmia; anophthalmia; elevated α-fetoprotein in midtrimester; association with Mayer-Rokitansky-Küster syndrome; etc.; (d) autosomal recessive inheritance; the Meckel syndrome with multiple congenital anomalies mapped to 17q21–q24.

Radiologic Manifestations: (a) *brain dysgenesis: encephalocele;* hydrocephalus; etc.; (b) *polydactyly* (usually postaxial); short limbs; bowing of the long tubular bones; (c) *renal cystic dysplasia.*

Note: Diagnostic triad: *occipital encephalocele, polycystic kidneys, and polydactyly* (present in about 60% of the cases).

MECONIUM PLUG SYNDROME

Clinical Manifestations: Abdominal distension; vomiting of green-stained material; *passage of meconium plug,* usually followed by clinical improvement; ileal meconium plug (white plug) associated with a high incidence of complications; association with other diseases: cystic fibrosis; Hirschsprung disease; exocrine pancreatic insufficiency; intussusception (in ileal meconium plug); small left colon syndrome; maternal and postnatal hypermagnesemia.

Radiologic Manifestations: *Small-bowel and large-bowel distension; mottled or bulky intraluminal colonic meconium masses;* presacral "mass" on a lateral radiogram of the abdomen (intraluminal rectal plug); air-fluid levels in the bowel uncommon; contrast enema (*meconium cast in the colon;* long narrow segment of bowel [small left colon]); prenatal ultrasound (progressive dilatation of intestines).

MEGACYSTIS-MEGAURETER SYNDROME

Clinical Manifestations: *Vesicoureteral reflux with constant recycling of large volumes of refluxed urine:* fever, abdominal pain, failure to thrive; infrequent voiding; urinary retention; enuresis; weak urinary stream; urinary tract infection in about three fourths of cases.

Radiologic Manifestations: (a) *large-capacity, smooth, and thin-walled bladder; massive vesicoureteral reflux; no bladder outlet or urethral obstruction;* (b) prenatal diagnosis by ultrasonograph: bilateral hydroureteronephrosis; a large, smooth, thin-walled bladder; normal volume of amniotic fluid.

MEIGE-NONNE-MILROY DISEASE

Clinical Manifestations: (a) *lymphedema,* often of the lower limbs; (b) miscellaneous abnormalities: congenital chylous ascites; protein-losing lymphangiectasia of the bowel; pleural effusion; susceptibility of affected tissues to infection; acute nephritis; (c) autosomal dominant inheritance.

Radiologic Manifestations: *Hypoplasia or absence of lymphatic channels;* dermal lymphatic filling in feet on visual and roentgenographic lymphangiograms; weakness of the lymphatic wall resulting in extravasation; absence of lymphatic valves.

MEIGS SYNDROME (DEMONS-MEIGS SYNDROME)

Clinical and Radiologic Manifestations: (a) *benign or malignant ovarian tumor; pleural effusion,* spontaneously disappearing after removal of ovarian tumor; *ascites*; (b) miscellaneous abnormalities: serous ade-nofibroma of ovary presenting with a diaphragmatic pleural nodule (mesothelial hyperplasia and lymphatic duct proliferation).

MENDELSON SYNDROME

Clinical Manifestations: (a) sudden postoperative appearance of pul-monary symptoms in patients with previously normal respiratory system: *tachypnea; tachycardia; wheezes (bronchoconstriction); rhonchi; crepi-tant rales;* fall in arterial oxygen tension; (b) miscellaneous abnormalities: pulmonary edema and shock; association with dermatomyositis.

Radiologic Manifestations: Irregular *patchy or confluent lung densi-ties* (frequently bilateral).

MÉNÉTRIER DISEASE

Clinical Manifestations: *Epigastric pain;* ulcerlike symptoms; anorexia; vomiting; diarrhea; hematemesis; melena; *hypoproteinemia; edema; ascites; large rugae (sometimes present throughout the stomach, others limited to various segments of the stomach, most prominent along the greater curvature).*

Radiologic Manifestations: (a) *enlargement of gastric rugae; thick gastric wall; mucus mixed with barium;* mucus cysts; (b) miscellaneous abnormalities: ascites; pleural effusion; bowel-wall edema; protein leakage into the bowel (detectable by Tc-99m–labeled human serum albumin).

Note: There is a significant difference between the disease in children and adults: association with cytomegalovirus infection and generally very good prognosis (benign, self-limited, and transient) in children; commonly chronic course in adults, with remission in some cases.

MICHELS SYNDROME

Clinical and Radiologic Manifestations: (a) short stature, growth deficiency; microcephaly; craniosynostosis; mental deficiency; blepharo-phimosis; blepharoptosis; epicanthus inversus; anterior chamber defects; ocular hypertelorism; abnormal eye motility; glaucoma; (b) probably auto-somal recessive inheritance.

MICROCEPHALIC OSTEODYSPLASTIC PRIMORDIAL DWARFISM

Classification and Differential Diagnosis: Refer to Tables SY-M-1 and SY-M-2.

Table SY-M-1   Clinical Features in the Differential Diagnosis of Primordial Dwarfism

	Seckel Syndrome Primordial Dwarfism	Osteo-dysplastic Primordial Dwarfism Type I	Osteo-dysplastic Primordial Dwarfism Type II	Osteo-dysplastic Primordial Dwarfism Type III	Microcephalic Osteodysplastic Dysplasia
General					
Low birth weight	+	+	+	+	-
Microcephaly	+	+	+	+	+
Intellectual deficits	+	+	+	+	+/-
Early death	-	+/-	-	+	-
Face					
Prominent eyes	+/-	-	+/-	+	+
Cataracts	-	-	-	-	+
Beaked nose	+	+	+	+	+
Micrognathia	+	+	+	+	+
Dysplastic ears	+/-	+	+	+	-
Skeletal					
Small anterior fontanel	+/-	+	+/-	+	-
Delayed closure of anterior fontanel	-	-	-	-	+
Limited extension at elbows	+/-	+/-	+/-	-	+/-
Clubfoot deformity	-	-	-	-	+
Pectus deformity	-	-	-	-	+

From Hersh JH, Joyce MR, Spranger J et al: Microcephalic osteodysplastic dysplasia, *Am J Med Genet* 51:194, 1994. Reprinted by permission of Wiley-Liss, Inc., a division of John Wiley & Sons, Inc. Copyright © 1994.

Table SY-M-2   Radiographic Signs in the Differential Diagnosis of Primordial Dwarfism

	Seckel Syndrome Primordial Dwarfism	Osteo-dysplastic Primordial Dwarfism Type I	Osteo-dysplastic Primordial Dwarfism Type II	Osteo-dysplastic Primordial Dwarfism Type III	Microcephalic Osteodysplastic Dysplasia
Steep base of skull	-	+/-	-	+	-
Platyspondyly	-	-	-	+	+
Irregularity of vertebral bodies	-	-	-	-	+
Odontoid hypoplasia	-	-	-	-	+
Hypoplasia of L1	-	-	-	-	+
Syrinx of spinal cord	-	-	-	-	+
Bowing of humeri/femur	-	+	-	-	-
Overtubulation of long bones	-	-	-	+	+
Dysplastic radial head	+/-	+	+/-	-	+/-
Large epiphyses	-	-	+	-	+
Coxa valga	-	-	-	-	+
"Dysplastic" hips	+/-	+	+/-	+	-
Metaphyseal irregularities	-	-	+ (distal femoral metaphyses)	+	+
Short metacarpals	-	-	+	-	+
Short metatarsals	-	-	-	-	+
Short phalanges	-	-	+	-	+
Coned and ivory epiphyses	-	-	-	-	+
Delayed bone age	+	+	+	+/-	-

From Hersh JH, Joyce MR, Spranger J et al: Microcephalic osteodysplastic dysplasia, *Am J Med Genet* 51:194, 1994. Reprinted by permission of Wiley-Liss, Inc., a division of John Wiley & Sons, Inc. Copyright © 1994.

Note: (a) the types I and III of microcephalic osteodysplastic primordial dwarfism are considered to be a single entity; some of the cases reported under the titles of types I and III have radiographic manifestations similar to cephaloskeletal dysplasia and may represent the same entity; (b) renal tubular leakage has been reported in type I/III of microcephalic osteodysplastic primordial dwarfism.

MIETENS-WEBER SYNDROME

Clinical Manifestations: (a) *mental retardation; growth failure;* small, narrow, and pointed nose with a depressed root; *bilateral opacity of the corneas; horizontal and rotational nystagmus; strabismus; flexion contracture of elbows;* atrophic calf muscles; (b) autosomal recessive or incompletely dominant inheritance.

Radiologic Manifestations: Dislocation of the head of the radius and absence of its epiphysis; abnormally short ulna and radius; clinodactyly; absent radii with radial deviation of the hands and flexed thumbs; absent fibula; clubfoot; pes valgus planus.

MIKULICZ SYNDROME

Definition: Any bilateral chronic enlargement of the salivary and lacrimal glands due to disease entities other than Mikulicz disease (benign lymphoepithelial lesions).

Clinical Manifestations: *Sialadenitis; sialosis* (nontender enlargement of the parotid glands); *multinodular enlargement of the gland; xerostomia;* absence or reduction of lacrimation.

Radiologic Manifestations: Sialographic findings of *ectasia of the ducts (sialadenitis); enlarged gland with sparse peripheral ducts (sialosis); decrease in the number of visualized duct radicles and displacement of ducts by granulomatous lesions;* destruction of the duct system in advanced stages.

MILLER-DIEKER SYNDROME (LISSENCEPHALY, TYPE I)

Clinical Manifestations: (a) *craniofacial dysmorphism:* microcephaly; hollow temples; dolichocephaly; micrognathia; anteversion of the nostrils; (b) *seizures* (generalized; infantile spasms-hypsarrhythmia); *poor reflexes; hypotonia; failure to thrive; poor motor development; inability to swallow; frequent pulmonary infections;* (c) chromosomal abnormalities: *deletion 17p13.3*; maternal cryptic translocation t(10;17)(q26.3;p13.3); etc.; (d) electroencephalography: high *alpha-beta* activity.

Radiologic Manifestations: *Microcephaly; smooth cortical surface (figure of eight shape) or decreased number of sulci; wide sylvian fissures; absence of insular opercularization; increased thickness of gray matter of the cortex; decreased white matter throughout the cerebral hemispheres; absence of or marked decrease in cortical-white matter interdigitations;* colpocephaly (localized dilatation of the atria and occipital horns); no infratentorial abnormalities or in some cases hypoplasia of the cerebellar hemispheres; mild hydrocephalus; round midline calcifications (in the septum pellucidum or genu of the corpus callosum); absence or hypoplasia of the corpus callosum; enlarged basal cisterns; Dandy-Walker anomaly.

MIRIZZI SYNDROME

Clinical Manifestations: *Obstructive jaundice;* cholecystitis; recurrent cholangitis; ultimately cholangitic cirrhosis.

Radiologic Manifestations: (a) *dilated intrahepatic duct associated with a normal-caliber distal duct and stone in the area of obstruction* (demonstrable by various imaging modalities); *delineation of the fistula and the obstructing stone* by endoscopic retrograde cholangiography; (b) miscellaneous abnormalities: liver atrophy; association with carcinoma (gallbladder; cystic duct).

MIXED CONNECTIVE TISSUE DISEASE (Sharp Syndrome)

Clinical Manifestations: (a) *fever; fatigue; weight loss; dyspnea; synovitis; swelling of the hands; polyarthralgia; dermatomyositis; myositis; Raynaud phenomenon; systemic lupus erythematosus–like rash;* rheumatoid-type nodules; (b) *high titer of IgM rheumatoid factors and antinuclear antibodies (directed against ribonuclear-sensitive nuclear antigens);* elevated sedimentation rate; anemia; leukopenia; thrombocytopenia; (c) pericarditis; asymmetric septal hypertrophy; left ventricular dilatation; progressive pulmonary deterioration; pulmonary hypertension; pulmonary vasculitis; pulmonary thromboembolic phenomena; (d) aspiration pneumonia; hypoventilatory respiratory failure; (e) dysphagia; *diminished esophageal motility;* diarrhea; (f) miscellaneous abnormalities: pneumatosis cystoides intestinalis and malabsorption syndrome; transverse myelopathy; diaphragmatic dysfunction.

Radiologic Manifestations: (a) diffuse or periarticular *osteoporosis; joint manifestations* (narrowing of joint spaces; erosion; bony ankylosis; subluxation; osteonecrosis); "penciling" of phalangeal tips; *resorption of the terminal tufts of the phalanges;* periarticular soft-tissue swelling; soft-tissue atrophy; soft-tissue calcification; (b) *esophageal dysfunction;* gastroesophageal reflux; (c) pulmonary infiltrates; pulmonary nodules; pulmonary infections; interstitial pulmonary fibrosis; pleural thickening; mediastinal adenopathy.

MÖBIUS SYNDROME

Clinical Manifestations: (a) *complete or partial cranial VII nerve paralysis;* unilateral or bilateral paralysis of other cranial nerves (III; IV; V; VI; IX; X; XII); (b) *limb malformations:* syndactyly; brachydactyly; absent digits; clubfoot; ectrodactyly; terminal transverse defects; digital contracture; etc.; (c) facial abnormalities: small palpebral fissures; epicanthal folds; hypertelorism; microstomia; bifid uvula; cleft palate; external ear deformity; micrognathia; (d) miscellaneous abnormalities: muscular involvement; neurobehavioral abnormalities; association with hypoglossia-hypodactylia anomalies; premature thelarche; crossed total hemihypertrophy; (e) most reported cases sporadic; considerable genetic heterogeneity (autosomal dominant, autosomal recessive, and X-linked recessive).

Radiologic Manifestations: (a) *motor disturbance of swallowing function;* chronic pneumonia; (b) *limb anomalies;* pectoral muscle deficiency; (c) central nervous system abnormalities: brain-stem hypoplasia/atrophy; unilateral cerebellar hypoplasia; small calcification in the pons and medulla (brain-stem nuclei); basal ganglia calcification; (d) fetal sonographic abnormalities: micrognathia, lack of normal fetal swallowing movements, and closed fist with the digits flexed over the thumbs.

Note: The term *Poland-Möbius* syndrome is used when the Möbius syndrome is associated with the absence of the pectoral major muscle and ipsilateral upper limb anomalies.

MOLDED BABY SYNDROME

Clinical and Radiologic Manifestations: *Plagiocephaly* (intrauterine molding); *pelvic obliquity associated with a unilateral (on the same side as the plagiocephaly) restriction of hip abduction in flexion;* scoliosis; torticollis; "bat" ears.

MORGAGNI-STEWART-MOREL SYNDROME (HYPEROSTOSIS FRONTALIS INTERNA)

Clinical Manifestations: Often occurring in women in the fifth decade of life: (a) *menstrual disorders; hirsutism; obesity;* (b) miscellaneous abnormalities: headaches; vertigo; fatigue; decrease in glucose tolerance; galactorrhea/hyperprolactinemia; violent headaches treated successfully with removal of the hypertrophic frontal bone; (c) familial cases have been reported; dominant (sex-limited autosomal or X-linked) transmission suggested.

Radiologic Manifestations: Gradual development of *symmetric internal hyperostosis of the calvaria,* most prominent in frontal region; bone scintigraphy (symmetric bifrontal high-uptake spreading laterally from and sparing the midline; "bull's eye" appearance in the frontal bone); indium-111 leukocyte imaging (uptake in the anterior portion of the calvarium); transient diminution of activity on early radionuclide images of brain with subsequent filling.

MORNING GLORY SYNDROME

Clinical Manifestations: (a) *strabismus; amblyopia; loss of visual acuity; refraction anomalies; enlarged, funnel-shaped, distorted, and excavated optic disc surrounded by an elevated annulus of chorioretinal atrophy and pigmentary changes;* (b) fluorescein angiography: *radially oriented exit of retinal vessels from the periphery of the disc;* (c) miscellaneous abnormalities: communication between the subretinal space and the vitreous cavity; association with midline craniofacial defect (cleft lip, cleft palate, sphenoethmoidal encephalocele, hypertelorism, bilateral dysplastic optic discs, and agenesis of the corpus callosum); association with coloboma of the optic nerve, porencephaly, and hydronephrosis in a newborn; association with chronic renal disease; association with basal encephalocele and progressive hormonal and visual disturbances.

Radiologic Manifestations: (a) *colobomatous area,* retinal detachment, cataract, thickened intraocular optic nerve and increased radiodensity in the postcontrast computed tomography; *normal retrobulbar optic nerve;* (b) miscellaneous abnormalities: enlarged retrobulbar optic nerve showing increased radiodensity on computed tomography and cavum vergae (case report); etc.

MOUNIER-KUHN SYNDROME

Clinical Manifestations: Congenital abnormality of trachea and main bronchi (absence or atrophy of elastic fibers and thinning of muscle): (a) *recurrent lower respiratory tract infection;* loud cough; hoarseness; dyspnea; copious purulent sputum production; (b) familial cases have been reported; autosomal recessive inheritance has been suggested.

Radiologic Manifestations: (a) *tracheobronchomegaly;* increase in lumen of the trachea with the Valsalva maneuver and narrowing with the Müller maneuver; (b) miscellaneous abnormalities: saclike recesses;

emphysema; pulmonary fibrosis, bullae; spontaneous pneumothorax; tracheomalacia with indentation of trachea anteriorly by the brachiocephalic artery.

MUIR-TORRE SYNDROME

Clinical and Radiologic Manifestations: (a) association of *single or multiple sebaceous gland tumor* (adenoma; epithelioma; carcinoma); and *internal malignancy* (colorectal, genitourinary; etc.); (b) miscellaneous abnormalities: association with acquired immunodeficiency syndrome; sebaceous carcinoma in an immunocompromised patient; metastatic carcinoma to retina in a patient with Muir-Torre syndrome; (c) autosomal dominant inheritance; variable penetrance.

MULIBREY NANISM

Clinical Manifestations: (a) prenatal growth deficiency; (b) *progressive growth failure;* hydrocephaloid head; *triangular face;* (c) *slenderness and muscular hypotonia;* (d) *peculiar voice;* (e) ocular abnormalities: *yellowish dots and pigment dispersion in the fundi; hypoplasia of the choroid;* strabismus; astigmatism, atrophy of the corneal epithelium; thickening of the Bowman membrane; (f) *hepatomegaly;* (g) *raised venous pressure;* cardiac lesions often associated with *pericardial constriction;* (h) cutaneous nevi flammei; (i) autosomal recessive inheritance.

Radiologic Manifestations: (a) dolichocephaly; J-shaped sella turcica; slightly increased basilar angle; *abnormally large cerebral ventricles and cisternae;* (b) cardiomegaly; pulmonary congestion; (c) ascites; (d) skeletal abnormalities; fibrous dysplasia of the tibia with progressive changes; fractures and pseudoarthrosis; thinness of long bones with a relative thickness of the cortex and very narrow or almost obstructed medullary channels.

Note: The acronym *MULIBREY* takes its origin from the names of the organs most prominently involved: *MU* (muscle), *LI* (liver), *BR* (brain), and *EY* (eyes).

MULTIPLE ENDOCRINE NEOPLASIA TYPE I (WERMER SYNDROME; MULTIPLE ENDOCRINE ADENOMATOSIS TYPE I)

Clinical Manifestations: Appear in most patients by the third or fourth decade of life: (a) *gastrinoma; severe peptic ulcer disease; insulinoma: hypoglycemia; VIPoma; glucagonoma; hypoaminoacidemia, weight loss; pancreatic polypeptide tumors; pituitary adenomas; Zollinger-Ellison syndrome* as a frequent component; (b) miscellaneous abnormalities: association with various tumors; presentation with hip fracture; (c) autosomal dominant inheritance; complete penetrance with variable expressivity.

Radiologic Manifestations: *Roentgenologic findings of endocrinopathy;* alimentary tract *ulcers in unusual locations* (duodenum and jejunum); marked enlargement of the mucosal folds of the stomach, duodenum, and jejunum; nodular defects of the intestinal wall; megaduodenum; *gastrointestinal dilatation and hypersecretion.*

MULTIPLE ENDOCRINE NEOPLASIA TYPE IIA (SIPPLE SYNDROME; MULTIPLE ENDOCRINE ADENOMATOSIS TYPE IIA)

Clinical Manifestations: (a) *medullary thyroid carcinoma (thyroid C cells) present in 100%; pheochromocytoma; multiglandular parathyroid hyperplasia or adenoma;* (b) autosomal dominant inheritance.

Radiologic Manifestations: (a) *thyroid tumor (calcification in the primary tumor and its metastases;* lack of concentration of ^{131}I by medullary thyroid carcinoma); (b) *pheochromocytoma;* (c) parathyroid hyperplasia; (d) miscellaneous abnormalities: bone metastases; chondrocalcinosis; abnormal haustral pattern; thickened mucosal folds and colonic diverticula in patients with ganglioneuromatosis; rapid transit of barium through the gastrointestinal tract; gastrointestinal ulceration; partial bowel obstruction by the ulcerating mass related to the metastatic lymph nodes.

MULTIPLE ENDOCRINE NEOPLASIA TYPE IIB (MUCOSAL NEUROMA SYNDROME; MULTIPLE ENDOCRINE ADENOMATOSIS TYPE IIB)

Clinical Manifestations: (a) *marfanoid body habitus;* muscle wasting; kyphosis; pectus excavatum; pes planus; pes cavus; (b) coarse facial features, pseudoprognathism; *neuromas of the eyelids, lips, and tongue;* (c) constipation and/or diarrhea; functional problems with swallowing; (d) delayed maturation; (e) autosomal dominant inheritance with very high penetrance and varying expressivity; new mutation in approximately 50% of cases.

Radiologic Manifestations: (a) *thyroid tumor;* (b) *pheochromocytoma;* (c) *alimentary tract manifestations associated with ganglioneuromas* (disturbed motility of the esophagus [segmental dilatation; tertiary contractions]; gastroesophageal reflux; distended stomach with a delayed emptying time; segmental dilatation of the small bowel with an increased or decreased transit time; abnormal colonic haustral pattern; "cornflake" mucosal pattern; megacolon; abnormal mucosal folds of the colon; diverticula of the colon in young patients); (d) musculoskeletal system abnormalities: pes cavus; slipped capital femoral epiphysis; joint laxity; poor muscle development.

MULTIPLE SYNOSTOSIS SYNDROME

Clinical Manifestations: (a) *facial dysmorphism* (low frontal hair implantation; wide nasal root; beaked nasal tip; alar hypoplasia; hemicylindric nose; thin upper lip; short philtrum; microstomia; strabismus); (b) *limitation of joint motions;* (c) *conductive hearing deficit* with an onset after adolescence; (d) short stature; failure to thrive; (e) autosomal dominant inheritance.

Radiologic Manifestations: (a) *progressive symphalangia: narrow distance between the proximal and middle phalanges in infancy, followed by progressive bony fusion;* deformity of the distal end of the metacarpals; (b) *other bony fusions:* middle-ear ossicles; radiohumeral; radioulnar; carpal; tibiotarsal; tarsal; vertebral; (c) other osteoarticular abnormalities: radial head subluxation; abnormal configuration of the carpal bones; shortness of the first metatarsals; short middle phalanges; pseudoepiphyses of the proximal phalanges; agenesis of the middle or distal phalanges of the hands and feet; disturbance in bone modeling of the phalanges; clinodactyly; syndactyly; pes planovalgus with a prominent lateral border; vertebral deformities; Scheuermann disease.

MURCS ASSOCIATION

Clinical and Radiologic Manifestations: Mayer-Rokitansky-Küster-Hauser syndrome in association with Klippel-Feil syndrome: *MU*llerian duct aplasia (congenital absence of the uterus and upper vagina, and normal fallopian tubes); *R*enal agenesis/ectopia; *C*ervical *S*omite dysplasia.

N

NAGER ACROFACIAL DYSOSTOSIS (Acrofacial Dysostosis)

Clinical Manifestations: A heterogeneous entity: (a) *hypoplasia of the zygomatic arches; hypoplasia of the mandible;* deformed external ear; downward slanting of the palpebral fissures; coloboma of eyelids; absent or sparse eyelashes; Robin anomaly; preauricular fistula; macrostomia; hearing defect (often bilateral; conductive; ossicular chain malformation); (b) *upper limb abnormalities, particularly hypoplasia of the radial aspect of the hand; short and deformed forearm; limitation of elbow extension;* (c) most cases sporadic; genetic heterogeneity (autosomal recessive; autosomal dominant); male-to-male transmission.

Radiologic Manifestations: (a) *mandibulofacial dysostosis (malar hypoplasia; mandibular hypoplasia);* (b) *preaxial limb anomalies:* radial hypoplasia or aplasia; proximal radioulnar synostosis; hypoplasia or aplasia of the thumb; duplication or triphalangeal thumbs; syndactyly of the first and second digital rays; hip dysplasia; limb reduction defects; (c) miscellaneous abnormalities: vertebral anomalies; rib anomalies; in utero ultrasonographic diagnosis (mandibulofacial deformities and limb anomalies).

NAIL-PATELLA SYNDROME

Clinical Manifestations: (a) *dysplasia of the nails; hypoplasia or absence of patellae;* palpable iliac horns; elbow deformity; flexion and contracture of other joints; (b) nephropathy of varying severity and manifestation: glomerulonephritis or nephrotic syndrome; (c) short stature; (d) ocular abnormalities: ptosis; abnormal pigmentation of the iris; glaucoma; microcornea; strabismus; microphthalmia; (e) musculoskeletal abnormalities: webbing of the elbows; scoliosis; foot deformities; (f) miscellaneous abnormalities: muscular anomalies; shoulder instability secondary to dysplasia involving the acromion and glenoid; diarrhea and hemolytic uremic syndrome associated with nail-patella syndrome; (g) autosomal dominant inheritance with complete penetrance and variable expressivity.

Radiologic Manifestations: (a) *iliac horns* arising from the central area of the outer surface of the iliac wings; the horns detectable by Tc-99m MDP bone scan (triangular; sharply demarcated areas of increased tracer activity); (b) elongated radius with *hypoplasia of the radial head* and subluxation or dislocation; *hypoplasia of the capitellum;* (c) *hypoplastic or absent patellae;* lateral dislocation or subluxation of hypoplastic patellae; *disproportionate prominence of the medial condyle of the femur;* sloped tibial plateaus; genu valgum; (d) miscellaneous skeletal abnormalities: asymmetric development of joints; degenerative arthritis; blocked full extension of elbows; increased carrying angle of elbows; clinodactyly; camptodactyly; laxity of finger joints; partial symphalangism of distal interphalangeal joints; calcaneovalgus deformity of the hindfoot; ball-and-socket ankle joint; forefoot supination and lateral subluxation of the tarsometatarsal joints; absent fibulae; clavicular horn and shoulder girdle dysplasia; (e) miscellaneous abnormalities: renal osteopathy; renal abnormalities; renal calculi.

NASOPALPEBRAL LIPOMA-COLOBOMA SYNDROME

Clinical Manifestations: (a) congenital symmetric upper lid and nasopalpebral lipomas; bilateral symmetric upper and lower palpebral colobomas located at the junction of the inner and middle third of the lids; telecanthus; etc.; (b) autosomal dominant inheritance.

Radiologic Manifestations: Normal interorbital distance; abnormal cephalometric measurements (shortness of the anterior cranial base; hypoplasia of the midface, particularly the maxillae).

NEPHROGENIC HEPATIC DYSFUNCTION SYNDROME
(Stauffer Syndrome)

Clinical Manifestations: *Hypernephroma; abnormal liver function test values, hepatomegaly,* regression of liver enlargement and abnormal liver function test results after nephrectomy (in some cases); nonspecific constitutional symptoms.

Radiologic Manifestations: *Renal tumor; hepatic arteriographic abnormalities* (pronounced hypervascularity; marked granularity during the capillary phase); *absence of liver metastases.*

NEPHRONOPHTHISIS

Clinical Manifestations: Onset of symptoms in first or second decade: (a) growth retardation; (b) *polyuria and polydipsia;* (c) *salt-wasting and progressive uremia;* (d) hypocalcemic tetany; (e) hypertension; (f) *fixed low specific gravity of urine;* (g) anemia; (h) variable numbers of cysts at corticomedullary junction; homogeneous thickening, splitting, reticulation, thinning, complete loss, granular disintegration, and collapse; (i) tapetoretinal degeneration; (j) autosomal recessive inheritance.

Radiologic Manifestations: (a) *small kidneys; nonvisualization or poor opacification of collecting systems* (excretory urography); (b) ultrasonographic abnormalities: disappearance of corticomedullary differentiation, with renal parenchyma either isoechoic or hyperechoic as compared with the liver or spleen; small medullary cysts (may not be detectable by ultrasound in some cases); (c) thin-section computed tomographic scan: medullary renal cysts.

NEPHROTIC SYNDROME

Clinical Manifestations: (a) anorexia; diarrhea; *edema;* (b) *albuminuria; hypoalbuminemia;* increase in serum concentrations of cholesterol, triglycerides, and low-density and very-low-density lipoproteins; low, normal, or elevated high-density lipoprotein concentrations; *lipiduria;* deficiency of prothrombin; elevated platelet counts and plasma fibrinogen levels; prolonged thrombin times; thrombotic complications; (c) miscellaneous abnormalities: association with familial hemophagocytic syndrome; association with Omenn reticulosis; association with Kimura disease; etc.; (d) autosomal recessive inheritance in the congenital type.

Radiologic Manifestations: (a) *ascites; pleural effusion;* intermittent mediastinal widening; (b) changing ultrasonic pattern: large, diffusely hyperechoic kidneys in the early stage; small kidneys with marked echogenicity of the deep cortex in the late phase of the disease; (c) stretching and narrowness of the intrarenal collecting system due to renal edema; (d) pericardial effusion; pulmonary edema; edema of the bowel wall; (e) abnormal renal parenchymal postcontrast enhancement; (f) thrombosis: renal vein; inferior vena cava; pulmonary artery; sagittal sinus; etc.

NEU-LAXOVA SYNDROME

Clinical Manifestations: (a) *craniofacial abnormalities:* microcephaly; slanted forehead; protuberant eyes; flattened nose; deformed ears; micrognathia; microphthalmia; cleft palate; (b) *limb anomalies:* hypoplastic fingers; syndactyly of the fingers and toes; *camptodactyly; clinodactyly;* rocker-bottom feet; (c) *generalized edema; lemon-colored and scaly ichthyotic skin;* (d) *short neck;* (e) autosomal recessive inheritance.

Radiologic Manifestations: (a) prenatal ultrasonographic abnormalities: intrauterine growth retardation; hypoechoic skeletal structures; kyphosis; feeble fetal activity; restricted limb movement; microcephaly with a receding forehead and prominent eyes; generalized edema; flexion deformities of the limbs; *swollen hands and feet causing the apparent absent digits; scalp edema; hydrothorax; hydramnios or oligohydramnios;* (b) short limbs; "sticklike" long bones; poor long bone cortex formation; undermineralization; thick calvaria; spina bifida; flat acetabular roofs; etc.

NEUROCUTANEOUS MELANOSIS SEQUENCE (ROKITANSKY–VAN BOGAERT SYNDROME)

Clinical Manifestations: (a) *pigmented cutaneous nevi; hairy nevi; rarely diffuse pigmentation without discrete nevi;* (b) *seizures; chronic meningeal irritation; cranial nerve palsies; increased intracranial pressure; myelopathy;* (c) miscellaneous abnormalities: association with malignant neoplasms; etc.

Pathology: *Excessive proliferation of melanin-producing cells in the skin and leptomeninges;* intracerebral melanotic pigmentation; truncal nevi association with intraspinal melanosis; intradural mass of the cervical canal.

Radiologic Manifestations: (a) *diffuse leptomeningeal enhancement after the administration of gadopentetate dimeglumine; intracerebral lesion (hyperintense on T_1-weighted sequence and hypointense on T_2-weighted sequence);* (b) miscellaneous abnormalities: ventriculomegaly; calcification in the suprasellar cistern, sylvian fissure, and occipital lobe; inferior vermian hypoplasia; Dandy-Walker complex; tumor; spinal cord distortion; intraspinal lipoma; syringomyelia.

NEUROFIBROMATOSIS I (VON RECKLINGHAUSEN DISEASE; NF-I)

Clinical Manifestations: A hamartomatous disorder (neurocristopathy, neuroectodermal and mesodermal dysplasia) with widespread multiple organ system involvement.

(A) SKIN: Café au lait spots; subcutaneous neurofibromas; elephantoid overgrowth of skin and soft tissues; miscellaneous (hemangioma, red-blue macules; pseudoatrophic lesions; giant hairy nevi; xanthogranulomas; hypomelanotic patches of skin and hair).

(B) NERVOUS SYSTEM: Neurofibromas of peripheral nerves; optic nerve involvement; central nervous system manifestations: macrocrania; learning disabilities; behavioral disturbances; mental retardation; seizures; childhood hypertensive stroke; difficulties in reading and writing; hyperactivity; urinary incontinence; paraparesis; infantile spasm; association of neurofibromatosis I, hemimegalencephaly, hemifacial hypertrophy, and intracranial lipoma.

(C) EYES: Lisch nodules (melanocytic hamartomas); eyelid neurofibroma; S-shaped ptosis of the lid; congenital glaucoma; buphthalmos; retinal detachment; retinal phakoma; hypertelorism; optic pathway tumors.

(D) SKELETAL SYSTEM: Bowing of the limbs; kyphoscoliosis; skull defects and deformities (temporal or frontal mass; pulsating or nonpulsating exophthalmos; displacement of the globe; edema of the eyelids and ptosis; disturbed vision); macrodactyly; pectus excavatum; pectus carinatum; genu valgum/varum; pes planus; association of neurofibromatosis with osseous fibrous dysplasia; postaxial polydactyly; osteomalacia (vitamin D–resistant, hypophosphoremic).

(E) ALIMENTARY SYSTEM: Pain; hemorrhage; nausea, vomiting; distension; constipation or diarrhea; perforation of the bowel; jaundice; hyperganglionosis of the distal bowel; sporadic cases of multiple intestinal neurofibromatosis without cutaneous features of von Recklinghausen disease; familial neuroblastoma–neurofibromatosis–Hirschsprung disease–jaw winking syndrome.

(F) CARDIOVASCULAR SYSTEM: Systemic arterial hypertension; idiopathic hypertrophic subaortic stenosis; congenital heart defects (pulmonary stenosis; aortic stenosis; ventricular septal defect; atrial septal defect; etc.); complete heart block; hypotension; aortic coarctation; coronary lesion associated with vasospasm and myocardial infarction; abdominal angina due to compression of the celiac and superior mesenteric arteries by plexiform neurofibromatosis; regressive hypertrophic cardiomyopathy in infancy; hemangiomas; lymphangiomatosis; presentation as a severe systemic vasculopathy; infantile gangrene.

(G) GENITOURINARY SYSTEM: Hypertrophy of the clitoral hood, clitoris, and labia; enlargement of the penis.

(H) ENDOCRINE AND METABOLIC DISORDERS: Hyperparathyroidism; sexual precocity; gigantism; osteomalacia; rickets; multiple endocrine adenomatosis; hypoglycemia; hyperprolactinemia; abnormalities of galactose metabolism; hypogonadism; irregular menses; infertility; ovarian cysts; early menopause.

(I) OTOLOGIC ABNORMALITIES: Abnormal hearing; neurofibromas of the external ear; middle ear neurofibromas.

(J) NEOPLASMS: (a) central nervous system: glioma; meningioma; malignant neurilemoma; etc.; (b) peripheral nervous system: neurosarcoma; neuromyxoma; etc.; (c) others: sarcomas; carcinomas; leukemia; lymphoma; sarcomatous degeneration of neurofibromas; nonossifying fibromas; melanoma; neuroblastoma; pheochromocytoma; rhabdomyosarcoma; adrenal cortical adenoma; leiomyosarcoma of the intestine.

(K) MISCELLANEOUS ABNORMALITIES: Overgrowth or undergrowth; breast enlargement; juvenile xanthogranuloma; sleep apnea; association with multiple endocrine neoplasia; occurrence of both neurofibromatosis I and II in the same individual (father with neurofibromatosis I and mother with neurofibromatosis II); association with monosomy 7; fragile X syndrome; coincidence of neurofibromatosis and myotonic dystrophy in a kindred.

(L) Autosomal dominant inheritance; mutation (about 50%); penetrance of almost 100%; the gene mapped to chromosome 17q21 band.

Radiologic Manifestations

(A) SKULL: Erosions and enlargement of foramina; bone defects, in particular in the posterior and superior orbital wall and along lambdoid sutures; enlarged orbit; mandibular abnormalities (hypoplasia with flattening of the external contour, thinning of the body and the ramus, widening of the medial and lateral coronoid spaces, bilateral coronoid hyperplasia); multiple frontobasal osseomeningeal defects (rhinoliquorrhea, meningoencephaloceles); lacunar-like skull.

(B) CENTRAL NERVOUS SYSTEM: (a) macrocephaly; (b) intraparenchymal manifestations: isointense or hyperintense foci (T_2-weighted sequences) in the brain stem, cerebellar white matter, dentate nucleus, basal ganglia, periventricular white matter, optic nerve, and optic pathways; isointense on T_1-weighted images, no mass effect (T_1 hyperintensities and mild mass effect in the globus pallidus lesions reported); deeply located high-signal-intensity lesions on T_2-weighted images more evident in young patients; (c) neoplasms: optic glioma (the most common lesion); glioma in the brain stem; diffuse gliomas of the cerebral hemispheres, cerebellum, and spinal cord; pilocytic astrocytoma; ependymoma; meningioma; hamartoma; ganglioglioma; (d) arterial occlusion or stenosis, moyamoya, aneurysms; (e) miscellaneous central nervous system abnormalities: hydrocephalus; aqueductal stenosis; prominent cerebrospinal fluid spaces;

plexiform neurofibromatosis of the orbit; dural ectasia affecting the optic nerve; enlarged internal auditory canals secondary to dural ectasia without associated acoustic neuromas; arachnoid cysts; arachnoid pouches; frontobasal meningoencephaloceles; nonneoplastic cerebral and cerebellar calcifications; choroid plexus calcification; agenesis of the corpus callosum in identical twins; hemimegalencephaly associated with hemifacial hypertrophy and intracranial lipoma.

(C) SPINE: Kyphoscoliosis, enlargement of intervertebral foramina; scalloping of vertebral bodies (anterior; posterior; lateral); prominent "erosive" changes at the apex of the kyphotic curve; agenesis or hypoplasia of pedicle(s); spondylolisthesis; spindling of transverse processes; widening of the gap between the zygapophyseal joints and the transverse processes of adjacent vertebrae (anteroposterior projections of the spine); increased distance between adjacent transverse processes; instability of spinal segments, leading to subluxation or dislocation; spine cleft; wedge-shaped vertebrae; thoracic lordoscoliosis; pseudoarthrosis and curve progression after spinal fusion; osteolysis; costovertebral dislocation.

(D) SPINAL CONTENTS: Dural ectasia; meningocele (cervical; thoracic; lumbar; sacral); intramedullary neurofibromatosis; stenosis of the neurocanal; cord compression and displacement; syringomyelia; spinal cord compression from atlantoaxial subluxation; intraspinal lesions with growth through foramen; spinal subarachnoid hemorrhage.

(E) LIMBS: Erosion of bones; S-shaped tortuousity of long bones; irregular periosteal thickening; hyperplasia or hypoplasia; intraosseous radiolucent defects; congenital bowing; pseudarthrosis (tibia most common with anterolateral bowing; other bones: ulna; femur; clavicle; radius; humerus); bone sclerosis; subperiosteal or cortical cysts; intramedullary neurofibromatosis; absence of a patella; dislocation of the radius and ulna; local overgrowth; subperiosteal hemorrhage; calcified hematoma; pathologic dislocation of the hip; association of nonossifying fibromas with neurofibromatosis; protrusio acetabuli; neuropathic arthropathy of the knee; nontraumatic dislocation of the hip.

(F) PERIPHERAL SOFT-TISSUE NEUROFIBROMATOSIS: Computed tomography of masses in the distribution of peripheral nerves (fusiform enlargement of the nerve; central areas of low attenuation; calcification); solid masses (paravertebral; laryngeal; mediastinal; abdominal; pelvis and ischiorectal fossae): rounded, clearly outlined masses with attenuation values of 30 to 40 Hounsfield units or widespread sheets of nodular tissues; segmental neurofibromatosis (a rare form of the disease in which cutaneous and neural changes are confined to one region of the body; monomelic neurofibromatosis).

(G) ALIMENTARY TRACT AND LIVER: Single or multiple tumors; submucosal or intraluminal filling defects; intestinal obstruction; volvulus;

intussusception; ulcerations; pseudo-Hirschsprung disease; hyperplastic esophagogastric polyp; tumor spread into the liver along the portal vein (infiltrative hypoechoic masses around the porta hepatis and intrahepatic portal branches; low attenuation masses on computed tomography); tubular colonic duplication.

(H) CHEST: Dumbbell neurofibroma; intercostal neurofibroma; rib penciling; "twisted ribbon" rib deformity; rib notching; mediastinal neurofibroma; spontaneous pneumothorax; hemothorax; fibrosing alveolitis (diffuse mottled densities changing to a strandy appearance and finally the formation of bullae and honeycomb lungs); interstitial fibrosis–associated pulmonary hypertension; pulmonary neurofibroma associated with arteriovenous shunting and hypoxemia.

(I) CARDIOVASCULAR SYSTEM: Acquired right ventricular outflow obstruction; aneurysm of the superior vena cava; renovascular hypertension resulting from neurofibromatosis of renal arteries (narrowing usually located in the proximal segment of the artery and optimally evaluated by Doppler ultrasound); spontaneous rupture of an artery (intercostal; renal; subclavian); abnormalities of the aorta and branches (stenosis; aneurysm) at various sites (renal; celiac; mesenteric; iliac; pulmonary; cerebral; etc.); extracranial vertebral artery aneurysm; lymphatic abnormalities (dilatation and tortuosity of lymphatic vessels and filling defects in the lymph nodes); left atrial wall aneurysm; arteriovenous fistula; obstruction of superior vena cava.

(J) URINARY TRACT: Bladder involvement (intrinsic mass or diffuse infiltrative process); involvement of the prostate, seminal vesicles, scrotum, penis, and ureter; hydronephrosis; hydroureter; displacement of the upper collecting system and bladder by the extrinsic mass(es); computed tomographic attenuation coefficient of the masses near soft-tissue density; markedly increased signal intensity on T_2-weighted magnetic resonance images and slightly increased signal intensity on T_1-weighted images (relative to muscular structures).

(K) SCINTIGRAPHY: Accumulation of ^{99m}Tc DTPA in the benign soft-tissue neurofibromatosis tumors.

(L) MISCELLANEOUS ABNORMALITIES: Osteomalacia (vitamin D–resistant; hypophosphoremic); buphthalmos; association with osseous fibrous dysplasia in a family.

Note

(A) The seven important clinical and radiologic manifestations of NF-I (National Institutes of Health Consensus Development Conference Statement) are: (1) *six or more café au lait macules (the greatest diameter more than 5 mm in prepubertal patients and more than 15 mm in postpubertal patients); (2) two or more neurofibromas or one plexiform neurofibroma; (3) axillary or inguinal freckling; (4) optic glioma; (5)*

two or more Lisch nodules (iris hamartomas); (6) a distinctive osseous lesion such as sphenoid bone dysplasia, cortical thinning of long bones with or without pseudarthrosis; (7) a first-degree relative with NF-I. Two or more of the seven criteria must be present to establish the diagnosis of NF-I.

(B) Approximately 85% of cases of the neurofibromatoses are of NF-I type; in addition to NF-II, some other types have been mentioned in the literature: mixed type; variant type; etc.

(C) The term *neurofibromatosis-Noonan syndrome* has been used for the cases of neurofibromatosis I with some features of Noonan syndrome: short stature; pectus excavatum; broad neck; congenital heart disease (in some cases); learning disability; etc.

(D) Overlap of the manifestations of Watson syndrome (pulmonary valvular stenosis, café au lait patches, dull intelligence, and short stature) and some of the manifestations of neurofibromatosis I (macrocephaly, Lisch nodules, and neurofibromas) has been reported.

(E) In the absence of accurate information, a definite diagnosis of "elephant man" has not been established; neurofibromatosis and Proteus syndrome have been considered as possibilities.

NEUROFIBROMATOSIS II (NF-II)

Clinical Manifestations: (a) *hearing loss related to acoustic schwannomas (acoustic neuroma);* tinnitus; abnormal vestibular function; (b) *presenile posterior subcapsular/capsular cataracts (85%); peripheral cortical lens opacities (frequently wedge-shaped);* combined pigment epithelial and retinal hamartomas; Lisch nodules; optic gliomas; (c) symptoms related to other intracranial and spinal cord tumors: meningioma (often multiple); cranial nerve (III to XII) schwannomas; tumors of glial cell origin; paraspinal dorsal nerve root tumors; (d) miscellaneous abnormalities: peripheral neuropathy; learning difficulties; papilledema; cutaneous lesions (café au lait macules; neurofibromas); occurrence of both NF-I and NF-II in the same individual (father with NF-I, mother with NF-II); combined hamartoma of the retina and retinal pigment epithelium; (e) autosomal dominant inheritance with high penetrance; sporadic; interfamily differences in disease severity and tumor susceptibility; the gene located in the chromosomal region 22q12; the assessment of carrier status of the at-risk individuals with chromosome 22 markers possible with a high degree of certainty.

Radiologic Manifestations: (a) *bilateral acoustic schwannomas* (neurinomas) in about 95% of the cases: hypointense or isointense to brain parenchyma on the short TR sequences and hyperintense on long TR sequences; homogeneous enhancement of the tumor following administration of gadolinium-DTPA except in the cases with central necrosis; (b) calcification within the necrotic center of tumors; (c) nontumoral intracranial calcified deposits: choroid plexus; cerebellar hemispheres; surface of the cerebral hemispheres; (d) spinal bony abnormalities secondary to tumors: enlargement of neural foramina; posterior vertebral scalloping; (e) intraspinal lesions (intramedullary masses [ependymomas]; intradural extradural masses [schwannomas, meningiomas]); (f) agenesis of the internal carotid artery.

Note: (a) the criterion proposed for the diagnosis of NF-II (National Institutes of Health Consensus Development Conference) is the presence of one of the following: (1) *bilateral eight nerve masses; (2) a first-degree relative with NF-II and either unilateral eight nerve mass or two of the following: neurofibroma; meningioma; glioma; schwannoma; juvenile posterior subcapsular lenticular opacity;* (b) acoustic schwannomas occur at an earlier age in NF-II (adolescents or young adults) as compared with those not affected with NF-II (over 40 years of age); (c) in sporadic nonfamilial acoustic schwannoma the tumor is unilateral, as compared with bilateral masses in NF-II; (d) complete audiologic assessment very helpful in an early detection of the disease among relatives; (e) NF-II has been subdivided into three types: the Gardner type (late onset), the Wishart type (early onset), and the Lee Abbott type (general meningiomatosis).

NOONAN SYNDROME

Clinical Manifestations: (a) *short stature; failure to thrive in infancy; delayed puberty;* (b) *facial dysmorphism:* increased midfacial height; hypertelorism; retrognathia; micrognathia; low nasal bridge and nasal root; wide mouth; prominent upper lip; highly arched palate; cleft palate; dental anomalies and malocclusion; micrognathia; (c) *eye abnormalities:* epicanthal folds; ptosis; hypertelorism; downward-slanting palpebral fissures; strabismus; myopia; proptosis; nystagmus; etc.; (d) low-set, excessively folded auricular helices; hearing loss; nerve deafness; (e) *short neck;* low posterior hairline; (f) *flat/shieldlike chest;* funnel chest deformity; pectus excavatum and/or carinatum; (g) cardiovascular abnormalities; (h) genital abnormalities: small, undescended testicles; penis abnormalities (small; large); hypospadias; deficient spermatogenesis and sterility; (i) musculoskeletal abnormalities: cubitus valgus; rounded shoulder; clino-brachydactyly; blunt fingertips; joint hyperextensibility; joint contractures; talipes equinovarus; (j) skin and appendage abnormalities: hyperelastic skin; nevi; moles; dystrophic nails; curly hair; thick hair; (k) neurobehavioral manifestations: mental retardation and microcephaly; hypotonia; recurrent convulsions; unexplained peripheral neuropathy; autistic disorder; (l) lymphatic system abnormalities: lymphedema; lymphangiectasis; cystic hygroma; chylothorax; (m) miscellaneous abnormalities: bleeding diathesis; neoplasms; immune disorders; etc.; (n) genetic heterogeneity; sporadic; autosomal dominant inheritance; variable expressivity.

Radiologic Manifestations: (a) craniofacial abnormalities: hypertelorism; biparietal foramina; dolichocephaly; microcephaly; macrocephaly; bitemporal bulging; steep inclination of the anterior fossa; micrognathia; (b) dental abnormalities: malocclusion; odontogenic keratocysts; (c) thoracic abnormalities: anterior bowing of the sternum at various levels; elongation of the manubrium and shortness of the body of the sternum; premature fusion of ossification centers of the body of the sternum; caudal slope of the ribs, cervical ribs; (d) limb anomalies: genu valgum; pes planus; short or long fingers; syndactyly; camptodactyly; clinodactyly of the fifth fingers; congenital dislocation of the radial head; scapula alata; talipes equinovarus; polydactyly; radioulnar synostosis; (e) spinal abnormalities: kyphosis, scoliosis; Klippel-Feil syndrome; fusion of vertebrae; (f) cardiovascular anomalies: pulmonary stenosis; hypertrophic cardiomyopathy; septal defects; mitral valve anomalies; etc.; (g) lymphatic abnormalities: peripheral lymphedema; hypoplastic peripheral lymph vessels; hypoplastic lymph nodes; chylothorax; pulmonary lymphangiectasis; (h) urinary system abnormalities: obstructive uropathy; duplication of the collecting system; renal hypoplasia; polycystic renal disease; (i) gastrointestinal tract abnormalities: lymphangiectasis; diverticulosis of the small intestine and incomplete rotation of the bowel; (j) fetal sonography: fetal edema; cystic hygroma; polyhydramnios; cardiomyopathy; (k) *skeletal maturation retardation.*

Note: The term *neurofibromatosis-Noonan syndrome* has been used for the cases of neurofibromatosis I with some features of Noonan syndrome: short stature, pectus excavatum, broad neck, congenital heart disease (in some cases), learning disability, etc.

NOONAN-LIKE/MULTIPLE GIANT CELL LESION SYNDROME

Clinical Manifestations: (a) short stature; (b) ocular hypertelorism; posteriorly angulated ears; mandibular prognathism; short webbed neck; (c) low-normal intelligence or developmental delay; (d) miscellaneous abnormalities: pulmonary stenosis; other congenital heart anomalies; oculomotor disturbances; sensorineural hearing loss; multiple lentigines; cutaneous hemangiomas; hyperextensibility; limitation of motion; cubitus valgus; scoliosis.

Radiologic Manifestations: *Cystlike giant cell lesions* (maxilla; mandible; tubular bones; ribs; joints; soft tissues).

O

OCULO-AURICULO-VERTEBRAL SPECTRUM (GOLDENHAR SYNDROME; GOLDENHAR-GORLIN SYNDROME)

Clinical Manifestations: Marked clinical variability: (a) *maxillary and/or mandibular hypoplasia;* insufficient closure of the jaw; temporo-mandibular joint anomalies; macrostomia associated with a lateral facial cleft; facial muscular hypoplasia; downward slanting of the palpebral fissures; (b) *epibulbar dermoid and/or lipodermoid; coloboma of the upper eyelid;* coloboma of the iris and choroid; (c) *ear anomalies: hypoplasia or atresia of the external auditory meatus and canal; preauricular tags and/or a blind fistula;* middle-ear and inner-ear anomalies; deafness; (d) dental anomalies; (e) central nervous system abnormalities; (f) usually sporadic; autosomal dominant inheritance in some cases.

Radiologic Manifestations: (a) *hypoplasia of the mandible, maxilla, and temporal bones;* (b) *vertebral anomalies;* rib anomalies; (c) craniofacial asymmetry; cranium bifidum; platybasia; hypoplasia of the petrous and ethmoid bones; absence of the internal auditory canal; cleft lip; cleft palate; (d) microcephaly; hydrocephalus; aqueductal stenosis; encephalocele; agenesis of the corpus callosum; agenesis of the vermis; holoprosencephaly, porencephaly; cerebral hypoplasia; Arnold-Chiari malformation; lissencephaly; lipoma of corpus callosum; calcification of the falx; hypoplasia of the external carotid artery; absence of internal carotid artery; (e) miscellaneous abnormalities: velopharyngeal insufficiency; alimentary tract malformations; genitourinary anomalies; cardiovascular anomalies; respiratory system anomalies; limb anomalies (radial limb anomalies; hypoplastic distal phalanges; polydactyly; terminal/paraxial hemimelia).

OCULO-DENTO-OSSEOUS DYSPLASIA (OCULO-DENTO-DIGITAL DYSPLASIA)

Clinical Manifestations: (a) *characteristic facial features:* narrow nasal bridge, pinched nose, thin anteverted nares, prominent columella, prominent epicanthal folds, narrow palpebral apertures, and pseudohypertelorism; (b) *ocular abnormalities:* microphthalmos; microcornea; glaucoma; iris anomalies; eccentric pupils; etc.; (c) *small teeth; generalized enamel hypoplasia; gross dental caries;* (d) *syndactyly;* (e) neurologic manifestations; (f) autosomal dominant inheritance with variable expressivity; new mutation in about 50% of the cases.

Radiologic Manifestations: (a) *bilateral syndactyly and camptodactyly of the fourth and fifth fingers;* clinodactyly of the fifth finger; hypoplasia of the middle phalanx of the index finger or other fingers;

hypoplasia or absence of the middle phalanges of some toes; (b) *amelogenesis imperfecta and microdontia;* (c) central nervous system abnormalities: basal ganglia calcification; diffuse abnormal T_2 signal hyperintensity involving the internal capsule; T_2 signal hypointensity in the globus pallidus, substantia nigra, red nucleus, and parietooccipital cortex; spinal cord atrophy; (d) miscellaneous abnormalities: small orbits; undertubulation of the long bones, especially the femur; widening of the ribs and clavicles; etc.

ODONTO-TRICHO-MELIC SYNDROME

Clinical and Radiologic Manifestations: (a) *extensive tetramelic reductions;* (b) *oligodontia; conical crowns;* (c) *ectodermal dysplasia:* thin, dry, and shiny skin; onychodysplasia; reduced scalp hair, body hair, eyebrows, and lashes; hypoplastic or absent areolae; (d) miscellaneous abnormalities: a peculiar face; cleft lip; cleft palate; deformed pinnae; large nose; protruding lips; mental retardation; hypogonadism; excess of tyrosine and/or tryptophan in the urine; etc.; (e) autosomal recessive inheritance.

OGILVIE SYNDROME

Clinical Manifestations: Most common in geriatric patients: *Atypical signs and symptoms of acute large-bowel obstruction.*

Radiologic Manifestations: *A pattern of colonic dilatation in the absence of an obstructing lesion* (colonic dilatation may involve the cecum and varying lengths of the colon distal to the cecum); few air-fluid levels; a gradual transition to the collapsed bowel; normal gas and fecal pattern in the rectum.

OPHTHALMO-MANDIBULO-MELIC DYSPLASIA

Clinical Manifestations: (a) *corneal opacities; mandibular deformity leading to difficulty in mastication; short and bowed forearm; flexion deformity of the fingers;* (b) autosomal dominant inheritance.

Radiologic Manifestations: (a) *absence of the coronoid process; obtuse mandibular angle; temporomandibular ankylosis;* (b) *upper-limb anomalies:* shallow glenoid fossa; aplasia of the lateral condyle of the humerus; abnormal trochlea; absent olecranon and coronoid processes of the ulna; absent radial head; dislocation of the radius at the elbow; bowed radial shaft; absent distal segment of the ulna; hypoplasia of the carpal bones; (c) *lower-limb anomalies:* coxa valga; hypoplasia of the lateral femoral condyle; shortness of the proximal portion of the fibula.

OPITZ BBBG SYNDROME (BBB/G SYNDROME; HYPERTELORISM-HYPOSPADIAS SYNDROME; G SYNDROME; BBB SYNDROME)

Clinical Manifestations

(A) **BBB VARIETY:** *Telecanthus or apparent hypertelorism; hypospadias;* cryptorchidism; mental retardation; etc.

(B) **G VARIETY:** *Dolichocephalic skull; prominent parietal eminences and occiput; large anterior fontanelle; hypertelorism; flattened nasal bridge; anteversion of nostrils; narrow palpebral fissures; epicanthal folds; strabismus; micrognathia; auricular abnormalities; hoarse cry; swallowing/respiratory difficulties; hypospadias;* chordee; cryptorchidism; etc.

(C) Autosomal dominant inheritance.

Radiologic Manifestations: (a) *hypospadias;* (b) neuromuscular disorder with *incoordination in swallowing and esophageal function;* (c) miscellaneous abnormalities: aspiration pneumonia; cerebellar vermal hypoplasia; Dandy-Walker anomaly; enlarged cisterna magna; enlarged fourth ventricle; absent or hypoplastic corpus callosum; cerebral atrophy; ventriculomegaly; wide cavum septum pellucidum; laryngo-tracheo-esophageal cleft (three children in one family); etc.

Note: (a) the acronym *BBB* represents the initials of the last name of each of the original reported families, and the acronym *G* is the initial of the first reported family with the syndrome; (b) there is overlapping of the clinical manifestations of types BBB and G; some of the manifestations listed under BBB variety may be present in G variety, and vice versa.

OPITZ TRIGONOCEPHALY SYNDROME (C SYNDROME)

Clinical Manifestations: Clinical variability: (a) *short stature at birth;* (b) *craniofacial dysmorphism:* trigonocephaly; microcephaly, broad nasal bridge; epicanthus; short nose; upward-slanting palpebral fissures; micrognathia; thick anterior alveolar ridges; multiple oral frenula; low simple philtrum; macrostomia; abnormal ear (abnormal shape, reduced cartilage; low-set and/or posteriorly rotated); anterior "cowlick"; strabismus; (c) *limb anomalies;* (d) most likely autosomal recessive inheritance.

Radiologic Manifestations: (a) *trigonocephaly;* "heaped-up" sagittal and metopic cranial sutures; incomplete bony fusion; bone defect between the orbits; microcephaly; (b) miscellaneous abnormalities: anomalous ribs; fused sternal ossification centers; scoliosis; hypoplasia of the metacarpals and phalanges; polydactyly; syndactyly; radial head dislocation; hip dislocation; cupping of the metaphyses of the metacarpal bones; skeletal maturation retardation; terminal transverse limb reduction; etc.

OPSOCLONUS-MYOCLONUS SYNDROME

Clinical and Radiologic Manifestations: Almost half of the published cases of infantile myoclonic encephalopathy have been associated with neuroblastoma, ganglioneuroblastoma, or ganglioneuroma: *ataxia; somatic myoclonus; opsoclonus;* etiologic factor detection by various imaging modalities.

ORO-FACIO-DIGITAL SYNDROMES (ORAL-FACIAL-DIGITAL SYNDROMES; OFDS)

Classification: These heterogeneous syndromes have in common oral, facial, and digital anomalies.

(A) OFDS I (PAPILLON-LEAGE AND PSAUME SYNDROME): (a) oral abnormalities: tongue clefts, frenula, missing teeth, and highly arched palate; (b) facial dysmorphism: telecanthus or hypertelorism, median cleft lip, and alar hypoplasia; (c) hand anomalies: clinodactyly; brachydactyly; syndactyly; (d) foot anomalies: preaxial polydactyly; (e) miscellaneous abnormalities: alopecia; miliary skin lesions; polycystic kidneys; brain dysgenesis; trembling; (f) X-linked dominant inheritance.

(B) OFDS II (MOHR SYNDROME): (a) oral abnormalities: tongue nodules, tongue clefts, frenula, and highly arched or cleft palate; (b) facial dysmorphism: bifid nose tip, and median cleft lip; (c) hand anomalies: clinodactyly, brachydactyly, syndactyly, preaxial or postaxial polydactyly; (d) foot anomalies: preaxial or postaxial polydactyly; (e) miscellaneous abnormalities: coarse hair; porencephaly; hydrocephaly; congenital heart defect; (f) autosomal recessive inheritance.

(C) OFDS III: (a) oral abnormalities: tongue nodules, tongue clefts, supernumerary teeth, small teeth, and cleft uvula; (b) facial dysmorphism: hypertelorism, bulbous nose, and low-set ears: (c) hand anomalies: postaxial polydactyly; (d) foot anomalies: postaxial polydactyly; (e) miscellaneous abnormalities: seesaw winking; myoclonic jerks; hyperconvex nails; short sternum; (f) autosomal recessive inheritance.

(D) OFDS IV: (a) oral abnormalities: tongue nodules, lobed tongue, frenula, and highly arched and/or cleft palate; (b) facial dysmorphism: epicanthal folds, micrognathia, and low-set ears; (c) hand anomalies: preaxial or postaxial polydactyly, brachydactyly, clinodactyly, and syndactyly; (d) foot anomalies: preaxial and postaxial polydactyly; (e) miscellaneous abnormalities: short stature; pectus excavatum; hypoplastic tibiae; porencephaly; cerebral atrophy; (f) autosomal recessive inheritance.

(E) OFDS V: (a) oral abnormalities: frenula; (b) facial dysmorphism: median cleft lip; (c) hand anomalies: postaxial polydactyly; (d) foot anomalies: postaxial polydactyly; (e) autosomal recessive inheritance.

(F) OFDS VI: (a) oral abnormalities: lobed tongue, tongue nodules, frenula, and highly arched and/or cleft palate; (b) facial dysmorphism: hypertelorism, cleft lip, and broad nasal tip: (c) hand anomalies: postaxial polydactyly, brachydactyly, clinodactyly, and syndactyly; central polydactyly; (d) foot anomalies: preaxial polysyndactyly; (e) miscellaneous abnormalities: renal agenesis/dysplasia; heart defect; cerebellar anomalies; (f) autosomal recessive inheritance.

(G) OFDS VII: (a) oral abnormalities: tongue nodules, frenula, and highly arched and/or cleft palate; (b) facial dysmorphism: hypertelorism, cleft lip, and facial asymmetry; (c) hand anomalies: clinodactyly; (d) miscellaneous abnormalities: preauricular skin tag; hydronephrosis; (e) possibly autosomal dominant inheritance.

(H) OFDS VIII: (a) oral abnormalities; lobed tongue, frenula, tongue nodules, highly arched palate, and absent teeth; (b) facial dysmorphism: cleft lip, telecanthus, and broad/bifid nose; (c) hand anomalies: polydactyly, and duplicated hallux; (d) foot anomalies: preaxial polydactyly; (e) miscellaneous abnormalities: tibial and radial defects; hypoplastic epiglottis; (f) X-linked recessive inheritance.

(I) OFDS IX: (a) oral abnormalities: lobed tongue, frenula, tongue nodules; cleft lip; (b) synophrys; (c) hand anomalies: brachydactyly and syndactyly; (d) foot anomalies: big toes; (e) miscellaneous abnormalities: retinochoroidal lacunae; short stature; (f) X-linked recessive or autosomal recessive inheritance.

(J) OFDS X: A case report of an infant with OFDS having mesomelic limb shortening, oligodactyly, and fibular aplasia may represent a new variant.

(K) OTHER SYNDROMES

1. Mohr-Majewski syndrome: (a) oral abnormalities: lobed tongue, frenula, and highly arched palate; (b) facial dysmorphism: hypertelorism, midline cleft lip, micrognathia, and low-set ears; (c) hand anomalies: postaxial polydactyly; syndactyly; (d) foot anomalies: preaxial and postaxial polydactyly; clubfoot; (e) miscellaneous abnormalities: deafness; tracheal or laryngeal defects; Dandy-Walker malformation; hypoplastic or absent tibiae; (f) autosomal recessive inheritance.

2. Egger-Joubert syndrome: (a) lobed tongue; micrognathia; preaxial or postaxial hand polydactyly; foot polydactyly; cerebellar anomalies; (b) autosomal recessive inheritance.

OROMANDIBULAR-LIMB HYPOGENESIS

Classification: Syndromes and anomalies of mandible, tongue, and maxilla associated with reductive limb anomalies.

Description

1. Charlie M syndrome: Ocular hypertelorism, facial paralysis (in some), cleft palate, absent or conically crowned incisors, and hypodactyly of the hands and feet.

2. Glossopalatine ankylosis syndrome: Linguopalatine adhesion, highly arched palate, cleft palate, hypoplastic mandible, hypodontia, temporomandibular ankylosis, facial paralysis, and variable degrees of limb anomalies (oligodactyly; peromelia; polydactyly; syndactyly; bilateral apodia); facial paralysis in some; mild clefting of the tip of tongue in some; sporadic.

3. Hanhart syndrome: Micrognathia, microstomia, hypodontia, delay in appearance of the teeth, deformed teeth, and variable limb anomalies (peromelia of the upper limbs or of all four limbs; oligodactyly; short digits).

4. Hypoglossia-hypodactylia syndrome.

5. Möbius syndrome.

Note: Oromandibular-limb hypogenesis syndrome has been reported following chorionic villus sampling.

OSTEOARTHROPATHY, FAMILIAL IDIOPATHIC (CURRARINO SYNDROME)

Clinical Manifestations: Onset of symptoms in infancy: (a) *eczematous skin eruption;* increased perspiration of the palms and soles; *clubbing of the fingers;* thickening of the arms and legs; synovial fluid containing few mononuclear cells (noninflammatory joint effusion); chronic periarticular swelling; pain; recurrent joint effusion; low-grade fever; mildly increased serum alkaline phosphatase level; (b) autosomal recessive inheritance.

Radiologic Manifestations: *Soft-tissue clubbing; periosteal elevation and subperiosteal new bone formation;* joint effusion; *widely open sutures and fontanelles;* wormian bones; *delayed closure of the cranial sutures.*

OSTEOLYSIS CLASSIFICATION

1. Phalangeal: several forms.

2. Carpal and tarsal: (a) Francois and others (autosomal recessive); (b) with nephropathy (autosomal dominant).

3. Miscellaneous: (a) Hajdu-Cheney form (autosomal dominant); (b) Winchester form (autosomal recessive): (c) Torg form (autosomal

recessive); (d) mandibuloacral dysplasia; (e) familial expansile osteolysis; (f) Gorham syndrome; (g) primary idiopathic terminal phalangeal osteolysis (sporadic); (h) others.

OSTEOLYSIS, FAMILIAL EXPANSILE

Clinical Manifestations: (a) *bone pain* (limbs only) with onset varied from the teenage years to middle age; some lesions painless; pathologic fracture; (b) *deafness;* hereditary incus necrosis; (c) miscellaneous abnormalities: progressive tooth mobility; spontaneous tooth fracture; pulpitis; high serum alkaline phosphatase levels; normal serum calcium and phosphorus values; elevated urinary hydroxyproline; (d) autosomal dominant inheritance.

Radiologic Manifestations: (a) bone changes before any localized lesions: slight modeling abnormality of the long bones; distorted trabecular pattern (tightly meshed appearance); (b) *focal expanding bone lesions;* (c) bone scintigraphy: greater uptake of the isotope in the tibiae as compared with the femora; focal increase in uptake at the site of the radiographic abnormalities; (d) cervical and/or apical root resorption.

OSTEOLYSIS WITH NEPHROPATHY

Clinical Manifestations: Onset of symptoms in early childhood: (a) multifocal *progressive deformities;* shortening of the extremities; *chronic progressive nephropathy;* micrognathia; highly arched palate; corneal opacity; valvular pulmonary stenosis; (b) sporadic; autosomal dominant inheritance.

Radiologic Manifestations: *Progressive disappearance of bones, in particular carpals and tarsals;* partial resorption of adjacent tubular bones ("sucked candy" appearance of the tubular bones); shortening and bowing of tubular bones; flattening/loss of normal curvature and osteoporosis of carpal and tarsal bones before the development of osteolysis.

OSTEOLYSIS WITHOUT NEPHROPATHY (CARPAL AND TARSAL OSTEOLYSIS)

Clinical Manifestations: Onset of symptoms in early childhood: (a) *arthritic complaints; swelling of joints and soft-tissue thickening followed by a period of progressive deformity; collapse in the wrists, ankles, etc.;* (b) autosomal dominant or X-linked dominant inheritance; less commonly reported as recessive; sporadic.

Radiologic Manifestations: *Demineralization in the early stage; collapse, sclerosis, and bone resorption* (carpals; tarsals; elbows; shoulders);

magnetic resonance imaging in carpal and tarsal osteolysis: absence of the bones; replacement by fibrocartilaginous tissue; arteriography: occlusion of the radial artery.

OSTEOMA CUTIS, FAMILIAL

Clinical Manifestations: (a) *subcutaneous areas of thickening* at various sites; subcutaneous mobile lumps; normal values for serum calcium, phosphorus, and alkaline phosphatase; (b) miscellaneous abnormalities: primary osteoma cutis associated with café au lait spots, wooly hair, and intrauterine growth deficiency; congenital platelike osteoma (a rare variant of osteoma cutis); (c) dominant trait.

Radiologic Manifestations: *Ectopic bone masses.*

OSTEOPOROSIS-PSEUDOGLIOMA SYNDROME

Clinical Manifestations: Clinical variability: (a) *blindness with onset in infancy: microphthalmos; iris, lens, and anterior chamber abnormalities; vitreoretinal abnormalities; cataracts;* (b) *short stature;* (c) *muscular hypotonia; hyperextensible joints; spontaneous fractures;* (d) miscellaneous abnormalities: elbow limitation of motion; short spine; barrel chest; kyphoscoliosis; thin/sparse hair; seizures; obesity; discolored teeth; mental retardation; microcephaly; etc.; (e) autosomal recessive inheritance; assigned to chromosome region 11q12–13.

Radiologic Manifestations: (a) *osteoporosis* with onset in childhood; narrow diaphyses; wide metaphyses; thin cortices; coarse trabecular structure; *fractures; long bone deformities; platyspondyly; "cod-fish vertebrae";* (b) *smallness of the ophthalmic fossa; lens and orbital calcifications; structural abnormalities of the eye;* (c) miscellaneous abnormalities: wormian bones; mild skeletal maturation retardation; ventricular septal defect.

OTO-PALATO-DIGITAL SYNDROME TYPE I (OPD-I SYNDROME; TAYBI SYNDROME)

Clinical Manifestations: (a) *short stature (most);* (b) characteristic craniofacial features: *frontal bossing; prominent occiput; prominent supraorbital ridges; flat face; broad nasal root; downward slanting of the palpebral fissures; microstomia; cleft palate;* (c) *conductive deafness;* (d) *short, broad thumbs and great toes,* and broad terminal phalanges of the other digits; (e) miscellaneous abnormalities: limited elbow motion; syndactyly of the toes; nail dystrophy; dental anomalies; omphalocele; (f) X-linked with lesser expression in females; most patients male.

Radiologic Manifestations: (a) *thick and dense base of the skull; prominence of the supraorbital ridges; steep clivus; poor pneumatization of the frontal and sphenoid sinuses;* delayed closure of the anterior fontanelle; small mandible; *poor development of the mastoids; dense middle-ear ossicles;* (b) posterior defect of the neural arch of the vertebrae; (c) dislocation of the radial heads; flat acetabulum; coxa valga; mild lateral bowing of femora; *carpal anomalies* (transverse capitate; comma-shaped trapezoid; carpal fusions; supernumerary carpal bones); *tarsal anomalies* (fusion; anomalous fifth metatarsal; extra calcaneal ossification center); *short thumbs and great toes;* large cone-shaped epiphysis of the distal phalanx of the thumbs and great toes; partial anodontia; (d) impacted teeth; (e) miscellaneous abnormalities: bowing of the long bones; widened lower thoracic and lumbosacral spinal canal; small pedicles; hip and elbow subluxation.

OVARIAN VEIN SYNDROME

Clinical and Radiologic Manifestations: *Obstruction of the distal part of the ureter by the ovarian vein;* symptoms often in parous women and exceptionally in children or nulliparous women: *abdominal pain;* abdominal colic; pain in the sacral area and thighs; nausea and vomiting; pyelonephritis; obstructive nephropathy; *ovarian vein (unilateral; occasionally bilateral) dilatation;* rapid improvement following embolization of the ovarian vein.

P

PACHYDERMOPERIOSTOSIS (TOURAINE-SOLENTE-GOLÉ SYNDROME)

Clinical Manifestations: Onset of symptoms around puberty: (a) *coarsening of facial features (thickening and folding of the skin); spade-like enlargement of the hands and feet; digital clubbing;* cylindric thickening of the legs and forearms; *furrowing, thickening, and oiliness of the skin;* excessive sweating; *cutis verticis gyrata* ("bulldog" scalp); (b) miscellaneous abnormalities: arthralgia, arthritis; involvement of the connective tissue of the eyelids; presentation as acromegaly-like syndrome; carpal and tarsal tunnel syndromes; calcification of the Achilles tendon; chronic leg ulcerations; (c) autosomal dominant and autosomal recessive modes of inheritance have been suggested; 85% of reported cases in males.
Radiologic Manifestations
(A) EARLY STAGE: *symmetric excessive subperiosteal new bone formation of the long bones, metacarpals, metatarsals, and proximal phalanges.*

(B) ADVANCED STAGE: (a) *diffuse subperiosteal bone formation;* ossification of the ligaments and tendons; joint effusion; *joint ankylosis;* acro-osteolysis; (b) scintigraphic abnormalities: diffuse uptake along the cortical margins of the long bones; (c) arteriographic abnormalities of limbs: sluggish flow; vascular stasis; tortuosity; segmental narrowing; (d) miscellaneous abnormalities: cortical thickening of the skull; absence of fatty bone marrow of the skull; cortical new bone formation of vertebrae; compression of the spinal cord.

PAGET-SCHROETTER SYNDROME

Clinical Manifestations: Rapid or gradual onset of pain, redness, tenderness, and increased venous pressure in an upper limb; cordlike masses in the axilla; marked venous collateral circulation of the arm and shoulder (infrared photography).

Radiologic Manifestations: (a) venographic demonstration of venous obstruction (subclavian-axillary vein, subclavian-innominate vein, or both) and collateral circulation; (b) color Doppler is recommended as screening method; not as informative as venography.

PALLISTER-HALL SYNDROME

Clinical Manifestations: (a) *panhypopituitarism;* (b) *craniofacial anomalies:* flat nasal bridge; short nose; ear anomalies; microglossia/micrognathia; buccal frenula; palatal anomalies; (c) *postaxial polydactyly/oligodactyly; nail dysplasia/hypoplasia; imperforate/anteriorly placed anus;* (d) miscellaneous abnormalities: endocrine disorders (adrenal aplasia/dysplasia; hypoadrenalism; testicular hypoplasia; thyroid aplasia/dysplasia; hypothyroidism); cryptorchidism; micropenis; etc.; (e) most reported cases sporadic; reported in sibs; autosomal dominant inheritance.

Radiologic Manifestations: (a) *hypothalamic hamartoblastoma; pituitary aplasia/dysplasia;* (b) *postaxial polydactyly/oligodactyly;* (c) miscellaneous abnormalities: central nervous system anomalies (microcephaly; holoprosencephaly; deficient olfactory bulbs/tracts; leptomeningeal cyst; absent corpus callosum; polymicrogyria; Dandy-Walker cyst; heterotopias; encephalocele); genitourinary anomalies (renal dysplasia; renal ectopia); polydactyly and asymptomatic hypothalamic hamartoma in mother and son (a variant of the syndrome); overlap of clinical manifestations with Kaufman-McKusick syndrome.

PALLISTER-KILLIAN SYNDROME (TETRASOMY 12P)

Clinical Manifestations: (a) *craniofacial dysmorphism:* coarse facial appearance; broad, high forehead; epicanthal folds; broad bridge of nose;

small nose; long and simple philtrum; prominent upper lip; bitemporal alopecia; sparse scalp hair, eyelashes, and eyebrows; hypertelorism; exophthalmos; macrostomia; abnormal ears; cleft lip; cleft palate; lip pit; small mandible in infancy; macroglossia/prognathia in older children and adolescents; (b) short neck; webbed neck; (c) hypotonia in newborn; hypertonia and *contractures in older children and adolescents;* (d) *isochromosome 12p mosaicism;* prenatal and postnatal false-negative test possible; (e) *mental and motor retardation; seizures; behavioral disorders;* (f) ocular abnormalities: microphthalmia; keratoconus; pinpoint pupils; aniridia; hypopigmentation of the fundi; (g) skeletal abnormalities: small and broad hands and feet; short finger and toes; tapering fingers; postaxial polydactyly of toes; (h) genitourinary abnormalities: ambiguous genitalia; hypoplasia of labia majora; absent upper vagina; absent uterus; cryptorchidism; small scrotum; (i) cardiovascular anomalies.

Radiologic Manifestations: (a) *distal digital hypoplasia; shortness of the long bones;* (b) miscellaneous abnormalities: urogenital sinus anomaly; imperforate anus; ventriculomegaly; cerebellar hypoplasia; hypoplastic corpus callosum; skeletal maturation retardation; diaphragmatic hernia; cystic kidneys; dysplastic kidneys; etc.

PANCOAST SYNDROME

Clinical Manifestations: *Pain* in the shoulder region with radiation into the axilla, toward the scapula, and along the ulnar aspect of the arm; *muscular atrophy* and weakness of the muscles of the hand; *Horner syndrome;* compression of blood vessels causing edema; hoarseness.

Pathology: Destructive lesion of the thoracic inlet (neoplastic; traumatic; inflammatory; etc.) with involvement of the brachial and sympathetic plexus nerves.

Radiologic Manifestations: *Apical thoracic density in the form of a cap or a mass;* bone destruction (ribs; vertebrae); indentation of the esophagus by a mass; displacement and encasement of subclavian and/or brachiocephalic arteries (magnetic resonance angiography).

PAPILLON-LEFÈVRE SYNDROME

Clinical Manifestations: Onset of symptoms in infancy: (a) *hyperkeratosis of the palm, sole, ankle, elbow, and knee; centripetal extension of the keratoses to the limbs and trunk; periodontopathy,* gingival swelling and erythema; loosening of the teeth; deep periodontal pockets of infection; loss of teeth; abnormally thin cementum; extensive destruction of the periodontal ligament; early eruption of permanent teeth; (b) autosomal recessive inheritance.

Radiologic Manifestations: (a) *marked destruction of supporting alveolar bone, with teeth soon becoming mobile and prematurely lost* (deciduous and permanent teeth); atrophy of the alveolar process following a period of bone destruction; almost completely edentulous by the age of 17 years; (b) miscellaneous abnormalities: skeletal maturation retardation; osteoporosis; acro-osteolysis; dural and choroidal calcifications.

PARINAUD SYNDROME

Etiology: Extraaxial pineal region masses; intrinsic midbrain masses; multifocal glioma; hydrocephalus; ischemic lesions; metabolic disorders; drug-induced; degenerative diseases; multiple sclerosis; infections; inflammations.

Clinical Manifestations: *Diplopia; ptosis or separation of the eyelids; paralysis of conjugate upward movement of the eye without paralysis of convergence; retraction; nystagmus; wide pupils; papilledema.*

Radiologic Manifestations: Demonstration of the etiologic factors.

PEHO SYNDROME (PROGRESSIVE ENCEPHALOPATHY–HYPSARRHYTHMIA–OPTIC ATROPHY)

Clinical Manifestations: (a) *hypotonia at birth; infantile spasms with hypsarrhythmia; psychomotor retardation; severe hypotonia with brisk tendon reflexes;* (b) *subcutaneous nonpitting edema;* (c) electroencephalographic abnormalities: focal or generalized epileptiform activity; (d) *visual failure; pale optic discs; optic atrophy;* (e) *microcephaly;* (f) apparently autosomal recessive inheritance.

Radiologic Manifestations: *Abnormal myelination; progressive brain atrophy; abnormal gyral formation; cerebellar and brain-stem atrophy in most cases.*

PENDRED SYNDROME

Clinical Manifestations: (a) *congenital perceptive hearing loss;* (b) *goiter* (thyroid dyshormonogenesis; intrinsic defect in thyroid iodine organification); (c) *pathologic perchlorate test findings;* (d) autosomal recessive inheritance; maps to chromosome 7q21–34.

Radiologic Manifestations: *Goiter; Mondini defect* (malformation of the cochlea: partial aplasia resulting in 1 to 1.5 coils instead of the normal 2.5 to 2.75 coils, with the middle and apical coils sharing a common cloaca).

PERISYLVIAN SYNDROME (CONGENITAL BILATERAL)

Clinical Manifestations: (a) *neurologic manifestations:* seizures; dysarthria; dysphagia; drooling; restriction of tongue movements; absent gag reflexes; pyramidal signs; delayed motor and language development; mild to moderate mental retardation; (b) miscellaneous abnormalities: congenital unilateral perisylvian syndrome (unilateral widening and verticalization of the sylvian fossa associated with an abnormal ipsilateral perisylvian cortex).

Radiologic Manifestations: *Bilateral perisylvian and perirolandic malformations: thick cortex; shallow sulci; broad gyri; exposed insula.*

PERLMAN SYNDROME

Clinical Manifestations: (a) *facial dysmorphism* (round, full, and hypotonic with open mouth; long, inverted V-shaped upper lip; micrognathia; serrated upper alveolar edge; upsweep of the anterior scalp hairline); *macrosomia;* etc.; (b) autosomal recessive inheritance.

Radiologic Manifestations: *Nephroblastomatosis/Wilms tumor;* renal hamartomas; nephromegaly; renal dysplasia.

PERSISTENT MÜLLERIAN DUCT SYNDROME

Clinical and Radiologic Manifestations: A form of *male pseudohermaphroditism with persistence of müllerian derivatives in phenotypic males* (defect in the synthesis or action of anti-müllerian hormone): (a) *unilateral or bilateral cryptorchidism (testes); normal external genitalia; inguinal hernia containing female genital organs (uterus and fallopian tubes);* typically 46,XY; azoospermia; testicular degeneration; etc.; (b) autosomal recessive inheritance.

PERSISTING MESONEPHRIC DUCT SYNDROME

Clinical and Radiologic Manifestations: The triad: (a) persistence of the mesonephric duct: *genitourinary anomalies;* (b) *rectal anomalies:* imperforate anus; anal stenosis; H-type urethroanal fistula; anteriorly displaced anus; (c) *anomalies of renal ascent or morphology:* pelvic kidney; hydronephrosis; multicystic kidney; crossed renal ectopia; retroiliac artery ureter; unilateral absence of kidney.

PEUTZ-JEGHERS SYNDROME

Clinical Manifestations: (a) *brown or black pigmentations of the lips, buccal mucosa, face, palms, and soles;* (b) *hamartomatous polyps;* malignant degeneration of the polyps (rare); (c) miscellaneous abnormalities: increased incidence of ovarian cysts and tumors (5%) (sex cord tumor); high risk of development of neoplasms (18 times greater than in the general population); pericentric inversion of chromosome 6; etc.; (d) autosomal dominant inheritance; incomplete penetrance.

Radiologic Manifestations: (a) *alimentary tract polyposis* (stomach; small bowel; colon); (b) extragastrointestinal polyps (urinary tract; bronchus; nose; gallbladder; bile duct); (c) miscellaneous abnormalities: appendiceal intussusception due to an appendiceal polyp.

PFEIFFER SYNDROME (ACROCEPHALOSYNDACTYLY, PFEIFFER TYPE)

Clinical Manifestations: (a) *craniofacial dysmorphism:* acrocephaly; brachycephaly; hypertelorism; downward slant of the palpebral fissures; strabismus; proptosis; beaked nose; highly arched palate; (b) *soft-tissue syndactyly of fingers and toes; brachydactyly; broad thumbs and great toes; ulnar deviation of thumbs; tibial deviation of great toes;* (c) miscellaneous abnormalities: mental deficiency (in some); etc.; (d) autosomal dominant inheritance; genetic heterogeneity: mapped to chromosome 8 centromere and a second locus on chromosome 10q25.

Radiologic Manifestations: (a) *premature closure of the sagittal and coronal sutures; hypertelorism; shallow anterior cranial fossa; flattened nasal bridge;* (b) hand abnormalities: *broad thumbs; mild soft-tissue syndactyly* (2-3; 3-4); varus deformity of the thumbs; brachydactyly; brachymesophalangy; absent middle phalanges; clinodactyly; symphalangism; fusion of carpal bones; fusion of the proximal end of metacarpals; (c) feet abnormalities: *broad great toes; mild soft-tissue syndactyly of the toes;* varus deformity of the great toes; brachymesophalangy; absent middle phalanges; malformed proximal phalanx of the great toes; short and deformed first metatarsals; duplication of the first metatarsal; accessory secondary ossification center of great toes and first metatarsals; partial duplication of the great toes; symphalangism; fusion of tarsal bones, fusion of the proximal end of metatarsals.

PHALANGEAL MICROGEODIC SYNDROME (MICROGEODIC PHALANGEAL SYNDROME)

Clinical Manifestations: *Swelling, redness, heat, and minimal pain in the fingers;* spontaneous regression of clinical manifestations within a few months; unknown cause.

Radiologic Manifestations: *Small lacunae in the middle and distal phalanges of affected fingers; mild widening of involved phalanges.*

PIBI(D)S SYNDROME

Clinical Manifestations: (a) *P*hotosensitivity, mild noncongenital *I*chthyosis, *B*rittle cystine-deficient hair, *I*mpaired intelligence, *D*ecreased fertility (in some), and *S*hort stature; (b) miscellaneous abnormalities:

dysarthria; spasticity with pyramidal signs; hyperreflexia; intention tremor; neurosensory hearing loss; nystagmus; jerky eye movements; cataracts; peripheral neuropathy; intermittent hair loss and trichothiodystrophy; (c) autosomal recessive inheritance.

Radiologic Manifestations: (a) mild ventriculomegaly; ventricular asymmetry; diffuse high signal throughout the cerebral white matter on T_2-weighted magnetic resonance images; (b) axial osteosclerosis.

PICKWICKIAN SYNDROME

Clinical Manifestations: (a) *marked obesity; somnolence;* excessive diurnal fatigue with psychotic symptoms; (b) *cardiorespiratory insufficiency with decreased alveolar ventilation;* intermittent cyanosis; periodic respiration; decreased hypoxic ventilatory drive; sleep apnea; arrhythmias; serious elevation of both pulmonary and systemic pressures; secondary polycythemia; myoclonic twitching; right ventricular hypertrophy; right ventricular failure (in an advanced stage).

Radiologic Manifestations: *Cardiomegaly; narrow oropharynx;* normal or prominent pulmonary vasculature.

PLUMMER-VINSON SYNDROME

Clinical Manifestations: Most patients middle-aged white women: glossitis; mucosal changes in the mouth, pharynx, and proximal segment of the esophagus *(webs; bands; mucosal folds)* causing dysphagia; *simple hypochromic anemia;* achlorhydria.

Radiologic Manifestations: *Web in the hypopharynx or cervical esophagus;* spasm in the pharynx and esophagus.

POEMS SYNDROME (Takatsuki Syndrome; Crow-Fukase Syndrome)

Clinical Manifestations: A complex multisystem disorder: (a) *polyneuropathy* (often sensorimotor); papilledema; increased cerebrospinal fluid protein concentration; (b) *hepatomegaly; splenomegaly; renomegaly; lymphadenopathy;* (c) *endocrinopathy:* gynecomastia; impotence; amenorrhea; glucose intolerance; adrenal insufficiency; hypothyroidism; (d) *M protein in the serum;* (e) *skin changes: hyperpigmentation; thickening; hirsutism; hyperhidrosis;* verrucous angiomas; (f) *bone lesions containing plasma cells and amyloid;* (g) peripheral edema; ascites; pleural effusion; (h) miscellaneous abnormalities: pericardial effusion; finger clubbing; white fingernails; yellow nails; etc.

Radiologic Manifestations: (a) various patterns of bone lesions: *single or multiple sclerotic ringlike lytic or mixed sclerotic and lytic bone lesions* *(most common in the spine, pelvis, and ribs; also reported in the skull and long bones); coarse bony trabeculae; cortical thickening; lacelike or "mulberry" nonhomogeneous pattern of bone sclerosis with sharply defined, spiculated contours; diffuse calvarial thickening;* "ivory vertebra"; compression fracture of thoracolumbar spine with or without sclerotic or lytic lesions; uptake on radionuclide bone scan (uncommon); (b) miscellaneous abnormalities: enlarged, echogenic kidneys; infiltrative orbitopathy; premature vascular calcification; thrombocythemia and arterial thrombosis; elevated intracranial pressure and diffuse white matter edema (magnetic resonance imaging).

Note: *POEMS* is an acronym for *P*lasma cell dysplasia-polyneuropathy, *O*rganomegaly, *E*ndocrinopathy, *M* protein, and *S*kin changes.

POLAND SEQUENCE

Clinical Manifestations: (a) *partial or complete absence of pectoralis muscles; anomalies of the ipsilateral upper limb;* posterior shoulder girdle abnormalities; association with malignancies; (b) sporadic; very few familial cases have been reported (mother and daughter; siblings; cousins).

Radiologic Manifestations: (a) *syndactyly;* polydactyly; hypoplasia of the arm and hand; absence of metacarpals and phalanges; (b) *relative hyperlucency of the ipsilateral hemithorax,* absence of a normal axillary fold on the affected side; *muscular and skeletal anomalies of shoulder and chest wall;* (c) breast hypoplasia or absence: three-dimensional computed tomography used as adjunct for planning chest-wall and breast reconstruction; (d) miscellaneous abnormalities: axillary web or band; lung herniation.

Association with Other Syndromes/Anomalies: Möbius (Poland-Möbius syndrome); Adams-Oliver syndrome; limb body wall disruption defect; frontonasal dysplasia; morning glory syndrome; oculo-auriculo-vertebral spectrum.

POLYCYSTIC KIDNEY DISEASE (PKD)

Classification
1. Dominant PKD (adult PKD)
2. Recessive PKD (infantile PKD)
3. Familial hypoplastic glomerulocystic kidney disease, autosomal dominant
4. Juvenile nephronophthisis–medullary cystic disease complex
   • Juvenile nephronophthisis, autosomal recessive
   • Medullary cystic disease, autosomal dominant
5. Cystic kidneys in syndromes: tuberous sclerosis; von Hippel–Lindau syndrome; Meckel syndrome; asphyxiating thoracic dysplasia; Ivemark syndrome (cystic kidneys, hepatic and pancreatic fibrosis); familial polycystic kidney-cataract-blindness

6. Medullary sponge kidneys (less than 5% inherited)
7. Congenital hypernephronic nephromegaly with tubular dysgenesis

POLYPOSIS SYNDROMES

1. Familial adenomatous polyposis: (a) very high risk (approaching 100%) of colon carcinoma; occult radiopaque jaw lesions, which are good predictors of polyp development in kindred with adenomatous polyposis and jaw lesions; extracolonic tumors; (b) autosomal inheritance
2. Familial juvenile polyposis coli; autosomal dominant inheritance
3. Familial gastric polyposis
4. Familial polyposis of the entire gastrointestinal tract (often juvenile type)
5. Cowden syndrome
6. Cronkhite-Canada syndrome
7. Gardner syndrome
8. Intestinal polyposis with exostoses (a family report)
9. Peutz-Jeghers syndrome
10. Ruvalcaba-Myhre-Smith syndrome
11. Turcot syndrome

POLYSPLENIA SYNDROME

Clinical Manifestations: (a) *cardiovascular anomalies;* (b) *noncardiac polysplenia type (biliary atresia/polysplenia)* with the manifestations of biliary atresia; (c) cyanosis due to intrapulmonary shunting.

Radiologic Manifestations: (a) *levoisomerism:* two lobes in each lung, bilateral hyparterial bronchi; (b) *cardiovascular anomalies* in about 90% of the cases: *interruption of the inferior vena cava with azygous or hemiazygous continuation;* bilateral superior vena cava; *cardiac defects; diffuse pulmonary arteriovenous malformation; etc.;* (c) *hepatic symmetry; absent gallbladder;* (d) alimentary system anomalies; (e) *biliary atresia/polysplenia type:* intrapulmonary shunting and reversal after liver transplantation; (f) *a common celiac-mesenteric artery and multiple spleens.*

Note: Noncardiac polysplenia type (biliary atresia/polysplenia): polysplenia reported in approximately 10% of children with biliary atresia.

POPLITEAL ARTERY ENTRAPMENT SYNDROME

Clinical Manifestations: Unilateral or bilateral *intermittent claudication* (foot; calf muscles) usually in young adult males; *numbness, tingling, or coolness of the foot relieved by leg position changes; ischemic symp-*

toms after vigorous exercises; absent or decreased ankle pulses; diminished resting ankle/brachial pressure index.

Radiologic Manifestations: (a) *arteriographic demonstration of segmental occlusion and medial displacement of the popliteal artery;* stress runoff technique (active plantar flexing against a foot board) may be necessary to show the obstruction; (b) magnetic resonance imaging demonstrating the abnormality of the popliteal artery course and its relationship to the musculotendinous structure of the popliteal fossa; (c) Doppler ultrasonographic demonstration of circulatory disorders; thrombosis; peripheral embolization; poststenotic aneurysm formation; (d) miscellaneous abnormalities: bony exostosis as the etiologic factor; leg muscle scintigraphy with ^{99m}Tc MIBI and single photon emission computed tomography in evaluation of vascular obstruction.

POSTAXIAL ACROFACIAL DYSOSTOSIS, MILLER TYPE

Clinical Manifestations: Phenotypic variability and changes with age: (a) *malar hypoplasia, lower lid ectropion, micrognathia, cleft palate, cleft lip, cup-shaped ears, low-set ears,* hypotelorism, and upward slant of short palpebral fissures; (b) *absence of the fifth digital rays of the four limbs* with or without associated forearm anomalies; (c) the majority of the cases sporadic; autosomal recessive inheritance in several families; autosomal dominant inheritance less likely.

Radiologic Manifestations: (a) *absence of the fifth digit; aplasia or hypoplasia of the fifth ray of the hand (unilateral or bilateral);* shortened forearm; ulnar hypoplasia; *absent fifth toes;* absent third and fourth toes in some; (b) miscellaneous abnormalities: preaxial anomalies (oligodactyly; short radius; proximally inserted thumbs); radioulnar synostosis; rib anomalies; vertebral segmentation anomalies; hypoplasia of femora; defective pelvic bone ossification; renal anomalies; midgut malrotation; gastric volvulus.

POSTCARDIOTOMY SYNDROME (POSTPERICARDIOTOMY SYNDROME)

Clinical Manifestations: Onset of symptoms weeks or months after a surgical procedure (closed or open heart surgery): *chest pain; fever;* muscle and joint pain; cough; *pericardial friction rubs;* dyspnea; elevated leukocyte count and erythrocyte sedimentation rate; relief of symptoms with salicylates or corticosteroids; high titer of heart reactive antibody; etc.

Radiologic Manifestations: *Pericardial effusion* (serous or serosanguineous); pleural effusion; basilar pulmonary infiltrates; noncardiac pulmonary edema; absence of frank congestive heart failure; cardiac tamponade; constrictive pericarditis.

POSTCHOLECYSTECTOMY SYNDROME

Clinical Manifestations: *Recurrence of symptoms* present prior to cholecystectomy (abdominal pain; nausea; vomiting; etc.)

Radiologic Manifestations: *Detection of abnormalities undiagnosed prior to cholecystectomy* (retained stones; ampullary stenosis [stenosis of the sphincter of Oddi, papilla of Vater stenosis, or papillary stenosis]; juxtapapillary diverticula; benign stricture; cancer of the bile duct; pancreatic disease; dysfunction of the sphincter; retained broken T-tube); *diagnosis of conditions not related to the biliary system undetected prior to surgery.*

POSTCOARCTECTOMY SYNDROME

Clinical Manifestations: Onset of symptoms usually after the second postoperative day: *abdominal pain; tenderness; distension; ileus; vomiting; melena;* fever; hypertension; leukocytosis.

Pathology: Related to postoperative paradoxical hypertension: hemorrhagic areas in the bowel wall; arterial and venous thrombosis; necrosis and ulceration of the bowel; perforation; inflammatory cellular infiltrate of the bowel wall; rupture of inferior phrenic artery aneurysm (a complication of mesenteric arteritis).

Radiologic Manifestations: *Adynamic ileus,* with dilated bowel loops seen on plain film; contrast study demonstrating *edema of the bowel with thickening of mucosal folds;* stenosis of the bowel at the site of scarring as a late sequela; vasoconstriction: beading, segmental constriction, dilatation, and stretching; delayed distal progression of the contrast.

POSTGASTRECTOMY SYNDROMES

Types
- Afferent loop syndromes (acute; chronic)
- Alkaline gastritis (reflux gastritis)
- Dumping syndromes (early and late)
- Efferent loop syndrome
- Malabsorption syndrome
- Postvagotomy-functional syndrome
- Small gastric pouch syndrome

Complications: Anemia; osteomalacia; osteoporosis; hypoglycemia; vitamin B_{12} deficiency; bezoar; jejunogastric intussusception; weight loss; diarrhea; cancer of the gastric remnant.

POSTMYOCARDIAL INFARCTION SYNDROME (Dressler Syndrome)

Clinical Manifestations: Onset usually after a *latency period* of one to several weeks following myocardial infarction: *chest pain; fever; polyserositis* (pericardium, pleura); increased erythrocyte sedimentation rate; leukocytosis; tendency to recur; heart-specific antibodies.

Radiologic Manifestations: *Enlargement of the cardiopericardial shadow; pleural effusion; pulmonary infiltrates* (in some); noncardiac pulmonary edema; widening of the upper portion of the mediastinum (one third of cases); pericardial effusion.

POSTPNEUMONECTOMY SYNDROME

Clinical Manifestations: Development of symptoms within the first year after right pneumonectomy: *dyspnea; recurrent pulmonary infections.*

Radiologic Manifestations: *Mediastinal shift; herniation of lung anteriorly into right hemithorax; rotation of heart and great vessels (counterclockwise); compression and deformity of trachea or left main bronchus (descending aorta, pulmonary artery, ligamentum arteriosum, and spine causing the pressure on the tracheobronchial tree).*

POTTER SEQUENCE

Clinical Manifestations: (a) *Potter facies:* flattened facies, widely spaced eyes, low-set large and floppy ears, micrognathia, a prominent fold that arises at the inner canthus and extends downward and laterally below the eyes; (b) *excessively lax skin in some;* (c) *limb-positioning defects:* rocker-bottom feet; etc.; (d) *fetal growth deficiency;* (e) autosomal recessive, autosomal dominant, and X-linked recessive patterns of inheritance have been suggested.

Radiologic Manifestations: (a) prenatal diagnosis by ultrasonography: *severe oligohydramnios; renal agenesis or dysplasia; limb deformities; fetal growth retardation;* (b) *pneumothorax; pneumomediastinum; decreased thoracic volume; bell-shaped thorax; poorly expanded and "structureless" lung (pulmonary hypoplasia);* (c) *absent kidneys; cystic kidneys; small bladder;* (d) ultrasonography in renal tubular dysgenesis: indistinct corticomedullary differentiation of the kidneys with cortical echogenicity equal to the liver; (e) miscellaneous abnormalities: large adrenal glands mimicking the presence of kidneys; clubfeet; etc.

PRADER-WILLI SYNDROME

Clinical Manifestations: Table SY-P-1

Table SY-P-1 Diagnostic Criteria for Prader-Willi Syndrome*

Major criteria
1. Neonatal and infantile central hypotonia with poor suck, gradually improving with age.
2. Feeding problems in infancy with need for special feeding techniques and poor weight gain/failure to thrive
3. Excessive or rapid weight gain on weight-for-length chart (excessive is defined as crossing two centile channels) after 12 months but before 6 years of age; central obesity in the absence of intervention
4. Characteristic facial features with dolichocephaly in infancy, narrow face or bifrontal diameter, almond-shaped eyes, small appearing mouth with thin upper lip, down-turned corners of the mouth (3 or more required)
5. Hypogonadism—with any of the following, depending on age:
   a. Genital hypoplasia (male: scrotal hypoplasia, cryptorchidism, small penis and/or testes for age [< 5th percentile]; female: absences or severe hypoplasia of labia minora and/or clitoris)
   b. Delayed or incomplete gonadal maturation with delayed pubertal signs in the absence of intervention after 16 years of age (male: small gonads, decreased facial and body hair, lack of voice change; female: amenorrhea/oligomenorrhea after age 16)
6. Global developmental delay in a child younger than 6 years of age; mild to moderate mental retardation or learning problems in older children
7. Hyperphagia/food foraging/obsession with food
8. Deletion 15q11–13 on high resolution (>650 bands) or other cytogenetic/molecular abnormality of the Prader-Willi chromosome region, including maternal disomy

Minor criteria
1. Decreased fetal movement or infantile lethargy or weak cry in infancy, improving with age
2. Characteristic behavior problems—temper tantrums, violent outbursts and obsessive/compulsive behavior; tendency to be argumentative, oppositional, rigid, manipulative, possessive, and stubborn; perseverating, stealing, and lying (5 or more of these symptoms required)
3. Sleep disturbance or sleep apnea
4. Short stature for genetic background by age 15 (in the absence of growth hormone intervention)
5. Hypopigmentation—fair skin and hair compared to family
6. Small hands (< 25th percentile) and/or feet (< 10th percentile) for height age

From Holm VA, Cassidy SB, Butler MC et al: Prader-Willi syndrome: consensus diagnostic criteria, *Pediatrics* 91:398, 1993. Used by permission.
*Scoring: Major criteria are weighted at one point each. Minor criteria are weighted at one-half point. Children 3 years of age or younger: Five points are required for diagnosis, four of which should come from the major group. Children 3 years of age to adulthood: Total score of eight is necessary for the diagnosis. Major criteria must comprise five or more points of the total score.

Continued

Table SY-P-1 Diagnostic Criteria for Prader-Willi Syndrome—cont'd

Minor criteria—cont'd
7. Narrow hands with straight ulnar border
8. Eye abnormalities (esotropia, myopia)
9. Thick viscous saliva with crusting at corners of the mouth
10. Speech articulation defects
11. Skin picking

Supportive findings (increase the certainty of diagnosis but are not scored)
1. High pain threshold
2. Decreased vomiting
3. Temperature instability in infancy or altered temperature sensitivity in older children and adults
4. Scoliosis and/or kyphosis
5. Early adrenarche
6. Osteoporosis
7. Unusual skill with jigsaw puzzles
8. Normal neuromuscular studies

From Holm VA, Cassidy SB, Butler MC et al: Prader-Willi syndrome: consensus diagnostic criteria, *Pediatrics* 91:398, 1993. Used by permission.

Radiologic Manifestations: (a) *acromicria;* (b) retarded skeletal maturation; (c) microcrania; increased sutural serration; wormian bones; short mandible with increased mandibular angle; small sella turcica area in the lateral projection; absent frontal sinuses; dental caries; (d) computed tomography of midthigh: higher ratio of fat to muscle in the patients with Prader-Willi syndrome as compared with obese patients without the syndrome, reflecting lesser development of the muscles in Prader-Willi syndrome; (e) slight ventricular dilatation; absence of posterior pituitary bright spot (magnetic resonance imaging).

PROGERIA (HUTCHINSON-GILFORD SYNDROME)

Clinical Manifestations: Onset of symptoms in the second year of life: (a) *typical facies* ("old man" appearance in childhood); frontal and parietal bossing; poor midface development; hypoplastic mandible; thin and beaked nose; (b) *dental abnormalities:* delayed/incomplete primary and secondary dentition; crowding; displacement; discoloration; anodontia; (c) *dwarfism; growth retardation; "horse riding" stance; wide-based gait;* (d) *scleroderma-like changes; brown pigmented areas on the trunk; thin skin with prominent superficial veins on face and scalp; midfacial cyanosis; alopecia with onset at occiput; generalized hypotrichosis; absent or sparse pubic hair; sparse or absent eyebrows and eyelashes;* nail abnormalities (*small, short, and thin*); (e) *joint deformity; muscular atro-*

phy; pointed end of short distal phalanges; (f) high and squeaky voice; (g) conductive hearing loss; fixation of the ossicular chain; (h) average or above average intelligence; (i) atheromatosis; systemic hypertension; myocardial infarction; congestive heart failure; (j) miscellaneous abnormalities: insulin resistance; hyperlipidemia; etc.; (k) *premature death;* (l) most reported cases sporadic; consistent with autosomal recessive inheritance in some cases.

Radiologic Manifestations: (a) *hypoplastic facial bones (in particular the mandible); bitemporal bossing; thin cranial vault;* sutural bones; strips of unossified membrane of the cranial vault; delay in closure of cranial sutures and fontanelles; (b) *slender long bones; coxa valga; genu valgum; pointed distal phalanges; progressive acro-osteolysis of the terminal phalanges;* (c) pyriform chest narrow at the apex; *short and thin clavicles; progressive thinning and resorption of the distal portions of the clavicles and ribs; thin ribs;* rib fracture; (d) osteoporosis; pathologic fractures; poor healing; (e) normal or delayed skeletal maturation; (f) miscellaneous abnormalities: ovoid vertebral body configuration in lateral projection; infantile vertebrae; progressive hip dislocation; avascular necrosis of femoral head; central lucent defects in tibia; kyphoscoliosis; etc.

PROTEUS SYNDROME

Clinical Manifestations: (a) *macrocephaly;* broad depressed nasal bridge and/or beaked nose; asymmetry; frontal bossing; skull abnormalities (called "Buckelschadel") with protuberances in the frontotemporal, parietooccipital, external auditory canals, periorbital, and the alveolar ridges regions; (b) *macrodactyly; partial gigantism of hands and/or feet; usually asymmetric involvement;* hemihypertrophy; (c) skin lesions: *epidermal nevi; hyperkeratosis; thickening of the skin and subcutaneous tissue of the palms and soles; nodular hypertrophy; lipomas; vascular anomalies; depigmentation; pigmented lesions;* (d) *limb asymmetry* (segmental; total); (e) eye abnormalities: strabismus; epibulbar tumor; enlarged eye; myopia; anisocoria; heterochromia irides; unilateral microphthalmos; cataracts; retinal detachment; chorioretinitis; nystagmus; ptosis; (f) miscellaneous abnormalities: enamel hypoplasia; gingival hyperplasia; neoplasms; cystic hygroma in a fetus; etc.

Radiologic Manifestations: (a) *macrocrania; "exostoses"; cranial hyperostosis;* wide subdural space; dilated ventricles; cerebral atrophy; (b) *limb abnormalities:* overgrowth of adipose tissues and bones (in particular in the hands and feet); macrodactyly; etc.; (c) very high or wide irregularly shaped vertebrae; intervertebral disc dystrophy; megaspondylodysplasia; long neck and/or trunk; kyphoscoliosis; cervical vertebral fusion; (d) abnormal ribs and scapulae (hypertrophy; etc.); (e) intraabdominal masses (lipoma; lymphangioma); (f) miscellaneous abnormalities: craniosynostosis; enchondroma; intracranial tumor; "Perthes-like" hip changes; hyperplastic/dysplastic joints; intraarticular osteocartilaginous bodies; progressive diffuse cystic emphysematous pulmonary disease; benign angiolipomatous tumor with intraspinal extension; hemimegalencephaly and associated brain anomalies.

PRUNE-BELLY SYNDROME

Clinical Manifestations: (a) *partial or complete absence of abdominal musculature;* (b) *dysplasia of the urinary tract;* (c) skeletal abnormalities: talipes equinovarus; limb deformities; (d) genital anomalies: *undescended testes;* aplasia of the external genitalia; ambiguous genitalia; megalourethra; (e) congenital heart disease; (f) an estimated male to female ratio of about 20:1 to 10:1; rare occurrence in siblings.

Radiologic Manifestations: (a) *flabby abdomen; bowel distension; bowel malrotation; fecal retention;* volvulus; atresia; stenosis; imperforate anus; (b) flared iliac wings; wide interpubic distance; (c) dysplastic kidneys; pyelocaliectasis; dilated and tortuous ureters; large bladder with an irregular contour; patent urachus; tapering of the base of the bladder extending to the posterior urethra; prostatic maldevelopment; megalourethra; dilated utricle; bladder wall calcification; renal calcification; urethral stenosis; urethral valve; (d) pulmonary hypoplasia; lobar atelectasis; pneumonias; recurrent bronchitis; rib cage narrowing; (e) musculoskeletal abnormalities: vertebral anomalies including sacral agenesis; meningomyelocele; scoliosis; torticollis; pectus carinatum; pectus excavatum; hip dysplasia; lower-limb hemimelia; digital hypoplasia; finger syndactyly; talipes equinovarus; valgus foot; toe syndactyly; metatarsus varus; polydactyly; flaring of costal margins; arthrogryposis; (f) intrauterine ultrasonographic findings: laxity of the abdominal wall; urinary system anomalies; ascites; fetal hydrops; limb anomalies; oligohydramnios or polyhydramnios.

PSEUDOTRISOMY 13 SYNDROME (HOLOPROSENCEPHALY-POLYDACTYLY SYNDROME)

Clinical and Radiologic Manifestations: (a) *holoprosencephaly;* (b) *postaxial polydactyly;* (c) *normal chromosomes;* (d) miscellaneous abnormalities: hydrocephalus; cerebellar hypoplasia; encephalocele; hypotelorism; microphthalmia; anophthalmia; median cleft lip; cleft palate; dysplastic/low-set ears; preaxial polydactyly; feet deformities; limb shortness; upper-limb defects; hemivertebra; cardiovascular anomalies; urogenital anomalies; gastrointestinal tract malformations; lung malsegmentation; etc.; (e) autosomal recessive inheritance.

PTERYGIUM SYNDROMES

Neck Pterygium (Webbed Neck)

ASSOCIATION WITH THE FOLLOWING: (1) chromosomal syndromes: trisomy 21; trisomy 13; trisomy 18; Turner syndrome; etc.; (2) Noonan syndrome; (3) Nielson syndrome: short stature, cleft palate, camptodactyly, and vertebral fusion; (4) Golden-Lakim syndrome: dolichocephaly, small mandible, pointed facies, bifid uvula, pectus excavatum, kyphoscoliosis, flexion deformity of the knees without webbing, pes cavus, and clubfoot; (5) LEOPARD syndrome; (6) fetal alcohol syndrome; (7) multiple pterygium syndrome; (8) pterygium colli medianum and midline cervical cleft; (9) Potter syndrome; (10) cardiovascular anomalies (hypoplastic left heart; coarctation of aorta; hypoplastic aorta; bicuspid aortic valve; aortic atresia; etc.); jugular lymphatic obstruction.

Pterygium Syndromes and Syndromes with Limb Pterygia

(A) POPLITEAL PTERYGIUM SYNDROME (FACIO-GENITO-POPLITEAL SYNDROME): (a) *lower lip pits; cleft lip and/or cleft palate;* micrognathia; ankyloblepharon filiforme; syngnathia; *popliteal web in severe cases extending from ischium to the heel (containing popliteal artery and the peroneal nerve); intercrural pterygium; genitourinary anomalies;* skeletal anomalies; nail anomalies; etc.; (b) autosomal dominant inheritance with variable expressivity and incomplete penetrance.

(B) ANTECUBITAL PTERYGIUM SYNDROME: (a) *web extending across the cubital fossa; other reported abnormalities* (subluxation of the radial head; maldevelopment of the radioulnar joint; aplasia of the trochlea of the humerus; cleft palate; association with nail-patella syndrome); (b) autosomal dominant inheritance with some reduction in penetrance.

(C) MULTIPLE PTERYGIUM–PTOSIS–SKELETAL ABNORMALITIES SYNDROME: (a) multiple pterygia; ptosis of the eyelids; antimongoloid slanting of the palpebral fissures; skeletal anomalies; (b) autosomal dominant inheritance.

(D) MULTIPLE PTERYGIUM SYNDROME (ESCOBAR SYNDROME): (a) *webbing of variable severity and distribution (neck; axilla; elbow; intercrural; knee; digits); short stature; orofacial anomalies* (epicanthal folds or hypertelorism; long philtrum; downward slanting palpebral fissures; low-set ears; micrognathia; eyelid ptosis; cleft palate; downturned corners of the mouth); *musculoskeletal abnormalities; genital anomalies; etc.;* (b) autosomal recessive inheritance.

(E) LETHAL MULTIPLE PTERYGIUM SYNDROME: Antimongoloid slant of the eyes; hypertelorism; cleft palate and lips; low-set ears; cutaneous syndactyly of the fingers; pterygium (neck; axilla; chin; antecubital; knee); genital abnormalities; various skeletal anomalies; etc.

(F) LETHAL PTERYGIUM SYNDROME WITH FACIAL CLEFT (BARTSOCAS-PAPAS SYNDROME): Low birth weight; microcephaly; ankyloblepharon; corneal ulceration; filiform band between the jaws; cleft palate and lips; hypoplastic nose; apparently low-set ears; lanugo hair; absent thumb/finger syndactyly; equinovarus/syndactyly of the toes; bilateral popliteal pterygium; hypoplastic nails; genital abnormalities; synostosis of the hands and feet.

Q

QUADRILATERAL SPACE SYNDROME

Etiology: Compression of the posterior humeral circumflex artery (PHCA) and axillary nerve in the quadrilateral space (fibrous bands; trauma).

Clinical Manifestations: Usual occurrence in young adults: *poorly localized shoulder pain; intermittent paresthesia in the upper limb during forward flexion, abduction, or both; aggravation of the symptoms with external rotation of the humerus.*

Radiologic Manifestation: : *Obstruction of the PHCA with the arm in abduction and external rotation; atrophy of one or both muscles (teres minor and deltoid) innervated by the axillary nerve* (demonstrable by magnetic resonance imaging).

R

RAEDER SYNDROME (PARATRIGEMINAL SYNDROME)

Clinical Manifestations: A lesion near the ascending sympathetic chain in the neck distal to the superior cervical ganglion: *unilateral migrainelike headache; pain in the distribution of the first* (V1) *and second* (V2) *divisions of the ipsilateral trigeminal nerve; an incomplete Horner syndrome:* miosis; ptosis; preserved facial sweating.

Radiologic Manifestations: Demonstration of the etiologic factors: sinusitis; vascular abnormalities; tumor; etc.

RAMON SYNDROME

Clinical Manifestations: (a) *cherubism; gingival fibromatosis; epilepsy; mental deficiency;* etc.; (b) consanguineous parents.

Radiologic Manifestations: *Fibrous dysplasia of the jaw:* "soap bubble," multilocular, with bone distension and thinning of the cortex of the maxilla and mandible.

RAMSAY HUNT SYNDROME

Clinical Manifestations: *Herpetic eruption on the external auditory meatus; tinnitus, vertigo, and deafness; facial paralysis.*

Radiologic Manifestations: Magnetic resonance imaging: abnormal enhancement of the labyrinth and the intratemporal cranial nerves; may mimic acoustic neuroma.

RASMUSSEN SYNDROME (RASMUSSEN ENCEPHALITIS)

Clinical Manifestations: Childhood onset in majority of the cases: (a) *progressive neurologic deficit, intractable seizures, progressive hemiparesis, decreased cognitive function, and mental retardation;* (b) electroencephalography in early stage: background slowing and diffuse epileptiform discharges; (c) pathologic findings compatible with viral disease; (d) miscellaneous abnormalities: growth retardation; uveitis; autoantibodies to glutamate receptor GluR3.

Radiologic Manifestations: *Cortical brain atrophy;* decreased cerebral blood flow (xenon computed tomography); hypometabolic brain state (positron emission tomography); axonal damage (magnetic resonance spectroscopy).

RAYNAUD SYNDROME

Definitions: (a) Raynaud phenomenon: episodic self-limited attacks of reversible, white color changes of the digits (ischemia), precipitated by cold, with symptoms of tingling, numbness or pain on recovery; (b) Raynaud syndrome: Raynaud phenomenon with no identifiable underlying cause or associated disease.

Clinical Manifestations: *Symptoms developing with exposure to cold or in association with emotional upset: symmetric involvement of hands; usually absence of gangrene, but if present, limited to the skin of the fingertips; normal pulse; absence of recognition of the underlying disorder as a cause of the symptom complex; recurrence of symptoms for at least 2 years without detection of the underlying cause;* prevalence of migraine and chest pain in patients with primary Raynaud disease.

Radiologic Manifestations: *Absence of filling of the distal parts of the digital arteries; diminished caliber of digital arteries;* reversible increased tracer uptake (methylene diphosphonate bone scintigraphy).

RECOMBINANT (8) SYNDROME (CHROMOSOME 8 RECOMBINANT SYNDROME)

Clinical and Radiologic Manifestations: (a) *unbalanced partial duplication–part deletion of chromosome 8;* (b) *unusual facies:* broad, square face; hypertelorism and/or telecanthus; high nasal bridge with prominent lateral nasal folds; thin upper lip; thick lower lip; malformed ears; (c) *mental retardation;* (d) *congenital heart disease* (about 90%); (e) miscellaneous abnormalities: genitourinary anomalies (cryptorchidism; hypoplastic scrotum; urinary tract anomalies; hypoplastic clitoris/labia); etc.

Note: This is an inherited chromosomal abnormality, with many cases reported in New Mexico and southern Colorado, in persons of Hispanic descent ("San Luis Valley syndrome").

REIFENSTEIN SYNDROME

Clinical and Radiologic Manifestations: (a) *hypospadias; postpubertal testicular atrophy; azoospermia and infertility; weak or absent virilization; gynecomastia;* high excretion of follicle-stimulating hormone; normal level of 17-ketosteroids; (b) testicular biopsy: Leydig cell hyperplasia, atrophic seminiferous tubules, and interstitial fibrosis; spermatogenesis in some; (c) miscellaneous abnormalities: prostatic utricle; Leydig cell neoplasia; (d) consistent with X-linked recessive inheritance; a single exchange of an alanine to a threonine at amino acid position 596 in the androgen receptor recognized as an inheritable trait in this syndrome.

REITER SYNDROME

Clinical Manifestations: (a) *urethritis;* (b) *arthritis;* (c) *conjunctivitis; iritis;* (d) *mucocutaneous lesions:* balanitis; keratodermia; buccal ulcerations; erythema; etc.; (e) miscellaneous abnormalities: diarrhea; myocarditis; pericarditis; cardiac conduction abnormalities; myocardial ischemia with narrowing of the coronary ostia, and aortic insufficiency; neuritis; association with HLA-B27 antigen; etc.

Radiologic Manifestations: (a) *bone erosion and joint effusion* (heels, toes, and sacroiliac joints in particular); massive synovial hypertrophy; *arthritis mutilans of the feet;* tendonitis with *periostitis* of or adjacent to sites of tendon insertions (plantar surface of the calcaneus, the major site); (b) miscellaneous abnormalities: aortic insufficiency; distal aortitis; lateral vertebral hyperostosis with bridging around the cartilaginous disc; cervical spine involvement rare; increased focal uptake of [99mTc] pyrophosphate; pseudothrombophlebitis due to an expansive popliteal cyst; epileptic seizures.

RELAPSING POLYCHONDRITIS

Clinical Manifestations: (a) fever; anorexia; weight loss; (b) *auricular chondritis;* painful erythematous swelling of the external ear; "cauliflower ear" deformity; conductive deafness; neurosensory deafness due to inner ear involvement; (c) *nasal chondritis;* swelling and tenderness; "saddle nose" deformity; (d) chest pain due to *costochondritis; hoarseness; cough; dyspnea; laryngeal and tracheal tenderness;* aphonia and airway obstruction due to edema; collapse of the trachea and cricoid rings; pulmonary function test abnormalities reflecting the upper airway obstruction; airway obstruction during both inspiration and expiration demonstrated by respiratory function test; (e) *arthralgia and arthritis* of large or small joints; tendinitis; (f) episcleritis; conjunctivitis; iritis; "salmon patch" conjunctival mass; exophthalmos; (g) myocarditis; dilatation of the cardiac valvular ring; aortic insufficiency; complete heart block; cardiovascular collapse; (h) confusion; disorientation; nystagmus; facial weakness; cerebral vasculitis; stroke; (i) association with the following: rheumatoid arthritis; subclinical Sjögren syndrome and phlegmon of the neck; Behçet syndrome in a patient with human immunodeficiency virus infection; myelodysplastic syndromes; antiphospholipid antibodies and recurrent venous thrombosis; (j) miscellaneous abnormalities: vasculitis; livedo reticularis; erythema nodosum; keratodermia; chondrosarcoma; etc.

Radiologic Manifestations: (a) *calcification of the external ear cartilage;* collapse of the cartilage of the nose; (b) *arthritis,* usually polyarthritis, with small and large joints involved; joint space narrowing; cartilage destruction; osseous erosions; arthritis mutilans; osteopenia; "periostitis" of the bones adjacent to involved joints; (c) cardiomegaly; aortic ring dilatation; aortic, mitral, and tricuspid insufficiency; aortic aneurysm; (d) *collapse of larynx and narrowing of trachea and main-stem bronchi (computed tomography; magnetic resonance imaging); bronchiectasis in segmental and subsegmental bronchi; severe chronic lung disease resulting from dissolution of the cartilaginous structure of air passages; deformity of the tracheobronchial tree; enlargement and irregularity of the cartilages of the larynx and tracheal rings; edema; fibrosis; calcification;* (e) radionuclide imaging (Tc-99m MDP bone scans and Ga-67 citrate): increased tracer concentration in the perinasal and periauricular areas and in the thyroid cartilage and the small joints of hands; (f) miscellaneous abnormalities: absence of mediastinal adenopathy; ureteral obstruction due to association with retroperitoneal fibrosis.

RENAL-GENITAL-EAR ANOMALIES

Clinical Manifestations: *Vaginal atresia; abnormal pinna, low-set ears, stenosis of the external auditory canal, and mild deafness;* etc.

Radiologic Manifestations: (a) *renal anomalies:* agenesis; dysgenesis; (b) middle ear: malformed ossicles; (c) skeletal anomalies: clinodactyly; short fourth metacarpals; congenital separation of the pubic symphysis; spina bifida occulta.

RENAL-HEPATIC-PANCREATIC DYSPLASIA (IVEMARK SYNDROME)

Clinical, Pathologic, and Radiologic Manifestations: (a) *renal malformations* (cystic dysplasia; abnormally differentiated ducts; deficient nephron differentiation); renal insufficiency; (b) *hepatic malformations* (enlarged portal areas containing numerous elongated biliary "profiles"; perilobular fibrosis; cholestasis; intrahepatic ductal dilatation); chronic jaundice; (c) *pancreatic anomalies* (fibrosis; cysts; diminution of parenchymal tissue); insulin-dependent diabetes mellitus; (d) miscellaneous abnormalities: reported in two brothers, one with hypertrophic cardiomyopathy and pancreatic exocrine insufficiency; (e) autosomal recessive inheritance.

RENDU-OSLER-WEBER SYNDROME

Clinical Manifestations: (a) *skin telangiectasis; epistaxis;* hematuria; upper and lower alimentary tract hemorrhage; hemoptysis; hemothorax; intracranial hemorrhage; intraocular hemorrhage; vaginal telangiectasias; (b) *symptoms related to pulmonary arteriovenous fistulae;* (c) miscellaneous abnormalities: seizures, motor/sensory deficit; hepatomegaly; hepatic bruit; high output failure due to hyperdynamic circulation; portal hypertension; portosystemic encephalopathy due to intrahepatic portosystemic shunts; presentation with polymicrobial brain abscess; etc.

Radiologic Manifestations: Pulmonary arteriovenous malformation; angiographic demonstration of *angiodysplasias;* dilated hepatic artery; abnormal echogenicity of the liver; etc.

RESTRICTIVE DERMATOPATHY

Clinical Manifestations: (a) *polyhydramnios; severe intrauterine growth retardation; reduced fetal movement late in pregnancy;* premature birth; (b) *characteristic facies:* hypertelorism, prominent eyes, thin nose, microstomia, and micrognathia; (c) *skin abnormalities:* taut and shiny; erythematous; superficial erosions; prominently visible subcutaneous vessels; thickened epidermis; thin dermis; (d) *features consistent with fetal akinesias deformation sequence;* (e) autosomal recessive inheritance.

Radiologic Manifestations: *Defective ossification and hypoplasia of clavicles and skull; overtubulation and modeling defects of the long bones;*

abnormal corticomedullary differentiation of the tubular bones; deficient phalangeal ossification of the hands; deficient ossification of radius and ulna.

RETT SYNDROME

Clinical Manifestations: Occurring exclusively in females: (a) *normal prenatal and perinatal period; normal psychomotor development through the first 6 months of life; normal head size at birth;* (b) *deceleration of head growth* (acquired microcephaly); *deterioration of higher brain function; abnormal electroencephalographic findings;* (c) miscellaneous abnormalities: refractive error; scoliosis; joint contracture; etc.

Radiologic Manifestations: (a) cerebral atrophy in some cases; (b) single photon emission computed tomography: *low global cerebral blood flow; markedly reduced flow in the prefrontal and temporoparietal association regions of the telencephalon;* (c) volumetric imaging study: markedly reduced brain volume; greater loss of gray matter in comparison to white matter; frontal region showing the largest decrease in size; reduced volume of the caudate nucleus; cerebellum and midbrain; (d) miscellaneous abnormalities: coxa valga; short fourth and/or fifth metacarpals and metatarsals; reduced bone density in the hands; etc.

REYE SYNDROME

Clinical Manifestations: (a) *history of recent viral infection or upper respiratory tract infection;* vomiting; (b) *encephalopathy;* (c) *hepatomegaly; acute liver failure; abnormal liver function test results;* (d) *hematologic and metabolic abnormalities:* increased leukocyte count, ammonia, serum aminotransferases, prothrombin time, creatine phosphokinase, serum short- and medium-chain fatty acids, amino acids, lactic acid, uric acid, blood urea nitrogen, amylase, cerebrospinal fluid glutamine and catecholamine; decreased serum and cerebrospinal fluid glucose levels and serum C1 and C1s complement activity; respiratory alkalosis; metabolic acidosis; (e) miscellaneous abnormalities: acute renal failure; acute pancreatitis; fatty degeneration of the liver and other viscera; central retinal vein occlusion.

Radiologic Manifestations: (a) *cerebral edema* presenting as a low density in deep white matter with subcortical sparing, effacement of sulci, and compression of the ventricles; (b) cerebral cortical laminar necrosis: (1) acute stage: T_2-weighted images showing laminar high signal, and contrast-enhanced T_1-weighted images showing laminar enhancement along the cerebral cortex; (2) chronic stage: unenhanced T_1-weighted image showing diffuse cortical laminar high signal; (c) *brain atrophy,* predominantly in the frontal lobe in the chronic phase; (d) proton magnetic resonance spectroscopy: cerebral metabolic imbalance during acute stage; (e) *fatty liver.*

RICHTER SYNDROME

Definition: Development of histiocytic lymphoma with generalized manifestations in a patient with chronic lymphocytic leukemia.

Clinical Manifestations: Abrupt onset of symptoms: fever; increasing lymphadenopathy; weight loss; abdominal pain; extranodal involvement; progression of hepatosplenomegaly; etc.

Radiologic Manifestations: *Marked lymphadenopathy; hepatosplenomegaly;* focal low-density lesions within the liver (computed tomography); lytic bone lesions.

RIGHT MIDDLE LOBE SYNDROME

Clinical Manifestations: *Cough, wheezing, and recurrent pneumonia;* bronchial narrowing may be detectable on endoscopy; association with the following: allergic bronchopulmonary aspergillosis and *Mycobacterium fortuitum.*

Radiologic Manifestations: (a) *total or partial atelectasis of the right middle lobe;* bronchial narrowing in some cases; (b) abnormal chest radiographs and respiratory function tests in the long-term follow-up in some patients with ongoing respiratory symptoms.

RIGID SPINE SYNDROME

Clinical Manifestations: (a) *restricted spinal flexion; overextended spine; fibrous shortening of the extensor muscles; reduced muscle size; loss of adipose tissue; myopathic pattern on electromyographic examination;* (b) miscellaneous abnormalities: elevated serum creatine phosphokinase level; muscle biopsy: variation in fiber size; hypertrophic nonobstructive cardiomyopathy; sinus venosus defect; (c) probably autosomal recessive inheritance.

Radiologic Manifestations: *Progressive limitation of flexion and extension of the cervical spine; wide separation of the laminae of C1 and C2 with the cervical spine in a neutral position.*

RILEY-DAY SYNDROME

Clinical Manifestations: (a) *dysautonomia:* fever; skin blotching; excessive sweating; cool extremities; reduced pain and taste sensation;

hypolacrimation; corneal hypoesthesia and corneal ulceration; episodic vomiting; abnormal esophageal motility; decreased lower esophageal sphincter pressure; oropharyngeal incoordination; difficulty in swallowing; regurgitation; etc.; (b) *motor incoordination; emotional lability;* (c) miscellaneous abnormalities: absence of fungiform papillae of the tongue; recurrent pneumonia; pulmonary function abnormalities; obstetric problems; abnormal brain-stem function shown by brain-stem auditory evoked potentials; spontaneous colonic ischemia and colocutaneous fistula; etc.; (d) autosomal recessive inheritance.

Radiologic Manifestations: (a) *swallowing difficulty:* incoordination in deglutition and closure of the larynx resulting in tracheal aspiration; delayed relaxation of the cricopharyngeus; incoordination between the esophageal peristaltic wave and the lower esophageal sphincter; dilatation and atonicity of the esophagus; poor emptying of the esophagus in the horizontal position; prolonged gastric emptying time; gastroesophageal reflux; small-bowel distension; megacolon; (b) aspiration; recurrent pneumonia; atelectasis; irregular pulmonary aeration; interstitial pulmonary fibrosis; peribronchial thickening; (c) miscellaneous abnormalities: retarded skeletal maturation; kyphoscoliosis; increased incidence of fractures and aseptic necrosis; neuropathic knee joint; hip dislocation; pes cavus; microcephaly; hydrocephalus; craniofacial disproportion; congenital heart disease.

RITSCHER-SCHINZEL SYNDROME (CRANIO-CEREBELLO-CARDIAC DYSPLASIA; 3C SYNDROME)

Clinical Manifestations: (a) craniofacial dysmorphism (macrocephaly, flat face, ocular hypertelorism, down-slanting palpebral fissures, anteverted nostrils, apparent low-set ears, narrow palate, and receding chin); congenital heart defects; etc.; (b) reported in siblings; reported in Canadian Native Indians.

Radiologic Manifestations: Hydrocephalus; vermis aplasia/hypoplasia; undermineralized skull; kyphoscoliosis; aberrant sternal ossification; skeletal maturation retardation; 11 pairs of ribs.

ROBERTS SYNDROME (SC-PHOCOMELIA SYNDROME)

Clinical Manifestations: Phenotypic variation and heterogeneity: (a) *low birth weight;* (b) *facial dysmorphism:* ocular hypertelorism, hypoplastic nasal alae, bilateral cleft lip/palate, protrusion of the intermaxillary portion of the upper jaw, abnormal pinnae, and micrognathia; (c) exophthalmos; cataracts; corneal opacity; colobomas of the eyelids; (d) *limb anomalies:* phocomelia; oligodactyly; flexion contractions; (e) *genital* *anomalies:* prominence of the phallus; cryptorchidism; enlarged clitoris; enlarged labia minora; cleft labia minora; septate vagina; hypospadias; (f) autosomal recessive inheritance; abnormal nuclear morphology and higher frequency of micronucleation than normal cells; the cytogenetic marker: premature centromere separation.

Radiologic Manifestations: (a) microbrachycephaly; wormian bones in the lambdoid sutures; (b) *hands and feet anomalies:* reduction anomalies of hands and feet; irregularity and reduction of the carpal bones; clinodactyly; fusion of the fourth and fifth metacarpals; polydactyly; talipes calcaneovalgus; soft-tissue syndactyly of the toes; (c) prenatal ultrasonographic demonstration of limb anomalies and hydrocephalus; (d) miscellaneous abnormalities: renal malformations; reduced rib numbers; heart defects; aneurysm of interatrial septum; etc.

ROBIN SEQUENCE (PIERRE ROBIN SYNDROME)

Clinical Manifestations: *Micrognathia; cleft palate (U-shaped); glossoptosis; upper airway obstruction;* multiple episodes of otitis media; cardiovascular anomalies; ocular abnormalities (esotropia; microphthalmia; glaucoma; etc.); mental retardation; growth retardation; etc.

Radiologic Manifestations: (a) *hypoplasia of the mandible; obtuse mandibular angle; cleft palate; upper airway obstruction;* (b) skeletal anomalies: amelia; congenital amputations; syndactyly; clubfoot; radiohumeral synostosis; oligodactyly; congenital hip dislocation; sickle-shaped scapulae; rib anomalies; sternal anomalies; combined occipito-atlanto-axial hypermobility with anterior and posterior arch defects of the atlas.

Robin Sequence Associated Syndromes/Anomalies: (1) amniotic band syndrome; (2) Andre syndrome: X-linked, abnormal facies, cleft palate, and generalized dysostosis; (3) arthrogryposis; (4) Beckwith-Wiedemann syndrome; (5) Brachmann–de Lange syndrome; (6) camptomelic dysplasia; (7) Carey-Fineman-Ziter syndrome: myopathy with Möbius syndrome and Robin sequence; (8) Catel-Manzke syndrome; (9) cerebro-costo-mandibular syndrome; (10) CHARGE association; (11) chromosomal abnormalities; (12) congenital myotonic dystrophy; (13) diastrophic dysplasia; (14) femoral hypoplasia; (15) femoral hypoplasia–unusual facies syndrome; (16) fetal alcohol syndrome; (17) fetal hydantoin syndrome; (18) fetal trimethadione syndrome; (19) hyperphalangism, clinodactyly of the index finger, and Robin sequence (possibly a new syndrome); (20) Joubert syndrome; (21) Möbius syndrome; (22) Marden-Walker syndrome; (23) Miller-Dieker syndrome; (24) Nager syndrome; (25) oto-palato-digital syndrome, type II; (26) Poland syndrome; (27) popliteal pterygium syndrome; (28) spondyloepiphyseal dysplasia congenita; (29) Stevenson syndrome: a digitopalatal syndrome with associated anomalies of the heart, face, and skeleton; (30) Stickler syndrome; (31) Treacher Collins syndrome; (32) velo-cardio-facial syndrome; (33) X-linked hydrocephalus; (34) Robin sequence associated with congenital thrombocytopenia, agenesis of the corpus callosum, distinctive facies, and developmental delay.

ROMBERG SYNDROME (PARRY-ROMBERG SYNDROME)

Clinical Manifestations: Progressive disease with an onset in childhood or early adult life: (a) *wasting of soft tissues on one side of the face,* with sharp vertical delineation between normal and abnormal sides (*coup de sabre*); predilection for left-sided involvement; misshapen and small ear; (b) alopecia; poliosis; focal pigmentary changes of the skin; (c) *neurologic disorders:* trigeminal neuralgia; ataxia; Horner syndrome; migraine; epilepsy; especially jacksonian motor and sensory types; abnormal electroencephalographic findings; (d) miscellaneous abnormalities: ocular complications; possible autoimmunity as a pathogenic factor.

Radiologic Manifestations: (a) *facial bone atrophy corresponding to sites of soft-tissue atrophy:* shorter body and ramus of the mandible and a delay in development of the angle; etc.; (b) delay in eruption of teeth on the involved side; (c) central nervous system abnormalities: cerebral hemisphere atrophy homolateral to the facial hemiatrophy; porencephaly; intracranial calcification; nonenhancing area of increased density in the parietal lobe; hyperdense areas in the brain (computed tomography); (d) miscellaneous abnormalities: basilar kyphosis of skull; salivary gland atrophy on the affected side.

ROTHMUND-THOMSON SYNDROME

Clinical Manifestations: (a) *erythema progressing to atrophy; depigmentation; hyperpigmentation; scaling; telangiectasia of the skin; a peculiar marmoration skin pattern; keratotic lesions after puberty; partial or total alopecia; defective nails;* (b) hypogonadism; (c) *defective teeth;* (d) hypersensitivity to light; (e) *cataract;* microphthalmia; microcornea; strabismus; glaucoma; (f) *short stature;* short distal portions of the limbs; (g) miscellaneous abnormalities: malignancies; myelodysplastic syndrome; malignant eccrine poroma; etc.; (h) autosomal recessive inheritance.

Radiologic Manifestations: Nonspecific findings: osteoporosis; osteosclerosis; short and broad phalanges, metacarpals, and metatarsals; absent thumb; mild epiphyseal dysostosis and metaphyseal sclerosis in some long bones; radial hypoplasia or agenesis; knee subluxation; phalangeal tuft resorption; flattened and elongated vertebral bodies; cystic bone changes; soft-tissue calcification; decreased subcutaneous tissues.

RUBINSTEIN-TAYBI SYNDROME

Clinical Manifestations: (a) *short stature;* (b) *facial dysmorphism:* small head, beaked or straight nose, nasal septum extending below the alae, apparent hypertelorism, and lateral downward slant of the palpebral fissures; abnormalities in position, rotation, size, or shape of the ears; (c) eye and eyebrow abnormalities: heavy or highly arched eyebrows; epicanthi; long eyelashes; nasolacrimal duct obstruction; strabismus; cataracts; glaucoma; colobomas; refractive errors; retinal detachment with high myopia; corneal "scar"; ankyloblepharon filiforme adnatum; Duane retraction syndrome; (d) oral manifestations: thin upper lip; pouting lower lip; small oral opening; retrognathia; micrognathia; highly arched and narrow palate; cleft uvula; cleft palate; (e) dental abnormalities: *talon cusps;* malpositioned teeth; crowded teeth; hypodontia; hyperdontia; microdontia; macrodontia; double rows of teeth; natal teeth; marked caries; (f) *broad thumb,* especially the distal phalanx; angulated thumb; broad fingers especially the distal phalanges; (g) *broad and large great toe;* angular deformity of the great toe; clinodactyly of the fourth or fifth toes; polydactyly of the little toe; (h) neurodevelopmental abnormalities: *mental, motor, social, and language retardation; difficulty with expressive speech skill;* peculiar grimacing smile; brisk reflexes; migraine headaches; seizures; electroencephalographic abnormalities; (i) congenital heart defects (about 30%); (j) genital abnormalities; (k) *tendency to keloid formation; excessive scar formation;* hypertrichosis; (l) miscellaneous abnormalities: overlapping toes; joint laxity; awkward gait; flatfeet; slight hip and knee flexion; endocrine disorders (premature thelarche; transient hypoglycemia with hyperinsulinemia in a newborn); neoplasms; monozygotic twins concordant for the syndrome and changing phenotype during infancy; etc.; (m) sporadic; very few familial cases; caused by mutations in the transcriptional co-activator CBP; submicroscopic interstitial deletions within 16p13.3.

Radiologic Manifestations: (a) hand abnormalities: *short and wide terminal phalanx of the thumbs;* a hole or distal notch in the distal phalanx that suggests an attempt at duplication; "delta deformity" of the proximal phalanx of the thumbs that causes angulation in about 40% of the cases; *short, wide, and tufted terminal phalanx of the fingers;* (b) feet abnormalities: short and wide terminal phalanx of the great toes; duplication in the proximal and/or distal phalanges of the great toes; "kissing delta phalanx" of the great toes in association with duplication (fused epiphyses); hallux valgus; (c) miscellaneous abnormalities: (1) large foramen magnum;

prominent forehead; large anterior fontanelle; parietal foramina; odontoid hypoplasia; C1-C2 instability; vertebral anomalies; sternal anomalies; rib anomalies; flaring of the ilia; dislocation of elbows; syndactyly; polydactyly; clinodactyly of the fifth finger; slipped capital femoral epiphysis; Calvé-Perthes disease; congenital dislocation of the patellae; skeletal maturation retardation; (2) gastroesophageal reflux; intestinal malrotation; megacolon; (3) urinary system abnormalities: double collecting system; vesicoureteral reflux; (4) nervous system abnormalities: absence of the corpus callosum; Dandy-Walker–like malformation; bilateral rolandic cortical clefts and diminished white matter; meningomyelocele; tethered cord.

RÜDIGER SYNDROME

Clinical and Radiologic Manifestations: (a) coarse facial features, flat nasal bridge, stubby nose, and protuberant upper lip; (b) thickened palms and soles with an abnormal dermatoglyphic pattern, short digits, palmar flexion contracture, and hypoplastic fingernails; (c) miscellaneous abnormalities: hydronephrosis due to ureteral stenosis; bicornuate uterus; inguinal hernia; low-pitched, hoarse voice; failure to develop motor control; bifid uvula; etc.; (d) possibly autosomal recessive inheritance.

S

SAETHRE-CHOTZEN SYNDROME

Clinical Manifestations: (a) craniofacial dysmorphism: *brachycephaly and/or acrocephaly;* facial asymmetry; visual defects; esotropia, exotropia; ptosis of the eyelids; lacrimal duct abnormalities; malformed ears; impaired hearing; flattened nasofrontal angle; beaked nose; cleft palate; highly arched palate; low-set frontal hairline; labial pits at the corners of the mouth; deviation of nasal septum; low-set ears; hypertelorism; strabismus; (b) mental subnormality in some cases; (c) *syndactyly (partial; soft tissue);* etc.; (d) autosomal dominant inheritance with marked penetrance and variable expressivity.

Radiologic Manifestations: (a) *variable degrees of craniosynostosis associated with plagiocephaly and facial asymmetry;* maxillary hypoplasia; microcephaly; absent or underdeveloped frontal sinuses and mastoids; abnormal cephalometric findings; dilatation of lateral ventricles; increased intracranial pressure; (b) *partial cutaneous syndactyly of fingers and toes;* (c) miscellaneous abnormalities: large sella turcica; parietal foramina; metopic suture synostosis; large fontanelles; delayed closure of fontanelles; calvarial ossification defect; cervical vertebral fusion; vertebral anomalies; small ilia and large ischia; coxa valga; short clavicles with distal hypoplasia; radioulnar synostosis.

SANDIFER SYNDROME

Clinical Manifestations: (a) *abnormal movement or positioning of the head, neck, and upper part of trunk during or after eating:* sudden extension, continual movement from side to side, and flexion of the upper portion of the trunk and neck; (b) *gastroesophageal reflux with or without hiatus hernia;* esophagitis; manometric demonstration of low amplitude and slow propagation of esophageal peristalsis; (c) miscellaneous abnormalities: vomiting; abdominal pain; occurrence in children with brain damage or metabolic defects; gastroesophageal reflux as a cause of torticollis in infancy.

Radiologic Manifestations: *With the clinically described contortions, the gastroesophageal junction rises, and the upper portion of the stomach enters the thoracic cavity (hiatal hernia).*

SATOYOSHI SYNDROME

Clinical Manifestations: *Painful muscle spasms with onset in childhood;* slowly progressive course; involving masticatory muscles and the muscles of neck, trunk, and limbs; *alopecia; diarrhea;* malabsorption; *short stature.*

Radiologic Manifestations: Irregularity and widening of the physes and a mixture of translucent and sclerotic areas in the metaphyses (mimicking metaphyseal chondrodysplasia); slipping of the epiphyses; acroosteolysis; osteolysis; cystic bone lesions; bone fragmentation at tendinous insertion sites; fatigue fracture; osteoarthrosis.

SCHINZEL-GIEDION SYNDROME

Clinical Manifestations: (a) *coarse facial features;* frontal bossing; wide sutures and anterior fontanelle; midfacial hypoplasia; orbital hypertelorism; short and upturned nose; low-set ears; (b) *seizures; profound motor and intellectual retardation;* (c) *genitourinary anomalies:* renal anomalies; hypospadias; hypoplastic scrotum; short penis; deep interlabial sulcus; hypoplasia of the labia majora or minora; hymenal atresia; (d) *clubfeet;* (e) *hypertrichosis;* (f) miscellaneous abnormalities: hypoplasia of the dermal ridges; hyperconvex nails; steatosis in the liver and lipid vacuolization of the zona fasciculata of the adrenals (case report); malignant neoplasms (embryonal tumors); syndactyly of hands; (g) probably autosomal recessive inheritance.

Radiologic Manifestations: (a) short and sclerotic base of the skull; poor skull vault mineralization; steep base of the skull; wide supraoccipital "synchondrosis"; multiple wormian bones; orbital hypertelorism; wide cranial sutures and fontanelles; (b) increased density of long tubular bones and vertebrae; broad ribs; long clavicles; wide distal metaphysis of femora; hypoplastic or aplastic pubic bones; moderate mesomelic brachymelia; short first metacarpals; hypoplasia of the distal phalanges in the hands and feet; (c) urinary system anomalies; (d) miscellaneous abnormalities: ventriculomegaly; agenesis of the corpus callosum in siblings (one with sacrococcygeal teratoma); etc.

SCHWARTZ-JAMPEL SYNDROME

Clinical Manifestations: Progressive disease with an onset of symptoms in infancy or childhood: (a) *"masklike" facies, blepharophimosis, microstomia, recessed chin, and full cheeks;* (b) *short stature; stiff posture; crouched stance; short neck; short trunk; waddling gait; pectus carinatum; kyphosis or kyphoscoliosis;* (c) *prolonged myotonic responses;* firm hypertrophic muscles; muscular weakness and wasting; depressed tendon reflexes; (d) *large-joint stiffness and contracture;* (e) high-pitched voice; (f) immunologic abnormalities; (g) manifestations in neonates: short stature; contractures; myotonia; muscle hypertrophy, muscle rigidity; choking; respiratory difficulty; apnea, abnormal facies; death due to asphyxia; (h) autosomal recessive inheritance; variable expressivity.

Radiologic Manifestations: (a) triangular deformity of the pelvis; flared iliac wings; (b) *hip disorders:* coxa vara or coxa valga; delay in appearance of femoral head ossification; fragmentation of the femoral head; flat femoral head; slipped capital femoral epiphysis; (c) miscellaneous skeletal abnormalities: slender diaphysis of the long bones; anterior bowing of the long bones; irregularity of the femoral and tibial epiphyses in the knee region; scoliosis; kyphoscoliosis; marked platyspondyly; coronally cleft vertebral bodies; failure of ossification of the anterior half of some vertebral bodies; basilar invagination; pectus carinatum; increased bone density in neonates.

Note: Two types: (1) classic type with late infantile or childhood onset of symptoms; (2) severe neonatal type with very poor prognosis (death due to respiratory complications).

SCHWARZ-LÉLEK SYNDROME

Clinical Manifestations: Normal at birth; onset in childhood: *enlargement of the head; marked frontal bossing; thick mandible; genu recurvatum.*

Radiologic Manifestations: *Marked hyperostosis and sclerosis of the skull,* in particular in the frontal and occipital regions; obliteration of the paranasal sinuses; *bowing of humeri and femora; widening of long bones* similar to that in Pyle disease.

SCIMITAR SYNDROME

Clinical Manifestations: May be asymptomatic or symptomatic: recurrent respiratory infection; decrease in breath sounds on the right side of the chest; small right hemithorax.

Radiologic Manifestations: The following represent the major components of the syndrome, with the first two being the most constantly occurring components: (a) *lobar aplasia or hypoplasia;* (b) *partial or total anomalous pulmonary venous drainage (scimitar-shaped vein located in the right supradiaphragmatic region and draining into the inferior vena cava; etc.);* (c) absence of a pulmonary artery; (d) pulmonary sequestration; (e) systemic arterialization of the lung; (f) absence of the inferior vena cava; (g) accessory diaphragm.

SCLERODERMA (Systemic sclerosis)

Clinical Manifestations: Scleroderma includes a group of heterogeneous connective tissue diseases ranging from localized scleroderma to progressive systemic sclerosis involving skin and internal organs.

(A) SKIN: *Edema, induration, and finally atrophy.*

(B) ALIMENTARY SYSTEM: Dysphagia; nausea and vomiting; constipation, or diarrhea; abdominal distension; intestinal pseudoobstruction; secondary malabsorption (abnormal intraluminal bacterial flora); fecalith formation associated with constipation; acute abdominal manifestation (obstruction; bowel perforation; peritonitis; ischemia; bowel infarction; hemorrhage due to telangiectasia).

(C) CARDIOVASCULAR SYSTEM: Pericardial disease (acute process with chest pain, dyspnea; fever, and a pericardial friction rub or a chronic picture of pericardial effusion); myocardial fibrosis (diffuse and patchy distribution; abnormalities of myocardial perfusion); disorders of cardiac rhythm and conduction; decreased right ventricular ejection fraction; decreased left ventricular ejection fraction; stress-induced reversible myocardial perfusion abnormalities; hypoxic pulmonary vasoconstriction; cold-induced reversible myocardial ischemia; pulmonary hypertension; cor pulmonale; *Raynaud phenomenon* (in about 60%), microangiopathy evaluated by dynamic fluorescence videomicroscopy; gangrene of the extremities.

(D) RESPIRATORY SYSTEM: Abnormalities of pulmonary function (restrictive ventilatory defect; airflow obstruction; depressed diffusing capacity for carbon monoxide); pulmonary hypertension.

(E) NEUROLOGIC MANIFESTATIONS: Autonomic dysfunction (parasympathetic impairment and sympathetic overactivity); peripheral nerve dysfunction; necrotizing encephalitis; brain abnormalities adjacent to the cutaneous manifestations.

(F) ANTINUCLEAR ANTIBODIES: Association of different types of sclerodermas with specific immunologic markers.

(G) MISCELLANEOUS ABNORMALITIES: Joint pain; skeletal myopathy; abnormal renal physiology (renovascular disease; elevated plasma renin activity; reduced para-aminohippurate); association of linear scleroderma and melorheostosis; scleroderma renal crisis; association with hypothyroidism or hyperthyroidism; impotence; etc.

Radiologic Manifestations

(A) SKELETAL SYSTEM: (a) *absorption of the distal phalanges;* absorption of carpal bones and the distal portions of the radius and ulna (rare); (b) periarticular soft-tissue swelling; *joint destruction;* (c) *soft-tissue calcification;* (d) generalized osteoporosis; (e) carpal synostosis; (f) periosteal new bone formation of the long bones; (g) thickening of the skin (ultrasonographic measurement of the finger: 3.3 ± 0.7 mm as compared with normal control subjects of 2.5 ± 0.2 mm); (h) other manifestations: ankylosis of the interphalangeal joints; intraarticular calcification associated with bone erosion; osteolysis of the calcaneus in a child with localized scleroderma; rib erosion; resorption of ribs and the medial ends of the clavicles.

(B) ALIMENTARY TRACT: (a) *wide and atonic esophagus with decreased peristalsis;* stricture; Barrett esophagus; (b) *atonic dilated stomach;* (c) gastroesophageal reflux; (d) *dilatation and sacculation of the small bowel* with decreased motility and peristaltic activity; prolonged transit time; increased fluid; diverticula; packed valvulae; (e) *areas of sacculation and narrowing of the colon* and thickened longitudinal folds in the narrowed segment; increased fluid; postevacuation residua; increased length; lack of haustrations; megacolon; (f) other manifestations: corrugated mucosal pattern of the esophagus; atypical wide-mouthed esophageal diverticula.

(C) HEART: Cardiomegaly; pericardial effusion.

(D) RESPIRATORY SYSTEM: *Small cystic areas in the lung; diffuse lung fibrosis; detection of interstitial lung disease* by high-resolution computed tomography (subpleural lines; honeycombing; parenchymal bands).

(E) MISCELLANEOUS ABNORMALITIES: Widening of the periodontal membrane; dilatation of the pulmonary artery and main branches in patients with pulmonary arterial hypertension; diffuse spotty lucencies on the nephrogram phase of renal arteriography; hyperintense areas adjacent to cutaneous and bony lesions (magnetic resonance imaging); intraspinous calcifications; pneumoperitoneum; mediastinal lymphadenopathy.

SEA-BLUE HISTIOCYTE SYNDROME

Clinical Manifestations: *Abnormal cells (histiocytes) containing large blue cytoplasmic granules in the bone marrow, skin, lung, gastrointestinal tract, nervous system, and spleen; splenomegaly; hepatomegaly;* progressive hepatic cirrhosis; lymphadenopathies; periodic hemorrhagic diathesis associated with thrombocytopenia; etc.

Radiologic Manifestations: Pulmonary nodular densities, hilar adenopathy; *hepatosplenomegaly.*

SECKEL SYNDROME (BIRD-HEADED DWARFISM)

Clinical Manifestations: (a) *low birth weight; dwarfism; mental retardation; craniofacial dysmorphism:* microcephaly; beaklike protrusion of the nose; hypoplasia of the cheek bones; prominent eyes; ocular hypertelorism; micrognathia; (b) probably autosomal recessive inheritance; three children in one family, all with chromosomal instability.

Radiologic Manifestations: (a) *microcrania; ocular hypertelorism; hypoplasia of the maxillae and mandible;* (b) hand and wrist abnormalities: ivory epiphyses; cone-shaped epiphyses in the proximal phalanges; disharmonic skeletal maturation; alteration in tubular bone length; small carpal bones; angular carpal bone configuration; normal or increased cortical thickness of the metacarpals; incurving of the distal phalanges; clubbing of fingers; hypoplastic thumb; (c) miscellaneous abnormalities: premature closure of cranial sutures; missing or atrophic teeth; kyphoscoliosis; sternal anomalies; absence of patellae; absence of tibiofibular joints; short fibulae; dislocations; rhizomelic shortening of the humeri and femora; cystic adenomatoid malformation of the lung; central nervous system malformations.

SENIOR SYNDROME (BRACHYMORPHISM-ONYCHODYSPLASIA-DYSPHALANGISM SYNDROME)

Clinical and Radiologic Manifestations: Short stature at birth; minute toenails (one or more small toes bilaterally); dysphalangism: hypoplasia/aplasia or fusion of the distal phalanges of the fifth finger and toe; brachymesophalangism V; incurving of the fifth fingers; etc.

SHAPIRO SYNDROME

Clinical Manifestations: (a) *episodic hyperhidrosis and hypothermia* (a central defect in temperature regulation); (b) miscellaneous abnormalities: abnormal electroencephalographic findings; acute renal failure; etc.

Radiologic Manifestations: *Agenesis of the corpus callosum.*

SHONE COMPLEX

Clinical and Radiologic Manifestations: *Parachute mitral valve* (all the mitral chords insert into one papillary muscle or muscle group); *supravalvular ring of the left atrium; subaortic stenosis; coarctation of the aorta.*

SHORT-BOWEL SYNDROME

Clinical Manifestations: (a) *diarrhea; steatorrhea; dehydration; malnutrition; failure to thrive; vomiting; gastric hypersecretion;* (b) miscellaneous abnormalities: metabolic acidosis due to D-lactic acidosis related to abnormal intestinal bacterial flora; encephalopathy due to D-lactic acidosis; oxaluria, oxalate nephropathy; noninfectious colitis associated with short gut syndrome and parenteral nutrition; parenteral malnutrition–induced liver disease.

Radiologic Manifestations: *Increased diameter of the small intestine; thickening and hypertrophy of the bowel wall.*

SHOULDER IMPINGEMENT SYNDROME (ROTATOR CUFF IMPINGEMENT SYNDROME)

Clinical Manifestations: Related to pressure on the supraspinatus tendon by the anterior portion of the acromion with the arm in abduction and/or forward flexion, resulting in edema and hemorrhage into the rotator cuff in the early stage followed by fibrosis, tendinitis, tears of the rotator cuff, and biceps tendon rupture: *pain during abduction and external rotation of the arm.*

Radiologic Manifestations: (a) *subacromial proliferation of bone, spurring of the interior aspect of the acromioclavicular joint, degenerative changes in the humeral tuberosities, and decreased coracohumeral distance;* (b) magnetic resonance imaging: *increased signal intensity in the tendinous portion of the rotator cuff* (due to degeneration and inflammation); *supraspinatus tear;* (c) dynamic sonography: fluid collection in subacromial-subdeltoid bursal system, with gradual distension of the bursa and lateral pooling of fluid to the subdeltoid portion while the arm is elevated.

SHPRINTZEN-GOLDBERG SYNDROME

Clinical and Radiologic Manifestations: (a) craniosynostosis; exophthalmos; maxillary and mandibular hypoplasia; soft-tissue hypertrophy of the palatal shelves; low-set, pliable auricles; (b) arachnodactyly; (c) miscellaneous abnormalities: abdominal hernias; obstructive apnea; mental retardation and developmental delay; joint contractures.

Note: Marfanoid-craniosynostosis syndrome (many clinical features of Marfan syndrome plus neurodevelopmental abnormalities) and Shprintzen-Goldberg syndrome are assumed to represent a single entity.

SHY-DRAGER SYNDROME

Clinical Manifestations: (a) *orthostatic hypotension* without acceleration of the pulse; *urinary and fecal incontinence;* abnormal urodynamic study results; *erectile impotence; anhidrosis;* (b) miscellaneous abnormalities: adductor vocal cord palsy; decrease in cerebellin and corticotropin-releasing hormone; association with the syndrome of inappropriate secretion of antidiuretic hormone and Gerhardt syndrome (paralysis of vocal cords); (c) possibly autosomal dominant inheritance.

Pathology: Symmetric degeneration in the tractus intermediolateralis, hypothalamus, caudate nuclei, and Onuf nucleus of the sacral cord.

Radiologic Manifestations: (a) decrease in signal intensity of the putamina, particularly along their lateral and posterior portions (T_2-weighted sequences and T_1-weighted spin-echo sequences); loss of signal intensity in the pallidum of moderate to marked degree; loss of signal intensity in the substantia nigra and, to a lesser degree in the red nucleus; (b) open vesical neck at rest.

SILVER-RUSSELL SYNDROME

Clinical Manifestations: (a) *low birth weight at full term; short stature;* (b) *partial or total asymmetry;* (c) *pseudohydrocephalic appearance with frontal bossing; small triangular face; small mandible; down-turned corners of the mouth;* (d) mental retardation in some cases; (e) metabolic-endocrine dysfunctions; renal tubular acidosis; (f) genitourinary system abnormalities: cryptorchidism; male with ambiguous genitalia; clitoromegaly; urinary tract infections; testicular cancer; (g) chromosomal abnormalities: trisomy 18 mosaicism; 47,XXY karyotype; translocation with breakpoint at site 17q25; deletion of the short arm of chromosome 18; ring chromosome 15; (h) the majority of the reported cases sporadic; familial cases (autosomal dominant; X-linked dominant; autosomal dominant mutation; autosomal recessive).

Radiologic Manifestations: (a) *clinodactyly; fifth digit phalangeal hypoplasia (middle or distal);* syndactyly, Kirner deformity; ivory epiphysis; second metacarpal pseudoepiphysis; (b) *skeletal maturation retardation;* difference in skeletal maturation of the two sides; (c) urinary system anomalies: horseshoe kidney deformity; hydronephrosis; enlarged kidneys; posterior urethral valve; anterior urethral valve; (d) miscellaneous abnormalities: abnormal craniometric and cephalometric studies; delayed dental age; enamel defect; slender long bones; hypoplasia or absence of phalanges; elbow dislocation; hip dislocation; irregularities of the end-plates of the vertebrae; hypoplasia of the sacrum and coccyx; Legg-Calvé-Perthes disease.

SIMPSON-GOLABI-BEHMEL SYNDROME

Clinical Manifestations: Great variability in the clinical manifestations and prognosis (mild to lethal form): (a) *prenatal and postnatal overgrowth;* (b) *psychomotor development ranging from normal to mildly retarded;* (c) *macrocephaly, "coarse" facial appearance, short and broad upturned nose, large mouth, macroglossia, submucous cleft lip and/or cleft palate, hypertelorism, grooved lower lip/tongue/gingiva, and malposition of teeth;* (d) miscellaneous abnormalities: highly arched palate; preauricular fistulae/pits; deafness; conduction defects; congenital heart defect; hydrops fetalis; (e) X-linked recessive inheritance; carrier females may show partial expression of the phenotype.

Radiologic Manifestations: (a) skeletal abnormalities: hypoplasia of the distal phalanges; syndactyly of the second and third fingers and toes; tibial clinodactyly of the second toes; ulnar clinodactyly of the second fingers; postaxial polydactyly; presence of two carpal ossification centers at birth; rib anomalies; pectus excavatum; vertebral anomalies, a tail bone; flared iliac wings and narrow sacroiliac notches in infancy; (b) miscellaneous abnormalities: congenital diaphragmatic hernia; bowel obstruction, Meckel diverticulum; large/cystic kidneys; renal dysplasia and embryonal tumor.

SINGLETON-MERTEN SYNDROME

Clinical Manifestations: *Fever of unknown origin in early infancy; muscular weakness; poor development; abnormal dentition;* normal serum calcium, phosphorus, and alkaline phosphatase levels.

Radiologic Manifestations: (a) *skeletal demineralization; expanded shafts of metacarpals and phalanges with widened medullary cavities;* (b) *cardiomegaly; intramural calcification of the proximal segment of the aorta* with extension into the descending aorta; aortic and mitral valve calcification; (c) miscellaneous abnormalities: shallow acetabular fossa; subluxation of the femoral head; coxa valga; soft-tissue calcification between the radius and ulna; hypoplastic distal radial epiphysis; constriction of the proximal part of the shaft of the radius; acro-osteolysis; equinovarus foot deformity.

SIRENOMELIA (MERMAID SYNDROME; SYMPUS APUS)

Clinical Manifestations: *Rotation and fusion of the lower limbs;* absence of anus; imperforate anus; defective or absent external genitalia; etc.

Radiologic Manifestations: *Skeletal anomalies (contracted lesser pelvis [small pelvic outlet syndrome]; sacral dysplasia; medial position, fusion, or absence of fibulae); genitourinary anomalies,* in particular renal agenesis; *gastrointestinal anomalies* (blind ending colon; imperforate anus; etc.); *oligohydramnios.*

SJÖGREN SYNDROME (GOUGEROT-SJÖGREN SYNDROME)

Clinical Manifestations: (a) *xerostomia; painless swelling of the parotid glands; pharyngolaryngitis sicca; rapid destruction of the teeth; rhinitis sicca; inflammation of labial salivary glands; keratoconjunctivitis; dry skin and vagina;* (b) *polyarthritis;* (c) respiratory system involvement; (d) central nervous system: the clinical picture resembling multiple sclerosis; aseptic meningoencephalitis; vasculitic neuropathy; psychiatric abnormalities; hemiparesis; transient aphasia; chronic progressive sensory ataxic neuropathy; peripheral neuropathy; concurrent cerebral venous sinus thrombosis and myeloradiculopathy; segmental anhidrosis in the spinal dermatomes; (e) miscellaneous abnormalities: immune disorders; endocrine and exocrine abnormalities; ulcerative colitis with selective IgA deficiency; etc.

Radiologic Manifestations: (a) *sialectasia* (punctate; globular; cavitary; destructive); atrophy of the salivary ducts; bilateral cystic lesions; parotid pseudotumors; salivary gland enlargement; heterogeneous attenuation having a multilocular appearance; salivary gland calcification; multiple hypointense mixed with hyperintense foci on T_1- and T_2-weighted images; hypoechoic areas 2 to 5 mm in diameter within the gland (homogeneous or nonhomogeneous) representing parotid lobules replaced by lymphocytic infiltration; (b) pulmonary reticular-nodular infiltrates; patchy infiltrate; hilar lymph node enlargement; bronchiectasis; enlarged mediastinal nodes; enlarged nodes with a foamy reticular pattern; (c) destructive juxtaarticular changes; (d) mucosal atrophy of the esophagus; achalasia of the cardia; gastric hypersecretion; (e) nonenhancing (computed tomography) lucencies in the brain in patients with clinical manifestations in the central nervous system; the lesions best detected by magnetic resonance imaging (predominantly within the subcortical and periventricular white matter).

Note: The diagnosis of Sjögren syndrome necessitates the presence of at least two of the following major manifestations: (a) *keratoconjunctivitis sicca;* (b) *xerostomia;* (c) *evidence of systemic autoimmune disease.*

SLEEP APNEA SYNDROME

Clinical Manifestations: (a) complaint of excessive sleepiness or insomnia; frequent episodes of obstructive breathing during sleep; loud snoring; morning headaches; dry mouth upon wakening; chest retraction during sleep in young children; (b) may be associated with other medical disorders: tonsillar enlargement, etc.; (c) miscellaneous abnormalities: increase in blood pressure associated with a decrease in heart rate and cardiac output during apneic episodes; nocturnal angina associated with heart failure and near-miss sudden death; nocturnal oxyhemoglobin desaturation; association with chronic renal disease; neuroendocrine dysfunction and reversal by continuous positive airways pressure therapy; depression; cognitive impairment.

Radiologic Manifestations: (a) airway obstruction; computed tomography: measurement of tongue size to evaluate its predictive value for the result of corrective surgery (uvulopalatopharyngoplasty); (b) pulmonary edema; (c) ultrafast spoiled GRASS magnetic resonance imaging of the pharyngeal airway: occlusion or narrowing; (d) altered intracranial hemodynamics shown by transcranial Doppler ultrasonography: increased cerebral blood-flow velocity during apnea, followed by a rapid decrease during snoring.

SLIT VENTRICLE SYNDROME

Clinical and Radiologic Manifestations: Impairment (excessive drainage) in shunted hydrocephalic patients; the recommended diagnostic triad: intermittent headaches lasting 10 to 30 minutes; smaller than normal ventricles on imaging studies ("slit ventricles"); slow refill of shunt-pumping devices.

SMALL LEFT COLON SYNDROME

Clinical Manifestations: *Symptoms of intestinal obstruction within the first 2 days of life;* high incidence of an association with maternal diabetes; etc.

Radiologic Manifestations: *Intestinal distension; significant narrowing of the colon extending from the splenic flexure to the anus;* intestinal perforation (small bowel; colon); association with meconium plug syndrome; increased subcutaneous fat thickness in infants of diabetic or gestational diabetic mothers.

SMITH-MAGENIS SYNDROME

Clinical and Radiologic Manifestations: (a) *growth failure;* (b) *brachycephaly; midfacial hypoplasia;* microcephaly; upward slant of palpebral fissures, upper lip turned at corner, prognathism; (c) *mental retardation; hyperactivity; self-mutilation; speech delay;* sleep disturbance; seizures; (d) *short and broad hands;* pronounced shortness of middle and distal phalanges; clinodactyly of fifth fingers; abnormal palmar creases; finger pads; (e) eye abnormalities: strabismus; Brushfield spots; high myopia; retinal detachment; iris dysgenesis; telecanthus; ptosis; cataracts; optic nerve hypoplasia; microcornea; microphthalmos; coloboma; (f) prenatal diagnosis of interstitial deletion of (17)(p11.2p11.2); (g) miscellaneous abnormalities: cardiac defect; genital anomalies; delayed dentition; malpositioned ears; hearing loss; hoarse/deep voice; mosaicism for deletion 17p11.2; infant born to a mother having a mosaic 17p11.2p12 deletion and minimal findings of Smith-Magenis syndrome; megacisterna magna due to cerebellar hypoplasia.

SNAPPING HIP SYNDROME (SNAPPING TENDON SYNDROME)

Etiology: Abnormalities of the fascia lata, gluteus maximus muscle, or iliopsoas tendon (snapping of the iliopsoas tendon over the iliopectineal eminence; etc).

Clinical Manifestations: Pain and an audible snapping of the hip with motion.

Radiologic Manifestations: Transient subluxation of the iliopsoas tendon: (a) ultrasonography (static and dynamic): thickening of the iliopsoas tendon, peritendinous fluid collection; abnormal motion of tendon associated with a painful palpable and audible sensation; (b) computed tomography: inflamed iliopsoas bursa; (c) magnetic resonance imaging: tendinitis; bursitis; excluding intraarticular pathology; (d) a negative defect impression of the ligament on the contrast-filled bursa is seen during hip motion at fluoroscopy; (e) tendinography and evaluation of the snapping with hip motion (fluoroscopic observation).

SNEDDON SYNDROME

Clinical Manifestations: (a) *generalized livedo* (skin changes often precede central nervous symptoms by a number of years); (b) *recurrent strokes;* long symptom-free intervals; most symptoms related to medium-sized cerebral artery occlusions; epileptic fits; (c) *mental deficiency associated with cerebral atrophy;* (d) miscellaneous abnormalities: systemic hypertension; Raynaud phenomenon; ischemic heart disease; disturbed sexual function in men; arteriooclusive nephropathy; mitral valve disease; endothelial antibodies.

Radiologic Manifestations: *Vascular occlusion;* irregularities of the vessel walls in the periphery; atypical moyamoya; disturbed regional cerebral flow shown before irreversible ischemic insults occur; lacunar infarctions in the basal ganglia and white matter; brain atrophy.

SOLITARY RECTAL ULCER SYNDROME (Rectal Ulcer Syndrome)

Clinical Manifestations: *Rectal bleeding; mucus discharge; anorectal pain; chronic constipation; prolonged straining; rectal prolapse; benign mucosal lesion in the distal wall of the rectum* (fibrous obliteration of the lamina propria; disruption of the lamina muscularis mucosae; extension of muscle fibers into the lamina propria).

Radiologic Manifestations: (a) granularity of the rectal mucosa, *thickened rectal folds;* rectal stricture; (b) defecography (evacuation proctography): *intussusception of the rectal wall; rectocele; rectal prolapse;* failure of relaxation of the puborectalis that prevents passage of a bolus; greater than normal perineal descent; (c) transrectal sonography: thick hypoechoic growth disrupting the echogenic margin of the perirectal fat.

SOTOS SYNDROME

Clinical Manifestations: (a) *large head; dolichocephaly; prominent forehead and supraorbital ridges; down-slant of palpebral fissures; ocular hypertelorism; prominent jaw; pointed chin; highly arched palate;* (b) *birth weight above average; very rapid growth in height and weight; long armspan; large hands and feet;* (c) *mental retardation; poor motor coordination; behavioral problems;* (d) absence of precocious sexual development; (e) miscellaneous abnormalities: chromosomal aberrations; neoplasms; urinary system anomalies; precocious puberty (case report); ocular abnormalities (presenile nuclear cataracts; megalophthalmos; exotropia; megalocornea; exophoria; iris hypoplasia); status epilepticus associated with absent corpus callosum; (f) sporadic in the majority of the cases; autosomal dominant and recessive modes of inheritance in some families.

Radiologic Manifestations: (a) *large dolichocephalic skull;* ocular hypertelorism; high-rising orbital roofs; normal-size sella turcica; (b) *disproportionately large hands and feet;* abnormal metacarpophalangeal pattern profile; (c) *advanced skeletal maturation, dysharmonic maturation of the phalanges and carpal bones* (the phalanges more advanced as compared with the carpals; delayed appearance of the scaphoid ossification); (d) enlarged subarachnoid space; dilated cerebral ventricles; cavum septum pellucidum, cavum velum interpositum; absent corpus callosum; (e) miscellaneous abnormalities: posteriorly inclined dorsum sella turcica; anterior fontanelle bone; vertebra plana; intervertebral disc herniation;

kyphosis or kyphoscoliosis; syndactyly; unequal leg length; pes planus; genu valgum; genu varum, valgoid feet; congenital hip dislocation.

SPLENOGONADAL FUSION/LIMB DEFORMITY

Clinical Manifestations: (a) *limb malformation:* amelia; peromelia; phocomelia; ectromelia; hemimelia; clubfoot; (b) *inguinal hernia; cryptorchidism; scrotal "mass";* (c) report of a child with the syndrome born to consanguineous parents.

Radiologic Manifestations: (a) ^{99m}Tc sulfur colloid imaging for *ectopic splenic tissue localization;* (b) demonstration of splenogonadal fusion by various imaging techniques; (c) *limb deformities;* hip dislocation.

SPLIT NOTOCHORD SYNDROME

Clinical and Radiologic Manifestations: (a) *spina bifida (anterior and posterior); spinal cord and nerve defects; split cord;* (b) *intestinal anomalies* including intestinal herniation through the dorsal cleft; (c) *neurologic deficit* associated with spinal cord anomalies; (d) *genitourinary anomalies;* (e) miscellaneous abnormalities: neuroenteric cyst; teratoma protruding through the lumbar cleft.

SPLIT-HAND/SPLIT-FOOT DEFORMITIES (LOBSTER-CLAW DEFORMITY; ECTRODACTYLY)

Definition: Defect in development of the central rays of the extremities; in the monodactylous type, the fifth digit is usually present.

Classification

(A) ISOLATED MALFORMATION: an autosomal dominant disorder with variable expressivity and reduced penetrance.

(B) SYNDROMIC: (1) acrorenal syndrome; (2) ADULT syndrome (*Acro-Dermato-Ungual-Lacrimal-Tooth* syndrome): ectrodactyly, excessive freckling, onychodysplasia, obstruction of lacrimal ducts, and hypodontia and/or early loss of permanent teeth; (3) anonychia with ectrodactyly; (4) EEC syndrome (*Ectrodactyly; Ectodermal dysplasia; Cleft lip/palate*); (5) chromosomal abnormalities: 7q21; Xq26; 10q24–q25; (6) Karsch-Neugebauer syndrome: split hand with congenital nystagmus, fundal changes, and cataract; (7) split hands/feet associated with other limb reduction defects (absence of long bones of upper and/or lower limbs); autosomal dominant in most families, with wide variability in expression; locus heterogeneity; (8) split hand/split foot with mandibulofacial dysostosis; (9) split hand with perceptive deafness.

SPONDYLO-CARPO-TARSAL SYNOSTOSIS SYNDROME
(CONGENITAL SYNSPONDYLISM)

Clinical Manifestations: (a) progressive scoliosis; short stature; hearing loss; flatfeet; clinodactyly of fifth fingers; cleft palate; (b) autosomal recessive inheritance.

Radiologic Manifestations: *Scoliosis; vertebral fusion; narrow intervertebral discs; unilateral unsegmented vertebral bar; carpal and tarsal fusion.*

SPONDYLOCOSTAL DYSOSTOSES (SPONDYLOTHORACIC DYSOSTOSIS; JARCHO-LEVIN SYNDROME)

Clinical Manifestations

(A) CLASSIFICATION: A heterogeneous disorder of vertebral segmentation anomalies: (1) *Jarcho-Levin syndrome* (spondylocostal dysostosis type I, spondylothoracic dysostosis): autosomal recessive inheritance; predominance in Hispanic families; (2) *autosomal dominant spondylocostal dysostosis;* variable gene expression; (3) *benign autosomal recessive:* most frequent type, variable gene expression.

(B) JARCHO-LEVIN SYNDROME: (a) *marked shortness of the neck and posterior aspect of the chest; increased anteroposterior diameter of the thoracic cage; protuberant abdomen;* (b) prominent occiput; broad forehead; wide nasal bridge; prominent philtrum; anteverted nares; inverted V-shaped mouth; (c) long, thin limbs with tapering digits.

(C) BENIGN AUTOSOMAL DOMINANT AND AUTOSOMAL RECESSIVE TYPES OF SPONDYLOCOSTAL DYSOSTOSIS: (a) *short trunk and neck; wide anteroposterior diameter of the chest; limited rotatory movement of the spine;* nerve root compression; (b) usually normal life expectancy.

Radiologic Manifestations: (a) *neurovertebral anomalies:* block vertebrae; hemivertebrae; butterfly deformity; sagittal clefts; widely open neural arches; missing vertebral bodies; diastematomyelia; meningocele; spinal cord anomalies; (b) *fan-shaped appearance of the ribs in the posteroanterior direction with posterior convergence of the ribs;* (c) congenital heart disease.

Note: (a) the distribution and severity of the costovertebral anomalies do not seem to be helpful in the differential diagnosis of the various genetic types of the disease because mild and severe clinical manifestations have been reported in the same family; (b) reported in monozygotic twins, discordant for spondylocostal dysostosis.

STAGNANT SMALL-BOWEL SYNDROME

Etiology: Small-bowel stenosis or stricture; gastrocolic fistula; ileocolic fistula; small-bowel diverticula; Crohn disease; blind loop (segment of the small intestine completely bypassed); blind pouch (side-to-side anastomosis associated with persistence of the residual afferent and efferent ends of the intestine).

Clinical Manifestations: *Weight loss; growth retardation; malnutrition; abdominal cramp; abdominal distension; malabsorption; macrocytic anemia; multiple vitamin deficiencies;* abnormal jejunal bile acid concentration due to abnormal bacterial flora; hypertrophy of the bowel wall, edema, inflammation, and ulceration; etc.

Radiologic Manifestations: Spherical, tubular, or club-shaped gas-containing structures on plain films of the abdomen; pseudotumor if filled with fluid or food debris; *demonstration of distended bowel by a contrast study of the bowel.*

STEELE-RICHARDSON-OLSZEWSKI SYNDROME

Clinical Manifestations: *Supranuclear ophthalmoplegia; pseudobulbar palsy; dystonia; axial rigidity; dementia* ("subcortical dementia"); cerebellar and pyramidal signs and symptoms minor or absent; absence of startle response to an unexpected auditory stimulus.

Radiologic Manifestations: Positron emission tomography: a global decrease in blood flow and oxygen utilization, more marked in the frontal region.

STERNAL MALFORMATION–ANGIODYSPLASIA ASSOCIATION

Clinical Manifestations: *Hemangiomas; telangiectasis* (face; scalp; neck; trunk; upper respiratory tract; abdomen); miscellaneous (skin changes over the sternal defect; absent pericardium; cleft lip; micrognathia).

Radiologic Manifestation: *Sternal defects:* complete or partial, including the cleft to the xiphoid.

STERNAL-CARDIAC MALFORMATIONS ASSOCIATION

Clinical Manifestations: *Sternal deformity (*pectus carinatum; anterior sternal defect; etc.); *congenital heart disease (*patent ductus arteriosus; ventricular septal defect; atrial septal defect; tetralogy of Fallot; transposition of the great arteries; etc.); etc.

Radiologic Manifestations: *Various sternal anomalies:* premature sternal fusion including chondromanubrial deformity; delayed ossification of the mesosternum; multiple manubrial ossification centers; sternal defects; etc.

STERNO-COSTO-CLAVICULAR HYPEROSTOSIS

Clinical Manifestations: Presentation between 30 and 50 years of age: (a) *pain in the upper part of the chest and shoulder; limitation of motion; exacerbation and remission;* (b) *palmoplantar pustulosis;* (c) moderate elevation of the sedimentation rate and C-reactive protein concentration; elevated serum globulin levels (α_1 and α_2); polyclonal gammopathy; mildly elevated serum alkaline phosphatase concentration; (d) biopsy: nonsuppurative acute and chronic inflammation of bones, muscles, and entheses; ligamentous fibrosis; ligamentous ossification; lymphocytes, plasma cells, and polymorphonuclear leukocytes within the wall of small vessels.

Radiologic Manifestations: (a) *hyperostosis and cortical thickening* (clavicles; sternum; upper ribs; etc.); sclerotic changes in the sacroiliac joint region; (b) *increased uptake on skeletal scintigraphy;* (c) miscellaneous abnormalities: pleural effusion, pulmonary infiltrates.

STEVENS-JOHNSON SYNDROME

Etiology: Various factors have been implicated: infections; drugs; collagen diseases; contactants; foods; visceral malignancies; radiation therapy.

Clinical Manifestations: (a) *erythema multiforme; vesicular lesions of the mucous membranes (stomatitis; urethritis; conjunctivitis);* (b) miscellaneous abnormalities: angular webbing; ulcerative colitis; ulcerative proctitis; nephritis; nephrotic syndrome; uremia, pericarditis; pericardial effusion; atrial arrhythmias; anonychia; oral mucosal scarring; chronic obliterative bronchitis; dysphagia; ocular cicatricial pemphigoid; blindness.

Radiologic Manifestations: Patchy atypical pneumonia; pneumothorax; pneumomediastinum; subcutaneous emphysema; chronic lung disease; bronchiolitis obliterans (shown by high-resolution computed tomography); pericardial effusion; calcification of the bladder wall; esophageal stricture; obliteration of the piriform sinus.

STEWART-TREVES SYNDROME

Angiosarcoma developing in chronic lymphedema.

STICKLER SYNDROME (ARTHRO-OPHTHALMOPATHY; WAGNER-STICKLER SYNDROME)

Clinical Manifestations: A connective tissue disease: (a) *typical facial features:* midfacial hypoplasia; broad nasal bridge; long philtrum; micrognathia; (b) *progressive myopia;* retinal detachment; glaucoma; amblyopia; astigmatism; strabismus; lenticular opacities; (c) *progressive sensorineural hearing loss;* (d) *enlarged wrist, knee, and ankle joints at birth;* hypermobility of the joints; limitation of mobility of the joints in some cases; joint pain; dislocated patella; marfanoid body build; (e) miscellaneous abnormalities: cleft palate (20%); Robin sequence in a newborn in association with hypotonicity and hyperextensibility of the joints; (f) genetic and clinical heterogeneity: autosomal dominant; phenotype variability in families; caused by mutations in the structural gene for collagen type II (COL2A1) in about 50% of cases; gene linked to chromosome 6.

Radiologic Manifestations

(A) INFANTS: *Rhizomelic limb shortening; wide metaphyses; vertebral coronal clefts.*

(B) CHILDREN AND ADOLESCENTS: (a) narrowness of the diaphyses of long bones; thin cortices; normal width of the metaphyses; *irregularity in ossification; flattening and underdevelopment of some epiphyses;* coxa valga; wide femoral neck; subluxation of the femoral head; protrusio acetabuli; hypoplasia of the iliac wings; arthritic changes; *irregularity of the end plates of the vertebrae;* Scheuermann-like changes; thoracic kyphosis; anterior wedging of the vertebral bodies; scoliosis; cervical spine stenosis and cervical cord myelopathy; (b) micrognathia; hypoplastic maxilla; short cranial base.

STIFF-MAN SYNDROME (MOERSCH-WOLTMANN SYNDROME)

Clinical Manifestations: An autoimmune disorder (heterogeneity related to autoantibodies): (a) *progressive symmetric muscle rigidity; painful muscle spasms* with profuse sweating and tachycardia that are precipitated by stimuli or movements; abnormal contractions of antagonistic muscles; exaggerated acoustic startle reflex in response to loud noise; increased tendon reflexes; *movement in block;* (b) paroxysmal autonomic dysfunctions; (c) *antibodies directed against glutamic acid decarboxylase;* organ-specific autoimmune disease (insulin-dependent diabetes mellitus; hyperthyroidism); (d) electromyographic abnormality: *continuous motor unit activity with superimposed bursts* that are abolished by nerve block, curare, general anesthesia, sleep, and benzodiazepines; (e) normal intellect.

Radiologic Manifestations: Fractures resulting from muscular spasm; hypertrophic arthropathy of the spinal column; brain atrophy.

STOKES-ADAMS SYNDROME

Clinical Manifestations: (a) *sudden change in heart rate with a transient and abrupt loss of consciousness* with or without convulsions; *decrease in cardiac output; fall in blood pressure; paleness; flushing of the face with resumption of heart beats;* (b) abnormal electrocardiographic and electrophysiologic studies confirming the diagnosis (c) reported as the first manifestation of rheumatic carditis.

Radiologic Manifestations: *Depend on etiologic factors:* congenital heart anomalies; myocarditis; acquired valvular diseases; myocardial infarction; metabolic diseases; infiltrative diseases of the myocardium; toxic agents; electrolyte disturbances; metastatic and primary neoplastic diseases.

STOLL-CHARROW-POZNANSKI SYNDROME (CEREBELLAR HYPOPLASIA–ENDOSTEAL SCLEROSIS)

Clinical Manifestations: (a) developmental delay, short stature; microcephaly; ataxia; (b) miscellaneous abnormalities: oligodontia, strabismus, nystagmus, congenital hip dislocation; (c) autosomal recessive inheritance.

Radiologic Manifestations: (a) hypoplasia of the vermis of the cerebellum; hypoplasia of the cerebellar hemisphere (less than that of the vermis); prominent sulci; (b) endosteal sclerosis with narrowness of the medullary space; metaphyseal sclerosis; vertebral sclerosis.

STRAIGHT BACK SYNDROME

Clinical Manifestations: (a) dyspnea (rare); (b) *ejection systolic murmur at the base of the heart or a late systolic murmur;* (c) right axis deviation, an rSr′ pattern in lead V_1; (d) pressure gradient between the right and main pulmonary arteries; (e) pectus excavatum; (f) miscellaneous abnormalities: mitral valve prolapse; bicuspid aortic valve.

Radiologic Manifestations: (a) *straight dorsal spine;* (b) *narrow anteroposterior diameter of the thoracic cage;* (c) *heart flattened* and displaced to the left; (d) prominent pulmonary artery segment, prominent right hilus and pulmonary vasculature in the right lower lung field; (e) pulmonary venous obstruction and dilatation (very rare).

STURGE-WEBER SYNDROME (STURGE-WEBER-DIMITRI DISEASE)

Clinical Manifestations: (a) *angiomatous lesions (port-wine nevi) of the face* in a trigeminal facial distribution, gingiva and alveolar ridges (a case reported without facial nevus); (b) *hemangiomas* of the conjunctiva, episclera, choroid, and retina; retinal vascular tortuosity; *glaucoma;* buphthalmos; iris heterochromia; retinal detachment; strabismus; (c) *contralateral hemiplegia;* homonymous hemianopia; (d) miscellaneous abnormalities: *seizures; mental retardation;* upper airway obstruction.

Radiologic Manifestations

(A) SKULL RADIOGRAPH: *Asymmetry* with a smaller hemicranium on the involved side; enlarged vascular channels of the skull; *double-contour gyriform patterns of intracranial calcification* in the subcortical region, primarily in the parietal and occipital regions.

(B) COMPUTED TOMOGRAPHY OF BRAIN: *Cerebral calcification* (unilateral or bilateral); *contrast enhancement of leptomeningeal angiomatosis; ipsilateral cortical atrophy;* enlargement of the ipsilateral ventricle; decreased volume of the ipsilateral hemicranium; enlarged subarachnoid space in cases with an enlarged ipsilateral hemicranium; enlargement and increased enhancement of the choroid plexus on the same side as the facial and intracranial lesions; ocular enhancement (choroid hemangioma).

(C) MAGNETIC RESONANCE IMAGING OF BRAIN AND MAGNETIC RESONANCE ANGIOGRAPHY: Thickened cortex with decreased convolutions; accelerated myelination in the abnormal cerebral hemisphere; cerebral atrophy; enlarged choroid plexus; cerebellar involvement (uncommon); enhancement in the brain cortex after contrast injection, which is considered to be due to blood-brain barrier breakdown; cerebral angiomas; pial angiomas; reduced flow of the transverse sinuses and jugular veins; prominent deep collateral venous system; lack of superficial cortical veins; reduced arterial flow signal; proptosis; abnormal ocular enhancement (choroid angioma).

(D) SCINTIGRAPHY OF BRAIN: Widened cap of radioactivity over the affected cerebral convexity; identical radioactivity in hemispheres in studies performed 1 to 3 hours following the injection of isotope material; regional cerebral hypoperfusion shown by Tc-99m HMPAO imaging and xenon-133 inhalation technique.

(E) ANGIOGRAPHY OF BRAIN: (a) arterial occlusion (rare); (b) *capillary or venous angiomatous stains;* (c) *various venous abnormalities:* nonfilling of the superior sagittal sinus; tortuosity; segmental ectasia; bizarre course of the cerebral veins and absence, deformity, and caliber irregularities of the deep veins; progressive venous occlusion in a neonate demonstrated with venography.

(F) POSITRON EMISSION TOMOGRAPHY OF BRAIN: Depressed local cerebral glucose utilization.

SUBCLAVIAN STEAL SYNDROME

Pathophysiology: Circulation to an arm via the vertebral artery in a patient with subclavian or innominate artery obstruction proximal to the origin of the vertebral artery with ischemia of the brain and/or arm as a result.

Etiology: Arteriosclerosis; thrombosis; tumor; Takayasu syndrome; congenital anomaly (hypoplasia, atresia, or isolation of the subclavian artery with a right or cervical aortic arch; vascular rings; coarctation of the aorta with obliteration of the subclavian artery orifice; coarctation of aorta and interrupted aortic arch); extravascular obstruction due to a fibrous band and surgically corrected congenital anomalies; granulation tissue secondary to cannulation of an artery; trauma; surgical procedure (Blalock-Taussig procedure); subclavian artery aneurysm; during extracorporeal membrane oxygenation; coronary-subclavian steal syndrome (post–coronary by-pass surgery); etc.

Clinical Manifestations: (a) *pain and numbness of the arm and hand, claudication;* (b) *dizziness; light-headedness; syncopal episodes; headache; vertigo;* visual defect; coldness; fatigue during activity; aphasia; hearing loss; etc.; (c) absent radial pulse; a difference in brachial artery pressure greater than 20 mm Hg; supraclavicular bruit; (d) congenital subclavian steal usually asymptomatic in childhood.

Radiologic Manifestations: (a) angiographic demonstration of *arterial obstruction to an arm and reverse direction of flow of contrast medium from the vertebral artery to the arm;* increased or decreased jugular vein opacity as compared with the opposite side; bidirectional and antegrade blood flow in the vertebral artery (case report); (b) Doppler sonography: *negative flow indicating backflow from brain;* (c) magnetic resonance angiography (phase encoded): demonstration of the normal and *abnormal flow direction in the vertebral arteries.*

SUPERIOR MESENTERIC ARTERY SYNDROME
(ARTERIOMESENTERIC DUODENAL COMPRESSION)

Definition: Compression of the third portion of the duodenum secondary to an increase in acuteness of the aorto-superior mesenteric artery angle.

Etiology: Rapid weight loss; anorexia nervosa; rapid growth without weight gain; hyperextension of the vertebral column (body brace; cast); duodenal hypotonia; familial; severe traumatic brain injury; spastic quadriparesis; as a complication of ileal pouch–anal anastomosis (total proctocolectomy).

Clinical Manifestations: *Postprandial epigastric fullness, nausea, vomiting, abdominal cramps, weight loss, and slender habitus.*
Radiologic Manifestations: (a) *dilatation of the duodenum proximal to a vertical linear extrinsic pressure defect of third portion of the duodenum;* marked "to-and-fro" peristaltic waves proximal to the obstruction; gastric dilatation (in some); relief of the obstruction in the prone position; (b) *narrow aorto-mesenteric angle* (10 to 12 degrees as compared with the normal of 45 to 65 degrees) and a *decrease in the aorto-mesenteric distance* (2 to 3 mm as compared with the normal of 7 to 20 mm); (c) computed tomography: duodenal distension and the close proximity of superior mesenteric vessels and aorta.

SWEET SYNDROME

Clinical and Radiologic Manifestations: (a) *fever; raised painful plaques on the extremities, face, and neck; dense dermal cellular infiltrate with neutrophils; polymorphonuclear leukocytosis;* (b) pulmonary infiltrates; (c) association with the following: malignancies (hematologic; metastatic breast carcinoma); drug induced (therapy with granulocyte colony–stimulating factor); infections; myeloproliferative disorders; lymphoproliferative disorders; myelodysplastic syndrome; Fanconi anemia; neuro-Behçet disease; chronic granulomatous disease of childhood; splenic irradiation for chronic myelogenous leukemia.

SWYER-JAMES SYNDROME (Macleod Syndrome)

Etiology: (a) sequela of various lung insults: bronchiolitis; bronchiolitis obliterans; measles; *Mycoplasma pneumoniae;* pertussis; adenovirus pneumonia; foreign-body aspiration; hydrocarbon pneumonia; radiotherapy; (b) idiopathic.
Clinical Manifestations: (a) *history of recurrent pulmonary infections in childhood;* (b) usually asymptomatic in adult life; however, the subject may have a cough, chronic and repeated pulmonary infections, decreased exercise tolerance, hemoptysis, and arterial blood desaturation; (c) miscellaneous abnormalities: bronchial asthma and spontaneous pneumothorax; association with Noonan syndrome (a case report).
Radiologic Manifestations: (a) *unilateral small, hyperlucent lung (or lobe);* (b) *poor air exchange* and change of lung density between inspiration and expiration; (c) *diminished pulmonary vasculature; small hilar shadow of the involved side;* (d) bronchographic demonstration of *dilatation of the bronchi and lack of alveolization of the contrast medium;* hyperdistensible bronchial diameter shown by functional bronchography (inflation under 50-cm water pressure); (e) angiographic demonstration of *diminished size and number of pulmonary vessels in the portion of the involved lung;* (f)

decreased perfusion and ventilation; (g) computed tomography: more accurate than plain chest radiography (in particular using ultrafast high-resolution method) in demonstration of the abnormalities including bilateral involvement *(hyperlucency; air-trapping; small pulmonary vessels).*

SYMPHALANGISM-SURDITY SYNDROME (Facio-Audio-Symphalangism Syndrome; WL Syndrome)

Clinical Manifestations: (a) *progressive conduction deafness with onset in childhood;* fixation of the foot plate of the stapes in the oval window; (b) *distinct facial features* (long and narrow face; broad and hemicylindric nose; lack of alar flare; broad nasal bridge; thin upper lip; low-set ears; asymmetric mouth; internal strabismus); (c) *proximal symphalangia of the fingers (2, 3, 4) and toes (2, 3, 4);* brachydactyly; clinodactyly; hypoplasia or aplasia of the distal segments of the fingers and/or toes and corresponding nails; hypoplasia of the thenar and hypothenar muscles; cutaneous syndactyly of the fingers (2, 3, 4) and toes (2, 3); (d) autosomal dominant inheritance; the gene for proximal symphalangism localized to chromosome 17q21–q22.

Radiologic Manifestations: (a) *proximal symphalangism:* progressive narrowing of the interphalangeal joints resulting in fusion of the phalanges (proximal interphalangeal joints of the fingers and distal interphalangeal joints of the toes usually involved); thumbs and great toes usually not affected; (b) brachydactyly; (c) miscellaneous abnormalities: short arm; cubitus valgus; humeroradial fusion; dislocated head of the radius; carpal and tarsal fusion; clinodactyly; hypoplastic/aplastic middle phalanx; hypoplastic/dysplastic distal phalanx; short legs; overtubulation of tibia and fibula; genu valgum; pes planovalgus; short foot; short hallux; pectus excavatum; short sternum; wide costochondral junctions; Klippel-Feil anomaly.

SYNDROME X

Clinical and Radiologic Manifestations: *Angina pectoris; ischemic-appearing result on exercise test; normal coronary arteriograms: no other explanation for the symptoms* (hypertension; valve disease; cardiomyopathy); neuroticism (anxiety; depression and somatic concerns); etc.

T

TABATZNIK SYNDROME (Heart-Hand Syndrome II)

Clinical Manifestations: (a) *cardiac arrhythmias; sloping shoulders, hypoplastic deltoid muscles, and short arm;* cryptorchidism; mild mental retardation; facial dysmorphism; (b) autosomal dominant or X-linked dominant inheritance.

Radiologic Manifestations: *Upper limb deformities:* flaring of lower end of humerus; flaring and obliquity of distal end of radius; absent styloid process of ulna; shortening and hypoplasia of fourth and fifth metacarpals; brachytelephalangy; accessory carpal bone; thumb polydactyly.

TAR SYNDROME (THROMBOCYTOPENIA–ABSENT RADIUS SYNDROME)

Clinical Manifestations: (a) *congenital deformity of the forearm and hand* (often bilateral) with the hand at right angles to the forearm; *thumb always present;* (b) hemorrhagic tendencies caused by *thrombocytopenia;* decrease in the number and severity of the thrombocytopenic episodes in most cases; (c) *myeloid leukemoid reactions* and eosinophilia; (d) *hypercellular bone marrow and congenital absence or marked reduction of megakaryocytes* without a reduction in other elements of the bone marrow; (e) miscellaneous abnormalities: congenital heart defects; increased cellular radiation sensitivity; (f) pattern consistent with autosomal recessive inheritance; great intrafamilial and interfamilial variability.

Radiologic Manifestations: (a) absent radius (bilateral) with or without other upper-limb anomalies (short and malformed ulna; absent ulna; abnormal humerus; absent humerus in 5% to 10% of cases with digits arising from the shoulder; hypoplastic digits; hypoplastic or fused phalanges; carpal bone hypoplasia or fusion; hypoplastic or absent middle phalanx of the fifth digit); (b) shoulder anomalies: absent or hypoplastic glenoid fossa, acromion, scapula, and clavicle; lateral clavicular hook; (c) lower-limb anomalies: hip dislocation; phocomelia; coxa valga; genu varum; subluxated knee; hypoplastic or absent patella; patellar dislocation; femoral and tibial torsion; abnormal tibiofibular joint; clubfoot deformity; abnormal toe placement.

TEEBI HYPERTELORISM SYNDROME

Clinical and Radiologic Manifestations: (a) *craniofacial dysmorphism:* round face; prominent forehead; pronounced ocular hypertelorism; mild downward slanting of the palpebral fissures; heavy and broad eyebrows; ptosis of the eyelids; broad and/or depressed nasal bridge; widow's peak; short nose with or without anteverted nostrils; hypoplastic maxilla; long, deep philtrum; dental malocclusion and/or overcrowded teeth; horizontal thin upper lip and/or pouty lower lip; prominent lower jaw; fleshy ear lobule and/or prominent anthelix; (b) slightly small broad hands; clinodactyly of the fifth finger; broad flatfeet with bulbous toes; mild interdigital webbing; (c) miscellaneous abnormalities: shawl scrotum; a child with ventricular septal defect, lipoma of the occipital area, and hypoplastic left hemisphere of the cerebellum; report of a mother and daughter (umbilical hernia/omphalocele, natal teeth, and minor craniofacial anomalies); (d) autosomal dominant inheritance.

TEL HASHOMER CAMPTODACTYLY SYNDROME

Clinical and Radiologic Manifestations: (a) short stature; (b) brachycephaly; *peculiar facies* (asymmetric; ocular hypertelorism; long philtrum; small mouth); *highly arched palate;* dental crowding; (c) *spindle-shaped fingers; camptodactyly; abnormal dermatoglyphics;* (d) *muscular hypoplasia of the chest, pelvis, and limbs;* (e) miscellaneous abnormalities: clubfeet; pes planus; joint hyperflexibility; joint dislocation; loose skin; inguinal hernia; mitral valve prolapse; atrial septal defect; humeroradial muscle aplasia; (f) autosomal recessive inheritance.

TETHERED CORD SYNDROME

Clinical Manifestations: Initial symptoms often in childhood: (a) *weakness; painful or numb lower limbs; spastic gait; muscle atrophy; neurogenic bladder; bladder dysfunction* (flaccid bladder; uninhibited bladder; mixed bladder dysfunction); *scoliosis; foot deformities;* (b) *external evidence of spinal dysrhaphia:* hypertrichosis; dermoids; subcutaneous lipomas; sinus tracts; (c) miscellaneous abnormalities: association of all types of imperforate anus with myelodysplasia (including those with normal spine radiographs); urogenital anomalies; VATER association; meningitis; etc.

Radiologic Manifestations: (a) *single or multiple vertebral bifid arches; wide interpediculate distances; kyphoscoliosis;* increased lumbar lordotic curve; (b) *wide dural sac; low filum terminale;* abnormal position and angle of the nerve roots; *cord splitting; tethering bands; tethering masses (dermoid; lipomatous tissue;* etc.); cavitary lesions/myelomalacia of the conus or the cord adjacent to the tethering lesions.

THALIDOMIDE EMBRYOPATHY

Clinical Manifestations: *Limb anomalies; ophthalmologic manifestations* (ocular mobility defects, mostly incomitant horizontal strabismus; aberrant lacrimation; microphthalmos; coloboma; congenital glaucoma; large refractive errors); etc.

Radiologic Manifestations: *Limb anomalies: preaxial reduction in size or number of skeletal elements:* amelia; proximal phocomelia; radial forearm anomalies; digits usually present; hip dislocation.

THEVENARD SYNDROME (ACRODYSTROPHIC NEUROPATHY)

Clinical Manifestations: Onset of symptoms often at puberty: (a) *peripheral sensory impairment; trophic changes and ulcer with the sole of the foot as the primary site; "elephant foot";* vasomotor disturbance; hypertrichosis; (b) autosomal dominant inheritance.

Radiologic Manifestations: Lesions often limited to the lower extremities: *acro-osteolysis; destruction of metatarsophalangeal joints;* Charcot arthropathy of the lower limbs with effusion; hemarthrosis; osteoporosis; pathologic fractures; dislocation.

THORACIC OUTLET SYNDROME

Clinical Manifestations: Brachial plexus–subclavian artery compression: *pain* (chest wall; shoulder; arm; hand); *numbness;* tetany of the hand; *skin color changes; claudications; bruit* in the supraclavicular or infraclavicular fossae; diminished pulse and lower blood pressure on the affected side; *wasting* of hand muscles; weakness and wasting in the forearm; functional abnormalities shown by sensory and motor conduction studies, quantitative electromyography, and somatosensory-evoked potentials.

Radiologic Manifestations: (a) arteriographic demonstration of the site and severity of *arterial obstruction;* venous obstruction (in some); (b) radioisotope demonstration of flow reduction; (c) color duplex sonography: doubling of peak systolic velocity or complete cessation of arterial flow with hyperabduction; complete cessation of the venous blood flow or loss of arterial and respiratory dynamics in the waveform of the subclavian vein with hyperabduction; (d) reported computed tomographic findings not seen on plain radiographs: impingement of the C7 transverse process on the scalene triangle or anteromedial aspect of the middle scalene muscle; (e) magnetic resonance imaging demonstration of deviation or distortion of nerves or blood vessels; band(s) compressing the neurovascular structures; cervical rib; posttraumatic callus of C7; hypertrophied serratus anterior muscle; (f) osteoporosis of the phalanges (in patients with emboli); (g) *bone abnormalities:* abnormal cervical transverse process; rudimentary rib; abnormalities of the first thoracic vertebra and corresponding rib; clavicular deformities; previous thoracoplasty.

THE 3-M SYNDROME (THREE M SYNDROME)

Clinical Manifestations: (a) *low birth weight; proportionate dwarfism;* (b) *craniofacial dysmorphism:* frontal bossing, hatched-shaped craniofacial configuration, large head for height, triangular face, flattened malar region, prominent ears, short nose with upturned nares, prominent mouth or full lips, long philtrum, small pointed chin, *V*-shaped dental arch, and malocclusion; (c) autosomal recessive inheritance.

Radiologic Manifestations: (a) *slender tubular bones;* slender ribs; short fifth digits; prominent heels; pes planus; decreased extension of the elbows; congenital hip dislocation; flaring iliac wings; shortened anteroposterior diameter of the lumbar vertebral bodies; irregularity of end-plates; spina bifida occulta; small pelvis; short femoral necks; (b) miscellaneous abnormalities: osteoporotic appearance; delayed bone age; intracranial aneurysms.

Note: *M* is the first letter of the last name of three of the authors of the original article.

TIETZE SYNDROME

Clinical Manifestations: Subacute or acute onset of *painful nonsuppurative tumefaction* at the costal cartilage; self-limiting and of unknown etiology; commonly involves the second right or left costal cartilages; pathologic examination: usually normal cartilage; some inflammatory change with fibrosis and ossification has been reported.

Radiologic Manifestations: Solitary lesion in about 80% of cases: (a) *soft-tissue swelling* in the tangential view; sclerosis of the sternal manubrium; (b) computed tomography: enlargement of the costal cartilage; ventral angulation of the involved costal cartilage; calcification within the cartilaginous mass; compression of the pectoralis muscle anteriorly and the pleura and lung parenchyma posteriorly; (c) scintigraphy: increased accumulation at the costochondral junction (Tc-99m MDP; Ga-67); (d) ultrasonography: thickened cartilage; inhomogeneously increased echogenicity; indistinct cartilage outline; hypoechoic halo.

TOLOSA-HUNT SYNDROME

Clinical Manifestations: (a) *recurrent or steady retroorbital pain of various intensity and duration; spontaneous remissions;* (b) *ophthalmoplegia:* third, fourth, and sixth nerves; first division of the fifth cranial nerve; periarterial sympathetic fibers; optic nerve; (c) *nonspecific inflammation (granulomatous) in the cavernous sinus or superior orbital fissure or at both sites;* (d) miscellaneous abnormalities: steroid-responsive pain; pseudotumor cerebri; association with autoimmune polyglandular syndrome; lesions extending from cavernous sinus to the intrasellar and juxtasellar regions.

Radiologic Manifestations: (a) orbital venography: *occlusion of the superior ophthalmic vein, collateral venous flow, and poor opacification or obliteration of the cavernous sinus;* (b) carotid arteriography: narrowing of the cavernous segment of the internal carotid artery, and arterial stationary wave phenomenon; (c) computed tomography: cavernous sinus inflammation, and high-density area in the orbit when the examination is performed more than 1 month after the onset of symptoms; (d) magnetic resonance imaging: abnormal signal and/or mass lesions in the cavernous sinuses (hypointense relative to fat and isointense with muscle on short TR/TE images and isointense with fat on long TR/TE scans) with extension into the orbital apex; (e) sellar erosion.

TORIELLO-CAREY SYNDROME

Clinical and Radiologic Manifestations: (a) postnatal growth retardation; microcephaly, telecanthus, short palpebral fissures, small nose, highly arched palate, cleft palate, micrognathia, and malformed ears; brachydactyly; soft-tissue syndactyly of toes; hypospadias; cryptorchidism; micropenis; agenesis/hypoplasia of the corpus callosum; cardiomyopathy; congenital heart defect; etc.; (b) autosomal recessive inheritance.

TOWNES-BROCKS SYNDROME

Clinical and Radiologic Manifestations: (a) *anorectal anomalies:* imperforate anus; anal stenosis; anteriorly located anus; (b) *thumb anomalies:* supernumerary; bifid; broad; triphalangeal; hypoplasia; ulnar deviation; (c) *ear anomalies:* overfolding of the superior helix; cup-shaped ears; microtia; preauricular tags or pits; pretragal sinus; large ears; (d) sensorineural deafness; malformed auditory ossicles; (e) foot deformities: flatfeet; rocker-bottom feet; absent or small third toe; syndactyly III/IV; clinodactyly of the fifth toe; fusion of the metatarsals; duplication of tarsal bones; overlapping of the second, third, and fourth toes; (f) autosomal dominant inheritance; intrafamilial variability; complete penetrance and variable expressivity.

TOXIC SHOCK SYNDROME

Clinical Manifestations: Association with infection by *Staphylococcus aureus* and some other organisms: (a) *intense myalgia;* (b) *high fever;* (c) *skin rash and desquamation;* (d) *vomiting and diarrhea;* (e) abnormal renal and liver function test findings; sterile pyuria; immature granulocytic leukocytosis; low platelet count; coagulation abnormalities; hypocalcemia; low serum albumin and total protein concentrations; elevation of blood urea nitrogen; alanine transaminase; bilirubin and creatine kinase levels; (f) *hypotension; syncope,* complete heart block; (g) *disorientation, alteration in consciousness without focal neurologic signs* when fever or hypotension are absent.

Radiologic Manifestations: (a) ultrasonography of the liver: increased brightness of portal vein wall echoes; diminished echogenicity of the liver parenchyma; (b) adult respiratory distress syndrome; pulmonary edema; cardiac failure.

TREACHER COLLINS SYNDROME (MANDIBULOFACIAL DYSOSTOSIS)

Clinical Manifestations: Abnormalities of the structures derived from the first and second pharyngeal pouch, groove, and arch: (a) *hypoplasia of the face with sunken cheek bones; malformed ear;* macrostomia; highly arched palate; cleft palate/lip; palatopharyngeal incompetence; blind fistulae between the auricle and the corner of the mouth; extra rudimentary ear tags; obliteration of the nasal frontal angle; narrow nares; hypoplasia of the alar cartilages; deficient elevator muscles of the upper lip; (b) *down-slanting of the palpebral fissure; coloboma in the outer portion of the lower lid* and, in some cases, the upper lid; (c) conductive deafness; (d) dental anomalies; malocclusion of the teeth; (e) autosomal dominant inheritance; genetic homogeneity; almost complete penetrance and wide variability in expression.

Radiologic Manifestations: (a) *hypoplasia of the malar bones;* defective lower margin of the orbits; agenesis of the malar bones; obtuse angle of the mandible; concave curvature of the horizontal ramus of the mandible; hypoplasia or aplasia of coronoid and condyloid processes; malocclusion; absence of palatine bones; cleft palate; *hypogenesis or agenesis of the mandible;* (b) *underdeveloped paranasal sinuses;* (c) *various ear abnormalities:* (1) hypoplasia or absence of the external auditory canal; (2) hypoplasia or absence of the tympanic cavity; closed middle-ear cavity by a thick osseous atretic plate; absent or dysplastic and rudimentary ossicles; presence of a single large conglomerate incudomalleal mass attached to the atretic plate, epitympanum or both; closed oval window; (3) hypoplasia or absence of the mastoid; (4) inner-ear abnormalities rare (deficient cochlea and vestibular apparatus); (d) abnormal course of the facial nerve canal; (e) progressive cranial basilar kyphosis associated with narrowing of the anteroposterior diameter of the pharynx and pharyngeal hypoplasia; (f) vertebral anomalies (in some); (g) prenatal sonographic diagnosis: fetal facial features (microcephaly; slanting forehead, micrognathia; microphthalmos); abnormal fetal swallowing; polyhydramnios.

TRICHO-DENTO-OSSEOUS SYNDROME

Clinical Manifestations: (a) *dark, very curly scalp hair* that straightens by the second decade of life; long eyelashes; *taurodontism of the mandibular first permanent molar; pitted dysplastic enamel; discoloration;*

eruption defects; nail defects: thinness of the nails; splitting of superficial layers of the nails; (b) autosomal dominant inheritance.

Radiologic Manifestations: *Sclerosis of the skull, in particular at the base;* nonpneumatization of the mastoids and paranasal sinuses; short mandibular rami; obtuse mandibular angles; *mild to moderate hyperostosis of the cortex of the tubular bones; sclerosis of the provisional zone of calcification; dental defects (*hypoplasia of the enamel; delayed formation and eruption of teeth; early loss of teeth; hypocalcification; enlarged pulp chambers; taurodontism of the molars; dental abscess).

TRICHORRHEXIS NODOSA SYNDROME (Pollitt Syndrome)

Clinical Manifestations: (a) *low birth weight; mental and physical retardation; brittle hair; sulfur deficient (cystine deficient); nail dysplasia;* etc.; (b) autosomal recessive inheritance has been suggested.

Radiologic Manifestations: Axial osteosclerosis; peripheral osteopenia; retarded skeletal maturation; kyphosis.

TRISMUS-PSEUDOCAMPTODACTYLY SYNDROME (Hecht Syndrome)

Clinical and Radiologic Manifestations: (a) *painless chronic trismus; pseudocamptodactyly* (short finger flexor tendons); short leg muscles producing *foot deformity* (talipes equinovarus; metatarsus adductus; hammer toes; claw toes; etc.); short stature; (b) autosomal dominant inheritance; more common in females.

TROELL-JUNET SYNDROME

Clinical and Radiologic Manifestations: Predilection for women: *acromegaly; toxic goiter* (usually nodular); *diabetes mellitus; hyperostosis of the vault of the skull.*

TUBEROUS SCLEROSIS (Bourneville-Pringle Syndrome)

Clinical Manifestations
(A) Skin Lesions: *Fibrous-angiomatous lesions* (adenoma sebaceum); "shagreen" patches; café au lait spots; forehead plaque; ash leaf–shaped depigmented macules; leathery skin in the lower part of the trunk; subungual fibroma.

(B) Neurologic Manifestations: Seizures; spasms in infancy; mental deficiency; developmental deficiency; increased intracranial pressure; psychiatric disorders, including autistic behavior and attention deficit.

(C) Cardiovascular Manifestations: (a) cardiac rhabdomyoma: 80% of cardiac rhabdomyomas associated with tuberous sclerosis; tumor-related symptoms (murmur; arrhythmias; heart failure); regression of tumor not uncommon; (b) aneurysms; (c) Wolff-Parkinson-White syndrome; extra systoles; conduction blocks; tachycardias; sinus bradycardia; (d) renovascular hypertension.

(D) Renal Manifestations: Renal enlargement (cysts; hamartoma; carcinoma); hematuria; renal and perirenal hemorrhage (may cause death); hypertensive crisis; chronic renal failure.

(E) Pulmonary Manifestations: Cor pulmonale; pneumothorax; chylothorax; lymphangiomatosis.

(F) Eyes: Retinal phakoma.

(G) Tumors: Cardiac rhabdomyoma or hamartoma; liver hamartoma; renal cell carcinoma; benign teratoma; lymphangioma; eosinophilic adenoma and acromegalic gigantism; sacrococcygeal chordoma; angiomyolipomas in the kidneys and less commonly in other internal organs; leiomyoma of colon; papillary adenoma of the thyroid gland.

(H) Miscellaneous Abnormalities: Hydrops fetalis; gynecomastia; sexual precocity; acanthosis nigricans; pitted enamel hypoplasia; isosexual precocity; hypothalamic endocrine disorders; macrodactyly; congenital hypothyroidism due to thyroid gland dysgenesis.

(I) Autosomal dominant inheritance with variable expressivity and genetic heterogeneity.

Radiologic Manifestations

(A) Central Nervous System: (a) computed tomography: *calcification (periventricular;* gyriform; cerebellar); subependymal nodules; parenchymal hamartomas (cortical tubers) with less attenuation than in the surrounding brain tissue; hyperdense lesions (rare); tubers not usually enhanced by contrast material; faint high-density areas that connect the ventricle to the cerebral surface; (b) magnetic resonance imaging: superior to computed tomography, particularly for cortical tubers, cystic lesions, and heterotopic clusters; subependymal nodules of intermediate signal intensity; parenchymal hamartomas with long T_1 and T_2 relaxation characteristics; high-signal lesions in the cerebellum; gadolinium-DTPA enhancement of subependymal nodules; linear abnormalities in the cerebral white matter connecting subependymal nodules to the subcortical lesions (as an area of hypointensity on T_1-weighted images and as an area of hyperintensity on T_2-weighted images); (c) ultrasonography: densely echogenic periventricular nodules; (d) positron emission tomography: hypometabolic cortical lesions; (e) early detection of brain lesion by I-123 IMP single photon emission computed tomography in neonate; (f) miscellaneous: hydrocephalus due to obstruction; neoplasm (giant-cell astrocytomas or higher-grade gliomas); arterial ectasia, and occlusion; reduced

Tc-99m HMPAO uptake in regions corresponding with magnetic resonance imaging–confirmed locations of cortical tubers; antenatal diagnosis by magnetic resonance imaging; gyriform enhancement of cerebellum simulating infarction; pachygyria.

(B) CARDIOVASCULAR SYSTEM: Cardiac rhabdomyoma or hamartoma; arterial aneurysm (aorta; intracranial; renal; peripheral); coarctation of the abdominal aorta and renal artery stenosis; cardiogenic emboli; cardiac failure.

(C) RESPIRATORY SYSTEM: Interstitial reticular infiltrates that may progress to honeycomb lung; cor pulmonale; pulmonary cyst; pulmonary lymphangioma; chylothorax; spontaneous pneumothorax; air trapping shown by dynamic ultrafast high-resolution computed tomography.

(D) URINARY SYSTEM: (a) angiomyolipomas: (1) ultrasonographic demonstration of a cluster of internal echoes at both low and high gain; (2) plain film and computed tomographic demonstration of intrarenal fat density; stretching of the calyces on excretory urography; (3) angiographic demonstration of hypervascularity and irregular outpouchings from interlobular and interlobar arteries; (b) renal cysts similar to adult polycystic disease (may present as the only initial manifestation of the disease in infancy); (c) renal cell carcinoma; Wilms tumor; (d) intratumoral and perirenal hemorrhage; (e) berry aneurysms of intrarenal arteries; spontaneous intraperitoneal rupture of a kidney.

(E) SKELETAL SYSTEM: Patchy localized sclerotic densities in the skull, vertebrae, pelvis, and long bones; cystlike defects in the phalanges, metatarsals, and metacarpals; localized periosteal thickening along the shaft of the tubular bones; rib expansion and sclerosis; exostosis and enostosis of the tubular bones; thinning of the occipital bone in association with a cortical tuber adjacent to the thinned bone (case report); clivus chordoma (case report); overgrowth (limb; digit; rib); kyphosis; scoliosis.

TURCOT SYNDROME

Clinical and Radiologic Manifestations: (a) *familial polyposis of colon;* (b) *primary neuroepithelial tumors of the central nervous system, particularly glioblastoma;* (c) miscellaneous abnormalities: sebaceous cysts; papillary carcinoma of the thyroid; leukemia; spinal cord neoplasm; concomitant occurrence with Gardner syndrome (polyposis coli, craniofacial exostosis, and astrocytoma); (d) autosomal recessive inheritance.

Note: "Glioma-polyposis" has also been reported in Gardner syndrome and in familial polyposis.

TURNER SYNDROME (ULLRICH-TURNER SYNDROME)

Chromosomal Abnormalities: Majority, 45,X (about 55%); less common: mosaicism (X/XX, X/XY, X/XX/XY); isochromosome X; ring X;

partial deletion of the X chromosome; 45,X/46,X,r(X)/46,X,dic(X). Occurrence in mother (45,X) and daughter (46,del(X)(p21).

Clinical Manifestations

(A) EXTERNAL PHYSICAL FEATURES: Growth failure with onset before birth; delayed spontaneous pubertal growth spurt; relatively small mandible; narrow palate; inner canthal folds; anomalous auricles; blue sclerae; strabismus; ptosis; cataract; webbed neck; low posterior hairline; appearance of a short neck; *transient lymphedema of the hands and feet in infancy; shield chest; widely spaced hypoplastic nipples;* wide arm span and *cubitus valgus;* cutaneous manifestations (hypoplastic nails; keloid and hypertrophic scars; dry skin; seborrheic dermatitis; abnormal dermatoglyphics; increased numbers of pigmented nevi; cutis laxa).

(B) CARDIOVASCULAR SYSTEM: *Coarctation of the aorta* and other congenital cardiovascular anomalies, including aortic aneurysm complicated with coarctation of aorta; systemic hypertension; intestinal telangiectasia; hemangiomas; lymphangiectasia.

(C) GENITAL SYSTEM: *Ovarian dysgenesis with primary amenorrhea;* infantile uterus, vagina, and breast; 5% have spontaneous menstruation; fertility rare and often associated with spontaneous abortion (structural and chromosomal defects of the fetus).

Radiologic Manifestations

(A) SKELETAL SYSTEM: (a) parietal thinning; brachycephaly; normal sellar volume or increase in size of the pituitary fossa with thinning of the posterior clinoids and dorsum sellae; double floor of the sella turcica; abnormal bony contour of the sella turcica; decreased dimensions of the mastoids; small facial bones; enlargement and increased thickness of the mandible; extensive calcification of petroclinoid ligaments; excessive pneumatization of sphenoid sinuses; increased angle of the base of the skull; thin cranial vault; craniosynostosis; (b) scoliosis; Scheuermann disease; vertebral fusion; cervical rib; thinness of the lateral aspect of the clavicle and posterior ends of the ribs; sternal anomalies (pectus excavatum; short sternum; premature fusion of the manubriosternal junction; premature fusion of mesosternum; decreased ratio of sternal body to manubrium; two ossification centers of the manubrium); (c) male configuration of the pelvic inlet; protrusio acetabuli; (d) *shortening of the fourth metacarpals;* fusion of the carpal bones; radiocarpal angulation; drumstick phalanges; disproportionately long phalanges in the fourth finger; coarse reticular patterns of the carpal bones; small carpal bone surface area; Madelung deformity; *depression of the medial tibial condyle;* exostosis of the tibia; recurrent dislocation of patellae; hypoplastic patellae; irregularity of the tibial metaphysis and epiphysis; tibiotalar slant; pes cavus; fusion of the tarsal bones; short fourth metatarsals; (e) skeletal maturation retardation; (f) osteoporosis.

(B) SEROSAL EFFUSIONS: Pleural-pericardial effusion and ascites in the neonatal period; chylous ascites.

(C) URINARY SYSTEM ABNORMALITIES (IN 33% TO 70% OF THE CASES): Horseshoe kidney; single renal cyst; multicystic dysplastic kidney; bifid pelvis; duplication; malrotation; retrocaval ureter.

(D) GENITAL ABNORMALITIES: Absence of ovaries in 45,X; from absent to infantile to normal adult-sized ovaries in the chromosomal mosaics; small uterus (sexual infantilism); small ovarian cysts.

(E) CENTRAL NERVOUS SYSTEM ABNORMALITIES: Significantly smaller than normal values in magnetic resonance imaging–measured volumes of hippocampus, caudate, lenticular, and thalamic nuclei, and parietooccipital brain matter; congenital anomalies (agenesis of the corpus callosum; Dandy-Walker anomaly; vein of Galen aneurysm; cortical dysplasia); occlusion of the internal carotid artery in a child.

(F) PRENATAL ULTRASONOGRAPHIC FINDINGS: Nuchal blebs or cystic hygroma (prenatal resolution in some cases); ascites; pleural effusion; fetal hydrops; small for gestational age.

Note: The subject of the case reported by Ullrich in 1930 was restudied at the age of 66 years and was found to have unequivocal 45,X chromosomal constitution in all cells examined.

TWIN-TO-TWIN TRANSFUSION SYNDROME (FETAL TRANSFUSION SYNDROME)

Clinical Manifestations: (a) one of the twins sharing placental circulation is *anemic,* and the other is *plethoric;* caused by twin-to-twin vascular anastomosis and an imbalanced placental circulation favoring one twin: (b) *disparity of body size, recipient twin being larger;* (c) polyhydramnios; (d) miscellaneous abnormalities: donor twin with blueberry muffin–like macules and papules associated with cutaneous erythropoiesis; fetal peripheral gangrene.

Radiologic Manifestations: (a) *cardiomegaly* and radiographic manifestation of *cardiac failure in the anemic twin;* (b) *cardiomegaly in the plethoric twin;* increased pulmonary vasculature; (c) fetal ultrasonography: *significant difference in the size of fetuses of the same sex; disparity in size between the amniotic sacs (polyhydramnios in the recipient's sac and oligoamnios in the donor's sac); disparity between the size or number of the vessels in the umbilical cords; a single placenta with areas of disparity in echogenicity; hydrops in either fetus or, very rarely, in both fetuses; enlarged heart; kidneys and muscular mass of the recipient fetus; difference in the urinary bladder size (full bladder in the recipient fetus and empty bladder in the donor fetus); tricuspid regurgitation and biphasic umbilical vein waveforms in recipient fetus; in utero cardiac dysfunc-*

tion in the recipient fetus; (d) miscellaneous abnormalities: reverse twin-to-twin transfusion after intrauterine death of the donor; lenticulostriate vasculopathy in the recipient of twin-to-twin transfusion; etc.

U

ULNAR-MAMMARY SYNDROME (SCHINZEL SYNDROME)

Clinical Manifestations: (a) *limb anomalies (digital, ulnar);* (b) *delayed growth and onset of puberty;* (c) *obesity;* (d) *hypogenitalism and diminished sexual activity;* (e) *hypoplasia of the nipples and apocrine glands; diminished ability to perspire;* (f) autosomal dominant inheritance with full penetrance and highly variable expression; gene mapped to 12q23–q24.1.

Radiologic Manifestations: (a) *limb anomalies:* short fifth finger; absence of fifth finger ray; absence of fourth finger ray (split-hand appearance); absence of fourth and fifth finger rays; absence of third to fifth finger rays; camptodactyly; hypoplastic/absent/deformed ulna; hypoplastic/absent/deformed radius; hypoplastic humerus, scapula, clavicle, and pectoralis major muscle; postaxial polydactyly; short fourth and fifth toes; (b) miscellaneous abnormalities: hypodontia and other dental anomalies; renal malformations.

URETHRAL SYNDROME IN WOMEN

Clinical Manifestations: (a) dysuria; retropubic pressure; dyspareunia; urinary frequency; (b) edematous and hyperemic external urethral orifice; narrowing of the urethral lumen; inflammatory changes of the trigone, bladder neck, and urethra; inflammation of paraurethral glands connected to the distal third of the urethra in prevaginal space (homologous to prostate); hypoestrogenism with resulting vaginal and urethral atrophy; pyelonephritis.

Radiologic Manifestations: Indentation at the base of the bladder; edematous pedunculated or sessile polyps most often located in the anterior aspect of the bladder neck; periurethral calcification.

UROFACIAL SYNDROME (OCHOA SYNDROME)

Clinical Manifestations: (a) *"inverse" facial expression when laughing* (crying appearance when smiling or laughing); (b) *diurnal and/or nocturnal enuresis; recurrent urinary tract infections;* (c) hypertension associated with urinary system disease; (d) cystometric studies: *hypertonic, hyperreflexic type of bladder with uninhibited contractions of the detrusor muscle in most patients;* (e) autosomal recessive inheritance.

Radiologic Manifestations: Vesicoureteral reflux (unilateral or bilateral); trabeculated bladder; spastic posterior urethra at the level of the external sphincter in most patients; significant residual urine after voiding; clubbing of the calices, hydronephrosis; scarring, small kidney size (manifestations of chronic pyelonephritis).

USHER SYNDROME

Classification: Type I: severe to profound hearing impairment, absent vestibular response, and pigmentary retinopathy; type II: moderate to severe deafness, normal vestibular response, and pigmentary retinopathy.

Clinical and Radiologic Manifestations: (a) *congenital sensorineural deafness; night blindness, retinitis pigmentosa;* vestibular dysfunction; (b) electroretinogram for detection of the syndrome before the onset of visual and funduscopic abnormalities; (c) miscellaneous abnormalities: mental retardation; psychosis; abnormal nasal cilia and sperm axonemes; bronchiectasis associated with chronic sinusitis and immotile nasal cilia in two brothers; a case with multiple sclerosis–like illness (magnetic resonance imaging: vermian atrophy and multiple white-matter lesions in the periventricular areas); (d) autosomal recessive inheritance; 100% penetrance; wide variability of expression; genetic heterogeneity; linkage to chromosomal region 11q13.5 in type I.

V

VATER ASSOCIATION (VACTEL; VACTERL; VACTER)

Definition: Association of some or all of the following anomalies:
V: *V*ertebral anomalies; *V*ascular anomalies.
A: *A*nal anomalies; *A*uricular defects.
C: *C*ardiovascular anomalies.
T: *T*racheoesophageal fistula.
E: *E*sophageal atresia.
R: *R*enal anomalies; *R*adial defects; *R*ib anomalies.
L: *L*imb anomalies.

Clinical and Radiologic Manifestations: High clinical variability: (a) vertebral anomalies: aplasia; dysplasia; hypoplasia; scoliosis; (b) vascular anomalies (cardiovascular anomalies): ventricular septal defect; patent ductus arteriosus; tetralogy of Fallot; single ventricle; transposition of the great arteries; (c) anorectal malformations: anal atresia most common; (d) tracheoesophageal fistula; (e) renal anomalies: aplasia; dysplasia; cysts; hydronephrosis; ectopia; persistent urachus; vesicoureteral reflux; uretero-pelvic junction obstruction; bilateral ureteral triplication with crossed ectopic fused kidneys; (f) radial dysplasia; hypoplasia of the thumb; triphalangeal thumb; radial polydactyly; radial aplasia; (g) other skeletal abnormalities: rib anomalies; sternal anomalies; Sprengel deformity; hypoplasia of the humerus; radioulnar synostosis; midline anomalies of the hand; absence of the pubis, femur, tibia, fibula, and two rays of the foot; clinodactyly; syndactyly; hypoplastic middle phalanx of the fifth digit; malposition of the digits; Klippel-Feil syndrome; vertebral hypersegmen-tation; cervical kyphosis.

VELO-CARDIO-FACIAL SYNDROME (SHPRINTZEN SYNDROME)

Clinical Manifestations: Considerable phenotypic variability: (a) *facial dysmorphism:* prominent nose with a broad, often squared root, narrow alar base; malar flatness; vertical maxillary excess; retrusion of the chin; mal-occlusion; narrow palpebral fissures; occasionally malformed auricles; (b) *cleft palate or occult submucous cleft;* (c) *cardiovascular malformations;* (d) *learning disability;* mental retardation; psychiatric disorders; (e) eye abnor-malities: tortuous retinal vessels; small optic discs; embryotoxon; cataracts; coloboma; unilateral microphthalmos; (f) autosomal dominant inheritance; intrafamilial variability; microdeletion at 22q11.2.

Radiologic Manifestations: (a) *cardiovascular malformations:* ven-tricular septal defect with or without a right-sided aortic arch; tetralogy of Fallot; hypoplastic pulmonary arteries; enlargement, medial displacement, and tortuosity of the internal carotid arteries; low carotid artery bifurca-tion; hypoplastic vertebral arteries; etc.; (b) miscellaneous abnormalities: platybasia; small posterior fossa; cysts adjacent to the frontal horns; cere-bellar atrophy; focal signal hyperintensities in the white matter on long TR images; small vermis.

Note: Some patients with this syndrome have manifestations of the DiGeorge sequence (hypocalcemia; hypoplastic or absent lymphoid tissue and T-cell deficiency; etc.); monosomy for the region of 22q11 has been reported in both conditions.

VOHWINKEL SYNDROME (KERATODERMA HEREDITARIA MUTILANS; MUTILATING KERATODERMA)

Clinical and Radiologic Manifestations: Onset usually in infancy: (a) *diffuse honeycombed hyperkeratosis of the palmar and plantar surfaces;*

star-shaped keratosis located on the dorsa of the digits; linear keratosis on the elbows and knees; ainhum-like constriction of the digits; autoamputation; (b) usually autosomal dominant inheritance; autosomal recessive inheritance and sporadic also reported.

VON HIPPEL–LINDAU SYNDROME (HIPPEL-LINDAU SYNDROME)

Clinical Manifestations: Onset of symptoms often in the third to fifth decades of life: (a) *ocular lesions:* hemorrhage; retinal detachment; glaucoma; uveitis; (b) *neurologic manifestations* related to cerebral, cerebellar, and spinal cord lesions; (c) polycythemia; hypertension; (d) autosomal dominant transmission with variable penetrance and delayed expression.

Pathology: (a) *retina: hemangioblastoma;* (b) *central nervous system: hemangioblastoma;* syringomyelia; meningioma; arteriovenous malformation of the cervical spinal cord; (c) kidney tumors (hemangioblastoma; hypernephroma; adenoma; cyst); bladder hemangioblastoma; epididymis tumors (cyst; clear-cell papillary cystadenoma of epididymis presenting as infertility; hypernephroid tumor); germ cell tumor of testis; testicular cyst; papillary cystadenoma of the broad ligament; (d) pancreatic tumors (hemangioblastoma; cyst; cystadenoma; islet cell adenoma, islet cell carcinoma); (e) liver tumors (angioma; cyst; adenoma); (f) splenic angioma; (g) adrenal gland tumors (pheochromocytoma; cyst); (h) lung cyst; (i) bone lesions (cyst; hemangioma); (j) skin and mucosa lesions (nevus; café au lait spots); (k) miscellaneous abnormalities: deafness due to endolymphatic sac tumor; omental cyst; mesenteric cyst; paraganglioma; posterior fossa epidermoid; carcinoid tumor of the common bile duct.

Radiologic Manifestations: *Masses* at various sites demonstrable by different imaging techniques: ultrasonography, computed tomography, magnetic resonance imaging (contrast enhanced), and angiography; calcification (orbit; brain).

Note: Pancreatic lesions (cysts; islet cell tumors; microcystic adenomas) may be the only abdominal manifestations (rarely causing bile duct obstruction), and may precede any other manifestation of the disease by several years (obstructive jaundice reported in siblings).

W

WAARDENBURG ANOPHTHALMIA SYNDROME

Clinical and Radiologic Manifestations: (a) *anophthalmia* (unilateral; bilateral); small orbit(s); (b) *distal limb anomalies:* syndactyly of the fingers; fused metacarpals; camptodactyly; syndactyly of the toes;

oligodactyly of the toes; clubfoot; (c) mental retardation; (d) consistent with autosomal recessive inheritance; parental consanguinity.

WAARDENBURG SYNDROME

Clinical Manifestations: (a) *pigmentary disturbance of the irides;* (b) *congenital partial or total sensorineural deafness;* (c) *pigmentary disturbance of the hair;* (d) *dystopia canthorum* (present in type I; absent in type II); broad, high nasal root; hypertelorism; hyperplasia of the medial segment of the eyebrows; confluent eyebrows; leukoderma; (e) autosomal dominant inheritance; variable expressivity; types I and III correlated with mutations in the human PAX3 gene on chromosome 2q37.

Radiologic Manifestations: (a) absence of oval window; thickened wall of the labyrinth; dysplasia of the semicircular canal; aplasia of posterior semicircular canal; (b) smaller than normal head circumference, clivus length and facial depth; narrow nose; nasal bone hypoplasia; short and retropositioned maxilla; (c) miscellaneous abnormalities: Sprengel deformity; rib anomalies; vertebral anomalies; syndactyly; gastric stasis.

Note: (a) Klein-Waardenburg syndrome ("Waardenburg syndrome type III"): features of Waardenburg syndrome type I phenotype plus musculoskeletal abnormalities; (b) Waardenburg-Shah syndrome: familial white forelock and white eyebrows and eyelashes, isochromia iridis, and long-segment Hirschsprung disease; parental consanguinity in some families; (c) in the type I, penetrance for dystopia canthorum is 99% and represents a homogeneous group; the type II is a heterogeneous group.

WALKER-WARBURG SYNDROME (HARD ±E Syndrome)

Clinical Manifestations: (a) *retinal dysplasia;* microphthalmia; glaucoma; iris hypoplasia; corneal opacity; cataracts; optic nerve hypoplasia; membranelike structure of the lens; (b) *congenital muscular dystrophy;* (c) autosomal recessive inheritance.

Radiologic Manifestations: (a) *type II lissencephaly or variant* (agyria; macrogyria; polymicrogyria; obstructive hydrocephalus; *vermis hypoplasia*); (b) antenatal sonography: ventriculomegaly; occipital encephalocele; cleft between cerebellar hemispheres; nonvisualization of the vermis; ocular abnormalities, including retinal nonattachment; (c) miscellaneous abnormalities: posterior encephalocele; Dandy-Walker anomaly; microcephaly; hypoplasia of corpus callosum and/or septum pellucidum.

Note: The acronym *HARD (E):* *H*ydrocephalus, *A*gyria, *R*etinal *D*ysplasia, *E*ncephalocele.

WALLENBERG SYNDROME (Lateral Medullary Syndrome)

Etiology: Occlusion of the vertebral artery or its branches (arteriopathy; chiropractic neck manipulation; self-induced manipulation; vertebral artery dissection; etc.); demyelinating diseases presenting as Wallenberg syndrome; rhombencephalitis with meningitis; being struck by lightening (embolism in the right lateral portion of the medulla).

Clinical Manifestations: Vertigo; nausea; vomiting; dysarthria; dysphagia; numbness either of the ipsilateral face or of the contralateral body, diplopia, blurred vision; nystagmus; facial weakness; loss of pain and temperature sensation on the contralateral face or ipsilateral face; *ipsilateral Horner syndrome; ipsilateral ataxia; contralateral hypalgesia.*

Radiologic Manifestations: (a) magnetic resonance imaging: *lateral medullary infarction;* (b) arteriography: vascular occlusion; angiographic findings of dissection.

WARFARIN EMBRYOPATHY

Clinical Manifestations: Maternal ingestion of vitamin K antagonist anticoagulant in the first trimester of pregnancy: (a) *craniofacial dysmorphism* (frontal bossing; underdeveloped nasal cartilages; small and up-turned nose; choanal stenosis; hypertelorism; poorly developed hypoplastic ears; large tongue); *low birth weight; short neck; short limbs; brachydactyly;* (b) miscellaneous abnormalities: blindness; optic atrophy; cataract; microphthalmos; prominent eyes; small eyelids; hypoplastic nails; respiratory difficulties; mental retardation.

Radiologic Manifestations: (a) *stippled calcification* (tubular bones; vertebrae; calcanei; ribs; pelvis; nose); tracheal cartilage calcification; (b) *short and broad hands; short distal phalanges; short long bones;* (c) *skull anomalies:* prominent occiput; extra fontanelles; frontal bossing; (d) miscellaneous abnormalities: radiodense skeleton; hydrocephalus; absent corpus callosum; intraventricular hemorrhage.

WATERHOUSE-FRIDERICHSEN SYNDROME

Clinical and Radiologic Manifestations: (a) fulminant bacterial sepsis, in particular, meningococcal septicemia; (b) disseminated intravascular coagulation; (c) shock; (d) anemia; leucocytosis; metabolic acidosis; (e) ultrasonography: bilateral adrenal hemorrhage; (f) reported as complication of colchicine overdose, posttraumatic asplenia, and primary biliary sepsis.

WEAVER SYNDROME (WEAVER-SMITH SYNDROME)

Clinical Manifestations: (a) *craniofacial dysmorphism:* round face in infancy; broad forehead; flat occiput; large ears; ocular hypertelorism; prominent or long philtrum; relative micrognathia; (b) *prenatal and postnatal growth excess;* (c) *a hoarse, low-pitched voice;* (d) limb abnormalities: large hands; prominent finger pads; camptodactyly; syndactyly; clinodactyly; broad thumbs; prominent toe pads; thin and deep-set nails; limited elbow or knee extension; foot deformities; (e) miscellaneous abnormalities: seizures; hypertonia; hypotonia; developmental delay (f) sporadic; reported in sibling; reported in twins and their mildly affected mother.

Radiologic Manifestations: (a) *dysharmonic accelerated skeletal maturation;* (b) skeletal abnormalities: small iliac wings; coxa valga; wide femoral necks; flared metaphyses, especially the distal femora and ulnae; mottled or irregular epiphyses; scoliosis; kyphosis; instability of the upper cervical spine associated with spinal cord impingement; short ribs; unilateral distally dislocated ulna; (c) miscellaneous abnormalities: dilatation of lateral ventricles; absent septum pellucidum.

WEBER-CHRISTIAN SYNDROME

Clinical Manifestations: Nonsuppurative nodular panniculitis: (a) *tenderness and skin redness followed by skin pigmentation and finally atrophy;* nodules; fever; arthritis/arthralgias; myalgia; (b) recurrent pneumonia; cardiac dilatation; congestive heart failure; abdominal symptoms related to mesenteric panniculitis; pancreatitis; hepatosplenomegaly; chronic active hepatitis; liver cirrhosis; acalculous cholecystitis; splenic vein occlusion; sterile splenic abscesses; nephrotic syndrome; (c) breast involvement; (d) miscellaneous abnormalities: elevated erythrocyte sedimentation rate; anemia; leukopenia; hypocomplementemia.

Radiologic Manifestations: (a) *calcifications of nodules; mammary calcifications;* (b) myocardosis with myocardial decompensation; coronary occlusion resulting from pericardial fibrosis; (c) pancreatitis; bone lesion related to pancreatitis (demineralization; destructive lesions in the hands and feet in association with periosteal reaction; pathologic fracture); (d) miscellaneous abnormalities: granulomatous pneumonitis; ileus caused by inflammatory changes of the bowel wall or mesentery; retroperitoneal fibrosis; sterile splenic abscess; xanthogranuloma of the dura and leptomeninges; sclerosing panniculitis of the mesentery; acinar cell carcinoma of the pancreas.

WEILL-MARCHESANI SYNDROME (SPHEROPHAKIA-BRACHYMORPHIA SYNDROME)

Clinical Manifestations: (a) *short stature with disproportionate shortening of the limbs, in particular, hands and feet;* (b) *stiff joints;* (c) *spherophakia (hyaloid degeneration of the lens fibers); microphakia; myopia;* ectopia lentis; glaucoma; (d) miscellaneous abnormalities: craniofacial dysmorphism (pug nose; depressed nasal bridge; broad head; mild maxillary hypoplasia; narrow palate); cardiovascular defects; (e) consistent with autosomal recessive inheritance.

Radiologic Manifestations: (a) *brachycephaly* or *scaphocephalic skull;* shallow orbits; hypotelorism; small maxillae and zygomatic arches; (b) *short metacarpals, metatarsals, and phalanges;* (c) skeletal maturation retardation; (d) miscellaneous abnormalities: short and wide diaphyses; thin cortices; mild epiphyseal deformities; slight anterior rounded appearance of the vertebrae; narrow spinal canal; thinness of disc spaces; widened ribs; thickening of the skull vault.

WEISMANN-NETTER SYNDROME

Clinical Manifestations: (a) *dwarfism; "saber shin" deformity of the legs,* usually bilateral, occasionally unilateral; (b) sporadic; familial cases (involvement over three generations through the female line); autosomal or X-linked dominant inheritance a good possibility.

Radiologic Manifestations: (a) *anterior bowing of the tibia and fibula with thickening of the posterior cortices* and distortion of the bony trabeculae in the midshafts; (b) miscellaneous abnormalities: bowing of long bones (radius; ulna; femur); thickening of the cortex of tubular bones; small pelvis with squaring of the iliac wings; kyphoscoliosis; dural calcification; exaggerated trabeculation of the carpals and epiphyses of the metacarpals and phalanges; thinness of the posterior aspect of the ribs and exaggerated downward angulation.

WERNER SYNDROME

Clinical Manifestations: (a) *premature aging* with an onset after adolescence; *juvenile cataracts; scleromatous skin changes; ischemic skin ulcerations; high-pitched voice; short stature* with a relatively large trunk and spindly extremities; *impotence and sterility; atherosclerosis; organic brain syndrome;* spastic paraparesis; peripheral neuropathy; coexistence of malignant tumors (in 10%); adult-type diabetes mellitus; somatic chromosomal aberrations in multiple tissues in vivo and in vitro; (b) autosomal recessive inheritance.

Radiologic Manifestations: (a) soft-tissue atrophy; soft-tissue calcification; (b) *osteoporosis localized to the extremities or generalized osteoporosis; osteosclerosis (endosteal thickening) of the phalanges;* (c) *atherosclerosis with calcification;* coronary artery disease; aortic stenosis; congestive heart failure; cardiomyopathy; valvular calcification; (d) osteoarthritis of the peripheral joints; spondylosis deformans; neurotrophic bone changes; (e) ventricular dilatation; brain atrophy; diffuse hypoperfusion shown by single photon emission computed tomography.

WERNICKE-KORSAKOFF SYNDROME

Clinical Manifestations
(A) WERNICKE DISEASE: The triad of *mental symptoms* (confusion, inattentiveness, and lethargy), *abnormal eye movements* (nystagmus, abducens and conjugate gaze palsies), and *truncal ataxia.*

(B) KORSAKOFF SYNDROME (KORSAKOFF PSYCHOSIS): *Abnormality of mentation, with learning and memory affected out of proportion with other cognitive functions.*

(C) WERNICKE-KORSAKOFF SYNDROME: *Survival after the acute illness (Wernicke disease) associated with the clinical manifestations of Korsakoff syndrome.*

Radiologic Manifestations: A characteristic topographic distribution of lesions (periventricular regions, the medial formations of the thalamus and mass intermedia, the floor of the third ventricle, the mamillary bodies, periaqueductal region at the level of the third cranial nerve nuclei, the reticular formation of the midbrain, and the posterior corpora quadrigemina): (a) computed tomography: symmetric, low-density lesions; (b) magnetic resonance imaging: (1) blood-brain-barrier disruption in acute Wernicke encephalopathy; hyperintense lesions during the acute phase of the disease, enhancement in the mamillary bodies and inferior quadrigeminal plate; (2) atrophy and dilatation of the third ventricle and aqueduct in the advanced phase; (c) resolution or diminution of the lesions following thiamin therapy.

WEST SYNDROME

Clinical Manifestations: An epileptic encephalopathy with onset in infancy or early childhood: (a) *brief and repetitive myoclonic seizures; interictal hypsarrhythmia;* (b) miscellaneous abnormalities: microcephaly, floppiness; spasticity; deafness; optic atrophy; mental retardation.

Radiologic Manifestations: (a) positron emission tomography: diffuse or focal transient hypometabolism (changing with clinical symptoms); (b) computed tomography and magnetic resonance imaging: brain atrophy; intracranial calcification; corpus callosum dysgenesis; cortical dysplasia; porencephaly; poor gray-white matter demarcation; delayed myelination; atypical gray matter heterotopia; (c) ACTH-induced adrenal enlargement in treated infants.

WEYERS ACRODENTAL DYSOSTOSIS (ACROFACIAL DYSOSTOSIS)

Clinical and Radiologic Manifestations: (a) *postaxial polydactyly of the hands and feet;* (b) *dental anomalies* (shape, number, and implantation of the upper and lower incisors); mandibular cleft; (c) miscellaneous abnormalities: radial clinodactyly and hypoplasia of the nails of the fifth fingers; partial syndactyly of the second and third toes; (d) autosomal dominant inheritance.

WEYERS OLIGODACTYLY SYNDROME

Clinical and Radiologic Manifestations: (a) *deficiency of the ulnar and fibular rays;* (b) miscellaneous abnormalities: antecubital pterygia; reduced sternal segments; renal anomalies; cleft lip/palate; hypoplasia of the maxilla; dental deformities.

WIEDEMANN-RAUTENSTRAUCH SYNDROME

Clinical Manifestations: (a) *intrauterine growth retardation; small for age; mental and motor retardation;* (b) *craniofacial dysmorphism:* progeroid face; apparent macrocephaly with frontal and biparietal bossing; widely open sutures; persistently open fontanelle; prominent scalp veins; sparse scalp hair; low-set ears; hypoplasia of the facial bones; beak-shaped nose; natal teeth; (c) *large hands and feet with long fingers and toes;* (d) *generalized paucity of subcutaneous fat; prominence of muscles and veins; paradoxical fat accumulation during infancy (buttocks; flanks; anogenital area);* (e) hypothyroidism; (f) autosomal recessive inheritance.

Radiologic Manifestations: (a) *large anterior fontanelle; wide cranial sutures; small viscerocranium; large neurocranium;* dilatation of cerebral lateral ventricles; cerebral atrophy; deficiency of mature myelin (a case report); (b) miscellaneous abnormalities: small, dense, and unerupted teeth; partially unossified atlas at birth; hypoplasia of the vertebral bodies; thin ribs; trident configuration of the acetabula; shortness of humeri and femora; irregular metaphyseal borders.

WILDERVANCK SYNDROME (CERVICO-OCULO-ACOUSTIC SYNDROME)

Clinical Manifestations: (a) *congenital perceptive deafness;* (b) *retraction of the bulb* in one or both eyes; *Duane retraction syndrome* (deficient abduction with retraction on adduction); *abducens paralysis;* (c) presentation with hemiparesthesia; (d) female-male ratio is 10:1.

Radiologic Manifestations: (a) *fused cervical vertebrae;* fused upper thoracic vertebrae; occipitocervical fusion; occipital vertebrae; spina bifida occulta; (b) constricted internal auditory meatus; underdevelopment of the bony labyrinth (cochlea and vestibular apparatus); often an absence of semicircular canals; Mondini deformity; stapes anomaly; inner-ear aplasia.

Note: The diagnostic triad: *Klippel-Feil anomaly, abducens nerve palsy, and congenital deafness.*

WILLIAMS SYNDROME (WILLIAMS-BEUREN SYNDROME)

Clinical Manifestations: (a) *craniofacial dysmorphism:* head circumference below normal; broad forehead; medial eyebrow flare; depressed nasal bridge; anteverted and small nose; full and heavy cheeks; long philtrum; pointed chin; widely opened mouth; pouting lips; prominent ears; periorbital fullness; (b) eye abnormalities: ocular hypotelorism; strabismus; blue eyes with a stellate pattern of the iris; cataracts; whitish anomalies in brown irides; vascular tortuosity of retina; ptosis; Marcus-Gunn phenomenon; (c) oral abnormalities: tongue thrusting; late dental eruption; microdontia; small roots; invagination of the incisors; malocclusion; anterior crossbite; deep or open bite; excessive interdental spacing; pathologic folding of the buccal mucosa; (d) *growth/developmental abnormalities:* short stature; mild to moderate mental retardation; overly affectionate, trusting, and outgoing personality; gross and fine motor deficiencies; delayed language development; talkative; good articulation skills; hypersensitive to sound; deep voice; moderate to severe degree of mental handicap in adults; (e) cardiovascular abnormalities: systemic hypertension secondary to peripheral vascular anomalies; myocardial infarction; progression of cardiovascular disease (hypertension, aortic stenosis, and pulmonary artery stenosis); (f) musculoskeletal manifestations: hypotonia in infancy; walking delay; joint contractures; scoliosis; increased exhaustion on exertion; lipid storage in muscles and increased variability of fiber size; (g) genitourinary abnormalities: voiding dysfunction (urinary frequency; daytime wetting; uninhibited detrusor contractions); small penis; renal insufficiency; cystadenoma of ovary; (h) *normocalcemia or hypercalcemia;* (i) sporadic in the majority of the cases; autosomal dominant inheritance in some; autosomal dominant transmission of isolated supravalvular stenosis is certain.

Radiologic Manifestations: (a) cardiovascular abnormalities: *supravalvular aortic stenosis;* shortening of the aortic segment between the coronary artery origins and the origin of the first brachiocephalic vessel; coarctation of the aorta; interrupted aortic arch; hypoplasia of the entire thoracic aorta; deformed aortic valve; stenosis of systemic arterial branches; renovascular hypertension; mitral valvular abnormalities; mitral regurgitation; ventricular septal defect; arterial septal defect; high bifurcation of the aorta; peripheral pulmonary stenosis; pulmonary valvular stenosis; tetralogy of Fallot; subaortic stenosis; aortic aneurysm; pulmonary artery sling; (b) dental abnormalities: enamel hypoplasia; small pulp chambers; bud-shaped molars; hypodontia; microdontia; osteosclerotic changes in the lamina dura; (c) skeletal system abnormalities: wide maxillary arch; widened mandibular angle; osteosclerosis; radioulnar synostosis; metacarpophalangeal pattern profile: small hands, and disproportionately large distal phalanx of the thumb; fifth-finger clinodactyly; camptodactyly, talipes equinovarus; kyphoscoliosis; pectus excavatum; (d) urinary system abnormalities: renal abnormalities; bladder diverticula; (e) nervous system abnormalities: reduced cerebral size; normal cerebellar size; enlargement of neocerebellar vermis, with low normal size in the paleocerebellar vermal lobules; large cerebellar tonsils; (f) miscellaneous abnormalities: craniostenosis; ectopic calcification associated with hypercalcemia.

WILLIAMS-CAMPBELL SYNDROME

Clinical Manifestations: Onset of symptoms often in the first year of life: *persistent cough; wheezy breathing;* gross increase in residual lung volume; severe impairment of maximum expiratory flow rates.

Radiologic Manifestations: Pulmonary hyperinflation; *bronchiectasis; ballooning of the bronchi during inspiration and collapse with expiration;* computed tomography: *areas of emphysematous lung parenchyma distal to dilated bronchi.*

WILSON-MIKITY SYNDROME

Clinical Manifestations: Usually occurs in premature or immature newborn infants; onset usually after a latent asymptomatic period of several days to weeks after birth: *tachypnea, retraction, cough, and transient cyanotic episodes;* fine rales; transient edema; hepatomegaly; long-term pulmonary sequelae.

Radiologic Manifestations: (a) early stage: *coarse streaky infiltrates and small "cystic" areas throughout the lung;* (b) later stage: *enlargement and coalescence of cystic foci ("bubbly lung"), in particular in the lower lobes, with overexpanded lower lobes and strandy densities in the upper lobes.*

WISKOTT-ALDRICH SYNDROME (ALDRICH SYNDROME)

Clinical Manifestations: An immunodeficiency disease with an onset in infancy or early childhood: (a) *eczema;* (b) *bloody diarrhea;* (c) *recur-*

rent infections: otitis media; sinusitis; pneumonia; viral infection; (d) purpura; congenital *thrombocytopenia;* decreased platelet survival; abnormal platelet function; increase in platelet counts following splenectomy; platelet counts and platelet size studies in midtrimester used in prenatal evaluation of the fetus at risk; (e) cellular and humoral immune deficiency; autoimmune hemolytic anemia; (f) *high tendency to the development of malignancy;* (g) nephropathy; (h) X-linked recessive inheritance.

Radiologic Manifestations: *Recurrent pneumonia, sinusitis, and mastoiditis;* absence of soft-tissue swelling in the region of the adenoids; hemorrhage (subperiosteal; soft tissues).

Note: The classic clinical triad consisting of *eczema, recurrent infections, and hemorrhage due to thrombocytopenia* is not always complete, and the clinical presentation may be atypical.

WOLFF-PARKINSON-WHITE SYNDROME

Clinical and Radiologic Manifestations: (a) *abnormal electrocardiographic pattern: short PR interval; widened QRS complex; initial delta wave;* (b) association with cardiac and noncardiac diseases (Ebstein anomaly of the tricuspid valve; idiopathic hypertrophic subaortic stenosis; congenitally corrected transposition of the great arteries; congenital hydrops; episodic appearance of supraventricular tachycardia; giant right atrial diverticulum); (c) abnormal echographic pattern of left ventricular posterior wall and interventricular septum motions; (d) three-dimensional localization of arrhythmogenic foci by radionuclide ventriculography (single photon emission computed tomography); (e) near miss sudden death in infancy.

WOLFRAM SYNDROME (DIDMOAD Syndrome)

Clinical Manifestations: Onset in childhood, highly variable clinical picture: (a) *diabetes insipidus;* (b) *diabetes mellitus;* (c) *optic atrophy;* (d) *sensorineural deafness;* (e) *neuropsychiatric manifestations:* ataxia; vertigo; tremor; dysphagia; dysarthria; hyporeflexia; seizures; hyposmia; strokelike episodes; psychiatric disorders; mental retardation; hyperreflexive neurogenic bladder with sphincteric dyssynergia; (f) eye abnormalities: ptosis; nystagmus; tonic pupils; pigmentary retinopathy; (g) endocrine disorders; (h) autosomal recessive inheritance; a gene linked to markers on 4p16.

Radiologic Manifestations: (a) *neurogenic bladder; bladder dilatation; hydronephrosis; hydroureter;* (b) magnetic resonance imaging: diffuse neurodegenerative process; brain atrophy.

Note: DIDMOAD syndrome: *D*iabetes *I*nsipidus, *D*iabetes *M*ellitus, *O*ptic *A*trophy, and *D*eafness.

WRINKLY SKIN SYNDROME

Clinical and Radiologic Manifestations: (a) *wrinkly skin of the dorsum of the hands and feet; increased palmar and plantar creases;* prominent vein pattern; skin hypoelasticity; dry skin; *wrinkled skin over the abdomen* (sitting position); (b) small for gestational age; failure to thrive; developmental delay; hypotonia; (c) microcephaly; brachycephaly; midface hypoplasia; (d) miscellaneous abnormalities: decreased muscle mass; winged scapulae; congenital hip "dysplasia"; joint hyperextensibility; mental retardation; facial asymmetry; kyphosis; lordosis; scoliosis; myopia; chorioretinitis; atrial septal aneurysm; (e) autosomal recessive inheritance most likely.

Y

YELLOW NAIL SYNDROME

Clinical Manifestations: Onset of symptoms in adult life; onset in childhood rare: (a) *thickened, smooth, and discolored (yellow or green) nails with transverse ridging and excessive curvature;* onycholysis; (b) *primary lymphedema;* (c) miscellaneous abnormalities: chronic cough; rhinitis and sinusitis (frequent association); association with the following: immunologic disorders; thyroid disorders; rheumatoid arthritis; tuberculosis; keratosis obturans; familial primary hypoplasia of lymphatics; malignancy.

Radiologic Manifestations: Recurrent pleural effusion, pericardial effusion, chylothorax; *bronchiectasis;* sinusitis; *hypoplasia of the lymphatic system;* lymphoscintigraphy: significantly reduced lymphatic drainage in the arms and legs.

Note: The typical components of the triad of *yellow discoloration of the nails, lymphedema, and chronic respiratory tract disease* may not be present, or they may appear at different intervals (months to years).

YOUNG SYNDROME (SINUSITIS-INFERTILITY SYNDROME; BARRY-PERKINS-YOUNG SYNDROME)

Clinical and Radiologic Manifestations: (a) *azoospermia* owing to bilateral epididymal obstruction; (b) *chronic and recurrent upper and lower respiratory infections* (sinusitis; bronchitis; etc.); bronchiectasis; (c) possibly autosomal recessive inheritance.

YOUSSEF SYNDROME

Clinical and Radiologic Manifestations: Vesicouterine fistula through the uterine isthmus; usually as a result of lower-segment cesarean section: *cyclic hematuria; absence of vaginal bleeding; urinary continence; demonstration of uterocystic communication by cystography or hysterosalpingography.*

Z

ZIMMERMANN-LABAND SYNDROME (GINGIVAL FIBROMATOSIS– ABNORMAL FINGERS)

Clinical and Radiologic Manifestations: (a) *gingival hypertrophy or fibromatosis;* (b) *bulbous soft nose; thick floppy ears;* (c) *nail hypoplasia/dysplasia; hypertrichosis*; (d) *clubbed "tree frog–like" fingers and toes; absence or hypoplasia of the terminal phalanges of the hands and feet*; (e) miscellaneous abnormalities: hepatosplenomegaly; epileptic seizures; skeletal abnormalities (hyperextensibility of the joints; contractures; asymmetry of the limbs; kyphosis; scoliosis; lumbar spondylodysplasia, osseous mandibular hypertrophy); (f) autosomal dominant inheritance.

2

Metabolic Disorders

A

ABETALIPOPROTEINEMIA (Bassen-Kornzweig syndrome)

Clinical Manifestations: (a) *degenerative nervous system disease* involving the cerebellum, long tracts, and peripheral nerves with Friedreich-like ataxia; *acanthocytosis (thorny red cells); atypical retinitis pigmentosa;* angioid streaks; *steatorrhea; malabsorption appearing in infancy; total plasma cholesterol level lower than 1.5 mmol/L (60 mg/dL); low levels of triglyceride with little increase after ingestion of fat; absent or greatly reduced β-lipoprotein demonstrable by immunoelectrophoresis;* etc.; (b) autosomal recessive inheritance; mutations of the microsomal triglyceride-transfer-protein gene; gene localized to chromosome 4q22–24.

Radiologic Manifestations: *Thickening of small-intestinal folds* (most marked in the duodenum and jejunum); thickening of the colonic haustra and abnormally prominent mucosal folds; *cardiac failure* in advanced cases (interstitial myocardial fibrosis); urolithiasis.

ACRODERMATITIS ENTEROPATHICA

Clinical Manifestations: An inborn error of metabolism resulting in *zinc malabsorption and deficiency:* (a) *acral and orificial vesicobullous, pustular, and eczematoid skin lesions;* recurrent infections of the skin and mucous membrane with *Candida albicans,* bacteria, or both; esophagitis; *hair loss; paronychia; ocular lesions* (blepharitis; conjunctivitis; corneal opacities; linear epithelial erosions); *diarrhea;* failure to thrive; emotional disturbances; *low serum zinc and alkaline phosphatase levels* (zinc-dependent enzyme); dramatic clinical response to zinc therapy; impaired enteral absorption of linoleic acid; low urinary zinc levels; etc.; (b) autosomal recessive inheritance; the mutation affects the zinc transport in human intestinal biopsies; the mutation affects zinc metabolism in human fibroblasts.

Pathology: (a) small-bowel biopsy: loss of villous architecture; flattening of villi; cuboid intestinal epithelial cells with enlarged nuclei and open chromatin distribution; (b) autopsy: pancreatic islet hyperplasia; absence of the thymus and germinal centers; plasmacytosis of the lymph nodes and spleen.

Radiologic Manifestations: Roentgenologic findings of *malabsorption syndrome; cerebral atrophy, reversible with zinc therapy; abnormal zinc absorption tests using scintigraphy.*

Note: The classic triad of *dermatitis, alopecia, and intractable diarrhea* is present in only 20% of cases; abnormal small-bowel biopsy showing the characteristic Paneth cell abnormalities may be present without diarrhea or failure to thrive.

ACROMEGALY AND GIGANTISM

Clinical Manifestations: (a) refer to Table ME-A-1; (b) sporadic; familial occurrence extremely rare: both autosomal recessive and autosomal dominant have been suggested.

Table ME-A-1   Acromegaly: Clinical and Metabolic Features

Local	
Visual field defects; cranial nerve palsy; headache	
Abdominal or chest mass	
Somatic	
Acral enlargement	Increased heel pad thickness, prognathism, hypertrophy of the frontal bones, malocclusion, macroglossia
Musculoskeletal	Arthralgias, hypertrophic arthropathy, carpal tunnel syndrome, acroparesthesias, proximal myopathy
Skin	Hyperhidrosis, skin tags, acanthosis nigricans
Colon	Polyposis, carcinoma
Cardiovascular	Left ventricular hypertrophy, asymmetrical septal hypertrophy, hypertension, congestive heart failure, arrhythmias, myocardial infarction
Sleep disturbances	Sleep apnea, narcolepsy
Visceromegaly	Salivary glands, liver, spleen, kidney
Metabolic and Endocrine	
Carbohydrate	Insulin resistance and hyperinsulinemia, impaired glucose tolerance, diabetes mellitus
Lipids	Hypertriglyceridemia
Mineral	Hypercalciuria, increased 1,25-dihydroxyvitamin D_3, increased urinary hydroxyproline
Electrolyte	Low renin, increased aldosterone
Gonadal	Menstrual abnormalities, galactorrhea, decreased libido, impotence, low testosterone-binding globulin
Thyroid	Thyromegaly, hyperthyroidism, low thyroid-binding globulin
Multiple endocrine neoplasia (I)	Hyperparathyroidism, pancreatic islet cell tumors

From Melamed S, Fagin JA: Acromegaly update: etiology, diagnosis and management, *West J Med* 146:328, 1987. Used by permission.

Radiologic Manifestations

(A) GIGANTISM: (a) tumor: sellar contour abnormality; bone erosion; low density and isodensity of the pituitary tumor on computed tomographic examination; focal areas of hypointensity on T_1-weighted images on magnetic resonance imaging; extrasellar extension; (b) *accelerated skeletal growth;* normal or retarded bone age; *delay in closure of the growth plate,* which may remain open into adult life; (c) increase in width of the tubular bones; (d) osteopenia (probably due to hypercalciuria).

(B) ACROMEGALY: (a) craniofacial findings: *enlarged sella turcica and bone erosion; enlargement of the paranasal sinuses and mastoid cells; hyperostosis of the calvaria in the frontal and occipital regions; elongation and widening of the mandible; widening of the mandibular angle;* (b) spine: *widening of the atlantoaxial joint; enlargement of vertebrae; scalloping of the posterior border of vertebral bodies; increase in the kyphotic curve of the thoracic spine; osteoporosis; osteophyte formation; spinal canal stenosis;* acute quadriplegia due to segmental compression of the spinal cord by intervertebral cervical disc protrusions; (c) ribs: *elongation and thickening; enlargement of costochondral junctions (the acromegalic rosary); sclerotic costal margins; wavy lower costal borders; calcification and ossification of the costal cartilages;* (d) limbs: *widening of joint spaces due to cartilage hypertrophy; thickening of the cortex of shaft of tubular bones, particularly in the hands and feet; spadelike appearance of the distal phalanges of the hands and feet; increase in number and size of the sesamoids of the hands and feet; metatarsal pencilling;* thickening of soft tissue (positive heel pad sign); (e) dual energy X-ray absorptiometry: increased bone mineral density in the lumbar spine and the proximal femur; (f) skeletal scintigraphy: enhanced activity in the costochondral junctions, calvarium, and appendicular skeleton; (g) miscellaneous abnormalities: (1) central nervous system: ectasia of cerebral arteries; enlarged cavernous portion of the internal carotid arteries with prolapse into the sella turcica ("kissing intrasellar arteries"); association with Chiari I malformation; (2) skeletal: association with polyostotic fibrous dysplasia; partial carpal fusion; Charcot joints; prominent phalangeal arteries; (3) respiratory: upper airway obstruction due to a significant increase in the thickness of the true and false cords; thickening of the bronchial wall; (4) calcification of the pinna; association with suprasellar and pulmonary hemangiopericytoma; (5) association with Zollinger-Ellison syndrome; (6) extraocular muscle enlargement; proptosis; noncongenital "hypertrophy" of upper extremities; (7) cardiomyopathy (left ventricular hypertrophy in particular); subclinical left ventricular dysfunction in some cases; (8) high prevalence of gallbladder stones; (9) multiple endocrine neoplasia type I associated with acromegaly (growth hormone–releasing hormone from pancreatic adenoma).

Complications: (a) high risk for development of various benign and malignant tumors (colon polyps; colon adenocarcinoma; gastric adenocarcinoma; breast adenocarcinoma; thyroid adenoma; thyroid papillary carcinoma; thymoma; parathyroid adenoma; uterine adenocarcinoma; cervical carcinoma; ovarian carcinoma; renal cell carcinoma; meningioma; neurinoma; osteosarcoma; multiple myeloma); the tumor screening programs for other high-risk patient groups have been recommended for patients with acromegaly; (b) significant intrathoracic airflow obstruction and nocturnal hypoxemia; (c) voice changes; (d) acute quadriplegia; (e) foot ulceration in association with severe peripheral neuropathy; (f) subclinical carpal tunnel syndrome.

ADDISON DISEASE (Adrenal Cortical Insufficiency)

Etiology: (a) primary: infarction associated with infection; hemorrhage; withdrawal from chronic glucocorticoid therapy; tuberculosis; fungal infections; sarcoidosis; hemochromatosis; amyloidosis; congenital and familial Addison disease; idiopathic; metastatic lesions (lung, kidney, colon, etc.); lymphoma; melanoma; acquired immunodeficiency syndrome; after bone marrow transplantation for Wiskott-Aldrich syndrome; etc.; (b) secondary (pituitary): Sheehan syndrome; neoplasms; tuberculosis; sarcoidosis; hemochromatosis; trauma; surgery; postirradiation; etc.; (c) autoimmune Addison disease: (1) association with chronic mucocutaneous candidiasis; acquired hypoparathyroidism; pernicious anemia; insulin-requiring diabetes mellitus; primary hypogonadism; immunoglobulin abnormalities; chronic active hepatitis; alopecia; vitiligo; spontaneous myxedema; Graves disease; chronic lymphocytic thyroiditis; (2) 21-hydroxylase, the major autoantigens involved in the pathogenesis of idiopathic Addison disease; (d) others: association with the following: X-linked adrenoleukodystrophy; osteoporosis; hyperthyroidism; myotonic dystrophy; achalasia and alacrimation (Addison-achalasia-alacrimation syndrome).

Clinical Manifestations: Chronic primary adrenal insufficiency (Addison disease): (a) *weakness and fatigability; weight loss;* (b) *digestive disorders* (anorexia; abdominal pain; vomiting; diarrhea or constipation); (c) *hyperpigmentation of the skin;* (d) pigmentation in the mucosa the mouth, vagina, and rectum; (e) salt craving; (f) anemia; (g) neuropsychiatric symptoms: irritability; confusion; delirium; (h) very low levels of plasma cortisol; hyponatremia; hyperkalemia; little or no increase in plasma cortisol in response to adrenocorticotropic hormone infusion; elevated percentage of circulating la-positive T cells; (i) the triad of *Addison-hypoparathyroidism-moniliasis;* association with different polyglandular autoimmune syndromes; (j) miscellaneous abnormalities: flexion contracture; sciatic-like pain; cardiac failure; adrenomyeloneuropathy presenting as Addison disease; precocious sexual development; association with bronchial asthma.

Radiologic Manifestations: (a) adrenal calcification (in about half of the patients with tuberculosis); (b) *microcardia;* (c) miscellaneous abnormalities: reduction in kidney size; splenomegaly; *calcification or ossification in the external ear;* increased incidence of gallbladder disease, dental caries, and perialveolar bone resorption; pituitary gland enlargement related to end-organ failure; reduced bone mineral density in females; (d) computed tomography: enlarged adrenal gland(s) in tuberculosis; inflammatory space-occupying lesions with central hypodensity and peripheral enhancement after contrast injection; partial or total calcified degeneration of the infected atrophied gland or enlarged gland showing irregular calcified degeneration and parenchymal caseation; small adrenal glands in disease of autoimmune origin, idiopathic, and in the pituitary form (the typical shape and density of the organ maintained); neoplasm; hemorrhage; necrosis.

ADRENAL HYPERPLASIA (CONGENITAL) (ADRENOGENITAL SYNDROME)

Clinical Manifestations: (a) the classic form recognized at birth or in early childhood: *virilization* (precocious pseudopuberty); *adrenal insufficiency;* (b) nonclassic adrenal hyperplasia (late onset): *hirsutism and/or menstrual irregularity;* (c) prenatal diagnosis of the salt-losing variant of 21-hydroxylase deficiency: amniotic fluid steroid analysis; early diagnosis by using chorionic villus sampling (detection of mutation in the steroid 21-hydroxylase gene); (d) genitourinary manifestations: low fertility rate in women with congenital adrenal hyperplasia; vaginal introitus inadequate for intercourse; male pseudohermaphroditism (a variant of congenital adrenal hyperplasia); bilateral testicular hypertrophy (11ß-hydroxylase deficiency); testicular tumors/nodules; testicular adrenal-like tissue; renal anomalies; (e) miscellaneous abnormalities: (1) acute adrenal crisis complicating congenital adrenal hyperplasia due to 11ß-hydroxylase deficiency; (2) physical appearance: male phenotype in genotypic females in the virilizing form of the disease; shield chest; (3) head and neck: hypertelorism; craniosynostosis; hydrocephalus; web neck; (4) unusual muscle strength in girls diagnosed later in childhood; (5) true precocious puberty in some cases: testicular enlargement in the boys; breast development in the girls; progressive pubic hair development; rapid growth; (6) others: hyperphosphatemic rickets; congenital hypothyroidism; learning disability; adrenal tumor; increased rate of left-handedness; short and curved fingers; syndactyly; association of nonclassic congenital adrenal hyperplasia with the polycystic ovarian syndrome; galactosialidosis presenting with congenital adrenal hyperplasia; reversible cardiomyopathy; (f) Autosomal recessive inheritance in 21-hydroxylase deficiency.

Radiologic Manifestations

(A) SIMPLE VIRILISM: (a) *advanced skeletal maturation;* (b) advanced pneumatization of the mastoids and paranasal sinuses; (c) premature calcification of the cartilage of the ribs and larynx; (d) *advanced tooth development;* (e) premature muscular development and osseous prominences; (f) premature development of skull diploe; (g) *genitography in females: different degrees of deviation from normal, including pseudohermaphroditism and true hermaphroditism;* (h) normal topography of the internal genitalia, small uterus, and normal or enlarged ovaries; urinoma of the fallopian tube related to a common urogenital sinus; hydrocolpos in virilizing congenital adrenal hyperplasia; (i) adrenal gland abnormalities: (1) infants with salt-losing form: mean length measurements of 20 mm or greater and mean width measurements of 4 mm or greater suggest the diagnosis of congenital adrenal hyperplasia (mean adrenal length is 14.4 mm and width is 1.9 mm in normal infants); "cerebriform pattern" of the adrenal glands on ultrasonographic examination; (2) untreated children: enlarged adrenal glands with preservation of normal configuration (enlargement predominantly cortical); (j) miscellaneous abnormalities: adrenal macronodules; adrenal adenoma and carcinoma; virilizing adrenocortical tumor superimposed on congenital adrenal hyperplasia; heterogeneous ultrasonographic pattern of testes in adolescents and young adults under long-standing treatment with glucocorticoids; testicular masses ("testicular tumors of adrenogenital syndrome") in pubertal and postpubertal patients (hypoechoic, unilateral or bilateral, multifocal).

(B) ADRENAL INSUFFICIENCY: Reduction in soft-tissue thickness due to dehydration; hyperlucent lungs; *microcardia;* paucity or absence of gastrointestinal gas simulating high gastrointestinal obstruction; cardiomegaly and even congestive heart failure (rare).

ADRENOLEUKODYSTROPHY AND ADRENOMYELONEUROPATHY

Classification: (a) X-linked, the most common form, a peroxisomal disease; (b) neonatal form with deficiency of peroxisomes; (c) deficiency of acyl-CoA oxidase with clinical manifestations similar to the neonatal form, but peroxisomes are present (reported in siblings).

Pathophysiology: Accumulation of a very long chain of saturated fatty acids with carbon length greater than C22 (from C24 to C30 with a peak of C26) in tissues and body fluids, particularly nervous system white matter and the adrenal cortex; widespread demyelination of cerebral white matter, inflammatory reaction, and atrophy of zona reticularis and fasciculata of the adrenal gland with ballooned, striated cells in the adrenal cortex; inability to break down very long chain fatty acid in the peroxisomes due to lignoceryl CoA synthetase deficiency.

Clinical Manifestations

(A) CHILDHOOD FORM (CLASSIC X-LINKED ADRENOLEUKODYSTROPHY; **XALD**): *Mild to moderate adrenal insufficiency that may be partially limited to elevated adrenocorticotropic hormone levels;* rapidly progressive cerebral syndrome with onset in childhood: behavioral problems; loss of memory; language and visual deterioration; loss of coordination; ataxia; dysarthria; seizures; hemiplegia; optic atrophy; development of vegetative state within a few years.

(B) NEONATAL FORM (**NALD**): *Hypotonia; poor feeding; failure to thrive;* absent grasp reflexes; pathologic changes that are different from XALD (cerebral heterotopia; micropachygyria; etc.); prenatal diagnosis by mutation analysis.

(C) ADRENOLEUKOMYELONEUROPATHY (**ALMN**): Symptoms usually presenting in young-adult period: *spastic paraplegia; distal symmetric peripheral neuropathy; adrenal insufficiency;* testicular insufficiency; etc.

(D) SYMPTOMATIC HETEROZYGOTE: *Chronic nonprogressive spinal cord syndrome: spastic paraparesis; peripheral neuropathy.*

(E) NERVOUS SYSTEM: Seizures; coma; frontal lobe syndromes; increased intracranial pressure (cerebral edema); encephalopathy preceding adrenal insufficiency; megaloencephaly; cerebral tumorlike presentation; Klüver-Bucy syndrome; ataxia in the adult variant; intellectual decline in adult variant; abnormal electroencephalographic findings.

(F) ENDOCRINE SYSTEM: Addison disease (males); sparse hair and multiple endocrine disorders (Addison disease, hypothyroidism, and Graves disease) in two women heterozygous for ALD; insulin-dependent diabetes mellitus.

(G) LABORATORY FINDINGS: High cerebrospinal fluid protein; pipecolic acidemia in NALD; carrier detection by determining *very long chain fatty acids in plasma and cultured skin fibroblasts.*

(H) MISCELLANEOUS ABNORMALITIES: Frequent alterations of visual pigment genes; Addison disease preceding neurologic symptoms by several years; XALD and hemophilia in the same kindred; NALD presenting as infantile progressive spinal muscular atrophy.

Radiologic Manifestations

(A) COMPUTED TOMOGRAPHY OF BRAIN: (a) *low-density white matter lesion originating in the occipital region and migrating forward into the temporal, parietal, and frontal lobes and cerebellum;* continuation of the process across the midline; sparing of gray matter; indistinctness of the ventricular wall due to low brain density; rim of enhancement at the periphery of the lesions on a contrast study; *progression to generalized central and cortical atrophy;* (b) atypical computed tomographic presentations such as lesions without opacification at the periphery after contrast enhancement, early frontal lobe involvement, ventricular and parietal lobe distortion suggestive of mass effect, cerebellar involvement, and central calcifications within the low attenuation lesions of white matter.

(B) MAGNETIC RESONANCE IMAGING OF BRAIN: More sensitive than computed tomography in the early phase of development of *demyelination; high signal intensity on T_2-weighted spin-echo sequences* (corresponding with the low attenuation seen on computed tomographic examination); *areas of very intense signals on T_2-weighted images, sometimes associated with decreased signals on T_1-weighted images in the same areas* (occipital, parietal, temporal, and frontal lobes; visual pathways; auditory pathways; motor pathways; corpus callosum; external capsule; etc.).

(C) SPINAL CORD: Decreased spinal cord diameter in individuals who are heterozygous for ALD-ALMN, in patients with ALD or ALMN, and in asymptomatic ALD-ALMN patients.

(D) SCINTIGRAPHY (^{99m}TC PERTECHNETATE): *Increased uptake in the involved brain regions.*

(E) MISCELLANEOUS ABNORMALITIES: Prominent veins in the white matter; unilateral cerebral abnormalities in XALD; cortical hypoperfusion demonstrated by ^{99m}Tc HMPAO single photon emission computed tomography in an 8-year-old boy.

AFIBRINOGENEMIA (CONGENITAL)

Clinical Manifestations: (a) provoked or spontaneous external or visceral *hemorrhages; absence of fibrinogen in plasma confirmed by chemical and immunoelectrophoresis;* normal or increased bleeding time; failure of blood clotting; etc.; (b) autosomal recessive inheritance.

Radiologic Manifestations: Hemarthrosis and "bone cysts" due to bleeding; visceral hemorrhage; pericardial hemorrhage; constrictive pericarditis.

ALDOSTERONISM (CONN SYNDROME)

Etiology: (a) aldosterone-producing adenoma (about 65% of the cases); (b) idiopathic hyperaldosteronism due to bilateral adrenal glomerulosa hyperplasia (about 30% of the cases); (c) glucosuppressive hyperaldosteronism; (d) adrenocortical carcinoma; (e) primary hyperplasia: hyperplastic adrenal glands with the morphology similar to that of idiopathic hyperaldosteronism but mimicking the aldosterone-producing adenoma (response to physiologic maneuvers and unilateral or subtotal adrenalectomy); (f) aldosterone-producing renin-responsive adenoma: morphology and response to unilateral adrenalectomy similar to aldosterone-producing adenoma; response to physiologic maneuvers similar to that of hyperplastic glands; (g) extraadrenal production of aldosterone by adrenal embryologic rest neoplasms within the kidney or ovary.

Clinical Manifestations: (a) *systemic arterial hypertension,* without edema; (b) *hyperaldosteronism* that is not suppressed appropriately during volume expansion; (c) *depression of plasma renin activity;* (d) *hypokalemic alkalosis;* (e) muscular weakness; muscle paralysis; polydipsia; polyuria; nocturia; paresthesia; tetany; headache; (f) miscellaneous abnormalities: renal failure caused by rhabdomyolysis; subarachnoid hemorrhage; postural hypotension; bradycardia; neonatal idiopathic hyperaldosteronism presenting with functional gastrointestinal symptoms associated with hypokalemia and hypertension.

Radiologic Manifestations: (a) *aldosterone assay of adrenal vein;* (b) selective retrograde epinephrophlebography of the adrenal veins demonstrating the *tumor displacing surrounding adrenal veins;* (c) arteriographic demonstration of a *sharply delineated avascular area within a densely opacified adrenal cortex;* faint homogeneous blush in some; (d) computed tomography more reliable for lesions over 10 mm in diameter; (e) magnetic resonance imaging: low-intensity mass; (f) scintigraphy (^{75}Se-selenomethyl-cholesterol) very useful (increased uptake in the abnormal gland); (g) miscellaneous abnormalities: adrenal myelolipoma; renal cysts; myocardial damage.

ALEXANDER DISEASE

Clinical Manifestations: (a) two broad clinical subgroups: (1) infantile form: *macrocephaly; regression; seizures;* (2) juvenile form: *bulbar signs as the major manifestations;* (b) possibly autosomal recessive inheritance; sporadic in most cases.

Radiologic Manifestations: (a) computed tomographic findings vary with progressive stage of the disease; typical findings in the advanced stage of the disease are as follows: *white matter lucency in the frontal lobe with extension into the peripheral zone; involvement of the external capsules; relatively lesser involvement of the internal capsules; increased density of the optic chiasm, optic radiations, columns of fornices, basal ganglia, subependymal rim and medial portions of the forceps minor; marked enhancement of the dense areas after contrast medium injection;* mild to moderate dilatation of the lateral and third ventricles; (b) ultrasonography: mild ventriculomegaly; abnormal increase in brain size; loss of definition of sulci; uniform appearance of cerebral tissues; (c) magnetic resonance imaging: *diffuse demyelination (increased signal intensity in T_2-weighted images; decreased signal intensity in T_1-weighted images); most marked in the frontal regions; coarsened pattern of sulci and gyri, suggesting diffuse infiltrating process;* (d) single photon emission computed tomographic scan: reduced cerebral metabolic activity; (e) miscellaneous abnormalities: small ventricles; hydrocephalus; cerebral calcifications (basal ganglia; cerebellum; periventricular white matter).

Note: Hereditary adult-onset Alexander disease has been reported with the following manifestations: palatal myoclonus, spastic paraparesis, and cerebellar ataxia.

ALKAPTONURIA

Enzyme Deficiency: Homogentisate 1,2-dioxygenase.

Clinical Manifestations: (a) *ochronosis:* brown or black pigmentation of the skin, oral mucosa, sclera, conjunctiva, limbic cornea, tendons, cartilage, cerumen, sweat, etc.; (b) *chronic arthropathy,* in particular, in the shoulder, hip, and knee joints; limitation of spinal motion; loss of height; etc.; (c) *alkaptonuria:* discoloration of the urine to brown or black on standing or on alkalinization; (d) renal stones; decreased kidney function; renal failure; prostatitis; prostatic enlargement; (e) cardiovascular ochronosis: cardiac valves; mitral anulus; mural endocardium; myocardium; arteriosclerotic plaques of aorta; epicardial coronary arteries; myocardial infarction; (f) upper respiratory symptoms (dryness of the pharynx; hoarseness); dyspnea; restriction of thoracic cage motions; gray airways (vocal cord, tracheal rings, and bronchial cartilage) seen on endoscopy; (g) association with the following: diabetes mellitus; Addison disease; polycythemia vera; hyperuricemia; ankylosing spondylitis; Parkinson disease; (h) autosomal recessive inheritance.

Radiologic Manifestations: (a) *spinal manifestations:* loss of lumbar lordosis; kyphosis; scoliosis; osteoporosis; narrowing of disc spaces; "vacuum" phenomena; disc calcification and ossification; ruptured intervertebral discs; osteophyte formation; calcification of the interspinous ligament; vertebral fusion; spinal fracture; (b) *extraspinal arthropathy:* cartilage calcification; effusion; loose joint bodies; articular and paraarticular calcification; joint narrowing, sclerosis; osteophytes; destruction of humeral and femoral heads; rupture of the Achilles tendon; etc.; (c) *renal calculi; nephrocalcinosis;* prostatic calculi; (d) miscellaneous abnormalities: calcifications (ear cartilage; aortic and mitral valves); root canal stenosis.

ALPHA$_1$-ANTITRYPSIN DEFICIENCY

Clinical Manifestations

(A) INFANTS AND CHILDREN: *Prolonged obstructive jaundice in infancy, liver cirrhosis, hepatosplenomegaly;* pulmonary disease; persistent hyperinflation of lungs in children with liver disease due to α_1-antitrypsin deficiency.

(B) ADULTS: Onset of symptoms often prior to 40 years of age: chronic bronchitis; *wheezing; progressive dyspnea; respiratory failure; cor pulmonale;* liver cirrhosis; asthenia; malnourished appearance.

(C) LABORATORY FINDINGS: *Almost complete absence of α_1-globulin;* very low serum trypsin inhibitory capacity; Pi typing (ZZ phenotype shown on crossed immunoelectrophoresis); chorionic villus samples used in prenatal diagnosis.

(D) Many genetic variants; inherited via two codominant autosomal alleles; PiM the most common genotype.

Radiologic Manifestations

(A) INFANTS AND CHILDREN: (a) hepatosplenomegaly; gastroesophageal varices; ascites; abnormal liver ultrasonogram (focal areas of heterogeneity simulating mass lesions; increased periportal echogenicity); gallbladder enlargement in the neonatal period; (b) hyperinflation of lungs; cystic degeneration of lung.

(B) ADULTS: (a) *hyperlucent lungs* with or without bullae; *emphysema more pronounced in the lower parts of the lungs;* bronchiectasis; areas of low density corresponding to parenchymal destruction and reduced perfusion (high resolution computed tomography); upper lung involvement shown by high-resolution computed tomography; bronchial wall thickening; spontaneous pneumothorax; (b) *marked homogeneous decrease in perfusion at the lung bases with increased flow in the upper portions of the lungs;* (c) cardiomegaly; cor pulmonale with a dilated pulmonary artery and proximal branches.

ALPHA-CHAIN DISEASE (IMMUNOPROLIFERATIVE SMALL INTESTINAL DISEASE)

Clinical Manifestations: (a) *chronic diarrhea, malabsorption, and progressive weight loss;* impaired absorption of vitamin B_{12}, glucose, lactose, and fat; *heavy-chain fragments of IgA; free of light chains (serum; urine; jejunal fluid);* (b) endoscopy: gastric erosion; edematous mucosa with enlarged villi; hyperplastic lymph follicles of terminal ileum; thickening of cecal mucosa; (c) miscellaneous abnormalities: leukemic manifestations, most commonly reported in young persons from Third World countries; nonsecretory alpha-chain disease involving stomach, small intestine, and colon (case report).

Pathology: Diffuse lymphoma type of proliferation with involvement of the mesentery and small bowel (peroral jejunal biopsy showing abnormal plasma cells).

Radiologic Manifestations: Small bowel: *thick circular folds; pseudostricture; pseudodiverticula; nodular mucosal pattern with a spiky and scalloped contour; segmental dilatation.*

ALUMINUM INTOXICATION (Aluminum-related Osteodystrophy)

Etiology: (a) chronic renal failure and hemodialysis-related disease: aluminum administered as a phosphate binder to uremic patients; aluminum pump used in hemodialysis; aluminum-containing dialysate owing to improper water treatment; aluminum in the diet or water supply; (b) aluminum hydroxide antacid; (c) parenteral nutrition-associated aluminum overload.

Clinical Manifestations: (a) *myopathy; muscle weakness;* (b) *bone pain;* (c) *poor response to vitamin D therapy;* (d) *encephalopathy* (dialysis dementia); (e) microcytic anemia not caused by iron deficiency; (f) normal to elevated serum calcium levels; normal or relatively low levels of immunoreactive parathyroid hormone and alkaline phosphatase activity; (g) bone histology: deposition of aluminum at the bone-osteoid junction; osteomalacia without features of osteitis fibrosa; severe mineralization defect; (h) miscellaneous abnormalities: prurigo nodularis in association with aluminum overload in maintenance hemodialysis; oxalosis associated with aluminum bone disease.

Radiologic Manifestations: *Osteoporosis; osteomalacia; rachitic bone changes;* pathologic nonhealing multiple *fractures* (rib; hip; vertebra; etc.); tumoral soft-tissue calcifications.

AMYLOIDOSIS

Clinical Manifestations: (a) weight loss; fatigue; dizziness; dyspnea; edema; (b) musculoskeletal system abnormalities: arthropathy; enlarged soft tissues around joints; myopathy; muscle stiffness; carpal tunnel syndrome; respiratory muscle weakness; trigger finger; flexor tendon contracture; spontaneous tendon rupture; (c) urinary system abnormalities: renal insufficiency; nephrotic syndrome: (d) cardiovascular system abnormalities: congestive heart failure; restrictive cardiomyopathy; decreased pulse pressure; arrhythmias; hypertension; orthostatic hypotension; constrictive pericarditis; low electrocardiographic voltage; conduction defects; (e) nervous system abnormalities: various motor and sensory deficits; autonomic nervous system symptoms; cranial nerve involvement; intracerebral hemorrhage; (f) skin abnormalities: scleroderma-like skin changes; hemorrhage; (g) alimentary system abnormalities: anorexia; abdominal pain; dysphagia; salivary gland involvement; changes in taste sensation; xerostomia; diarrhea; constipation; malabsorption; bleeding; esophageal motor dysfunction; gastroparesis; (h) hepatomegaly; progressive hepatic failure; splenomegaly; (i) respiratory system abnormalities: amyloidosis of the nasopharynx, larynx, tracheobronchial tree, and lungs; pulmonary hemorrhage; (j) miscellaneous abnormalities: macroglossia; lymphadenopathy; breast mass; Sjögren syndrome; association with hypogammaglobulinemia; hypersplenism; bleeding problems; etc.; (k) autosomal dominant inheritance in the familial form; high penetrance.

Laboratory Findings: (a) Congo red test; (b) biopsy: involvement of arterioles of the rectal mucosa; etc.; (c) albuminuria; cylindruria; hypoalbuminemia; hypercholesterolemia; electrophoresis and immunoelectrophoresis of serum and urine; (d) bone marrow biopsy: plasma cell dyscrasia; (e) prenatal diagnosis by chorionic villus sampling (familial amyloidotic polyneuropathy).

Radiologic Manifestations

(A) MUSCULOSKELETAL SYSTEM: Paraarticular soft-tissue nodules and swelling; amyloid myopathy (slight prolongation of muscle T_1 and T_2 relaxation times associated with marked reticulation of the subcutaneous fat); fluid collection within the joints and synovial spaces; joint subluxation; neuroarthropathy; subchondral cysts; avascular necrosis; osteoporosis; pathologic fractures; collapse of vertebral bodies; lytic lesions.

(B) URINARY SYSTEM: (a) enlarged, small, or normal-sized kidneys; irregular renal contour in the contracted type of kidneys; (b) reduced renal function on excretory urography; (c) angiography: normal or slightly decreased renal artery size; irregular narrowing and tortuosity of the interlobar arteries; nonvisualization of the cortical and interlobular arteries; renal vein thrombosis (frequently involving the segmental or interlobar veins); indistinctness of the corticomedullary junction; (d) ultrasonography: marked echogenicity of the cortex as compared with the liver and spleen; (e) miscellaneous abnormalities: localized amyloidosis of the renal pelvis, ureters, bladder, prostate, seminal vesicles, vas deferens, testes, penis, and urethra that mimics neoplastic lesions.

(C) CARDIOVASCULAR SYSTEM: (a) congestive heart failure; (b) ultrasonography: impaired left ventricular systolic contraction; prominence of the papillary muscles; highly refractile granular sparkling myocardial echoes on two-dimensional echocardiography; (c) computed tomography: low myocardial density on precontrast tomograms and diffuse myocardial thickening on postcontrast tomograms; (d) myocardial uptake of Tc-99m(V) DMSA; (e) magnetic resonance imaging: thickening of the myocardium; luminal irregularity and abrupt arterial caliber changes.

(D) ALIMENTARY SYSTEM: Dilatation of the intestine; thickening of mucosal folds; slow transit time; pseudoobstruction; bowel ischemia with ulceration; stricture; bowel perforation; mesenteric amyloidosis mimicking an abdominal tumor (stellate appearance on computed tomography); nodular wall lesions mimicking neoplasms; thumb printing; ileocecal valve enlargement; polypoid protrusions; pneumatosis cystoides intestinalis; pneumoperitoneum; ascites associated with portal hypertension, cardiac disease, and renal disease.

(E) LYMPHATIC SYSTEM MANIFESTATIONS: Lymphadenopathy, filling defect of the nodes shown by lymphangiography, periaortic lymph node enlargement and calcification.

(F) LIVER AND SPLEEN: Hepatomegaly; splenomegaly; space-occupying lesions in the liver demonstrated by radionuclide, ultrasonographic, and computed imaging techniques; low density that becomes more clearly visible on postcontrast injection computed tomographic examination; uptake of bone-seeking radiopharmaceuticals such as Tc-99m methylene diphosphonate and Tc-99m pyrophosphate; hepatic and splenic calcification.

(G) CENTRAL NERVOUS SYSTEM: Cerebral amyloid angiopathy (deposition of amyloid in medium and small arteries of the cerebral cortex and leptomeninges) causing intracerebral hemorrhage at atypical sites (cortical; multiple; bilateral); repeated episodes of bleeding; amyloidoma as a space-occupying lesion; vascular wall irregularity, and vascular occlusion shown by angiography; signal hyperintensity in the white matter on T_2-weighted spin-echo pulse sequence (leukoencephalopathy); subcortical punctate areas of hypointensity on the T_2-weighted images.

(H) RESPIRATORY SYSTEM: Laryngo-tracheo-bronchial lesions (computed tomography: soft-tissue thickening; plaques; amyloidoma; obstruction); pulmonary lesions in many forms (honeycomb, miliary, single or multiple nodules, diffuse alveolar septal, calcification, etc.); pulmonary edema (heart failure).

(I) MISCELLANEOUS ABNORMALITIES: Orbital and nasopharyngeal amyloidosis presenting as masses; extraskeletal uptake of bone tracer; mediastinal calcified amyloid tumor; breast masses simulating carcinoma; amyloid goiter; soft-tissue uptake of Tc-99m dicarboxy propane diphosphonate; etc.

ASPARTYLGLUCOSAMINURIA

Enzyme Abnormality: Deficiency of the lysosomal enzyme 1-aspartamido-ß-*N*-acetylglucosamine amidohydrolase (aspartylglycosaminidase, AGA, EC3.5.1.26).

Clinical Manifestations: Onset of symptoms at about 2 to 6 years of age: (a) *progressive psychomotor retardation;* epileptic seizures (more common in adults); (b) *facial dysmorphism,* very mild in early childhood, becoming more apparent at school age: gargoylelike features with a broad face, wide mouth, thick lips, large tongue, low nasal bridge, and anteverted nostrils; (c) *multivacuolated lymphocytes in the peripheral blood and bone marrow; increased urinary excretion of aspartylglycosamine; demonstra-*

tion of enzyme defect (aspartylglycosaminidase) in leukocytes and cultured fibroblasts; reduced number of neutrophils; decreased prothrombin activity; prenatal diagnosis by demonstrating enzyme deficiency in cultured cells from a midterm amniotic fluid sample; abnormal enzyme assays on cord blood lymphocytes; cultured cells from skin biopsy specimens and placental villi; (d) miscellaneous abnormalities: short neck; prominent thoracic kyphosis; scoliosis; bulging abdomen; hernias; poorly developed sex characteristics; hoarse voice; recurrent respiratory infections; recurrent diarrhea; malabsorption; systolic murmur; mitral insufficiency; joint hyperflexibility; muscular hypotonia; lens opacities; myoclonic seizures; angiokeratoma; macroorchidism; hepatosplenomegaly in early infancy; (e) autosomal recessive inheritance; high frequency in individuals of Finnish descent; a single nucleotide change in the gene encoding glucosamine responsible for the disease.

Radiologic Manifestations: (a) thick calvaria; microcephaly; underdeveloped frontal sinuses; small sella turcica; cerebral cortical atrophy; (b) osteochondrosis-type vertebral changes; flattening and anterior beaking of some vertebral bodies; spondylolysis and spondylolisthesis in early childhood; (c) cortical thinning of the tubular bones; osteoporosis; pathologic fractures; scoliosis; retarded skeletal maturation.

B

BEHR SYNDROME

Clinical Manifestations: (a) optic atrophy in infancy; ataxia; increased deep tendon reflexes; positive Babinski; pyramidal tract dysfunction; nystagmus; mental deficiency; urinary incontinence; (b) abnormal electroencephalographic findings; (c) abnormalities in free amino acid pool (plasma; cerebrospinal fluid); (d) clubfoot; (e) autosomal recessive inheritance.

Radiologic Manifestations: Magnetic resonance imaging: diffuse, symmetric white matter abnormalities of the cerebral hemispheres and brain stem (increased signal intensity on T_2-weighted images).

BIOTINIDASE DEFICIENCY

Clinical Manifestations: Biotinidase deficiency results in reduced activities of biotin-dependent carboxylases, with symptoms presenting in infancy: (a) *alopecia; seborrheic dermatitis;* (b) *conjunctivitis; mucositis; erythematous rash;* (c) *hypotonia; infantile spasms; seizures; hearing loss;*

ataxia; psychomotor regression; (d) eye abnormalities: infections; optic neuropathies and visual disturbances; optic atrophy; motility disturbances; retinal pigment changes; pupillary abnormality; (e) *lactic acidemia; a diagnostic urinary metabolite pattern of organic acids;* laryngeal stridor; favorable response to pharmacologic doses of biotin (clinical and radiologic, with reversal of "brain atrophy").

Radiologic Manifestations: *Diffuse cerebral and cerebellar atrophy.*

BLUE DIAPER SYNDROME

Clinical and Radiologic Manifestations: *Defect in intestinal absorption of L-tryptophan in association with increased tryptophan in feces and increased tryptophan derivatives in urine:* (a) failure to thrive; recurrent fever; irritability; constipation; susceptibility to infections; (b) *blue discoloration of diapers* (indican oxidized to indican blue on exposure to air); *hypercalcemia;* (c) miscellaneous abnormalities: microcornea; hypoplasia of the optic disc; abnormal eye movements; nephrocalcinosis; (d) autosomal recessive or X-linked recessive inheritance.

C

CALCINOSIS UNIVERSALIS

Clinical Manifestations: Onset usually before the age of 20 years; more common in females: fatigue; difficulty in locomotion; muscular pain; low-grade fever; *palpable calcific plaques in subcutaneous or deeper tissues;* high levels of γ-carboxyglutamic acid in involved tissues and urine.

Radiologic Manifestations: *Long bands of symmetric subcutaneous calcification with progressive spread to deeper connective tissues* (tendons; ligaments; nerve sheets); leak of calcium deposits through the skin; extraskeletal uptake of Tc-99m high-density polyethylene oxidronate.

Note: About one third of cases of calcinosis universalis are secondary to scleroderma or dermatomyositis.

CALCIUM PYROPHOSPHATE DIHYDRATE DEPOSITION DISEASE

Clinical Manifestations: (a) episodic acute or subacute *arthralgia with soft-tissue swelling* (knee, hip, shoulder, elbow, wrist, ankle, acromioclavicular, talocalcaneal, and metatarsophalangeal); *pseudorheumatoid arthritis* or *pseudoosteoarthritis symptoms;* (b) *CPPD (cal-*

cium pyrophosphate dihydrate) crystals within the joint and surrounding tissues; (c) miscellaneous abnormalities: fever; cervical myelopathy; tumoral CPPD mimicking a cervical spine neoplasm; pseudotumoral lesions; calcium pyrophosphate deposition in ligamentum flavum; spinal canal stenosis due to thickening of ligamentum flavum; associated with Coffin-Lowry syndrome; neurologic symptoms associated with hypertrophy and calcification of the ligamentum flavum or posterior longitudinal ligament in the cervical spine; (d) autosomal dominant inheritance (incomplete penetrance, variable expressivity) with onset in young adults; sporadic cases with onset usually in middle-aged and older patients.

Radiologic Manifestations: (a) *chondrocalcinosis;* (b) *paraarticular tendon and bursal calcification;* (c) *discrete subchondral rarefaction, articular space narrowing; bone sclerosis;* spine and paraspinal soft-tissue CPPD crystal deposition; spinal stenosis; atlantoaxial subluxation; calcification within soft tissues; spinal cord compression and cervical myelopathy (hyperintensity of the cord on magnetic resonance imaging); (d) miscellaneous abnormalities: massive soft-tissue calcification adjacent to the joint; destructive wrist arthropathy; Charcot-like joints; temporomandibular joint involvement; abnormal activity in the joint regions on scintigraphy (In-111–labeled leukocyte imaging).

CANAVAN DISEASE (CANAVAN–VAN BOGAERT–BERTRAND DISEASE)

Clinical Manifestations: A leukodystrophy with onset of symptoms in early infancy: (a) *megaloencephaly;* (b) *initial hypotonia followed by spasticity;* (c) *progressive psychomotor degeneration; blindness, deafness;* (d) biochemical heterogeneity: *increased N-acetylaspartic acid levels in urine, blood, and cerebrospinal fluid; marked aspartoacylase deficiency* shown in cultured skin fibroblasts and other tissues; (e) prenatal diagnosis: *assay for* N-acetyl-L-*aspartate in amniotic fluid; aspartoacylase activity evaluation using chorionic villus samples and/or amniocytes;* (f) proton nuclear magnetic resonance spectroscopy: reduced levels of choline and creatine; increased levels of lactate and inositol; (g) autosomal recessive inheritance; prevalent among Ashkenazi Jews; mutations in aspartoacylase leading to loss of enzymatic activity identified.

Pathology: A progressive degenerative disease with spongy changes predominantly affecting the white matter (lipid-filled glial cells), caused by the deficiency of aspartoacylase.

Radiologic Manifestations: (a) variable ultrasonographic picture: *increased sonolucency of the white matter; multiple anechoic cavitary lesions;* increased echogenicity in the periventricular gray matter; ventriculomegaly in more advanced cases; (b) *demyelination with white-*

matter disease in internal capsule, external capsule, genu of corpus callosum, subcortical white matter, and posterior fossa: (1) computed tomography: *diffuse symmetric decreased attenuation within the white matter without areas of abnormal contrast enhancement;* (2) magnetic resonance imaging: *marked prolongation of the T_1 and T_2 relaxation times, hyperintense signal from the lentiform nuclei and the head of the caudate nuclei on the T_2-weighted images;* (c) urine spectroscopy: high *N*-acetyl-aspartate concentration; (d) *brain atrophy;* (e) cholelithiasis.

CARBOHYDRATE-DEFICIENT GLYCOPROTEIN SYNDROME

Clinical Manifestations: Changing clinical picture according to age.

(A) INFANCY (MULTISYSTEM STAGE): Failure to thrive; psychomotor/ developmental delay; hypotonia; convergent squint; liver dysfunction; hepatomegaly; cardiomyopathy; pericardial effusion; lipodystrophic skin changes; joint restriction; inverted nipples; *olivopontocerebellar atrophy;* congenital cataracts; anterior horn neurons of spinal cord involvement; prenatal cardiomyopathy and pericardial effusion; familial brachydactyly.

(B) LATE INFANCY AND CHILDHOOD (ATAXIC–MENTAL RETARDATION STAGE): Mental deficiency; motor disability; lower neuron impairment; cerebellar ataxia; strokelike episodes.

(C) TEENAGE (LEG ATROPHY STAGE): Short stature; peripheral neuropathy with lower limb weakness and muscle atrophy; nonprogressive cerebellar ataxia; kyphoscoliosis.

(D) ADULT (STABLE DISABILITY STAGE): Slight facial dysmorphic features; short stature; protrusion of thorax; kyphoscoliosis; relatively long and thin limbs; permanent neurologic deficiencies; subcutaneous lipodystrophy; female hypogonadism; hepatic dysfunction; cataracts.

(E) LABORATORY FINDINGS: Hypoalbuminemia; hypocholesterolemia; decreased serum heptoglobin; decreased serum protein C; decreased blood coagulation activities; *highly raised serum concentrations of the biochemical marker carbohydrate-deficient transferrin.*

(F) Autosomal recessive inheritance.

Radiologic Manifestations: (a) *marked atrophy of the cerebellum and pons (olivopontocerebellar atrophy);* (b) renal microcysts (hyperechoic renal pattern); renal macrocyst; (c) miscellaneous abnormalities: kyphosis; scoliosis; osteoporosis of vertebrae; irregular and sclerotic end-plate of the lower thoracic and upper lumbar vertebrae with central tongue of the vertebral bodies.

Note: A subtype has been reported in two infants with microcephaly, epilepsy, absent psychomotor development, and no signs of liver dysfunction.

CARBONIC ANHYDRASE II DEFICIENCY (MARBLE BRAIN DISEASE; OSTEOPETROSIS–RENAL TUBULAR ACIDOSIS–CEREBRAL CALCIFICATION SYNDROME)

Clinical Manifestations: (a) *physical and developmental retardation;* (b) *facial appearance:* broad face, overhanging forehead, narrow nose, epicanthal fold, thin upper lip, poorly developed philtrum, everted lower lip, micrognathia, and dental malocclusion; (c) *renal tubular acidosis* (*proximal,* distal, or combined type): *hyperchloremic metabolic acidosis;* hypokalemia (in some); *deficiency of carbonic anhydrase II and protein levels in red blood cells;* (d) iliac crest biopsy: unresorbed calcified primary spongiosa; (e) miscellaneous abnormalities: muscle weakness; failure to thrive; short stature; psychomotor delay and mental subnormality; low levels of carbonic anhydrase in parents and sibling; osteomalacia; cranial nerve compression; (f) autosomal recessive inheritance.

Radiologic Manifestations: (a) *osteosclerosis and skeletal modeling defect* (may gradually resolve by adulthood); fractures; (b) *cerebral calcification:* basal ganglia; periventricular white matter.

CARCINOID SYNDROME

Clinical Manifestations: Carcinoid syndrome occurs when the humoral output of tumors (primary and metastases) exceeds the capacity of monoamine oxidase present in the liver and lung for metabolism of serotonin: (a) *flushing of the skin;* telangiectasia of the face and neck; (b) *episodes of diarrhea and abdominal cramps; motor dysfunction of the small bowel and colon;* digestive tract bleeding; bowel obstruction; (c) deficiency syndromes; (d) *attacks of wheezing;* (e) intractable right-sided *congestive heart failure;* valvular heart disease (usually right-sided); pericarditis; angina pectoris; hypoxia due to right-to-left shunt; (f) *hypertension; secretion of pharmacologically active substances* (serotonin, kallikrein, substance P, and prostaglandins); (g) familial cases reported in a father and daughter and in a brother and sister.

Pathology: Deposition of fibrous tissue on cardiac valves and endocardium resulting in tricuspid stenosis and insufficiency, pulmonary stenosis, and (rarely) left-sided valvular involvement; loss of trabeculation of the ventricle due to endocardial fibrosis.

Radiologic Manifestations: (a) small bowel is most common site of tumor: (1) *atypical intramural defect in earlier stage and intraluminal lobulated growth in later stage;* direct extension of tumor into the mesentery with a resultant fanlike appearance of the mucosa; bowel obstruction; intussusception; bowel perforation; rapid transit time of barium; (2) angiography: a stellate arterial pattern; narrowing of deep mesenteric branches; poor to moderate tumor stain, and lack of visualization of draining veins; (3) computed tomography: *demonstration of a mesenteric soft-tissue mass with radiating linear strands; primary tumor (often in the distal portion of the ileum); retroperitoneal lymph node enlargement; liver metastasis;* (b) bronchial tumor; (c) carcinoid heart disease: (1) *cardiomegaly, right-sided heart failure;* (2) echocardiography: *thickening, shortening, and immobility of the tricuspid valve leaflets in association with valvular regurgitation; thickening and doming of the tricuspid valve in association with stenosis;* no evidence of commissural fusion; *pulmonary valvular abnormalities similar to the tricuspid valve disease;* (3) cardioangiography: *tricuspid stenosis and insufficiency; pulmonary stenosis* (hourglass tapering toward the valve: proximal pulmonary artery and subvalvular right ventricular outflow tract); (d) scintiscanning with the use of ^{131}I MIBG: intense tracer uptake in the tumor and metastases; left ventricular uptake of a labeled somatostatin analog; (e) miscellaneous abnormalities: phalangeal and metacarpophalangeal arthropathy (juxtaarticular osteoporosis; multiple cystic areas; erosions of joint surfaces); pleural thickening.

CARNITINE DEFICIENCY SYNDROMES

Classification
(A) PRIMARY: (1) systemic: low levels of muscle, blood, and liver carnitine; (2) myopathic: muscle carnitine deficiency.

(B) SECONDARY: (1) genetic defects of intermediary metabolism: Acyl-CoA dehydrogenase deficiencies; organic acidemias; mitochondrial respiratory disorders; carnitine octanoyltransferase deficiency; methylenetetrahydrofolate deficiency; ornithine transcarbamylase deficiency; (2) other disorders: inadequate intake; total parenteral nutrition; kwashiorkor; loss of carnitine (renal failure; Fanconi syndrome; etc.); valproate therapy; liver cirrhosis; endocrine disorders (hypothyroidism; adrenal insufficiency; hypopituitarism); pregnancy; Reye syndrome; Rett syndrome; etc.

Clinical and Radiologic Manifestations
(A) SYSTEMIC: Usually affecting infants and children; *progressive muscle weakness; severe nonketotic hypoglycemia; hepatic encephalopathy; cardiomyopathy; congestive heart failure; ventilatory failure;* death in early childhood in untreated cases.

(B) MYOPATHIC: Onset of symptoms in older children and young adults, *slowly progressive muscular weakness, cardiorespiratory as late manifestation.*

(C) MISCELLANEOUS ABNORMALITIES: Hypoprothrombinemia; hyperammonemia; elevated levels of liver and muscle enzymes in serum; lipid excess in hepatocytes during the encephalopathic attacks (similar to Reye syndrome); muscle carnitine deficiency presenting as familial fatal cardio-myopathy; cardiomyopathy presenting as neonatal hydrops; a possible cause of gastrointestinal dysmotility (vomiting, delayed gastric emptying, infrequent bowel movements, and reduced lower esophageal sphincter pressure).

(D) Often sporadic; autosomal recessive inheritance in primary carni-tine deficiency; phenotypic variation among different families and within the same family.

CELIAC DISEASE

Clinical Manifestations: Gluten intolerance resulting in malabsorp-tion: (a) alimentary system: *pale, bulky, loose, greasy, and foul-smelling stools; distended abdomen; increased amount of fecal fat;* abnormal xylose absorption; *abnormal fat and glucose tolerance test findings; clinical and histologic recovery on a gluten-free diet;* (b) general symptoms: *anorexia, irritability; loss of subcutaneous fat; muscular hypotonia and wasting;* edema; bleeding tendency (vitamin K deficiency); *hypoproteinemia (pro-tein-losing enteropathy);* iron deficiency anemia; (c) immunologic abnor-malities: high levels of IgA and IgG antibodies against gliadin in patients on a gluten-containing diet; reduced number of T-lymphocytes; increased pro-duction of IgA and IgM antigliadin antibodies by cultured mucosal tissue of untreated patients; salivary IgA antigliadin antibody as a method of screen-ing for the disease before intestinal biopsy; (d) celiac crisis in infants: anorexia; depression; irritability; severe vomiting and diarrhea; dehydra-tion; large and watery stools; shocklike state; (e) miscellaneous abnormali-ties: (1) gastrointestinal tract: lymphocytic gastritis associated with elevated gastric permeability; esophageal and gastric intraepithelial lymphocytes; mononuclear cell inflammation in the small-bowel mucosa; constipation; rectal prolapse; megacolon; high risk of developing ulcerative colitis in the first-degree relatives; intestinal lymphangiectasia with intestinal protein loss; (2) nervous system: folic acid deficiency associated with epilepsy and cerebral calcifications; moderate to severe dementia and brain atrophy in adults; cortical vascular anomalies associated with epilepsy; neuromyopa-thy; cerebellar and posterior and lateral column abnormalities; (3) skin: der-matitis herpetiformis; chronic urticaria; erythema elevatum diutinum; cuta-neous vasculitis; abnormal dermatoglyphic patterns (more frequent whorls and less frequent ulnar loops than in controls); (4) malignancies: intestinal lymphoma; fibrosarcoma and IgA deficiency; carcinomas (esophagus; pharynx; etc.); fibrosarcoma; (5) endocrine disorders: transient hypopara-thyroidism; tetany; Graves disease; diabetes mellitus (insulin-dependent type); (6) respiratory system: asthma; chronic cough and airway obstruc-tion; (7) nutritional deficiencies: hypozincemia; vitamin D deficiency rickets; scurvy; copper deficiency; folic acid deficiency; (8) inflammatory diseases: pericarditis; polyarteritis; chronic hepatitis; glomerulonephritis; polymyositis; intraocular inflammation; (9) others: short stature; obesity; bone pain; enamel defects; occurrence in monozygotic twin; celiac disease as a cause of transient hypocalcemia and hypovitaminosis D; chromosomal instability in lymphocytes; Becker muscular dystrophy; high frequency of celiac disease in Down syndrome (8 of 115 patients with Down syndrome having positive laboratory tests).

Radiologic Manifestations: (a) *abnormal intestinal motor functions:* dilatation (width of the jejunum greater than 65% of the width of the third lumbar vertebra); decreased number of jejunal folds and increased number of ileal folds (jejunal-ileal fold reversal); transient small-bowel intussusception; delay in mouth-to-cecum transit time; *clumping and flocculation of barium in the small bowel; coarsening of mucosal folds;* jejunal fold separation; "bubbly" duodenal bulb (1 to 4 mm filling defects on air-contrast study); (b) ultrasonographic findings: abnormal bowel wall (narrow intestinal wall; absence of normal mucosal texture; hyperperistalsis); ascites; pericardial effusion; (c) cerebral calcifications (parietooccipital regions); brain atrophy; (d) miscellaneous abnormalities: mesenteric and paraaortic adenopathy with regression of the findings with clinical improvement; nonspecific intestinal ulceration (rare); bone demineralization; rickets; fractures; skeletal maturation retardation; gastric fundic gland polyposis; megacolon; aneurysmal bone cyst.

Note: It has been suggested that in patients with epilepsy and cerebral calcification of unknown cause, celiac disease should be excluded by intestinal biopsy.

CEREBROTENDINOUS XANTHOMATOSIS

Enzyme Deficiency: A lipid storage disease with defective activity of mitochondrial enzyme sterol 27-hydroxylase, resulting in the deposition of sterols in various tissues and organs (tendons; lungs; bones; central nervous system; etc.).

Clinical Manifestations: Often diagnosed in the third decade of life or later: (a) *cataracts;* (b) *tendon xanthomas;* (c) *low intelligence; pyramidal signs; cerebellar signs; peripheral neuropathy; abnormalities in electrophysiologic studies;* (d) *elevated serum cholestanol concentrations; excessive urinary excretion of bile alcohols;* (e) miscellaneous abnormalities: cerebrotendinous xanthomatosis without tendon xanthoma mimicking Marinesco-Sjögren syndrome; optic neuropathy; chronic diarrhea; (f) autosomal recessive inheritance; molecular diagnosis in presymptomatic stage; triplet with cerebrotendinous xanthomatosis, homozygous for mutant gene coding for the sterol 27-hydroxylase (case report).

Radiologic Manifestations: (a) central nervous system abnormalities: diffuse or focal *cerebral and cerebellar white matter disease* (low density lesion on computed tomography and high signal intensity on T_2-weighted magnetic resonance imaging); globus pallidus lesions; cerebral and cerebellar atrophy; (b) magnetic resonance of Achilles tendon: *diffuse enlargement of the tendon; multiple areas of hypersignals in T_1- and T_2-weighted images (lipid deposits);* (c) Ga-67 uptake in tendon (case report); (d) osteoporosis; fractures following minimal trauma.

CHOLESTEROL ESTER STORAGE DISEASE

Enzyme Deficiency: Lysosomal acid lipase (acid cholesteryl ester hydrolase); accumulation of cholesterol ester in most tissues, particularly in liver.

Clinical Manifestations: Onset in childhood to adulthood: (a) *premature atherosclerosis;* (b) *elevated plasma concentration of cholesterol; hyperlipidemia;* (c) *hepatomegaly* (deposition of cholesteryl ester and triglycerides in the hepatocytes and Kupffer cells; periportal infiltration by lymphocytes, plasma cells, and foamy macrophages; septal fibrosis); micronodular cirrhosis; portal hypertension; hyperbilirubinemia; *splenomegaly;* (d) muscle involvement; (e) autosomal recessive inheritance.

Radiologic Manifestations: *Hepatomegaly, splenomegaly, portal hypertension, and esophageal varices;* faint adrenal calcification (rare).

CHRONIC GRANULOMATOUS DISEASE OF CHILDHOOD
(BRIDGES-GOOD SYNDROME; NEUTROPHIL DYSFUNCTION SYNDROME)

Etiology: Phagocyte oxidase deficiency: a defect in the superoxide-generating system of neutrophils, monocytes, and eosinophils needed for killing catalase-positive bacteria by reduced by-products of oxygen. The "Variant X-linked CGD" is a milder form of the disease and is characterized by a decreased respiratory burst and cytochrome b content of phagocytes. Patients with autosomal recessive type usually have less severe disease and lack cytosolic factor necessary for the respiratory oxidative burst.

Clinical Manifestations: Granulomas composed of giant cells and pigmented, lipid-laden histiocytes: (a) infections: (1) agents: *Serratia, Klebsiella-Aerobacter; Pseudomonas, Escherichia coli; Proteus; Salmonella;* fungi; *Pneumocystis carinii; Staphylococcus;* (2) sites of infections: lungs; lymph nodes; bones; spleen; liver; brain; nose; eyes; mouth; pericardium; etc.; (b) *eczematoid dermatitis;* (c) dysuria; urinary retention; urinary tract infection; nonfunctioning kidney; chronic glomerulonephritis; cystitis; prostatitis; orchitis; balanitis; (d) vomiting; progressive esophageal obstruction; intestinal obstruction; diarrhea; malabsorption; (e) anemia; leukocytosis; elevated sedimentation rate; (f) miscellaneous abnormalities: short stature; ascites; selective IgA deficiency; paralysis due to epidural extension of intrathoracic infection (aspergillosis); association with 18q– syndrome and end-stage renal failure due to Henoch-Schönlein nephritis; ocular involvement (foci of granulomatous inflammation in choroid and sclera); crusted scalp nodules in an infant; (g) heterogeneous phenotypic disorder; X-linked recessive inheritance in about two third of patients; autosomal recessive inheritance in females and some males.

Radiologic Manifestations

(A) CHEST: (a) lung and mediastinum: *chronic and recurrent pneumonia;* persistent pneumatocele; honeycomb lung; emphysema, hilar adenopathy; mediastinitis; diffusion of mediastinitis into the vertebrae, ribs, and spinal canal; (b) heart and vessels: pericarditis; cardiac failure in children with mediastinitis; stenosis of the aorta and brachiocephalic vessels; mycotic pseudoaneurysm of the internal mammary artery.

(B) ABDOMEN: (a) hepatic granuloma (hypoechoic; poorly marginated areas without posterior enhancement); splenic granuloma; hepatosplenomegaly; (b) subdiaphragmatic and visceral abscesses; suppurative retroperitoneal lymphadenopathy; scrotal abscess; (c) alimentary system: esophageal obstruction; focal or diffuse gastric wall involvement; annular stenosis of the gastric outlet; intestinal obstruction; enterocolitis mimicking Crohn disease; progressive esophageal dysfunction; functional gastrointestinal obstruction; combined gastroduodenal involvement (thickened folds); (d) genitourinary system: hydronephrosis; destruction of papillae; abscess formation in the kidneys; cystitis; bullous edema of the bladder associated with reduced bladder capacity; ureteral stricture; prostatic cyst; urethral stricture; (e) *speckled calcific densities in the lungs, liver, spleen, and lymph nodes.*

(C) SKELETAL SYSTEM: Infection due to hematogenous spread or to direct spread from an adjacent focus (rib; vertebra; etc.).

CONGENITAL CHLORIDE DIARRHEA (DARROW-GAMBLE DISEASE)

Clinical Manifestations: (a) *absence of chloride bicarbonate exchange in the small bowel, resulting in osmotic diarrhea (stools containing high concentrations of sodium and chloride); dehydration; metabolic alkalosis; hypochloremia;* (b) undiagnosed and untreated: death in infancy, or survival complicated by dehydration, renal insufficiency, and neuromotor skill retardation; (c) autosomal recessive inheritance; the gene assigned to chromosome 7 by linkage in Finnish and Swedish families.

Radiologic Manifestations: (a) prenatal detection of intestinal distension (pseudoobstruction); polyhydramnios (due to diarrhea); (b) postnatal: bowel distension; air-fluid levels within bowel; active intestinal peristasis (ultrasonography).

COPPER DEFICIENCY

Etiology: Chronic diarrhea; chronic intestinal malabsorption; total parenteral nutrition treatments in infants and adults; long-term enteral nutrition; infants with prolonged liver damage; chronic draining biliary or enteric fistulae; protein loss; use of chelating agents; restricted cow-milk feeding in infants; use of milk formula low in copper in premature babies; excessive zinc ingestion.

Clinical Manifestations: (a) *depigmentation of the skin and hair;* (b) *psychomotor retardation; hypotonia;* apneic attacks; (c) *swelling of limbs* due to subperiosteal hemorrhage; (d) *distended blood vessels;* (e) association with rickets; (f) *sideroblastic anemia;* vacuolation of erythroid and myeloid bone marrow cells; iron deposition in some mitochondria and vacuoles; *leukopenia; neutropenia;* antineutrophil antibodies; (g) *low levels of ceruloplasmin, serum copper, and urinary copper.*

Radiologic Manifestations: (a) *osteoporosis* in the early stage; (b) *irregularity, increased density, and cupping of the provisional zone of calcification; sickle-shaped spur formation continuous with the provisional zone of calcification;* (c) miscellaneous abnormalities: multiple undisplaced fractures; epiphyseal separation; subperiosteal hemorrhage; periosteal elevation with subperiosteal calcification; soft-tissue calcification; retarded skeletal maturation.

CUSHING SYNDROME

Clinical Manifestations: (a) *"moon face"; "buffalo hump"; thinning of the skin; myopathy; wasting and muscle weakness; fragility of blood vessels, and a tendency to bruise; weight gain* and growth failure in juvenile Cushing syndrome; headaches; back pain; (b) mental changes; (c) *excessive endogenous excretion of cortisol and other adrenal steroids;* (d) laboratory tests to detect hypercortisolism: low- and high-dose dexamethasone suppression tests; the corticotropin-releasing hormone stimulation test; bilateral sampling of the inferior petrosal sinus before and after administration of corticotropin-releasing hormone; (e) association with other disorders: Zollinger-Ellison syndrome; multiple endocrine neoplasia (medullary thyroid carcinoma producing corticotropin-releasing hormone); obese patients with diabetes mellitus and poor glycemic control; hypergastrinemia; etc.

Radiologic Manifestations: (a) *osteoporosis; pathologic fractures;* heavy callus formation at the site of fractures (ribs; pelvis); cystic changes of the skeleton; aseptic necrosis of the epiphyses with secondary arthropathy; *compression fractures of the vertebrae* with marginal condensation of bodies; (b) enlargement and erosion of the sella turcica (in a few); empty sella turcica; pituitary imaging demonstrating microadenoma or macroadenoma; (c) petrosal sinus sampling to differentiate between pituitary and ectopic ACTH Cushing syndromes; (d) adrenal neoplasm; adrenal hyperplasia (the glands may be enlarged without a change in shape); (e) radionuclide scanning (19-iodo-cholesterol ^{131}I) helpful in evaluating gland physiology and in differential diagnosis of the neoplasm and hyperplasia; (f) ectopic occult ACTH syndrome: various imaging modalities used to localize the source (computed tomography of chest and abdomen most helpful); (g) miscellaneous abnormalities: advanced or retarded skeletal maturation; muscle atrophy; failure of bone scanning to detect fracture; lipomatosis; adrenal hemorrhage complicating ACTH therapy; adrenal calcification; nephrocalcinosis; pancreatic calcification in infants (after ACTH treatment); cortical atrophy of cerebral and cerebellar hemispheres; ectopic pituitary adenoma within the sphenoid sinus; loss of the lamina dura; rebound thymic hyperplasia after treatment of Cushing syndrome.

CYSTINOSIS (LIGNAC–DE TONI–FANCONI SYNDROME)

Pathophysiology: (a) cystine accumulation within cell lysosomes of various tissues: reticuloendothelial cells; meninges; choroid plexus; pineal gland; kidneys; ocular tissues; bone marrow; circulating leukocytes; pancreas; intestine; thyroid; etc.; (b) deficient tubular reabsorption of water; glucose; amino acids; phosphate; sodium; potassium; bicarbonate; etc.

Clinical Manifestations: Considerable clinical heterogeneity (infantile form; nephropathic form; adult form): (a) *failure to thrive;* (b) *dehydration;* (c) *polyuria; polydipsia;* (d) *renal tubular acidosis;* rickets; hypophosphatemia; (e) *hypokalemia;* (f) *renal glycosuria, chronic renal failure;* (g) hepatosplenomegaly; (h) *cystine crystals* in eyes; bone marrow; leukocytes; intestinal mucosa; lymph nodes; brain; etc.; (i) ocular manifestations (crystal deposits in the cornea, conjunctiva, uveal tract, retinal pigment epithelium, and extraocular muscles): recurrent corneal erosion; *photophobia;* retinal depigmentation; decreased visual acuity; (j) neurologic disorders: mild global intellectual deficits to marked mental deterioration; motor incoordination; hypotonia; dysphagia; swallowing dysfunction; voice volume reduction; difficulty in articulation; seizures; coma; (k) myopathy (late complication); (l) endocrinopathy: *hypothyroidism;* pancreatic endocrine (insulin-dependent diabetes mellitus) and exocrine insufficiencies; pituitary-testicular axis dysfunction; (m) heterozygote detection for cystinosis with measurement of the cystine content of purified preparations of polymorphonuclear leukocytes; diagnosis with use of placenta and cord blood; (n) autosomal recessive inheritance; gene locus mapped to the short arm of chromosome 17.

Radiologic Manifestations: (a) *severe resistant rickets;* (b) *secondary hyperparathyroidism;* (c) retarded skeletal maturation; (d) urinary system: radiolucent stone(s); acquired structural urinary tract abnormalities (megacystis and hydroureteronephrosis due to chronic high urine volume; renal cysts; hyperechoic kidneys; small kidney with cortical thinning; echoic foci in medullary pyramids consistent with nephrocalcinosis); (e) subcortical and cortical brain atrophy; multifocal cystic necrosis; dystrophic cerebral calcification (basal ganglia; periventricular); hydrocephalus; (f) miscellaneous abnormalities: thyroid atrophy; manifestations of hypothyroidism; diminished pancreatic size with increased echogenicity consistent with chronic pancreatitis.

CYSTINURIA

Etiology: *Inborn error of membrane transport of cystine, lysine, ornithine, and arginine in the intestinal tract and renal tubules.*

Classification: (1) type I (the most common type): no active transport of cystine or dibasic amino acids across the mucosal gradient; normal urine cystine values in heterozygous individuals; (2) type II: markedly reduced or absent cystine transport across the mucosal gradient; elevated urine cystine in heterozygous individuals (less than in homozygous); (3) type III: reduced intestinal absorption of cystine and dibasic amino acids; elevated urine cystine in heterozygous individuals (intermediate between types I and II).

Clinical Manifestations: Onset of symptoms in childhood or young adult life: (a) *nephrolithiasis-related symptoms* (6% to 8% of urolithiasis in pediatric population; about 50% of homozygotes develop cystine renal stone): abdominal colic and dysuria; (b) recurrent urinary tract infections; (c) hyperuricemia; (d) *cystine crystal in the urine; positive nitroprusside test reaction; thin-layer chromatography or high-voltage electrophoresis for identifying urinary amino acids;* intestinal transport defect demonstrated by oral loading tests and intestinal perfusion studies; renal tubular transfer defects demonstrated by clearance studies (cystine, lysine, arginine, and ornithine); (e) miscellaneous abnormalities: slight shortness of stature; anuria due to bilateral cystine urolithiasis; squamous cell carcinoma of the renal pelvis; association with congenital myotonic dystrophy; association with Jeune syndrome; (f) autosomal recessive inheritance with allelic mutation.

Radiologic Manifestations: *Urolithiasis:* single, multiple, staghorn configuration.

D

DEPRIVATION DWARFISM

Clinical Manifestations: (a) *adverse familial environment; emotional and behavioral disorders* (bizarre eating habits; depression; self-mutilation; sleep disturbances; lack of response to pain; enuresis; encopresis);

poor performance on cognitive tests; *developmental delay; short stature; small head size; rapid increase in head circumference on restoration of adequate nutrition* (catch-up growth); (b) miscellaneous abnormalities: associated with widening of cranial sutures, but without evidence of increased intracranial pressure; hormonal abnormalities (pituitary; thyroid; adrenal); reversibility of physiologic growth hormone secretion; elevated levels of sweat electrolytes; acute gastric dilatation.

Radiologic Manifestations: *Widening of cranial sutures during treatment;* computed tomography (*prominent cortical and interhemispheric sulci, suggestive of mild cerebral atrophy before treatment;* obliteration of sulci and various cisternae following treatment); skeletal demineralization; *retarded skeletal maturation.*

DIABETES INSIPIDUS

Classification

(A) CENTRAL DIABETES INSIPIDUS (NEUROHYPOPHYSEAL; CDI): (a) idiopathic; (b) lesions in the hypothalamic-neurohypophyseal axis *(defective synthesis or secretion of antidiuretic hormone [ADH]):* (1) trauma; postsurgical; aortocoronary bypass operation; (2) tumor; Langerhans cell histiocytosis; leukemia (CDI may precede, follow, or present concomitantly with leukemia); lymphoma; xanthoma disseminatum; (3) infections; sarcoidosis; congenital cytomegalovirus infection; systemic blastomycosis; necrotizing infundibulohypophysitis; (4) hypoxic brain damage; carbon monoxide poisoning; pituitary apoplexy; postpartum pituitary necrosis; brain death; (5) intracranial birth defect (septo-optic dysplasia; agenesis of the corpus callosum; etc.); (6) thrombotic thrombocytopenic purpura; dysplastic pancytopenia; vascular abnormalities; (7) miscellaneous: Wegener granulomatosis; amyloidosis; Erdheim-Chester disease.

(B) NEPHROGENIC DIABETES INSIPIDUS (ADH-RESISTANT DIABETES INSIPIDUS; NDI): Failure of response of the distal nephron cells to normal amounts of circulatory ADH (vasopressin-resistant hyposthenuria): pharmacologically induced (lithium carbonate; demeclocycline; methoxyflurane); electrolyte disorders (hypercalcemia; chronic hypokalemia); chronic renal insufficiency; adult polycystic disease; medullary cystic disease; obstructive uropathy; chronic pyelonephritis; sickle cell disease; Sjögren syndrome; etc.

Clinical Manifestations

(A) *Polyuria; polydipsia;* nocturia; failure to thrive; vomiting; constipation; excessive crying in infants; dehydration; intermittent fever; *hypotonic urine; normal or elevated serum osmolarity; unresponsiveness to ADH in the nephrogenic type.*

(B) ASSOCIATION WITH OTHER CONDITIONS AND DISEASES: (1) *central diabetes insipidus:* dysplastic pancytopenia; anterior pituitary dysfunction in the idiopathic form; amenorrhea-galactorrhea (posttraumatic after pituitary stalk rupture); etc.; (2) *nephrogenic diabetes insipidus:* central nervous system disorder (including hydrocephalus); cystinosis; transsphenoidal meningoencephalocele; etc.

(C) INHERITANCE: (a) familial CDI: autosomal dominant or X-linked recessive inheritance; (b) familial NDI: X-linked inheritance with a variable expression in carrier females; autosomal recessive.

Radiologic Manifestations

(A) CDI AND NDI: *Hydronephrosis, hydroureter, and megacystis.*

(B) CDI: (a) intracranial etiologic factors (tumor; trauma; infection; etc.); (b) thickened pituitary infundibulum; absence of high-intensity signal in the posterior pituitary lobe on T_1-weighted images; no or faint early enhancement of the posterior pituitary lobe after injection of gadopentetate dimeglumine; (c) miscellaneous abnormalities: empty sella; variable signal intensity of the posterior lobe of pituitary in the members of a single family (familial CDI).

(C) NDI: intracranial calcification (frontal, parietal, and occipital lobes; basal ganglia); absence of the normal high signal (T_1-weighted image) of the posterior lobe of the pituitary gland on magnetic resonance examination; pituitary stalk rupture (posttraumatic), etc.

DIABETES MELLITUS

Classification

(A) IDIOPATHIC DIABETES: (a) type I: insulin-dependent: familial occurrence in some; (b) type II: non–insulin-dependent: more common in males; strong familial history of diabetes mellitus.

(B) SECONDARY DIABETES: (a) pancreatic disease: congenital pancreatic hypoplasia; pancreatectomy; pancreatitis; hemochromatosis; neoplasms; etc.; (b) insulin receptor abnormalities; (c) hormonal disorders: acromegaly; Cushing syndrome; primary aldosteronism; pheochromocytoma; glucagonoma; etc.; (d) drugs: diuretics; oral contraceptives; glucocorticoids; phenytoin; phenothiazines; tricyclic antidepressants; etc.; (e) pregnancy; (f) genetic syndromes: Prader-Willi syndrome; myotonic dystrophy; hyperlipemias; leprechaunism; Friedreich ataxia; etc.

Clinical Manifestations

(A) MAJOR MANIFESTATIONS: *Polyuria; polydipsia; polyphagia;* weight loss; lethargy; leg cramps; *hyperglycemia* (increased hepatic glucogenesis and reduced tissue uptake); *glycosuria; elevated fasting blood glucose level; ketosis; acidosis; hyperlipoproteinemia;* lower than normal serum values of total and ionized calcium and magnesium.

(B) COMPLICATIONS: (a) *ocular:* blurring of vision; myopia; weakness of accommodation; cataract; lipemia retinalis; diabetic retinopathy; blue-yellow vision deficits; etc.; (b) genitourinary: pyelonephritis; nodular glomerulosclerosis; tubular dysfunction; hypernatremia; hematuria; hypercalciuria; erectile dysfunction; penile necrosis; etc.; (c) dermal: infections; eruptive xanthomatosis; necrobiosis lipoidica diabeticorum; thickening, tightening, and/or waxy quality of the skin; (d) digestive: motility disorders; vomiting; constipation; diarrhea; fecal incontinence; megacolon; esophageal dysfunction; congenital diabetes mellitus and fatal secretory diarrhea in newborn (absence of islets of Langerhans in the pancreas, and diffuse dysplastic changes in small and large intestinal mucosa); cholangitis *(Candida);* necrosis of ileum; (e) neurologic: peripheral neuropathy; cranial nerve dysfunction; autonomic nervous system dysfunction manifested by orthostatic hypotension; decreased sweating; hyperhidrosis; delayed gastric emptying; bowel and bladder distension; megacolon; (f) cardiovascular: hypertension; myocardial infarction; early onset of diabetes often associated with increased left ventricular mass, abnormal contractility, and high blood pressure; atherosclerosis; peripheral vascular disease (detectable by waveform analysis before the vasculopathy becomes clinically apparent).

(C) MISCELLANEOUS: Impaired respiratory function; abnormal zinc metabolism; carnitine insufficiency in children with type I diabetes mellitus; fibrous mastopathy; spontaneous muscular infarction; association with gouty arthritis; calcium pyrophosphate dihydrate deposition disease; ankylosing hyperostosis of the spine; congenital pancreatic agenesis (neonatal diabetes mellitus and pancreatic exocrine insufficiency).

Radiologic Manifestations

(A) SKELETAL SYSTEM: (a) noninfectious manifestations: osteoporosis; glenohumeral periarthritis; flexor tenosynovitis; Dupuytren contracture; carpal tunnel syndrome; neuroarthropathy; diabetic cheiroarthropathy (joint contractures of the fingers and some other joints associated with thickening of the skin); adhesive capsulitis of the hip joint; foot abnormalities (osteoporosis; osteosclerosis; osteolysis; juxtaarticular defects of the cortical bone; ischemic bone necrosis; new bone formation; spontaneous fracture and subluxation; neuropathic arthropathy); less than normal thickness of the heel soft tissues (ultrasonography); muscular infarction; (b) osteomyelitis; septic arthritis; (c) comparison of various imaging modalities in the differential diagnosis of osteomyelitis, neuroarthropathy, and soft-tissue ulcers of the foot: plain radiographs are most specific (83%) and least sensitive (43%); bone scans are most sensitive (93%) and least specific (43%); ^{111}In-labeled leukocyte scan is both sensitive (79%) and specific (78%); magnetic resonance imaging is helpful in differentiating neuroarthropathy from osteomyelitis.

(B) VASCULAR SYSTEM: Arterial calcification (soft tissue; visceral); arterial wall stiffness in insulin-dependent diabetes mellitus; narrowing and rugosities of the leg arteries.

(C) **Digestive System:** Abnormal esophageal function; gastric dilatation with impaired peristalsis; gastric retention; gastric bezoar; retained gastric contrast material on delayed radiographic examination; megacolon.

(D) **Urinary System:** Bilateral renal enlargement; "upside-down" contrast-urine level in glycosuria .

(E) **Central Nervous System:** Cerebral edema with increased intracranial pressure associated with diabetic ketoacidosis; intracerebral hematoma; high risk for metrizamide myelography; cerebral metabolic disturbances shown by proton magnetic resonance spectroscopy in patients with subacute and chronic diabetes mellitus; cerebral atrophy (from the sixth decade on; more common than in nondiabetic control group).

Syndromes Associated with Diabetes Mellitus

1. Alström syndrome: Diabetes mellitus, retinal degeneration, obesity, sensorineural deafness, acanthosis nigricans, male hypogenitalism, and some other abnormalities (renal disease; hyperuricemia; hypertriglyceridemia; kyphosis; baldness; hepatic dysfunction; hypothyroidism); autosomal recessive inheritance.

2. AREDYLD syndrome: *AcroRenal–Ectodermal DYsplasia– Lipo-atrophic Diabetes* syndrome: shortening of the fourth and fifth metacarpals; bowing of tibia; genitourinary abnormalities; hypotrichosis; anodontia; amastia; nonketotic insulin-resistant diabetes; etc.

3. Autosomal dominant insulin resistance syndrome due to a post-banding defect: Obesity, macroorchidism, acanthosis nigricans, hyperinsulinemia, and later overt insulin-resistant diabetes mellitus; curly scalp hair; deficient face and body hair.

4. Bruns-Garland syndrome: Diabetic amyotrophy.

5. Caudal dysplasia sequence (infant of diabetic mother).

6. Mendenhall syndrome (Robson-Mendenhall syndrome): Pineal hyperplasia, insulin-resistant diabetes mellitus associated with dysmorphism, dental precocity, hirsutism, acanthosis nigricans, abdominal protuberance, and phallic enlargement.

7. Primordial bird-headed nanism associated with progressive ataxia, early onset of insulin-resistant diabetes, goiter, and primary gonadal insufficiency.

8. Rosenbloom syndrome: Limited joint mobility, beginning usually in the fifth finger and extending laterally, affecting interphalangeal, metacarpophalangeal, and large joints in children and adolescents with diabetes mellitus.

9. Wolcott-Rallison syndrome: Infancy-onset diabetes mellitus and multiple epiphyseal dysplasia.

10. Wolfram syndrome (DIDMOAD syndrome): *Diabetes Insipidus, Diabetes Mellitus, Optic Atrophy*, and sensorineural *Deafness*;

autosomal recessive inheritance; a neurodegenerative disease; deletion of mitochondrial deoxyribonucleic acid (case report).

11. Familial (apparently autosomal dominant) pancreatic hypoplasia, diabetes mellitus, and congenital heart disease.

12. SHORT syndrome: *S*hort stature, *H*yperextensibility of joint, *O*cular "depression," *R*ieger anomaly, and delayed *T*eething; other manifestations: distinct facial features; partial lipodystrophy; nonketotic hyperglycemia; diabetes mellitus secondary to severe insulin resistance; intrauterine growth retardation; slow weight gain; etc.

DUBIN-JOHNSON SYNDROME

Clinical Manifestations: A defect in the porphyrin metabolism: (a) neonatal cholestasis; chronic or intermittent hyperbilirubinemia (conjugated types predominating); *persistent nonhemolytic hyperbilirubinemia; a black liver; lipochrome-like pigmentation of liver cells;* elevated sulfobromophthalein (Bromsulphalein) level after 2 hours; urinary excretion of coproporphyrin, mostly (80%) as isomer I instead of isomer III; normal total urinary coproporphyrin; (b) autosomal recessive inheritance.

Radiologic Manifestations: (a) computed tomography: increased liver density; (b) ^{99m}Tc HIDA cholescintigraphy: delayed visualization or nonvisualization of the gallbladder and bile duct in association with a prolonged, intense, and homogeneous visualization of the liver.

E

ERDHEIM-CHESTER DISEASE

Clinical Manifestations: Onset of symptoms often in the fifth to seventh decade of life: (a) xanthomatous patches of the eyelids; bone pain; chest pain; cough; sinus discharge; secondary infection; (b) cardiac failure; myocardial infiltration; pericardial infiltration; pulmonary infiltration; (c) miscellaneous abnormalities: hepatosplenomegaly; proptosis; diabetes insipidus; fever; weight loss; renal disease; hypopituitarism; cerebral manifestations with a picture similar to that of multiple sclerosis; progressive cerebellar dysfunction; breast involvement; muscle involvement; etc.

Pathology: *Lipogranulomatous lesion* in the skeletal system, the orbits, retroperitoneum, heart, lungs, kidneys, central nervous system, meninges, pituitary, etc.; bone biopsy (granular lipid-laden histiocytes in the bone marrow, thickened bony trabeculae, and extraosseous discharge of xanthomatous marrow).

Radiologic Manifestations: Appendicular skeleton often involved: (a) *progressive and widespread irregular patchy sclerosis of the medullary region; obliteration of the corticomedullary junction; thick cortices; coarse trabecular architecture;* subperiosteal reaction; epiphyses usually uninvolved or minimally involved; minimal vertebral changes; focal rib lesions (lipid granulomatosis of the ribs); (b) augmented uptake of ^{99m}Tc in the skeletal system at various sites; (c) retroperitoneal and visceral infiltration shown on computed tomographic examination; (d) cardiomegaly; pulmonary infiltration; pleural effusion; (e) retroorbital masses due to diffuse infiltration; proptosis; (f) central nervous system: magnetic resonance imaging: prolonged (weeks) enhancement of the lesions (intraaxial and extraaxial) after injection of gadolinium.

F

FABRY DISEASE (ANDERSON-FABRY SYNDROME)

Enzyme Deficiency: α-galactosidase A.

Clinical Manifestations: Onset of symptoms in childhood or at puberty (heterozygotes less symptomatic than hemizygotes): (a) *acroparesthesias; hypohidrosis;* (b) *angiokeratoma of the skin;* (c) *fever;* (d) *chronic gastrointestinal symptoms:* nausea; vomiting; abdominal pain; (e) *progressive azotemia and renal failure;* (f) varicosities; hemorrhoids; (g) *ocular manifestations:* corneal opacities; aneurysmal dilatation and tortuosity of conjunctival and retinal vessels; haziness or whorled streaks in the corneal epithelium; (h) recurrent hemoptysis; bronchitis; asthmatic wheezing; (i) *renovascular hypertension;* (j) mitral valve prolapse; left ventricular hypertrophy; myocardial infarction or ischemia; complete atrioventricular block; hypertrophic cardiomyopathy in late-onset variant; abnormal electrocardiographic findings (short PR interval; giant negative T waves; high-voltage QRS complexes in the left precordial leads); thromboembolism; (k) *cerebrovascular disease;* dizziness; vertigo; diplopia; dysarthria; aphasia; nystagmus; convulsions; memory loss; autonomic and sensory nerve involvement; etc.; (l) miscellaneous abnormalities: priapism; polyarteritis nodosa–like necrotizing vasculitis; small-bowel ischemia; psychiatric disorders; femoral head avascular necrosis; (m) X-linked recessive inheritance; heterozygous females may be symptomatic; new mutation.

Laboratory Findings: Anemia; proteinuria; azotemia; elevation of the erythrocyte sedimentation rate; urinary sediment containing casts, red cells, and glycolipids; enzyme deficiency (fibroblasts; kidney; heart; serum; leukocytes); prenatal diagnosis by a demonstration of deficient α-galactosidase in cultured cells from amniotic fluid; early diagnosis of enzyme deficiency on chorionic villi biopsies.

Pathology: Disorder of glycolipid metabolism due to a deficiency of the enzyme α-galactosidase A resulting in accumulation of glycosphingolipids in lysosomes of many cell types, particularly in the vascular epithelium (kidney; skin; heart; neural tissues; leukocytes; etc.); typical lamellar inclusions in the lysosomes.

Radiologic Manifestations: (a) *cardiomegaly;* congestive heart failure; highly refractile myocardial echoes very similar to those reported in amyloidosis; (b) hypertensive heart disease; (c) *poor renal function on excretory urography and radionuclide studies;* (d) bowel involvement resulting in thickened mucosal folds of the small bowel and a lack of normal colonic haustration; spasticity; dilatation of the bowel; granular pattern of the ileum; (e) chronic airflow obstruction; pulmonary ventilation and perfusion defects; hyperaeration; bullae; (f) deformities of the hands, wrists, ankles, and feet due to joint involvement; limitation of joint motions; avascular necrosis, particularly the femoral head and talus; (g) central nervous system: (1) magnetic resonance imaging abnormalities involving cerebrum, cerebellum, and brain stem: altered signal (increased; decreased); dilatation of the ventricles and cortical sulci; (2) elongated, ectatic, and tortuous vertebral and basilar arteries.

FAHR DISEASE (FERROCALCINOSIS)

Clinical Manifestations: (a) seizures; tetany; rigidity; tremors; physical retardation; mental deterioration; *progressive development of spasticity and sometimes athetosis,* with progression to a decerebrate state; (b) miscellaneous abnormalities: coincidence with phenylketonuria; twofold increase of cerebrospinal fluid homocarnosine (in autosomal dominant bilateral striopallidodentate calcinosis); mitochondrial myopathy associated with calcification of basal ganglia and endocrine deficits; (c) sporadic; autosomal dominant inheritance in some.

Pathology: Cerebral and cerebellar calcification in the vessel walls and the perivascular spaces of arterioles, capillaries, and veins (basal ganglia; periventricular white matter of the cerebral hemispheres; dentate nuclei of the cerebellum); laser spectroscopy has shown, in addition to calcium, the presence of mucopolysaccharides, zinc, phosphorus, chlorine, iron, aluminum, magnesium, and potassium.

Radiologic Manifestations: (a) *bilateral symmetric calcification of the striatum, pallidum, and dentate nucleus* as the major sites, and the thalamus, cortex, and cerebral and cerebellar white matter as minor sites; (b) magnetic resonance imaging: *varying degrees of signal intensity from the calcified regions* ("black to white"), probably reflecting the different stages of the disease or different metabolic states at the sites of calcium deposition.

FANCONI SYNDROME (DE TONI–DEBRÉ–FANCONI SYNDROME)

Classification: (a) idiopathic; (b) genetic diseases: cystinosis; tyrosinemia; Lowe syndrome; galactosemia; fructose intolerance; Wilson disease; glycogen storage disease; familial nephrosis; defect in complex III of the respiratory chain; (c) acquired diseases: amyloidosis; nephrotic syndrome; multiple myeloma; Sjögren syndrome; renal transplantation; drugs; heavy metals (mercury; lead; etc.); malignant neoplasms; etc.

Clinical Manifestations: Triad of *glycosuria, generalized aminoaciduria, and hypophosphatemia* (due to a defect in phosphate reabsorption and phosphaturia): (a) dwarfism; muscle weakness; anorexia; vomiting; inanition; photophobia with cystine deposits in the cornea; chronic acidosis; uremia; hypouricemia; hypokalemia; (b) miscellaneous abnormalities: hypercalciuria; elevated serum 1,25-dihydroxyvitamin D concentration; acute neurologic deterioration resembling Leigh syndrome; muscle cytochrome *c* oxidase deficiency; mitochondrial myopathy with lactic acidemia; ifosfamide-induced Fanconi syndrome and rickets in children with Wilms tumor; deletion of the mitochondrial deoxyribonucleic acid in a case of association of Fanconi and Pearson syndromes.

Associations with Fanconi Syndrome: (1) hepatic failure, lactic acidemia, and defective activity of hepatic succinate: cytochrome *c* reductase; (2) diabetes mellitus and idiopathic Fanconi syndrome; (3) familial Fanconi syndrome associated with hypoglycemia, progressive liver failure, neurologic deterioration, and mitochondrial phosphoenolpyruvate carboxykinase deficiency; (4) familial Fanconi syndrome with malabsorption and galactose intolerance; (5) acute tubulointerstitial nephritis with uveitis syndrome presenting as multiple tubular dysfunction, including Fanconi syndrome; (6) ichthyosis, dysmorphism, jaundice, and diarrhea.

Radiologic Manifestations: (a) *rickets or osteomalacia resistant to vitamin D in the usual dose;* (b) poor renal uptake of Tc99m DMSA and high urinary concentration of the tracer.

FARBER DISEASE (LIPOGRANULOMATOSIS)

Enzyme Deficiency: Deficiency of lysosomal enzyme acid ceramidase resulting in tissue storage of ceramide (subcutaneous; kidney; brain; etc.).
Clinical Manifestations: Symptomatic in the first few months of life:

(a) failure to thrive; cachexia; projectile vomiting; cutaneous pigmented lesions over bony prominences; xanthoma-like lesions on the face and hands; *nodular masses mainly over the wrist and ankles; hoarseness* and later laryngeal obstruction; hyperesthesia; *joint swelling and contracture;* hepatosplenomegaly; *mental and neurologic deterioration;* (b) *ceramidase activity deficiency in various tissues* (skin; fibroblasts; white blood cells; liver; chorionic villi; etc.); (c) miscellaneous abnormalities: diarrhea; cholelithiasis; transient proteinuria; increased urinary total sialic acids; hydrops fetalis; (d) autosomal recessive inheritance.

Radiologic Manifestations: (a) *generalized demineralization; nodular tumefaction about the peripheral joints; joint capsular distension;* subluxation of hip joints due to distension; *juxtaarticular bone erosions;* flaring of costochondral junctions; (b) *muscle atrophy;* (c) miscellaneous abnormalities: *pulmonary interstitial finely nodular infiltrates;* internal hydrocephalus.

FLUOROSIS

Clinical Manifestations

(A) CHRONIC POISONING: (a) *skeletal manifestations:* painful limbs; joint deformities; knock-knee; bowlegs; saber shins; limited joint motions; stiffness and rigidity of the spine; thoracic kyphosis; (b) myelopathy caused by compression of the spinal cord; (c) *dental mottling;* (d) abdominal pain; atrophic gastritis, loss of microvilli, and cracked-clay appearance and surface abrasions on the mucosal cells; (e) decreased testosterone concentrations in male patients with skeletal fluorosis; (f) increased total body calcium (neutron activation analysis).

(B) ACUTE POISONING: Nausea, vomiting, diarrhea, abdominal pain, and paresthesia.

Radiologic Manifestations

(A) CHILDREN: Ground-glass density of the calvaria; lack of a normal distinct diploic space; sharp borders of the cranial sutures; absence of the lamina dura; wide vertebral bodies and dense end-plates; relative thickening of intervertebral disc spaces; a combination of a radiologic picture of osteomalacia, osteoporosis, and osteosclerosis; thickened ribs; serrations along the iliac crests.

(B) ADULTS: Thickened and dense skull, particularly at the base; irregularity and hypercementosis of dental roots; resorption of periodontal bone; sclerosis of the vertebrae; calcification of the spinous ligaments; osteophytosis of vertebral bodies; generalized skeletal sclerosis associated with narrowing of thickened bony trabeculae; periostitis deformans; needlelike calcific projections at sites of attachment of the intercostal muscles; calcification of the interosseous ligaments and joint capsules; osteoporosis as the earliest detectable radiographic change; intense skeletal uptake of 99Tc MDP.

FUCOSIDOSIS

Enzyme Deficiency: A lysosomal storage disorder caused by deficiency of α-L-fucosidase enzyme leading to an accumulation of fucosyl compounds (glycolipids, lipoproteins, oligosaccharides, and polysaccharide) in almost all organs; prenatal diagnosis of enzyme deficiency from cultured amniocytes.

Clinical Manifestations: (a) *Hurler-like clinical features* with a coarse facies, prominent forehead, hypertelorism, broad and flattened nose, heavy eyebrows, large tongue, thick lips, dental anomalies (number, morphology), broad thorax, lumbar hyperlordosis, hepatosplenomegaly, and recurrent respiratory infections; (b) *deteriorating psychomotor achievements; peripheral neuropathy;* amyotrophy; muscular weakness; hypotonia changing to hypertonia, spastic quadriplegia; decorticate and/or decerebrate rigidity; (c) *angiokeratoma corporis diffusum;* thick skin; thin dry skin; (d) recurrent respiratory infections; (e) autosomal recessive inheritance; disease-causing mutations.

Laboratory Findings: (a) histochemical and ultrastructural abnormalities on the biopsy specimens (skin; conjunctiva; rectal mucosa): abnormal macrophages filled with fucose-rich granules; characteristic inclusions in the endothelial cells, fibroblasts, and Schwann cells; (b) prenatal diagnosis of enzyme deficiency from cultured amniocytes.

Radiologic Manifestations: (a) skull: progressive thickening of the diploic spaces, particularly over the frontal and supraorbital region; early synostosis of one or more cranial sutures; absent or poorly developed paranasal sinuses; (b) spine: short odontoid; cervical platyspondyly; kyphosis at the thoracolumbar junction; anterior beaking of the lower thoracic and lumbar vertebrae; scoliosis; small fifth lumbar vertebra; vacuum discs; short sacrum with square-shaped vertebrae; absent or rudimentary coccyx; (c) chest: medial widening and slight shortening of the clavicles; spatulated ribs; slightly widened and poorly developed glenoids; (d) pelvis and limbs: sclerosis; scalloping and widening of the acetabular roofs; flattening and irregularity of the femoral heads; enlargement and shortening of femoral necks; coxa valga; widening of the shaft of long bones; thin cortex; (e) retarded skeletal maturation; (f) cerebral atrophy.

G

GALACTOSEMIA

Enzyme Deficiency: One of the three enzyme deficiencies: galactose-1-phosphate uridyltransferase (the most common); galactokinase; epimerase.

Clinical Manifestations: (a) neonate: symptoms develop with milk feeding: *lethargy; hypotonia; vomiting; diarrhea; failure to thrive; jaundice; hepatomegaly;* renal tubular damage; susceptibility to infection; signs of increased intracranial pressure (cerebral edema); cataracts developing within the first month of life; *hypoglycemia; elevated galactose metabolites in urine; galactosuria;* assays for demonstrating enzyme deficiency (red cells; leukocytes; etc.); prenatal diagnosis from cultured amniotic fluid cell or chorionic villi (galactose-1-phosphate uridyltransferase deficiency); (b) childhood (untreated patients; occasionally also in treated patients): *mental retardation; physical retardation; tremor; cerebellar dysfunction; verbal dyspraxia; spasticity; cataracts; progressive hepatocellular damage; liver dysfunctions; liver cirrhosis;* ovarian hypofunction; *galactosuria;* (c) adulthood: late onset of neurologic symptoms: cerebellar disorders; generalized seizures; progressive apraxia; etc; (d) autosomal recessive inheritance.

Radiologic Manifestations: *Cerebral edema* in newborns; multiple small hyperintense lesions in the cerebral white matter on T_2-weighted images; absence of normal drop-off in peripheral white-matter signal intensity on intermediate- and T_2-weighted images (children over 1 year of age without measurable transferase activity); *cerebral atrophy, cerebellar atrophy;* diminished bone mineralization.

GALACTOSIALIDOSIS

Enzyme Deficiencies: Combined ß-galactosidase and *N*-acetyl-neuraminidase.

Clinical Manifestations: Phenotypic variations: (a) early infantile type: mild to severe course (similar to that of GM_1 gangliosidosis): *hydrops fetalis; ascites; coarse face; cherry-red macular spot; hepatosplenomegaly;* early death; (b) late infantile form (onset at 6 to 12 months of age): *dysmorphism; organomegaly; cherry-red spot; mental retardation;* myoclonus; hazy cornea; pyramidal tract signs secondary to white-matter disease; abnormalities of electroencephalogram and evoked potentials; (c) childhood-adulthood presentation: *corneal clouding; cherry-red spot; various neurologic symptoms; myoclonus; mental retardation;* (d) laboratory findings: anemia; proteinuria; reduced amount of 32 kDa phosphoglycoprotein associated with ß-galactosidase and α-neuraminidase in lysosomes; heterogeneity of carboxypeptidase activity in infantile-onset galactosialidosis; biochemical findings suggesting a variant of galactosialidosis associated with congenital malformations, including complex cyanotic congenital heart disease; dense granular inclusions (conjunctival biopsy in adult form in two siblings); (e) miscellaneous abnormalities: *Hurler-like picture;* cardiomyopathy; mitral and aortic valvular disease; kidney enlargement;

hernias; hypotonia; frequent infections; presentation with congenital adrenal hyperplasia; (f) autosomal recessive inheritance.

Radiologic Manifestations: (a) *dysostosis multiplex* in most severe cases; (b) *organomegaly;* increased renal echogenicity; congenital adrenal hyperplasia; (c) central nervous system: white-matter disease; increased thalamic density (computed tomography); delayed myelination; mild to moderate global brain atrophy.

Note: The terms *Goldberg syndrome* and *Goldberg-Wenger syndrome* refer to the child-adult form of this metabolic disorder.

GAUCHER DISEASE (CEREBROSIDE LIPIDOSIS)

Enzyme Deficiency: Absence or severe deficiency of glucocerebrosidase (the enzyme necessary for the hydrolysis of glucosylceramide to glucose and ceramide), resulting in accumulation of insoluble glucocerebroside in the reticuloendothelial cells of the liver, spleen, and bone marrow. Very rarely, a deficiency of saposin, a cofactor needed for the catalytic function of glucocerebrosidase, may cause the disease.

Classification: Three types representing different allelic disorders with different mutations in the structural gene of the deficient enzyme:

(A) TYPE 1 ("ADULT FORM"; CHRONIC NONNEUROPATHIC): Most common type; clinical presentation at any age; skin pigmentation, bone lesions, hypersplenism, and pingueculae; about 99% of all the cases of Gaucher disease are the type 1.

(B) TYPE 2 (ACUTE NEUROPATHIC FORM): Onset of symptoms in infancy and the clinical picture of pseudobulbar palsy.

(C) TYPE 3 (SUBACUTE NEUROPATHIC; JUVENILE FORM): Onset usually in childhood; slow and progressive neurologic manifestations (hypertonicity; seizures; gait problems; mental retardation; etc.).

Clinical Manifestations: (a) *bone and joint pain; bone tenderness;* fever; purpura; epistaxis; hemorrhagic infarcts; hematuria; conjunctival pigmentation; abnormal skin pigmentations; abdominal fullness; *hepatosplenomegaly;* hypersplenism; pulmonary function abnormalities (airway obstruction with reduced expiratory flow; reduced lung volume; alveolar-capillary diffusion abnormality); (b) anemia; thrombocytopenia; leukopenia; (c) *Gaucher cells in the bone marrow; acid β-glucosidase activity deficiency in fibroblasts and circulating white blood cells;* (d) increased risk of cancer in late adulthood; especially hematopoietic in origin; (e) autosomal recessive inheritance; genetic heterogeneity within and among subtypes; the gene of glucocerebrosidase located in the region of q21 of chromosome 1.

Radiologic Manifestations

(A) BONES: (a) *resorption of bone trabeculae; coarse foamlike appearance; moth-eaten pattern; pathologic sclerotic changes; expansion of bones (Erlenmeyer flask deformity of the femora); periosteal reaction with a solid or lacelike type of subperiosteal new bone formation;* pathologic fractures; collapse of the femoral head; enlarged phalangeal nutrient foramina; small tubular hands and feet involvement similar to those of thalassemia major (osteoporosis, reticulated trabecular pattern, widening of the medullary cavity, and thinned cortex); collapse of the vertebrae; thinning and deformity of the ribs and slender long bones in neonatal disease; degenerative articular changes; extradural compression of the spinal cord associated with vertebral collapse in type 1; rare involvement of the skull; (b) computed tomography in type 1: abnormal cortical density; expansion of the marrow space; abnormal attenuation of the marrow cavity; calcification in the marrow cavity; decreased trabecular bone mass and diminished bone marrow fat shown by quantitative computed tomography; (c) magnetic resonance imaging: nonhomogeneous reduction in both T_1- and T_2-weighted marrow signals, with increased T_2 signals during avascular episodes; (d) scintigraphy: peripheral expansion of normal marrow; greater marrow expansion with patchy areas lacking uptake, or a greater loss of uptake with retention of the nuclide in other reticuloendothelioid organs and circulation; imaging in "bone crisis" in type 1 (decreased uptake of radionuclide at the onset of the crisis, followed by formation of a ring of increased uptake after 6 weeks, and return to "normal" in about 6 months); (e) In-111 leukocyte imaging: hepatomegaly; lack of central marrow activity; extensive lymph node uptake; etc.

(B) **SPLEEN:** *Splenomegaly;* hypoechoic lesions (focal homogeneous clusters of Gaucher cells); hyperechoic lesions (Gaucher cells; fibrosis); splenic nodules with varied signal intensity (isointense on T_1-weighted and hypointense on T_2-weighted images); subcapsular fluid collection; infarction; obstruction of the splenic vein.

(C) **LIVER:** *Hepatomegaly;* lobulation of the liver surface; increased echogenicity of the liver; central areas of decreased attenuation (computed tomography); focal areas of signal intensity (stellate or segmental) (magnetic resonance imaging).

(D) **LUNGS:** Reticulonodular densities; pulmonary hypertension.

(E) **MISCELLANEOUS ABNORMALITIES:** Combined portal and vena caval hypertension; exaggerated anterior vertebral notching; central depression of multiple vertebral end-plates; bone lesions simulating osteomyelitis; intramedullary hemorrhage associated with "bone crisis"; mitral valve involvement (stenosis; regurgitation; calcification); aortic valve involvement (thick; restricted motion; stenosis); intrathoracic extramedullary hematopoiesis.

GILBERT SYNDROME

Enzyme Deficiency: Reduction in the activity of hepatic bilirubin UDP-glucuronosyltransferase.

Clinical and Radiologic Manifestations: (a) fatigue; weakness; abdominal pain; *jaundice due to low-grade unconjugated hyperbilirubinemia;* normal liver biopsy findings; normal biliary system in the presence of jaundice; association with chronic fatigue syndrome; (b) autosomal dominant inheritance; isolated sporadic cases; caused by heterozygous missense mutation in the gene for bilirubin UDP-glucuronosyltransferase.

GLUCAGONOMA SYNDROME

Clinical Manifestations: Pancreatic α-cell tumor (glucagonoma): (a) *necrolytic migratory erythematous rash; angular stomatitis; painful glossitis; cheilitis;* (b) *normochromic normocytic anemia;* (c) *diabetes mellitus;* (d) *tumor identification: immunocytochemistry with glucagon antibodies;* low level of serum amino acids; hypoproteinemia; (e) miscellaneous abnormalities: tendency to thrombosis; weight loss; neuropsychiatric disorders; high plasma glucagon concentration.

Radiologic Manifestations: Demonstration of *pancreatic tumor* by various imaging techniques (ultrasonography; computed tomography; magnetic resonance imaging; arteriography); selective sampling of glucagon concentration at various locations in the pancreatic vein.

GLUTARIC ACIDURIA TYPE I

Enzyme Deficiency: Glutaryl-coenzyme A dehydrogenase deficiency.

Clinical Manifestations: Onset of symptoms usually in infancy: (a) *macrocephaly,* present at or shortly after birth, often preceding the neurologic disease; *acute encephalopathic episode; progressive dystonia and dyskinesia; spastic paralysis; mental, psychomotor, and social developmental delay;* (b) *excessive levels of glutaric and 3-hydroxyglutaric acids in urine; absence of demonstrable functional levels of glutaryl-CoA dehydrogenase in fibroblasts and leukocytes;* reduced serum carnitine; (c) prenatal diagnosis by testing for glutaric acid concentration in amniotic fluid and glutaryl-CoA dehydrogenase activity in cultured amniotic cells; (d) improvement after dietary therapy and prevention of catabolism during febrile illness; (e) autosomal recessive inheritance; clinical variability among homozygous individuals.

Radiologic Manifestations: *Generalized cerebral atrophy or hypoplasia, most prominent in the frontal and temporal lobes;* bilateral symmetric progressive demyelination; hypodensity of the lenticular nuclei (computed tomography), hypodensity of caudate; enlargement of the subarachnoid space (external hydrocephalus); *dilatation of the insular cisterns; "bat wing" dilatation of the sylvian fissures; bilateral arachnoid cysts of the temporal fossa.*

Note: Glutaric aciduria type II: multiple acyl-CoA dehydrogenase deficiency; hepatopathy, encephalopathy, cardiopathy, renal and brain malformations, including fetal polycystic kidneys, and symmetric hypoplasia of the temporal lobes.

GLYCOGEN STORAGE DISEASE TYPE I (VON GIERKE DISEASE)

Classification: (a) type Ia: glucose-6-phosphatase deficiency in liver, kidney, and intestine: hepatomegaly, nephromegaly, hypoglycemia, lactic acidemia, and hyperuricemia; (b) type Ib: glucose-6-phosphate translocase deficiency (T1); (c) type Ic: phosphotranslocase deficiency (T2): hepatomegaly.

Clinical Manifestations: Onset of symptoms in infancy: (a) failure to thrive; (b) *massive hepatomegaly;* (c) convulsions; repeated episodes of *hypoglycemia and acidosis;* hyperlipidemia; hyperuricemia; gouty arthritis; abnormal renal function; (d) miscellaneous abnormalities: hemorrhagic pancreatitis; familial bleeding tendency; recurrent infections; peliosis hepatis in type Ia; hyperlipidemia; vasoconstrictive type of pulmonary hypertension (a fatal complication); chronic renal disease, proteinuria, and urolithiasis (case report); amyloidosis; (e) autosomal recessive inheritance.

Type Ib Manifestations: Growth failure; hepatomegaly; splenomegaly; nephromegaly; hypoglycemia; lactic acidosis; neutrophil deficiency (impaired neutrophil chemotaxis and metabolism); inflammatory diseases; hyperlipidemia; generalized amyloidosis; ocular changes (delayed appearance of the choroidal flush on fluorescein angiography; atrophy of the retinal pigment epithelium and choriocapillaries; etc.).

Radiologic Manifestations: (a) *hepatomegaly;* variable attenuation coefficient of liver on computed tomographic examination depending on simultaneous glycogen deposition and fatty infiltration; liver tumor (adenoma; carcinoma; hepatoblastoma); liver focal nodular hyperplasia; (b) *progressive enlargement of the kidneys;* increased attenuation coefficient of the renal cortex due to glycogen deposition (computed tomographic); echogenic kidneys; nephrocalcinosis in type Ia; renal calculi; (c) skeletal changes: retarded bone maturation; multiple growth arrest lines; overconstriction of the long bones; pseudo-Madelung deformity; widening of distal aspects of the metacarpals; coxa valga; anteriorly scalloped vertebral bodies; Schmorl nodes; exaggerated lumbosacral lordosis; scoliosis; osteoporosis; pathologic fracture; gouty changes; (d) radionuclide study: hepatomegaly with diminished radionuclide accumulation; splenomegaly with increased uptake; (e) miscellaneous abnormalities: smooth-walled, slightly narrow colon and absence of haustrations; moyamoya; acute or chronic pancreatitis (pseudocyst formation) in type Ia; polycystic ovaries.

GLYCOGEN STORAGE DISEASE TYPE II (POMPE DISEASE)

Enzyme Deficiency: Deficiency of acid α-D-glucosidase, demonstrable in the liver, muscle, fibroblasts, and chorionic villi.

Clinical Manifestations: Generalized involvement, particularly the heart, nerves, and muscles.

(A) TYPE IIA (INFANTILE FORM): (a) hypotonicity; difficulty in sucking; dyspnea; diaphragmatic paralysis in infancy; circumoral cyanosis; irritability; failure to thrive; macroglossia; (b) cardiac involvement: Wolff-Parkinson-White syndrome; supraventricular tachycardia; ventricular fibrillation; left-axis deviation; short PR interval; huge QRS complexes; T-wave inversion; (c) rapid progression of disease, with the development of firm muscles, loss of deep tendon reflexes, respiratory infections, and cardiac failure; (d) oligosaccharide excretion.

(B) TYPE IIB (JUVENILE FORM): Muscular involvement (weakness with a clinical picture similar to pseudohypertrophic muscular dystrophy; firm muscles); intercostal muscle disease predisposing to recurrent pneumonia; oligosaccharide excretion.

(C) TYPE IIC (ADULT FORM): Progressive myopathy (striated muscles); diaphragmatic paralysis; oligosaccharide excretion.

(D) Autosomal recessive inheritance; extensive heterogeneity; mutations and deletions.

Radiologic Manifestations: (a) *moderate to massive cardiomegaly* with normal pulmonary vasculature or vascular congestion in some; (b) echocardiography, cardioangiography, and magnetic resonance imaging: *marked thickening of the ventricular wall; significant obstruction of the left ventricular outflow region;* pronounced systolic anterior motion of the anterior mitral valve leaflet; irregular inhomogeneous appearance of the myocardium; (c) radionuclide cardiography: muscular hypertrophy; hypokinesis of the ventricles; (d) muscular abnormalities: diaphragmatic paralysis; atrophy of posterior paraspinal and psoas muscles.

GLYCOGEN STORAGE DISEASE TYPE III (CORI DISEASE; FORBES DISEASE)

Enzyme Deficiency: Amylo-1,6-glucosidase.

Clinical and Radiologic Manifestations: Phenotypic variability: (a) short stature; protuberant abdomen; hepatomegaly; hepatic cirrhosis (rare); splenomegaly; portal hypertension; (b) hypoglycemia with failure to respond to glucagon; ketoacidosis; hyperlipidemia; (c) myopathic pattern; "mixed" (neuromyopathic) pattern; peripheral neuropathy; (d) hypertrophic cardiomyopathy; ventricular tachycardia; (e) debranching enzyme deficiency in liver, muscle, red and white blood cells, fibroblasts, etc.; (f) prenatal diagnosis: quantitative assay for debranching enzyme activity, and immunoblot analysis with a polyclonal antibody prepared against purified porcine-muscle debranching enzyme; (g) skin biopsy: glycogen storage in epithelial secretory cells of eccrine sweat glands and in the smooth muscle fibers of the erector pili; (h) miscellaneous abnormalities: deficient cranio-facial development; narrow upper jaw; taurodontism of the primary denti-tion; polycystic ovaries; (i) autosomal recessive inheritance.

GLYCOGEN STORAGE DISEASE TYPE IV (ANDERSEN DISEASE; AMYLOPECTINOSIS)

Enzyme Deficiency: The branching enzyme (α–1,4-glucan:α–1,4-glu-can 6-glycosyltransferase).

Clinical and Radiologic Manifestations: Onset in early infancy, vari-able clinical manifestations: (a) hepatomegaly; splenomegaly; *progressive hepatic cirrhosis;* portal hypertension; ascites, esophageal varices; (b) *fail-ure to thrive;* (c) hypotonia; (d) *enzyme deficiency* demonstrable in cul-tured skin fibroblasts and leukocytes; (e) miscellaneous abnormalities: congenital variant (fetal hypokinesia sequence with arthrogryposis and lung hypoplasia); a mild juvenile variant; progressive cardiac failure fol-lowing orthotopic liver transplantation (cardiac amylopectinosis); hepato-cellular adenoma; nonprogressive liver form; three point mutations in the glycogen-branching enzyme.

GLYCOGEN STORAGE DISEASE TYPE V (MCARDLE DISEASE)

Enzyme Deficiency: Myophosphorylase.

Clinical Manifestations: The disease usually becomes evident in childhood or adolescence: (a) *severe muscle cramps; inability to sustain exercise; muscle wasting;* low back pain; myofascial pain dysfunction syn-drome; intermittent claudication of the masseter muscles; *acute oliguric renal failure;* (b) *myoglobulinuria and creatinuria after vigorous exercise; failure of venous lactate to increase after exercise;* (c) *muscle biopsy: excess glycogen; decreased muscle phosphorylase activity;* (d) leukocyte testing diagnostic in about 90% of patients; hyperuricemia; hypogamma-globulinemia; (e) genetically heterogeneous: autosomal recessive inheri-tance; dominant transmission occasionally.

Radiologic Manifestations: (a) computed tomography: *posterior paraspinal muscle atrophy,* psoas muscles usually spared; (b) renal angiog-raphy: preferential diffuse reduction in cortical perfusion; attenuation of distal interlobar and arcuate arteries; absence of cortical nephrogram; delayed clearing of contrast medium through the renal parenchyma; (c) ^{31}P nuclear magnetic resonance test: *no drop in intramuscular pH; excessive* *reduction in phosphocreatine in response to exercise; failure of glycogen breakdown and formation of lactic acid;* (d) magnetic resonance imaging: much less increase in T_2 of the muscle after exercise (as compared with normal subjects).

GM₁ GANGLIOSIDOSIS (Gangliosidosis GM₁; Norman-Landing Disease)

Enzyme Deficiency: Lysosomal acid ß-galactosidase.

Clinical Manifestations: A generalized sphingolipidosis; storage of GM_1 ganglioside and oligosaccharides in the brain and viscera.

(A) GM₁ Gangliosidosis Type I (Infantile): (a) *retarded psychomotor development from birth;* (b) *abnormal facial features:* frontal bossing; depression of the nasal bridge; large low-set ears and a long upper lip; (c) *hepatosplenomegaly;* (d) *dorsal kyphoscoliosis;* enlarged and stiff wrist and ankle joints; *short and stubby fingers with flexion contracture;* (e) cherry-red macular changes; (f) vacuolized lymphocytes and marrow cells; normal levels of urinary mucopolysaccharide; increased GM_1 ganglioside in the brain and ganglioside and mucopolysaccharide levels in the viscera; deficiency of ß-galactosidase activity in leukocytes, urine, brain, liver, or cultured skin fibroblasts; enzyme assays of cultured amniotic fluid cells; detection of galactosyl-oligosaccharides in amniotic fluid with high-performance liquid chromatography; (g) anomalous eosinophil granulocytes in the blood and bone marrow; etc.

(B) GM₁ Gangliosidosis Type II (Juvenile): Onset of symptoms in the first 2 years of life: (a) mental and motor retardation; spasticity; ataxia; seizures; dystonia; dementia; absence of Hurler-like features; slight to moderate organomegaly; (b) foam cells in the bone marrow; vacuolated cells in the liver, spleen, and glomeruli; deficient ß-galactosidase activity in leukocytes, brain, liver, and cultured fibroblasts.

(C) Adult GM₁ Gangliosidosis: Onset of clinical manifestations usually in the teens; wide range of clinical manifestations: *gait and speech disturbances caused by persistent muscle hypertonia; dystonic postures and movements; facial grimacing; parkinsonian manifestations;* seizures; near-normal intellect to severe intellectual impairment.

(D) Autosomal recessive inheritance.

Radiologic Manifestations

(A) GM₁ Gangliosidosis Type I (Infantile): (a) *gibbus deformity; beaking and hypoplasia of the vertebral bodies; thin cortices* of the tubular bones; coarse trabecular pattern; *marked subperiosteal new bone formation of the humeri and medullary expansion; widened ribs; flaring and cupping of the metaphyses (wrists, knees, and ankles in particular); stippled calcific densities in the ankle and some other joint regions;* (b) miscellaneous abnormalities: neonatal ascites; brain atrophy; areas of decreased attenuation in the white matter (computed tomography); thalamic hyperdensity on computed tomography; short trachea.

(B) GM$_1$ Gangliosidosis (Juvenile and Adult Types): Variable skeletal abnormalities (normal or dysplastic): (a) cortical thinness of the long bones; dysplasia of the femoral head; hypoplasia of the vertebral bodies; flatness of the vertebral bodies; osteosclerosis of the skull; etc.; (b) miscellaneous abnormalities: *hyperintensity lesions in the putamen on T$_2$-weighted and proton density images;* ventriculomegaly; brain atrophy; atrophy of the caudate nuclei.

GM$_2$ GANGLIOSIDOSIS

Enzyme Deficiencies: (a) Tay-Sachs disease (the B variant; GM$_2$ gangliosidosis type I) with *N*-acetyl-ß-hexosaminidase A deficiency; (b) Sandhoff disease (the 0 variant) with deficiency of both ß-hexosaminidase A and B; (c) type AB, with deficiency of GM$_2$ activator protein; (d) B$_1$ variant type, which has an altered substrate specific of ß-hexosaminidase A.

Clinical Manifestations

(A) Tay-Sachs Disease and Sandhoff Disease (Infantile Form): Onset of symptoms during the first 6 months of life: (a) normal-appearing at birth; *"doll-like" appearance (Tay-Sachs disease) in infancy; apathy; hypotonia; developmental arrest followed by regression; exaggerated startle response to noise; seizures; decerebrate rigidity;* (b) *blindness; cherry-red macular spot; optic atrophy;* (c) *enzyme deficiency in serum and tissues;* (d) prenatal diagnosis made by measuring the enzyme in amniotic fluid, cultured amniocytes, or chorionic villi samples; immunofluorescence analysis of ganglioside GM$_2$ in cultured amniocytes by confocal laser scanning microscope; deoxyribonucleic acid–based test as an adjunct to screen carriers; hepatosplenomegaly (in some cases of Sandhoff disease).

(B) Tay-Sachs Disease and Sandhoff Disease (Juvenile and Adult Forms): (a) significant clinical and enzymatic heterogeneity; lower motor neuron, pyramidal tract, and cerebellar deterioration; (b) miscellaneous abnormalities: late-onset Tay-Sachs disease presenting as catatonic schizophrenia; adult form of Sandhoff disease with atypical manifestations (progressive spinal muscular atrophy of the limb-girdle type, sensory polyneuropathy, and cerebellar ataxia).

(C) Autosomal recessive inheritance; a predilection for Ashkenazi Jews in Tay-Sachs disease; no racial preference in Sandhoff disease.

Radiologic Manifestations: Variable computed tomographic and magnetic resonance imaging manifestations in different phases of the disease and in different types: (a) involvement of the white matter, caudate nucleus, thalamus, and putamen in the early phase of the disease: high signal intensity on T_2-weighted images, starting from the occipital and temporal regions; (b) later phase: involvement of thalamus, basal ganglia, and the white matter everywhere in the brain: (1) hyperintensity in the basal ganglia, thalamus, and along the cortical layer of the cerebrum on T_1-weighted images that appear hypointense on T_2-weighted images; enlarged caudate nuclei protruding into lateral ventricles; brain atrophy; (2) computed tomography: thalamic hyperdensity; (c) ultrasonography: increased echogenicity of thalamus.

GOUT

Classification: Idiopathic; associated with other metabolic disorders; drug-induced.

Clinical Manifestations: Acute gouty arthritis or chronic tophaceous gout (deposition of monosodium urate crystals in tissues from supersaturated extracellular fluid): (a) *arthritis* involving various joints, with a predilection for joints of the lower limbs (shoulders, sacroiliac joints, and spine rarely involved); soft-tissue swelling and nodular masses in the paraarticular regions; (b) *hyperuricemia, deposition of monosodium urate crystals in joints and periarticular tissues;* (c) *gouty renal disease;* renal failure; nephrolithiasis; (d) miscellaneous abnormalities: most gouty arthritis in women is postmenopausal and often associated with renal insufficiency; neuropathy; carpal tunnel syndrome (gouty tenosynovitis); finger pad tophi; Charcot-like joint in tophaceous gout; (e) in some familial cases autosomal dominant factors have been suggested and, in others, X-linked factors suggested.

Radiologic Manifestations: (a) *soft-tissue swelling; nodular paraarticular densities; calcification or ossification of tophi;* (b) *arthritis:* preservation of the articular space in the early stage of disease; narrowing of joints in the advanced stage; intraarticular milk of calcium in saturnine gout; (c) *bone erosions in articular and/or periarticular regions;* expansile bone lesions with bony spurs extending into periosseous soft tissues; osteophytosis; cyst-like or punched-out bone lesions surrounded by minimal sclerotic changes; enlarged ulnar styloid process; club-shaped deformity of the metacarpal, metatarsal, and phalangeal heads; thickening of the diaphyses; pseudotumor of the outer end of the clavicle (saturnine gout); isolated or dominant lesions of patella; pathologic fracture of the patella; intraosseous calcification in tophaceous gout; recurrent atraumatic hemarthrosis; (d) miscellaneous abnormalities: narrowing of intervertebral disc spaces; erosion of endplates; erosion of the odontoid process; subluxation of the atlas; sacroiliac joint lesions with bone erosion; osteoporosis.

Note: Renal stone formation and crystal nephropathy in infants and children may result from inherited deficiencies of purine salvage enzymes (hypoxanthine-guanine phosphoribosyltransferase and adenine phosphoribosyltransferase) or the catabolic enzyme xanthine dehydrogenase.

H

HALLERVORDEN-SPATZ DISEASE

Clinical Manifestations: Onset often in adolescence; onset in childhood and adulthood less common: (a) progressive pyramidal and extrapyramidal signs, predominantly in the lower limbs; *generalized dystonia with predominance of oromandibular involvement; muscular rigidity; involuntary movements; choreoathetosis; tremor; behavioral changes; progressive loss of verbal communication; dementia; retinal degeneration;* (b) autosomal recessive inheritance.

Pathology: A degenerative disorder with excess deposition of iron-containing pigments within the globus pallidus, pars reticularis of the substantia nigra, and red nuclei; pallidal demyelination and focal axonal swellings in the pallidonigral system and the cortex; accumulation of ceroid-lipofuscin and neuromelanin; osmiophilic deposits in cytosomes (bone marrow biopsy; electron microscopy of the buffy coat); sea-blue histiocytes and cytoplasmic inclusions in circulating lymphocytes.

Radiologic Manifestations: (a) computed tomography: *cerebral atrophy; symmetric areas of increased density in the globus pallidus; flattening of caudate nuclei heads; basal ganglia mineralization;* (b) magnetic resonance imaging: *decreased signal intensity of the basal ganglia; changing pattern on T_2-weighted images of pallidi during the progressive course of the disease: increased signal intensity; decreased signal intensity (iron deposition); the eye-of-the-tiger sign (area of loose tissue with vacuolization);* ferrokinetic evaluation (increased uptake of ^{59}Fe in the basal ganglia).

HEMOCHROMATOSIS

Classification: (a) *primary (hereditary hemochromatosis):* four types: (1) classic type, with elevated transferrin saturation, serum ferritin levels, and liver iron content; (2) severe iron overload presenting at an early age; (3) elevated total-body iron stores, normal serum ferritin levels, and transferrin saturation; (4) markedly elevated transferrin saturation and serum ferritin levels, minimal elevation in total-body iron stores; (b) *secondary:* multiple blood transfusions; refractory anemia; liver cirrhosis; chronic excessive iron intake; portal-to-systemic venous shunts; (c) *neonatal* *hemochromatosis* (reported in sibs): pathologic similarities to hereditary hemochromatosis as seen in adults, but the human leukocyte antigen associations seen in adult hemochromatosis are absent.

Clinical Manifestations: Onset of symptoms in primary hemochromatosis is usually between 40 and 60 years of age, rarely in childhood or young adulthood: (a) *bronze pigmentation of the skin;* (b) *liver cirrhosis;* hepatomegaly; splenomegaly; (c) diabetes mellitus (bronze diabetes); (d) *cardiac arrhythmias;* congestive heart failure, cardiac dysfunction as a presenting manifestation of the disease in some cases; ventricular abnormality on echocardiography and blood pool imaging (ventricular size and function); sick sinus syndrome; early death due to cardiac dysfunction; (e) *arthralgia,* particularly of the second and third metacarpophalangeal joints; (f) hypogonadotropic hypogonadism: loss of libido; impotence; amenorrhea, absence of spermatozoa in the seminal fluid; impaired spermatogenesis shown by testicular biopsy; (g) *increased serum iron levels; almost complete saturation of iron-binding capacity;* (h) neuromuscular disorders: weakness; decreased hearing; confusion; dementia; rigidity; myoclonic jerks; ataxia; peripheral neuropathy; syndrome of hepatocerebral degeneration; (i) prenatal-perinatal manifestations: nonimmune hydrops; fetal death; neonatal cirrhosis; neonatal hemochromatosis associated with maternal autoantibodies against Ro/SS-A and La/SS-B ribonucleoproteins; association with minor congenital anomalies; (j) autosomal recessive inheritance; genetic heterogeneity.

Radiologic Manifestations: (a) *generalized arthropathy;* thinning of cartilage; subchondral sclerosis; cyst formation; *fibrocartilage calcification; osteoporosis;* (b) *cardiomegaly;* congestive heart failure; "restrictive" type of cardiomyopathy; (c) liver neoplasm as a complication; (d) computed tomography: increased attenuation (liver; spleen; lymph nodes) due to iron deposition; (e) magnetic resonance imaging: short T_1 and T_2 values; T_2 relaxation time in the 15 to 30 ms range (normal, 52 ± 8 ms) resulting in the image-labeled "black" liver; (f) prenatal diagnosis using magnetic resonance imaging (comparing fetal liver signal intensity with that of mother's liver signal intensity or fetal fat signal intensity).

HEMOPHILIA

Clinical Manifestations: (a) *bleeding at various sites;* (b) *deficiency of factors VIII (hemophilia A) or IX (hemophilia B);* (c) miscellaneous abnormalities: leukemia; Burkitt lymphoma; generalized lymphadenopathy and T-cell abnormalities; septic arthritis; progressive liver disease in patients who received factor VIII or IX concentrates; association with pulmonary valve stenosis; coronary artery disease; acquired hemophilia due to the production of antibody against factor VIII coagulant activity; transfusion-related acquired immunodeficiency syndrome; splenic rupture; (d) X-linked recessive inheritance (hemophilia A and B).

Radiologic Manifestations

(A) MUSCULOSKELETAL SYSTEM: (a) *joint distension* with active bleeding episodes; *cartilage and subchondral bone erosions; subchondral cysts; narrowing of joint spaces; synovial irregularities;* chondrocalcinosis; increased articular and periarticular tissue density; epiphyseal necrosis; *premature closure of the growth plates;* limb shortening; *accelerated growth maturation; epiphyseal overgrowth;* slipped epiphysis; widening of the radial notch of the ulna; widening of the femoral intercondylar notch; flattening of the inferior border of the patella; *squared appearance of the patella;* patellar length-to-width rates over 2; (b) *pseudotumor* at sites of tendinous attachments, and in muscles with large periosteal attachment, in subperiosteal or intraosseous locations: hematoma with thick fibrous capsule, filled with coagulum, calcified or ossified; bone erosion or destruction with periosteal elevation and new bone formation; intraosseous cyst; (c) others: osteopenia; bony ankylosis; hip joint dislocation complicating repeated hemarthrosis; joint contractures (ankle; knee; elbow); cervical spine abnormalities in adults (cystic changes or end-plate irregularity within one or more vertebral bodies; increased atlantodens interval of 5 mm).

(B) GASTROINTESTINAL TRACT: Intramural hemorrhage; thickening and shortening of small-bowel mucosal folds; thickening of the bowel wall; pseudotumor of the stomach.

(C) URINARY SYSTEM: Filling defects due to blood clots; nonfunctioning kidney; chronic obstructive renal enlargement; distorted upper collecting system due to compression; calculus; renal papillary necrosis; hemorrhage into the bladder wall.

(D) CHEST: Hemopneumothorax; hemomediastinum; pulmonary scarring and fibrosis; pleural thickening; hyperinflation.

(E) CENTRAL NERVOUS SYSTEM: (a) *intracranial hemorrhage;* congenital intracranial hemorrhage; single or multiple high signal intensity (T_2-weighted images) within the white matter; intraspinal bleeding (intraaxial or extraaxial); (b) congenital lesions: posterior fossa collection of cerebrospinal fluid.

(F) OTHER REPORTED SITES OF BLEEDING: Sublingual; laryngeal; pharyngeal; peritoneal; retroperitoneal; splenic (calcifying hematoma); perineal; into a choledochal cyst.

(G) MISCELLANEOUS ABNORMALITIES: Cholelithiasis; computed tomographic changes of liver disease (chronic active hepatitis; cirrhosis); increased periarticular uptake on bone scintigraphy (in the initial stage of synovial hypertrophy and the late stages of the disease).

HEMOSIDEROSIS (IDIOPATHIC PULMONARY) (IDIOPATHIC PULMONARY HEMOSIDEROSIS)

Clinical Manifestations: Onset of symptoms in infancy or childhood: (a) *cough; dyspnea; hemoptysis;* fever during acute attacks; *remissions* lasting months to years; (b) *microcytic hypochromic anemia; hemosiderin-laden macrophages in sputum and gastric washings;* (c) miscellaneous abnormalities: decreased dismutase activity of erythrocytes associated with easy peroxidability of the erythrocytes; association with enteropathy and jejunal villous atrophy; circulating immune complex; (d) some familial cases have been reported (mother and son; siblings).

Pathology: *Recurrent intrapulmonary bleeding with hemosiderin deposition in the lungs;* pulmonary fibrosis in the late stage; increased number of mast cells in the lung.

Radiologic Manifestations: Findings most marked in perihilar and basilar regions: (a) *small nodules; diffuse ground-glass infiltrates; fine patchy stippling;* marked clearing and *changing pattern* during periods of clinical recovery; reticulostriate pattern of *interstitial fibrosis* after recurrent episodes of acute hemorrhages subside; cor pulmonale with cardiomegaly in some cases; hilar lymphadenopathy; (b) accumulation of radiolabeled red cells in the lung on a scan image; (c) magnetic resonance imaging of lungs: increased signal intensity on T_1-weighted images, and reduced signal intensity on T_2-weighted images.

HERMANSKY-PUDLAK SYNDROME

Clinical Manifestations: Lysosomal ceroid storage disease: (a) *tyrosinase-positive oculocutaneous albinism;* (b) *bleeding diathesis caused by abnormal platelet function;* (c) *pigmented reticuloendothelial cells; pigment-laden macrophages;* (d) *deposition of ceroid-like material in tissues* (granulomatous colitis; cardiomyopathy; restrictive lung disease; kidney failure); ceroid pigment deposition in circulating blood monocytes and T-cell lymphocytes; (e) ocular findings: *albinotic retina with macular hypoplasia;* reduced visual acuity; *congenital nystagmus; strabismus;* esotropia; exotropia; hypertropia; embryotoxon; Axenfeld anomaly; iris pigmentation ranging from minimal to normal; (f) increased urinary excretion of dolichols in patients with evidence of ceroid storage in the kidneys; (g) autosomal recessive inheritance; most prevalent in Puerto Rico and in an isolated village in Swiss Alps.

Radiologic Manifestations: *Progressive, diffuse, bilateral interstitial pulmonary fibrosis;* honeycomb cystic lung pattern; bullous lung changes; diffuse colitis: asymmetric pattern of focal, superficial, and deep ulcerations.

HOMOCYSTINURIA

Enzyme Deficiency: Cystathionine ß-synthase.

Clinical Manifestations: (a) marfanoid features (in one third); *cutaneous malar flush;* patchy erythematous blotches; fine, sparse, dry, and fair hair; (b) *lens dislocation;* cataract; optic atrophy; cystic degeneration of the retina; retinal detachment; glaucoma; (c) *high levels of plasma homocystine and methionine, homocysteine, and a mixed disulfide of cysteine and homocysteine;* persistent urinary excretion of homocystine; raised levels of homocystine and methionine in amniotic fluid (amniocentesis); decreased enzyme activity in cultured fibroblasts; positive urinary cyanide-nitroprusside test (false negatives reported); (d) miscellaneous abnormalities: abnormal clotting tendency; presentation with sagittal sinus thrombosis in infancy; homocysteine-induced epithelial damage with platelet involvement; factor VII deficiency; cerebral and cardiovascular atherosclerosis and thromboses; abdominal pain due to vascular occlusion; pancreatitis due to vascular occlusion; presentation with stroke; hypertensive encephalopathy; pulmonary embolism; joint contractures; joint laxity; pes planus; pes cavus; pectus carinatum; pectus excavatum; kyphoscoliosis; increased carrying angle at the elbows; hepatomegaly; inguinal hernia; omphalocele; narrow palate; highly arched palate; generalized dystonia associated with basal ganglia lesions; arterial hypertension (thromboembolic changes in the segmental renal artery branches); etc.; (e) autosomal recessive inheritance; mutations in the cystathionine ß-synthase gene.

Radiologic Manifestations: (a) *osteoporosis;* "codfish" vertebrae; scoliosis; kyphosis; *dolichostenomelia with a tendency to bowing or fracture;* humerus varus; bowed radius and ulna; enlarged carpal bones; metaphyseal spicules; elongated talus; retarded ossification of the lunate; accelerated skeletal maturation; genu valgum; short fourth metacarpal; (b) microcephaly; overdevelopment of the paranasal sinuses; thick calvaria; hyperostosis frontalis interna; wide diploic space; dural calcification; prognathism; (c) pectus carinatum or excavatum; (d) vascular abnormalities: calcification; intimal striation of the arteries with a rippled appearance on arteriography; thromboembolic episodes; atheromatous lesion; vascular narrowing or total obstruction; saccular expansion; moyamoya; (e) computed tomography and magnetic resonance: demonstration of vascular occlusion manifestations (small and large vessels); multiple small areas of increased intensity in the white matter on T_2-weighted images.

Note: (a) other forms of enzyme deficiency causing homocystinuria: *5,10–methylenetetrahydrofolate reductase; methionine methyltransferase* (methionine synthase); (b) heterozygosity for homocystinuria is a risk factor for premature cerebrovascular disease in children and adults.

HYDROXYAPATITE DEPOSITION DISEASE (CALCIUM HYDROXYAPATITE CRYSTAL DEPOSITION DISEASE)

Etiology: *Calcium hydroxyapatite crystal deposition in periarticular tissue;* in some cases associated with intraarticular deposition of the crystals.

Clinical Manifestations: Onset of symptoms usually between the ages of 40 and 70 years: (a) *monoarticular or polyarticular pain; limitation of joint motion; swelling;* tenderness; (b) miscellaneous abnormalities: tender nodule(s); mild fever; elevated sedimentation rate; association with renal failure and hemodialysis; etc.

Radiologic Manifestations: *Periarticular calcification (tendon; capsule; bursa); abnormality of adjacent osseous structures (osteoporosis; osteosclerosis; cystic lesions; irregularity of the bony contour).*

Note: The calcific deposits are often variable in size and shape (mostly ovoid in form; some with linear or triangular configurations; smooth margins); tendinous calcifications are usually located near the site of tendon insertion.

HYPERAMMONEMIC DISORDERS

Etiology: Organic aciduria; urea cycle defect (ornithine transcarbamylase deficiency, an X-linked disorder, the most common heritable urea cycle defect); amino acid transport defect; fatty acid metabolic disorders (short-chain and medium-chain acyl-CoA dehydrogenase deficiencies); hepatic failure; Reye syndrome; drug-induced (sodium valproate, etc.); primary systemic carnitine deficiency; transient hyperammonemia of the newborn; congenital portosystemic shunt; essential amino acid supplements; short bowel syndrome with chronic renal failure; in heterozygotes with ornithine-transcarbamylase deficiency; etc.

Clinical Manifestations: Symptoms in primary hyperammonemia related to the level of ammonia: (a) neonates: onset of symptoms hours or days after birth: *lethargy; poor feeding; vomiting; hyperventilation; grunting respiration; seizures; diaphoresis; coma;* (b) children: *anorexia; vomiting; irritability; ataxia; hyperactivity; combativeness; stupor; delirium; coma; increased intracranial pressure;* (c) late onset: symptoms depend on the degree of enzymatic deficiency: less severe signs or symptoms than the aforementioned; *cyclic vomiting; migrainous headaches; cognitive impairment; mental retardation;* etc.

Radiologic Manifestations: *Cerebral edema;* cerebral cortex hypodensity (computed tomography); demyelination and incomplete peripheral myelination (magnetic resonance imaging); *cerebral atrophy;* magnetic resonance imaging and computed tomographic findings resembling brain infarct.

Note: HHH syndrome (*H*yperammonemia, *H*yperornithinemia, and *H*omocitrullinuria): an autosomal recessive disorder that may present in the neonatal period or later with variable clinical severity: protein intolerance; vomiting; lethargy; growth failure; neurologic abnormalities (seizures; incoordination; pyramidal signs; decreased vibration sense; bucco-facio-lingual dyspraxia; learning difficulties; subnormal intelligence; anomalies of peripheral nerve conduction velocity and evoked potentials; retinal depigmentation and chorioretinal thinning; coma); hepatomegaly; elevation of transaminases; coagulopathy; abnormal white matter (magnetic resonance imaging).

HYPERINSULINISM

Etiology: Nesidioblastosis (focal and diffuse types); beta cell hyperplasia; beta cell adenoma; Beckwith-Wiedemann syndrome; leucine sensitivity; thyrotoxic hypokalemic periodic paralysis; transient hyperinsulinism in newborn; familial hyperinsulinism; hyperinsulinism and polocytic ovaries in adults in association with hepatic glycogen storage diseases (types Ia and II).

Clinical Manifestations: Frequently diagnosed in the newborn or infant; also reported in adults.

(A) Transient hypoglycemia in infants of diabetic mothers and infants with erythroblastosis fetalis.

(B) Nesidioblastosis; adenoma: (a) persistent hypoglycemia; elevated plasma insulin levels; intravenous glucose infusion rate of more than 15 mg/kg/min to maintain a blood glucose level over 2 mmol/L; low blood ketones; a glycemic response to glucagon; (b) clinical manifestation of hypoglycemia (*tremors; jitteriness; apnea; cyanosis; seizures; central nervous system damage*); (c) reversible hypertrophic cardiomyopathy; (d) autosomal recessive inheritance (in persistent hyperinsulinemic hypoglycemia of infancy or nesidioblastosis).

Radiologic Manifestations: (a) noninvasive imaging techniques (ultrasonography; computed tomography; magnetic resonance imaging) to detect the lesion; (b) arteriography for localizing islet cell adenomas; (c) measurement of insulin concentration in the pancreatic venous effluent; (d) localization of insulinomas with selective injection of calcium into the artery supplying the tumor (an abrupt increase in serum levels of insulin); (e) abnormal fat thickness (above normal in neonates with nesidioblastosis).

HYPERLIPOPROTEINEMIAS (HYPERLIPIDEMIA)

Classification: Table ME-H-1.

Table ME-H-1   Summary of the Hyperlipoproteinemias

Type	Occur in Children/ Adolescents	Laboratory Findings	Clinical Manifestations
I	Yes	Normal Chol, ↑ trig	Eruptive xanthomas, abdominal pain, pancreatitis, lipemia retinalis
II Heterozygote	Occasionally	IIa ↑Chol, normal trig IIb ↑ Chol, ↑trig	Tendinous xanthomas, xanthe-lasma palpebrum, tuberous xanthomas, arcus corneae, premature CAD
II Homozygote	Yes	IIa ↑ Chol, normal trig IIb ↑ Chol, ↑ trig	Tendinous xanthomas, intertrigi-nous xanthomas, xanthelasma palpebrum, tuberous xan-thomas, arcus corneae, premature CAD
III	Rare	↑Chol, ↑trig	Palmar xanthomas, tuberous xan-thomas, premature CAD
IV	Rare	Normal Chol, ↑ trig	Eruptive xanthomas, palmar xan-thomas, tuberous xanthomas, premature CAD
V	Rare	↑ Chol, ↑ trig	Eruptive xanthomas, abdominal pain, pancreatitis, lipemia retinalis

From Maher-Wiese VL, Marmer EL, Grant-Kels JM: Xanthomas and the inherited hyperlipopro-teinemias in children and adolescents, *Pediatr Dermatol* 7:166, 1990. Reprinted by permission of Blackwell Scientific Publications.
Chol, Cholesterol; *trig,* triglycerides; *CAD,* coronary artery disease.

I. TYPE I HYPERLIPOPROTEINEMIA (FAMILIAL HYPERCHYLOMICRONEMIA)

Clinical and Radiologic Manifestations: Onset of symptoms in infancy or childhood: (a) *recurrent abdominal pain, recurrent episodes of pancreatitis, lipemia retinalis, and eruptive xanthomas;* (b) *lipoprotein lipase deficiency or apolipoprotein C-II deficiency; serum with lactescent appearance due to massive accumulation of chylomicrons; triglyceride levels of over 1000 mg/dl;* (c) miscellaneous abnormalities: hep-atosplenomegaly; no predisposition to premature atherosclerosis; (d) auto-somal recessive inheritance; frequency of less than 1/100,000 live births.

II. TYPE II HYPERLIPOPROTEINEMIA (HYPERCHOLESTEROLEMIA)

Clinical and Radiologic Manifestations: Two subtypes: type IIa, with deficiency in cell membrane receptor for low density lipoprotein, causing high levels of circulating low density lipoproteins, and type IIb, with accumulation of low density lipoproteins and very low density lipoproteins: (a) *arcus corneae;* (b) *eruptive xanthomas;* (c) *tuberous xanthomas* (subcutaneous water-density masses over the extensor surfaces, particularly in the elbow, hand, buttocks, knee, and ankle regions; rare occurrence of soft-tissue calcification); (d) *tendinous xanthomas:* ultrasonography of Achilles tendon: tendon enlargement; hypoechoic or hyperechoic lesions; magnetic resonance imaging of Achilles tendon: increased signal intensity within xanthoma; (e) *bone involvement* either by an extrinsic effect of xanthomas (multiple well-defined periarticular cortical erosions with intact cortices, most common in the small bones of the hands and feet) or primary bone lesions due to subperiosteal xanthomas and intramedullary lesions (scalloping of the external cortical surface; small and round or oval lytic medullary defects; honeycomb appearance; endosteal erosion; subchondral collapse; juxtaarticular defects; pathologic fractures); increased uptake on bone scan using ^{99m}Tc pyrophosphate; (f) cardiovascular involvement: *coronary artery disease; calcific atherosclerosis of the aortic root;* calcification of the aortic arch; narrowing of the ascending aorta; left ventricular outflow obstruction; aortic valve stenosis; arterial segmental vasoconstriction; (g) *elevated serum cholesterol levels; elevated plasma triglyceride levels; clear serum;* (h) nephrocalcinosis; (i) autosomal codominant inheritance (intrafamilial variability): (1) homozygotes, 1/1,000,000 live births; more severe clinical form with onset of symptoms in early childhood; (2) heterozygotes, 1/500 live births; onset of symptoms in most cases in the third or fourth decade of life.

III. TYPE III HYPERLIPOPROTEINEMIA (DYSBETALIPOPROTEINEMIA; BROAD BETA-TYPE HYPERLIPOPROTEINEMIA)

Clinical and Radiologic Manifestations: Usually diagnosed in the fourth to sixth decades of life: (a) *tuberous or tuberoeruptive xanthomas; palmar crease xanthomas; tendinous xanthomas;* (b) *premature atherosclerosis; coronary artery disease;* (c) *osseous xanthomas;* (d) *opalescent serum, elevated levels of chylomicron and very low density lipoprotein remnant particles due to modification or absence of apoprotein E* (responsible for the hepatic clearance of chylomicron and very low density lipoprotein remnant particles); *elevated cholesterol levels over 300 mg/dl with elevated very low density lipoprotein fraction and triglycerides;* hyperuricemia; (e) obesity; (f) autosomal recessive inheritance.

IV. TYPE IV HYPERLIPOPROTEINEMIA (HYPERTRIGLYCERIDEMIA)

Clinical and Radiologic Manifestations: Often diagnosed after the second decade of life: (a) *xanthomas (eruptive; tuberous; palmar);* (b) osseous xanthomas; (c) *premature coronary artery disease;* (d) *opalescent serum; hypertriglyceridemia;* normal or elevated serum cholesterol levels;

(e) miscellaneous abnormalities: lipemia retinalis; pancreatitis; arthralgia; arthritis; hepatosplenomegaly; obesity; insulin resistance; glucose intolerance; hyperinsulinemia; hyperuricemia; peripheral vascular disease; coronary artery calcification; (f) autosomal dominant inheritance.

V. TYPE V HYPERLIPOPROTEINEMIA

Clinical and Radiologic Manifestations: Usually detected in the third decade of life: (a) *eruptive xanthomas;* (b) *recurrent bouts of abdominal pain; pancreatitis;* hepatosplenomegaly; paresthesia; (c) *lipemia retinalis;* (d) coronary artery disease; (e) *opalescent plasma; fasting chylomicronemia; hyperglyceridemia; hypercholesterolemia;* hyperuricemia; (f) autosomal dominant inheritance.

HYPERPARATHYROIDISM

I. NEONATAL HYPERPARATHYROIDISM

Classification: (a) primary type; (b) infant born to a mother with poorly controlled hypoparathyroidism or pseudohypoparathyroidism.

Clinical Manifestations: (a) *respiratory difficulty; poor feeding; hypotonia; failure to thrive; seizures; polydipsia; polyuria; constipation;* vomiting; swallowing difficulty; (b) splenomegaly; hepatomegaly; (c) *hypercalcemia; hypophosphatemia; hypercalciuria; hyperphosphaturia; aminoaciduria; normal levels of serum alkaline phosphatase; elevated levels of serum immunoreactive parathormone;* anemia; (d) miscellaneous abnormalities: association with alkaptonuria; occurrence in twins; chest wall deformity; limb deformity; craniotabes; facial dysmorphism; bulging fontanelle; absent reflexes; hyperreflexia; heart murmur; (e) sporadic; familial (hypocalciuric hypercalcemia present in the majority of familial cases).

Radiologic Manifestations: (a) *severe generalized bone demineralization; coarse bony trabeculae; subperiosteal bone resorption; metaphyseal cupping;* periodontal osteoporosis; osteitis fibrosa cystica; *pathologic fractures;* (b) renal calcinosis.

Note: (a) two types of familial hyperparathyroidism have been reported: autosomal dominant inheritance (usually associated with endocrine adenomatosis) and autosomal recessive inheritance (neonatal severe primary hyperparathyroidism); (b) neonatal hyperparathyroidism may be associated with familial hypocalciuric hypercalcemia (autosomal dominant inheritance).

II. PRIMARY HYPERPARATHYROIDISM

Etiology: Parathyroid adenoma; parathyroid hyperplasia; parathyroid carcinoma; multiple endocrine neoplasia syndromes; nonparathyroid tumors secreting a parathormone-like substance.

Clinical Manifestations: (a) *bone and joint pain and tenderness;* (b) *symptoms related to hypercalcemia* (psychologic disorders; hypotonicity of smooth and skeletal muscles; nausea; vomiting; polyuria; polydipsia); (c) abnormal electrocardiographic findings (short ST-segment duration; increased amplitude of the QRS complex; prolonged T-wave duration); (d) *renal stones;* terminal uremia; (e) *systemic hypertension; ventricular hypertrophy;* (f) *limb deformities;* decreased stature; finger clubbing; (g) *high levels of serum calcium; depressed serum phosphate levels; elevated urine calcium and phosphate levels; elevated serum alkaline phosphatase levels; elevated circulating parathyroid hormone levels; positive phosphate resorption and calcium infusion tests;* (h) miscellaneous abnormalities: anemia; pancytosis; pancreatitis; peptic ulcer disease; thymic carcinoid tumors; thyroid carcinoma; colonic carcinoma; parathyroid cancer; Graves disease; familial hyperparathyroidism caused by solitary adenomatosis; hungry bone syndrome (migration of calcium and phosphorus ions into the bones, causing extreme hypocalcemia) following resection of parathyroid adenoma; myotonic dystrophy; hypertrophic cardiomyopathy; arrhythmia; convulsion and hypocalcemia in newborn due to maternal hyperparathyroidism; paraplegia due to osteitis fibrosa; (i) sporadic; familial (autosomal dominant inheritance), with and without other components of multiple endocrine neoplasia syndromes.

Radiologic Manifestations

(A) SKELETAL SYSTEM: (a) *demineralization; brown tumor* (sharply marginated bone lesion that may expand the cortex); bone resorption (particularly in the radial margin of the middle phalanges, medial and lateral ends of the clavicle, ribs, sacroiliac joint, tarsal bones, ischial tuberosity, humerus, iliac crest, scapula, and lamina dura); erosive arthritis; demineralization of calvaria (homogeneous, mottled, granular, or ground-glass patterns); (b) patchy sclerosis of the calvaria; basilar invagination; biconcave deformity of the vertebral bodies; kyphosis; scoliosis; deformed pelvis; pathologic fractures; slipped capital femoral epiphysis; osteosclerosis (rare); (c) increased ^{99m}Tc pyrophosphate uptake; in vivo single photon emission computed tomographic quantitative bone scintigraphy (^{99m}Tc MDP) demonstrating significantly increased values; (d) hypervascularity on arteriography and computed tomography.

(B) URINARY SYSTEM: *Renal calculi; nephrocalcinosis.*

(C) PATHOLOGIC CALCIFICATIONS: Vessels; articular cartilages; periarticular soft tissues; lung; heart valves; myocardium; kidneys (nephrocalcinosis); prostate; pancreas; salivary glands; conjunctiva; etc.

(D) PARATHYROID ADENOMA: Double-phase scintigraphy used for detection of the parathyroid tumor.

(E) MISCELLANEOUS ABNORMALITIES: Peptic ulcer; pancreatitis; gallstones; parathyroid mass; thymoma as a cause of true ectopic hyperparathyroidism.

Note: Hypohyperparathyroidism refers to a disorder with the following features: (a) renal resistance to exogenous parathyroid hormone; (b) hypocalcemia; hyperphosphatemia; elevated serum alkaline phosphatase levels; elevated level of serum parathyroid hormone; (c) no evidence of renal disease or malabsorption; (d) subperiosteal bone resorption; metaphyseal changes; epiphyseal displacement (particularly slipped capital femoral epiphysis); brown tumor; (e) bone biopsy finding of hyperparathyroidism.

III. SECONDARY HYPERPARATHYROIDISM (OSTEITIS FIBROSA CYSTICA; RENAL OSTEODYSTROPHY)

Etiology: (a) pronounced parathyroid hyperplasia secondary to chronic renal disease; common occurrence in hemodialysis patients; (b) miscellaneous: long-term furosemide therapy in infants; oral contraceptives; idiopathic hypercalciuria; gluten enteropathy.

Clinical Manifestations: Bone and joint pain and tenderness; limb deformities; digital clubbing; distal phalangeal brachydactyly; renal failure; *elevated serum phosphate levels and low ionized serum calcium levels;* etc.

Radiologic Manifestations

(A) SKELETAL SYSTEM: (a) *subperiosteal bone resorption* (phalangeal tufts; radial aspect of the proximal and middle phalanges of the fingers; margins of the ribs; lamina dura; medial margin of the proximal segments of the humerus, femur, and tibia); (b) *intracortical bone resorption* (cortex of the metacarpals); (c) *endosteal bone resorption* (phalanges of the digits); (d) *subligamentous bone resorption* (humeral and ischial tuberosities; trochanters; inferior margin of the distal portion of the clavicle; inferior surface of the calcaneus); (e) *subchondral bone resorption* (sternoclavicular; acromioclavicular and sacroiliac joints; discovertebral junctions; pubic symphysis; shoulder); (f) *erosive arthropathy*; (g) *brown tumor at various sites, including* vertebral brown tumor as an expansive mass associated with paraplegia; sellar and parasellar destructive lesions; brown tumor of the facial bones; (h) *fractures:* epiphyseal displacement due to metaphyseal fracture; cold fracture on nuclear bone imaging; (i) *osteosclerosis:* spine (rugger-jersey pattern), pelvis, ribs, epiphyses, and metaphyses; (j) *periosteal neostosis;* osteoporosis; (k) osteomalacia; increased bone radiotracer uptake.

(B) ABNORMAL CALCIFICATION AT VARIOUS SITES: Tumoral calcifications; bone erosion associated with tumoral calcinosis; chondrocalcinosis (pyrophosphate dihydrate crystal deposition); vascular calcification; pulmonary calcified nodule (increased radionuclide uptake using ^{99m}Tc methylene diphosphate, and chest radiography); cerebral subcortical calcification; soft-tissue calcification layering; cardiac calcification; breast calcification.

(C) ENLARGED PARATHYROID GLANDS

(D) Miscellaneous Abnormalities: Distal phalangeal brachydactyly secondary to healed renal osteodystrophy; retarded skeletal maturation; "lateral Blount disease" (lateral angulation of the proximal tibial epiphyses and genu valgum); rapid progressive mitral and aortic stenosis; jaw enlargement.

Note: The combination of two pathologic processes is responsible for the clinical and radiographic manifestations of renal osteodystrophy: *hyperparathyroidism from an excess of parathyroid hormone and rickets/osteomalacia due to a deficiency of 1,25-dihydroxycholecalciferol.*

HYPERPHOSPHATASIA (Juvenile Paget Disease; Familial Osteoectasia)

Clinical Manifestations: Onset of symptoms in infancy or early childhood: (a) dwarfism; *progressive enlargement of the head;* saddle nose; short neck; *bowed limbs; pigeon breast deformity; muscular weakness; swelling of the extremities; premature shedding of deciduous teeth;* (b) *high levels of serum acid and alkaline phosphatases;* high levels of urinary excretion of hydroxyproline; elevated activity of serum aminopeptidase; increased uric acid levels in serum and urine; etc.; (c) autosomal recessive inheritance.

Radiologic Manifestations: Progressive skeletal deformities: (a) *enlargement and thickening of the skull,* widening of the diploic space, indistinct outer table, and uneven mineralization of the calvaria; platyspondyly; kyphoscoliosis; biconcave vertebral bodies; enlarged disc spaces; osteomalacic type of pelvic deformity; protrusio acetabuli; coxa vara; long-bone deformities (curved; thickened; cylindric transverse trabeculae; narrowed or dilated medullary cavity; meshed radiolucent bone texture); thickened metacarpals, metatarsals, and phalanges; (b) scintigraphy: intense uptake of radionuclide by the skeleton.

HYPERPROLACTINEMIA

Clinical Manifestations: Usually in young women; may or may not be associated with pregnancy: (a) *galactorrhea; amenorrhea;* delayed puberty or, very rarely, precocious puberty in males; (b) *elevated prolactin levels* that fail to respond to phenothiazines, thyrotropin-releasing hormone, or hypoglycemia; normal or, more often, low plasma gonadotropin levels; (c) miscellaneous abnormalities: acromegaly and hyperprolactinemia associated with polyostotic fibrous dysplasia.

Radiologic Manifestations: More than half of tumors are *microadenomas* (less than 1 cm in diameter): (a) normal sella turcica size in most cases; abnormal sellar contour (asymmetry and erosion of sellar floor); granular calcific deposits in the anterior part of sella turcica; (b) computed tomography: focal hypodense lesion; sellar floor erosion; infundibulum displacement; gland height greater than 8 mm; abnormal diaphragm sellae configuration; (c) magnetic resonance imaging: upward convexity of a pituitary gland containing a low-intensity lesion; contralateral deviation of the stalk; hemorrhage; (d) progressive trabecular osteopenia in women with hyperprolactinemic amenorrhea.

HYPERTHYROIDISM (Graves Disease; Maladie de Basedow)

Etiology: Graves disease (diffusely enlarged gland); thyroid nodule; thyroiditis; chorionic thyroid-stimulating hormone (TSH); congenital; transient neonatal hyperthyroidism caused by transplacental transport of pituitary TSH receptor antibodies; ovarian carcinoma.

Clinical Manifestations

(A) NEWBORN: Hyperactivity; irritability; tachycardia; tachypnea; vomiting; diarrhea; hypertension; delayed cerebral development; periorbital edema; exophthalmos; high-output cardiac failure; association with hyperviscosity syndrome; abnormally high levels of long-acting thyroid-stimulating hormone.

(B) CHILDREN AND ADULTS: (a) weight loss, increased appetite; muscular weakness; palpitation; intolerance to heat; sweating; (b) cardiovascular manifestations: arrhythmias; angina; congestive heart failure; cardiac tamponade; thyroid-related coronary artery spasm; mitral valve prolapse; pulmonary hypertension; fatal thyrotoxic heart disease; (c) digestive system manifestations: diarrhea; rapid gastrointestinal transit time; (d) endocrinopathy: goiter; thyroid bruit; tumor of the thyroid gland; menstrual irregularities; decreased libido; impotence; gynecomastia; (e) ophthalmopathy: exophthalmos; subconjunctival edema; extraocular muscle paralysis; lid lag; (f) urinary system: micturition frequency; nocturia; adult enuresis; (g) neuromuscular manifestations: tremor; nervousness; corticospinal tract disease; periodic paralysis; psychosis; coma; (h) thyroid acropachy: soft-tissue swelling of the hands and feet; digital clubbing; (i) skin manifestations: localized thickening of the skin, usually in the pretibial area; Plummer nails (onycholysis); (j) associations with the following: Down syndrome; thyroid cancer; mixed connective tissue disease; myasthenia gravis; combined thymic hyperplasia and lymphoid hyperplasia; del(18p) syndrome; McCune-Albright syndrome with Cushing syndrome; (k) miscellaneous abnormalities: rhabdomyolysis in thyroid storm; presentation in children with seizures and coma; increased right to left shunt in congenital cyanotic heart disease; esophageal atresia and tracheoesophageal fistula in infants born to hyperthyroid women receiving methimazole during pregnancy.

Laboratory Findings: Elevated thyroxine levels and triiodothyronine (T_3) levels; radioactive iodine (^{131}I) uptake test; T_3 suppression test; leukopenia, lymphocytosis, anemia, thrombocytopenia; elevated alkaline phosphatase levels; hypercalcemic hypercalciuria.

Radiologic Manifestations

(A) SKELETAL SYSTEM

1. Infants and children: *Advanced skeletal maturation;* premature closure of cranial sutures; cone-shaped epiphyses; brachydactyly; asymmetric shortening of the metacarpals and phalanges; osteopenia; early costochondral calcification in adolescents.

2. Adults: *Osteoporosis,* particularly involving the spine and pelvis; spontaneous fractures following minor traumas; thyroid acropachy (periosteal new bone formation in the diaphyses of tubular bones, particularly involving metacarpals, metatarsals, and proximal and middle phalanges, with a "bubbly" or "lacy" appearance); anterior marginal osteophytes of the cervical vertebrae and straightening or reversal of cervical lordosis; increased bone metabolism shown by Tc-99m MDP uptake (using in vivo single photon emission computed tomographic quantitation).

(B) CHEST: Cardiomegaly; thymic enlargement.

(C) OPHTHALMOPATHY (UNILATERAL OR BILATERAL): Proptosis; bowing of the medial lamina papyracea; venous engorgement (compression of orbital venous drainage); conjunctival and eyelid swelling; enlargement of the lacrimal gland and the optic nerve with compression at the orbital apex causing decreased vision; swelling of the extraocular muscles, sparing the tendons, with long T_2 relaxation time measurement with magnetic resonance imaging.

(D) THYROID IMAGING: (a) scintigraphy: semiquantitative 30-minute Tc-99m methoxy-isobutyl-isonitrile thyroid uptake used for rapid diagnosis of hyperthyroidism; (b) magnetic resonance imaging: moderate to marked diffuse increase in signal intensity; (c) computed tomography: demonstration of intrathoracic goiter.

(E) MISCELLANEOUS ABNORMALITIES: Cerebral developmental abnormalities: ventriculomegaly; increased space in the interhemispheric fissure; exaggerated gyral pattern.

Note: Marine-Lenhart syndrome is a variant of Graves disease with the following criteria: enlarged thyroid gland; poorly functioning, histologically benign thyroid nodules with the nodules that are TSH-dependent, with TSH-independent paranodular tissue; return of function to the nodules following endogenous or exogenous TSH stimulation.

HYPOPARATHYROIDISM

Classification

(A) IDIOPATHIC: More common in females.

(B) SECONDARY: Postoperative; hypomagnesemia; iron overloading (particularly with hemolytic anemias).

(C) NEONATAL: Maternal hyperparathyroidism; transient neonatal hypoparathyroidism (premature infants; infants of diabetic mothers; infants with birth asphyxia).

(D) FAMILIAL: X-linked; autosomal recessive; autosomal dominant.

(E) ASSOCIATION WITH OTHER ENDOCRINOPATHIES: Polyglandular autoimmune syndrome with the clinical manifestations of mucocutaneous candidiasis, vitiligo, alopecia, etc.

(F) ASSOCIATION WITH OTHER DISEASES AND SYNDROMES: Pernicious anemia; steatorrhea; Kearns-Sayre syndrome; Wilson disease; hemochromatosis; tumor metastasis to the parathyroids; rickets; congenital lymphedema; nephropathy; congenital anomalies derived from branchial arches and pouches (DiGeorge syndrome; velopharyngeal musculature incompetence); conotruncal cardiac defects (normocalcemia with normal constitutive level of parathyroid hormone, but deficient parathyroid hormone secretory reserve; chromosome 22q11 deletions in some); thymoma; Klippel-Feil syndrome; POEMS syndrome; etc.

Clinical Manifestations: (a) neuromuscular hyperirritability: *carpopedal spasms; tetany; paresthesia of the limbs and/or around the mouth; laryngeal stridor; hyperreflexia; positive Chvostek and Trousseau signs; seizures;* psychosis; parkinsonism; mental retardation; dysarthria; dysphagia; dementia; sensorineural hearing loss; (b) diarrhea; steatorrhea; (c) dental defects; (d) cataracts; (e) congestive heart failure; prolonged QT interval; (f) ectodermal disorders: eczema; alopecia; skin moniliasis; etc.; (g) short stature; (h) *hypocalcemia; hyperphosphatemia; phosphate diuresis following the administration of parathyroid hormone; low or undetectable serum immunoreactive parathyroid hormone level;* (i) miscellaneous abnormalities: hypocalcemic myopathy; partial monosomy 10p; congenital pulmonary valve defects; pseudotumor cerebri; concurrent renal hypomagnesemia and hypoparathyroidism with normal parathormone responsiveness; coexistence with celiac disease; transient hypoparathyroidism in a patient with fever of unknown origin.

Radiologic Manifestations

(A) SKELETAL SYSTEM: Thickening of calvarial tables; homogeneous thickening of petrous bones; thickening of facial bones; generalized or focal areas of increased bone density; greater than normal bone mass (photon absorptiometry); demineralization (very rare); premature closure of the epiphyseal growth plates; undertubulation of the metacarpals; bandlike irregular area of increased density in the metaphyseal regions, iliac crest, and vertebral bodies; spinal changes simulating those of ankylosing spondylitis; periosteal reaction; hyperostosis frontalis interna associated with spike-wave stupor (case report).

(B) **TEETH:** Hypoplasia of enamel and dentine; blunting of dental roots; delayed or failure of eruption; thickening of the lamina dura; prominence of the dental membrane.

(C) **SOFT TISSUE:** Calcification in skin, muscle, etc.

(D) **CENTRAL NERVOUS SYSTEM:** Widening of the cranial sutures due to increased intracranial pressure; brain edema associated with a clinical picture of pseudotumor cerebri; intracranial calcification (basal ganglia; cerebellum; choroid plexus; vascular and perivascular in the white matter of the cerebral and cerebellar hemispheres; depth of the sulci).

(E) **MISCELLANEOUS ABNORMALITIES:** Gastrointestinal hypersecretion; bowel spasm, intestinal pseudoobstruction; cardiomegaly; congestive heart failure.

HYPOPHOSPHATASIA (RATHBUN DISEASE)

Clinical Manifestations

(A) **SEVERE CONGENITAL FORM:** *Globular "boneless" skull; severe deformities and shortness of the limbs;* skin dimple over the sites of long-bone angulation; blue sclerae; *stillbirth or often death soon after birth;* some may survive and fall into the pattern of group B; manifestations present at birth.

(B) **INFANTILE FORM:** *Anorexia; vomiting; constipation; failure to thrive; fever of unknown origin; irritability; convulsions; cyanotic episodes; loud cries; dehydration; wide cranial sutures; bulging fontanelle; angulation of limbs;* onset of symptoms after the first month of life.

(C) **CHILDHOOD FORM:** *Delayed onset of walking; myopathy (pain, weakness, and stiffness); dental caries; premature loss of deciduous teeth* (as the first presenting manifestation); often discovered in early childhood.

(D) **ADULT FORM:** Bone pain; *tendency to fractures.*

(E) Autosomal dominant inheritance; autosomal recessive inheritance (the severe form); a structural abnormality in the tissue-nonspecific alkaline phosphatase gene.

Laboratory Findings: Characterized by deficient activity of tissue-nonspecific (liver/bone/kidney) isoenzyme of alkaline phosphatase: (a) *low or absent serum alkaline phosphatase activity* (total and bone fraction); (b) *increased blood and urine levels of phosphoethanolamine and inorganic pyrophosphate;* (c) hypercalcemia in severe forms; (d) prenatal diagnosis: first-trimester diagnosis with a monoclonal antibody to the liver/bone/kidney isoenzyme of alkaline phosphatase (chorionic villus sample); alkaline phosphatase in amniotic fluid cell culture; mutational analysis of the fetus at risk.

Radiologic Manifestations

(A) PRENATAL: *Failure to observe a fetal head by 16 weeks' gestation;* increased echogenicity of the falx cerebri in association with poor mineralization of the skull; *shortness and bowing of the poorly mineralized tubular bones; fractures;* increased amniotic fluid volume; various femoral deformities (chromosome-like; camptomelic-like; shortening with or without metaphyseal cupping or irregularities).

(B) SEVERE CONGENITAL FORM: *Marked retardation of skeletal ossification;* variability in ossification of the various parts of the skeleton; partial or complete absence of calcium deposits in the cranial vault; partial ossification of the base of the skull and facial bones; poor and irregularly ossified skeleton with some bones not ossified at all; spurs in the midportion of the long bones of upper and lower limbs ("Bowdler spur"); dense vertebral bodies; platyspondyly; vertebral clefts; *multiple fractures.*

(C) INFANTILE FORM: *Defective skeletal mineralization,* particularly in the growing ends of bones, with *irregular ossification of the metaphyses* and a coarse trabecular pattern; *wide cranial sutures.*

(D) CHILDHOOD FORM: Mild to moderate *rachitic changes;* premature closure of sutures rare.

(E) ADULT FORM: *Osteoporosis.*

(F) MISCELLANEOUS ABNORMALITIES: Slender bones; defect in the central metaphyseal region of the distal femoral segments; epiphyseal defects; S-shaped configuration of the tibiae; abnormal configuration of the distal phalanges; partial premature fusion of the epiphyses; wedging of the lower thoracic and upper lumbar vertebrae; premature closure of cranial sutures (early scintigraphic detection by a demonstration of increased abnormal activity along the suture lines); *loss of the lamina dura; premature tooth loss;* nephrocalcinosis; articular chondrocalcinosis; calcification of the ligaments and intervertebral discs; reduced bone mineral density and low parathyroid hormone levels in patients with the adult form of the disease.

HYPOPITUITARISM (ANTERIOR LOBE)

Classification
1. Hypothalamic lesions.
2. Destruction of the gland (trauma; surgery; tumor; infection; granulomas; irradiation; fibrosing pseudotumor of the sella and parasellar area); amyloidosis; hemochromatosis (hypogonadotropic hypogonadism); peripartum lymphocytic hypophysitis.

3. Vascular diseases: infarction; postpartum necrosis; diabetes mellitus; collagen vascular lesions; sickle cell disease; aneurysm of the internal carotid artery.
4. Idiopathic.
5. Familial (autosomal recessive and X-linked recessive).
6. Congenital absence of pituitary gland.
7. Association with midline brain anomalies.

Hormones

(A) HYPOTHALAMIC: Corticotropin-releasing hormone; thyrotropin-releasing hormone; gonadotropin-releasing hormone; growth hormone–releasing hormone; dopamine; somatostatin; vasopressin; oxytocin.

(B) PITUITARY: Somatotrope: growth hormone; lactotrope: prolactin; thyrotrope: thyroid-stimulating hormone; gonadotrope: follicle-stimulating hormone, luteinizing hormone; corticotrope: adrenocorticotropic hormone (ACTH).

Clinical Manifestations: Various combinations of hormonal deficiencies may be present with corresponding clinical manifestations:

(A) CONGENITAL ABSENCE OF THE PITUITARY GLAND: *Apnea; cyanosis; prolonged hypoglycemia; microphthalmos;* micropenis; cryptorchidism; absence or hypoplasia of the sella turcica; hyperbilirubinemia.

(B) PREPUBERTAL (LORAIN-TYPE DWARFISM): *Short stature; normal body proportions; infantile cranial proportions; high-pitched voice; poor dentition, crowding and impaction of teeth; underdevelopment of secondary sex characteristics.*

(C) ADULTS: ACTH deficiency (weakness; weight loss; dizziness; headaches; hair loss; hypotension; dehydration; hypoglycemia; etc.); thyroid-stimulating hormone deficiency (tiredness; paresthesia of the extremities; hair loss; dry skin; constipation; etc.); gonadotropins (amenorrhea; decreased libido; impotence; skin wrinkles; hair loss; etc.); pituitary apoplexy (symptoms simulating meningitis or subarachnoid hemorrhage).

(D) ASSOCIATION WITH SYNDROMES: (1) de Morsier syndrome; (2) Möbius syndrome; (3) primary empty-sella syndrome; (4) Turner syndrome; (5) Silver-Russell syndrome; (6) Rieger syndrome; (7) Pallister-Hall syndrome; (8) Rothmund-Thomson syndrome; (9) Fleischer syndrome (X-linked hypogammaglobulinemia and isolated growth hormone deficiency); (10) the syndrome of mental retardation, facial anomalies, hypopituitarism, and distal arthrogryposis in siblings; (11) microphthalmia with single central incisor and hypopituitarism; (12) Brachmann–de Lange syndrome; (13) hereditary sensory and autonomic neuropathy with growth hormone deficiency; (14) Sheehan syndrome.

(E) ASSOCIATION WITH MALFORMATIONS: Microphthalmia; postaxial polydactyly; dental malformations (upper incisors); midline facial anomalies; cleft palate/lip; holoprosencephaly.

(F) MISCELLANEOUS ABNORMALITIES: Cardiac structural and functional abnormalities in adult patients with growth hormone deficiency (improved left ventricular function after growth hormone replacement); myocardial dysfunction in treated adult hypopituitarism; increased cardiovascular mortality; Creutzfeldt-Jakob disease in pituitary growth hormone recipients; sensorineural deafness; association with choroideremia (an X-linked, progressive, and degenerative disease of the retina and choroid); neonatal hypoglycemia caused by hypopituitarism in infants with congenital syphilis; isolated growth hormone deficiency associated with combined immunodeficiency; association with other endocrinopathies (adrenal; thyroid) .

Radiologic Manifestations

(A) PREPUBERTAL: (a) *relatively large cranial vault* in relation to the facial bones; small sella turcica volume; large sellar volume (empty sella); (b) *marked delay in eruption of teeth;* (c) skeletal manifestations: (1) *retarded skeletal maturation,* with more severe retardation seen in carpal bones than in the epiphyses of the tubular bones; (2) absence of growth lines in the tubular bones; (3) osteoporosis (in growth hormone deficiency); (4) delayed ossification of the marginal epiphyses of the vertebrae; relative platyspondyly; slipped capital femoral epiphysis; (d) computed tomography and magnetic resonance imaging in growth hormone deficiency: pituitary gland of varying volume (aplasia; hypoplasia); *attenuation or transection of the pituitary stalk;* extreme elongation of the pituitary stalk; *absence of the usual intrasellar location of the posterior pituitary gland's high-intensity signal on T_1-weighted images;* neurohypophysis located near median eminence ("ectopic" posterior lobe with hyperintense signal); (e) associated abnormalities: Arnold-Chiari malformation; degenerative plaques around posterior horn of lateral ventricle and parietal area, infarcts in caudate nucleus and putamen; craniovertebral malformation with basilar impression.

(B) ADULT: (a) pituitary stone; enlarged sella turcica related to a tumor; (b) calcification of the auricular cartilage; (c) rudimentary, hypoplastic, or aplastic olfactory sulci in idiopathic hypogonadotropic hypogonadism; (d) reduced bone mineral density in untreated growth hormone deficiency during puberty.

HYPOTHYROIDISM

I. ADULT HYPOTHYROIDISM

Clinical Manifestations: (a) *neuropsychiatric symptoms:* depression; mental retardation; sensory neuropathy; deaf mutism; spastic motor neuropathy; ataxia; dysarthria; myxedema coma; (b) *myxedema;* (c) bloating; flatulence; constipation; paralytic ileus, pseudoobstruction; megacolon with features of ischemic and pseudomembranous colitis; (d) *cardiac man-*

ifestations: (1) pericardial effusion; cardiac tamponade; (2) myocardiopathy: abnormal left ventricular function; low cardiac output; reduced stroke volume; depressed contractility; reduced left ventricular ejection time and prolonged preejection period; asymmetric thickening or hypertrophy of the interventricular septum; reduced left ventricular internal dimensions and outflow dimensions; reduced systolic septal excursion; (3) silent myocardial ischemia; (e) *myopathy* of various degrees of severity (delay in tendon reflexes; respiratory muscle weakness); Hoffmann syndrome (increased muscle mass; muscle stiffness and weakness; low levels of serum thyroxine); (f) *joint effusion* with rheumatic signs; viscous joint fluid containing calcium pyrophosphate crystals; (g) *thyroid function abnormalities:* low levels of serum thyroxine; high levels of thyroid-stimulating hormone; increased levels of serum creatinine phosphokinase; (h) miscellaneous abnormalities: restless leg syndrome; urticaria in association with hypothyroidism; anemia (normochromic normocytic, hypochromic microcytic, or macrocytic); pseudotumor cerebri; abnormal gonadal function (infertility; impotence; etc.); hyponatremia; increased plasma arginine vasopressin level; reduced micturition frequency; macroglossia; increased prevalence of hypothyroidism in patients with gout; hypothyroidism following radiosurgical treatment of cancer of the hypopharynx (elevated thyroid-stimulating hormone levels).

Radiologic Manifestations: (a) *skeletal system abnormalities:* joint effusion; chondrocalcinosis; popliteal cyst; rheumatoid manifestations; radiographic findings similar to juvenile hypothyroidism in adult cretinism; (b) *gastrointestinal tract abnormalities:* hypotonicity; acute or chronic paralytic ileus; loss of colonic haustrations (smooth colon); pseudoobstruction, particularly of the colon; (c) cholestasis; biliary cirrhosis; (d) serosal manifestations: ascites; pleural effusion; pericardial effusion; cardiac tamponade; (e) pituitary gland: *pituitary hyperplasia secondary to thyroid failure, regression of hyperplasia after thyroid hormone therapy;* (f) central nervous system: cerebellar calcification; basal ganglia calcifications; magnetic resonance imaging abnormalities of globus pallidus and substantia nigra (hyperintensity on T_1-weighted images and hypointensity on T_2-weighted images).

Note: Thyroid hormone resistance syndrome: an autosomal dominant disorder caused by mutations in the thyroid hormone receptor ß gene.

II. JUVENILE HYPOTHYROIDISM

Clinical Manifestations: (a) *sluggish behavior; growth retardation; infantile appearance; myxedema;* recurrent respiratory infections; (b) *small face; large fontanelle; relative macrocephaly; widely separated eyes; puffy face; prognathism; underdeveloped jaw; delay in shedding of primary teeth and eruption of permanent teeth; macroglossia; thick* *neck;* (c) *endocrinopathy:* failure of development of secondary sex characteristics or precocious sexual development; vaginal bleeding; adnexal masses (cystic ovaries); irregular menses; galactorrhea; gynecomastia; bloody discharge from breasts; testicular enlargement; apparent "ambiguous genitalia"; (d) *metabolic disorders:* hypersensitivity to vitamin D; increased calcium absorption from the gastrointestinal tract; hypercalcemia; nephrocalcinosis; dystrophic calcium deposits; (e) heart: pericardial effusion; cardiomyopathy; asymmetric septal hypertrophy; myocardial dysfunction (echocardiography); (f) nervous system: *neurologic disorders;* ataxic syndrome; mental retardation; (g) laboratory findings: *low levels of thyroxine and triiodothyronine; high levels of thyroid-stimulating hormone;* elevated cholesterol level; carotenemia; flat glucose tolerance curve; anemia; depressed renal function; (h) association with (1) chronic lymphocytic thyroiditis; (2) cystinosis (due to accumulation of cystine crystals in the thyroid gland and tissue atrophy); (3) Down syndrome; (4) genetic factor in a limited number of familial cases; (5) reversible hypocalciuric hypercalcemia; (6) sensorineural hearing loss in sporadic congenital hypothyroidism; (7) association with acquired von Willebrand disease; (8) nephrotic syndrome; (i) Kocher-Debré-Sémélaigne syndrome: association of cretinism with muscular hypertrophy; (j) miscellaneous abnormalities: rheumatic symptoms; transient hypothyroidism in infants following contrast angiocardiography; vasculitis associated with anemia and pulmonary cavitation during antithyroid drug therapy; pseudotumor cerebri following treatment of hypothyroidism; hypertrichosis; blunted growth hormone secretion associated with hypertrichosis and pituitary enlargement in primary hypothyroidism; central hypothyroidism in some patients with end-stage renal disease; elevated sweat chloride in autoimmune hypothyroidism; association with cystic fibrosis.

Radiologic Manifestations: (a) *skull abnormalities:* brachycephaly; flat forehead; wide sutures; late appearance of the diploic space and vascular markings; large fontanelle in infants; multiple wormian bones; short base of the skull; dense skull, particularly at the base; sclerosis in the periorbital region; diminished angle between the nasal bones and frontal bone; enlarged sella turcica, often with a round appearance and well-defined margins ("cherry" sella); truncated anterior clinoid processes; vertical clivus; delayed closure of the synchondrosis at the base; delayed development of sinuses and pneumatization of the mastoids; premature craniosynostosis (a complication of thyroid replacement therapy); prominent obtuse mandibular angle; (b) *skeletal system abnormalities:* (1) spine: flattened and hypoplastic vertebral bodies and wide disc spaces (oligosymptomatic hypothyroidism presenting as apparent spondyloepiphyseal dysplasia); dorsolumbar kyphosis; gibbous deformity associated with beaking of the lower dorsal and upper lumbar vertebrae; (2) sternum: persistent segmentation into adulthood; (3) pelvis: narrow pelvis with decreased pubic angle; vertical iliac wing; wide acetabular roof corresponding to a deformed femoral head; (4) limbs: epiphyses ("cretinoid epiphyseal dysgenesis" [irregular granular pattern of ossification; widening and flattening of the epiphyses]; delayed closure of the growth plates; osteochondroses; irregular ossification and fragmentation of the femoral head); metaphyses/diaphyses (shortening of long bones; associated thickening of the cortex and narrowing of the medullary canal; thick transverse bands in the shaft and metaphyses of long bones; increased density of the provisional zone of calcification; humerus varus; short femoral neck; coxa vara); hands and feet (normal, stubby, or slender tubular bones of the hand; distal extension of an osseous projection from the midportion of the distal phalangeal metaphyses; low calcaneal arch; shortened calcaneus; changes in the tubular bones of the foot similar to those in the hand); delayed appearance and retarded growth of secondary ossification centers; (c) *central nervous system abnormalities:* hyperplasia or microadenoma of the pituitary gland; empty sella; cerebral atrophy in young congenital hypothyroid subjects; delayed maturation of brain and improved myelination of white matter in response to thyroid hormone treatment; (d) renal manifestation: nephrocalcinosis; (e) gonads: ovarian cysts resolving in response to treatment of hypothyroidism; (f) teeth: primary teeth less affected; *delayed shedding of primary teeth; delayed formation of secondary teeth;* multiple dental caries; (g) heart: pericardial effusion; dilatation of the cardiac chambers; muscular hypertrophy; (h) scintigraphy: (1) *iodine-123 scintigraphy is helpful in distinguishing anatomic from functional causes of hypothyroidism and in locating the thyroid gland in patients with neck masses;* (2) ectopic thyroid tissue detected (midline of the neck, between the base of the tongue and aortic arch) in a high percentage of infants and children with hypothyroidism; (i) thyroid gland sonography: (1) no thyroid seen: *agenesis or ectopic gland;* (2) *large gland:* goitrous hypothyroidism; (3) *small or normal gland:* mild or transient forms of hypothyroidism and hyperthyrotropinemia.

Note: (a) the overlap syndrome: advanced isosexual maturation relative to bone age may be associated with multicystic ovaries; (b) the radiologic manifestations of oligosymptomatic hypothyroidism may be mistaken for spondyloepiphyseal dysplasia; (c) hypothyroidism and associated pituitary hyperplasia may be complicated by intracranial hypertension; (d) hypothyroidism in young children often caused by chronic autoimmune thyroiditis, rarely occurring before 3 years of age; (e) thyroid hormone resistance syndrome: an autosomal dominant disorder caused by mutations in the thyroid hormone receptor ß gene.

III. INFANTILE HYPOTHYROIDISM

Etiology: Thyroid agenesis or dysgenesis; congenital goiter due to maternal drug ingestion; genetic defects in thyroid hormone synthesis or metabolism; abnormal thyroxine-binding globulin synthesis; congenital endemic goiter; familial transient hypothyroidism secondary to transplacental thyrotropin-blocking antibodies; transient primary hypothyroidism in sick premature newborns; familial (autosomal recessive) thyroid-stimulating hormone deficiency.

Clinical Manifestations: (a) *lethargy; respiratory distress; nasal stuffiness; noisy respiration; hoarse cry; stridor (soft-tissue myxedema; goiter); feeding problems; constipation; intermittent cyanosis; persistent neonatal jaundice; distended abdomen; umbilical hernia; myxedema; hair and nail abnormalities; hypotonia; hyporeflexia; persistent infantile reflexes;* organic brain damage; (b) *facial features:* narrow forehead, puffy eyes, puffy cheeks, depressed nasal bridge, pug nose, and protruding tongue; small mandible; delayed fontanelle closure; sparse hair; thick neck, redundancy of the neck skin; (c) heart: *bradycardia; hypotension;* congenital heart block; increased circulation time; heart murmur; diminished T, P, and R waves; asymmetric septal hypertrophy; (d) thyroid function tests: *low levels of thyroxine and triiodothyronine and high levels of thyroid-stimulating hormone in cord serum;* serum thyroglobulin assay (good correlation with thyroid scintigraphy and ultrasonography) in athyroid infants; *depressed basal metabolic rate;* (e) association with congenital anomalies: cardiovascular; central nervous system; skeletal; genitourinary; etc.; (f) syndromes: (1) congenital hypothyroidism; spiky hair, cleft lip and palate, choanal atresia, hypoplastic epiglottis and larynx, long tortuous eyelashes, and undetectable thyroid tissue on scintigraphic scan ("spiky hair syndrome"); (2) chromosomal abnormalities: trisomy 9; trisomy 21; 46,XX/69.XXX diploid-triploid mixoploidy; (3) association with congenital nephrosis and hypoadrenocorticism; (4) abnormal facies, hypothyroidism, postaxial polydactyly, and severe retardation; (5) telangiectasia, unclassified spondyloepiphyseal dysplasia, hypothyroidism, and retinal detachment; (g) miscellaneous abnormalities: galactorrhea; infantile hypothyroidism in siblings (an unusual presentation of pseudohypoparathyroidism, type Ia); hypercalcemia; polycythemia; hip dislocation; association with cystic fibrosis; goitrous cretinism manifesting as newborn stridor.

Radiologic Manifestations: (a) skeletal system: normal or slightly retarded bone age at birth; *delayed skeletal maturation and long-bone growth in the postnatal period;* epiphyseal dysgenesis; increased bone density; poor cortical bone differentiation; congenital vertebral anomalies (partial absence of the vertebral bodies; hemivertebrae; abnormal rib-vertebral articulations); abnormal rib segmentation; (b) endocrine gland imaging: (1) thyroid gland sonography: no thyroid seen—agenesis or ectopic gland; large gland—goitrous hypothyroidism; small or normal gland—mild or transient forms of hypothyroidism and hyperthyrotropinemia; fetal goiter (demonstration of high flow pattern); (2) *thyroid scintigraphy: localization of ectopic tissue, absence of thyroid activity,* absence of salivary gland activity on the ^{99m}Tc images; (3) sonographic detection of fetal ovarian cysts; (4) pituitary gland enlargement regressing in response to thyroid hormone therapy; (c) miscellaneous abnormalities: thickening of precervical soft tissues; mild cardiomegaly.

I

IRON DEFICIENCY ANEMIA

Clinical Manifestations: (a) *tiredness, easily fatigued, palpitations, dyspnea, syncope, irritability, headache, light-headedness, numbness, tingling, poor physical and psychomotor development, difficulty in feeding, and impaired intellectual capacity and work performance;* (b) *pallor;* angular stomatitis; glossitis; gastritis; nail abnormalities (thinning; brittleness; longitudinal ridging; spoon nails; etc.); (c) hemic murmurs; cardiomegaly; cardiac hypertrophy; congestive heart failure; (d) hepatosplenomegaly; (e) papilledema associated with increased intracranial pressure; (f) *hypochromic microcytic anemia; low mean cell volume; decreased serum ferritin level; increased serum iron binding capacity;* increased red cell distribution width, increased red cell protoporphyrin level; (g) increased hemoglobin concentration after iron therapy; (h) miscellaneous abnormalities: blue sclerae; susceptibility to infections; thrombocytosis; hypoproteinemia; anemia caused by a transferrin receptor antibody; papilledema; recurrent benign intracranial hypertension (pseudotumor cerebri); cranial nerve palsy; cardboard-induced iron deficiency anemia; iron deficiency in children with cyanotic congenital heart disease due to relative anemia; transient ischemic attacks; association with Prasad syndrome.

Radiologic Manifestations: (a) skull: *widening of the diploic space* (frontal, parietal, occipital), thinning of the outer table, vertical striation, small sella turcica; (b) hands: *widening of tubular bones due to expansion of the medullary space, thin cortices;* (c) osteoporosis.

K

KEARNS-SAYRE SYNDROME

Clinical Manifestations: Onset of symptoms often before the age of 20 years: (a) *progressive external ophthalmoplegia;* (b) *retinitis pigmentosa;* corneal edema; corneal clouding; (c) *cardiac conduction defects* (first-degree AV block; fascicular blocks; complete heart block; nonspecific ST segment and T-wave abnormalities; sinus node dysfunction); dilated cardiomyopathy; cardiovascular dysfunction resulting in death; cerebral infarction related to cardiomyopathy; (d) cerebellar ataxia; somnolence; lethargy; neurosensory hearing loss; seizures; mental retardation or dementia; abnormal electroencephalographic findings; (e) renal disorders: renal tubular involvement mimicking Bartter syndrome; Fanconi syndrome; renal tubular acidosis; manifestations of Lowe syndrome associated with those of Kearns-Sayre syndrome; (f) elevated cerebrospinal fluid protein levels; reduced plasma and cerebrospinal fluid folate; reduced levels of coenzyme Q10 in serum and in the mitochondrial fraction of skeletal muscle; a defect in complex II of the respiratory chain; deletion of the mitochondrial deoxyribonucleic acid in muscle, spinal cord, and brain; (g) endocrine disorders: diabetes mellitus; hypoparathyroidism; pseudohypoparathyroidism; fatal hyperglycemic acidosis; (h) miscellaneous abnormalities: occurrence in twins; short stature; delayed sexual maturation; muscle weakness; cervical dysphagia (due to involvement of the pharyngeal muscles, sphincter, and proximal esophageal striated muscles); anhidrosis; sideroblastic anemia; pernicious anemia and hypoparathyroidism (case report).

Pathology: Mitochondrial (mitochondria–deoxyribonucleic acid deletion) and muscle fiber abnormalities (ragged-red fibers); spongiform degeneration of white matter; fibrotic lesions in the His bundle and proximal bundle branches; progressive cytochrome *c* oxidase deficiency; fatty infiltration of the pancreas.

Radiologic Manifestations: (a) central nervous system: (1) *microcephaly;* cerebellar hypoplasia; (2) *leukoencephalopathy:* computed tomography: scattered areas of decreased attenuation within the white matter; cerebral calcification (basal ganglia; thalami; cerebral hemispheres); magnetic resonance imaging: high signals in the white matter on T_2-weighted images; low signals on T_1-weighted images; (b) metaphyseal dysplasia.

Note: (a) the diagnostic triad of Kearns-Sayre syndrome: *progressive external ophthalmoplegia, heart block, and retinitis pigmentosa;* (b) cases with external ophthalmoplegia and signs of a mitochondrial encephalomyopathy but without retinal degeneration or heart block are classified under ophthalmoplegia-plus syndrome.

KOCHER-DEBRÉ-SÉMÉLAIGNE SYNDROME

Clinical Manifestations: *Myxedema;* retarded intellectual, physical, osseous, and dental development; constipation; bradycardia; peculiar facies; large tongue; coarse hair and skin; *generalized increase in muscular mass* ("Herculean appearance," "prizefighter," "athletic appearance," "pseudoathletic"); congenital nystagmus.

Radiologic Manifestations: *Retarded skeletal and dental maturation; large muscle mass.*

KRABBE DISEASE (Globoid Cell Leukodystrophy)

Enzyme Deficiency: Lysosomal enzyme galactocerebroside ß-galactosidase.

Clinical Manifestations: A progressive degenerative disease of the central and peripheral nervous system (leukodystrophy): (a) classic infantile type: *unexplained fever; irritability; hypertonia; feeding problems; myoclonic seizure; quadriparesis; progression to a decerebrate state;* early slowing and arrest of growth; failure to thrive; microcephaly; onset in the first year of life; (b) late infantile–juvenile: *visual failure; cerebellar ataxia; spasticity; polyneuropathy; dementia; psychosis; abnormal visual, auditory, and somatosensory evoked potentials;* considerable biochemical and clinical variations in this type; (c) autosomal recessive inheritance.

Pathology: Severe degree of oligodendroglia loss; marked demyelination in the cerebral hemispheres, cerebellum, brain stem, and spinal cord; segmental demyelination of the peripheral nerves; presence of globoid cells (considered to be macrophages containing galactocerebroside); globoid cell leukodystrophy inclusions in sweat gland epithelial cells.

Radiologic Manifestations: (a) computed tomography: (1) *increased density in the thalami, corona radiata, and cerebellar cortex in the early stage of the disease;* (2) *low density in the white matter, and calcification-like, symmetric, and punctate high-density areas in the corona radiata in the advanced stage;* (3) *brain atrophy;* (b) magnetic resonance imaging: (1) *plaque-like, high signal intensity in the periventricular region and cerebellar white matter on T_2-weighted images in the early stage;* (2) *high signal intensity in T_2-weighted images and low signal intensity in T_1-weighted images in the white matter in the advanced stage; an enhancing rim between the demyelinated white matter and the unaffected arcuate fibers in the post–contrast-administration images;* (3) *brain atrophy;* (c) miscellaneous abnormalities: paraventricular calcification; late-onset Krabbe disease mimicking an infiltrating glioma; optic nerve hypertrophy.

KWASHIORKOR

Clinical Manifestations: (a) *failure to thrive* (usually after weaning); *mental apathy; weak cry; diarrhea; skin pigmentation and dryness; change of color of the hair from black to brown and then to red; edema;* (b) hypokalemia; hyponatremia; hypochloremia; low serum albumin levels; mild anemia; endotoxemia (the lipopolysaccharide toxic component of the cell wall of gram-negative bacteria); (c) trace elements (zinc; copper; selenium) deficiency; vitamin A deficiency (conjunctival xerosis; Bitot spot; corneal xerosis; keratomalacia); (d) electrocardiographic changes (sinus tachycardia; low QRS amplitude; prolonged QTc intervals or short QTc intervals; prolonged PR intervals); (e) abnormal brain-stem auditory evoked potentials.

Radiologic Manifestations: (a) *markedly abnormal motor function of the intestine:* abnormal transit time; temporary stoppage of barium suspension; uneven diameter of the intestinal lumen; (b) *severe cerebral shrinkage* (widened cortical sulci; widened interhemispheric fissures and cerebellar folia; enlarged ventricles, particularly the frontal horns of lateral ventricles); resolution of "brain atrophy" after nutritional rehabilitation; (c) *microcardia* due to decreased muscle mass (echocardiography); (d) *osteoporosis; retarded skeletal maturation.*

Note: *Kwashiorkor* is a term originally used by the Krobo-Ga-Adangbe megatribe of the Gold Coast of Africa (now Ghana); described as a nutritional disease of children by Cicely Williams in 1935.

L

LACTASE DEFICIENCY (Lactose Intolerance)

Enzyme Deficiency: intestinal ß-galactosidase (lactase) activity.

Classification: (1) primary: may not manifest itself until adulthood; (2) secondary: caused by diseases damaging the enterocytes.

Clinical Manifestations: Intolerance to milk-containing foods: (a) *abdominal cramps, bloating, and diarrhea due to a shift of water into the intestinal tract;* positive lactose-H_2 breath test; reduction in clinical symptoms and in breath hydrogen excretion after co-ingestion of lactose and lactase-containing tablets; (b) lactase deficiency in early infancy: medullary nephrocalcinosis associated with hypercalcemia; (c) autosomal recessive inheritance; most common in American Indians, African Americans, and Asians; less common in Caucasians.

Radiologic Manifestations: (a) stress test with the use of lactose produces symptoms and radiologic abnormalities of *barium dilution, bowel* *dilatation, and an extremely rapid transit time;* (b) medullary nephrocalcinosis in infancy.

LARON SYNDROME

Clinical Manifestations: A primary growth hormone resistance disease; heterogeneous (growth characteristics, biochemical features, and genetic defects): (a) *dwarfism;* upper to lower body segment ratio more than 2 SD above the normal mean; (b) *craniofacial features:* decreased head circumference; relative prominence of the calvaria in relation to facial structures; protruding forehead; increased biparietal-bicondylar ratio; saddle nose; small chin; (c) *marked growth retardation; delayed puberty and maturity;* adult height between 110 and 138 cm; (d) *high levels of circulating growth hormone; low levels of serum insulinlike growth factor; resistance to the effects of endogenous or exogenous growth hormone* (defect in growth hormone receptors); hypoglycemia; (e) miscellaneous abnormalities: small hands and feet; obesity; small muscle mass; small genitalia; high-pitched voice; sparse hair; decreased sweating; retinal atrophy; (f) autosomal recessive inheritance; mutation of growth hormone receptor; more commonly reported in children of Jewish, Arab, Oriental, Spanish, Portuguese, and Italian descent.

Radiologic Manifestations: (a) *retarded skeletal maturation* (retarded for chronologic age, but advanced for the patient's height); (b) craniofacial disproportion: prominent forehead with thick frontal bone; elongated posterior fossa; large anterior fontanelle; poorly pneumatized mastoids; hypoplastic facial bones; (c) miscellaneous abnormalities: posteriorly wedged lumbar vertebrae; thin tubular bones; multiple growth arrest lines; slipped femoral epiphysis; Legg-Calvé-Perthes disease; prominent fat associated with poorly developed muscles.

LEIGH DISEASE (Subacute Necrotizing Encephalomyelopathy)

Clinical Manifestations: A biochemically heterogeneous multisystem disease with onset of symptoms usually in infancy or early childhood (juvenile and adult onset rare): (a) *regressive psychomotor development; feeding difficulties; somnolence; hypotonia; ataxia; bulbar paresis; nystagmus; cortical blindness; deafness; abnormal eye movements; seizures; vegetative state; autonomic respiratory failure; cranial nerve palsies; movement disorders (dystonia; rigidity; tremor; chorea; hypokinesia; myoclonus; tics);* (b) inborn errors affecting mitochondrial energy metabolism: defects in one or more of the respiratory chain enzyme complexes (respiratory chain complex IV most common; respiratory chain complex I second most common); pyruvate dehydrogenase complex deficiency; (c) *lactic acidemia;* pyruvic acidemia; alaninuria; fumaric aciduria; (d) miscellaneous abnormalities: peripheral neuropathy; renal disease; hypertrophic cardiomyopathy, cardiac mitochondrial dysfunction; myopathy; (e) autosomal recessive inheritance (not in all cases); mitochondrial deoxyribonucleic acid point mutation.

Pathology: Focal symmetric necrosis (thalamus; hypothalamus; putamen; dentate nuclei; cerebellum; optic chiasm; spinal cord); demyelination; vascular proliferation; astrocytosis.

Radiologic Manifestations: (a) variable and widespread distribution of necrotic lesions of the gray and white matter in the brain, brain stem, and spinal cord: (1) computed tomography: *low attenuation lesions with no enhancement of the lesions following the intravenous administration of contrast medium;* (2) magnetic resonance: *delayed myelination; demyelination; T_1 and T_2 prolongation in corpora striata, thalami, substantia nigra, inferior olivary nuclei, periaqueductal gray matter, and cerebral cortex;* (3) ultrasonography: *hyperechoic lesions in the putamen and caudate nucleus* detectable in the preclinical stage; progressive ventriculomegaly; (b) *brain atrophy;* (c) pathologic lactate production shown by magnetic resonance volume selective proton spectroscopy of basal ganglia.

LEPRECHAUNISM (DONOHUE SYNDROME; DYSENDOCRINISM)

Clinical Manifestations: (a) *prenatal and postnatal growth retardation; grotesque facial features:* elfin facies; low-set and malformed ears; widely spaced and deep-set eyes; broad nose; thickened lips; micrognathia; *acanthosis nigricans; enlarged genitalia;* rugation of the labioscrotal folds; polycystic ovaries; breast hyperplasia; brachydactyly; *large hands and feet; lack of subcutaneous fat and muscle mass; severe insulin resistance with paradoxical hypoglycemia;* etc.; (b) prenatal diagnosis by mutational analysis of insulin receptor gene in deoxyribonucleic acid from amniotic cells; (c) autosomal recessive inheritance.

Radiologic Manifestations: Nonspecific: microcephaly; wide sutures; cerebral atrophy; asymmetric ventricles; thin corpus callosum; osteopenia; "osteosclerosis"; retarded bone age; miscellaneous abnormalities (enlarged kidneys; ovarian enlargement; ovarian cysts; medullary renal cystic disease).

LESCH-NYHAN SYNDROME

Enzyme Deficiency: Hypoxanthine guanine phosphoribosyltransferase deficiency resulting in the overproduction of purine and consequently uric acid.

Clinical Manifestations: (a) *self-mutilation,* probably caused by dopaminergic denervation; altered central nervous system dopamine metabolism; (b) *mental and growth retardation; motor dysfunction;* spasticity; choreoathetosis; *microcephaly; cerebral palsy;* (c) *tophaceous gout;* (d) miscellaneous abnormalities: failure to thrive; hyperuricemia; polydipsia; polyuria; crystal nephropathy; urinary calculi; renal insufficiency in infancy; transient neonatal hypothyroidism; recurrent coma; reduction of larger myelinated nerve fibers and lipidlike inclusions in the cytoplasm of Schwann cells; megaloblastic anemia; partial deficiency of the enzyme hypoxanthine-guanine phosphoribosyltransferase; (e) X-linked recessive inheritance (Xq26–q27); very rarely reported in females.

Laboratory Findings: (a) *high concentration of uric acid in blood and urine;* low dopamine ß-hydroxylase activity and diminished sympathetic response to stress and posture; carriers detected by analysis of hair roots for enzyme activity (agarose gel electrophoresis and autoradiography); first-trimester diagnosis by chorionic biopsy (radiochemical assay of hypoxanthine phosphoribosyltransferase activity and fetal sexing); reduced enzyme activity in cultured amniotic fluid cells; (b) detection of the carrier state and prenatal diagnosis by mutation detection and linkage analysis.

Radiologic Manifestations: (a) *changes secondary to self-mutilation:* amputation of fingertips and phalanges; (b) radiolucent or faintly radiopaque *urinary stones* (hypoxanthine; xanthine; uric acid); *markedly echogenic cortices; echo poor medullary pyramids containing streaks of echogenicity in the early stage of the disease; spotty increased renal parenchymal echogenicity due to many tiny calculi* (some stone formation related to allopurinol treatment, resulting in xanthinuria and oxypurinoluria); small kidneys with poor function on excretory urography; (c) miscellaneous abnormalities: microcephaly; brain atrophy; bone erosions; calcareous deposits of gout; retarded skeletal maturation; peripheral manifestations of cerebral palsy (coxa valga, hip subluxation or dislocation).

LIPODYSTROPHIES (LIPOATROPHY)

Classification
(A) PROGRESSIVE PARTIAL LIPODYSTROPHY (BARRAQUER-SIMONS SYNDROME): Usually sporadic; familial incidence rare; strong predilection for females (4/1).

(B) FAMILIAL PARTIAL LIPODYSTROPHY (KÖBBERLING-DUNNIGAN SYNDROME): Probably X-linked dominant mode of inheritance with lethality in males.

(C) CONGENITAL TOTAL LIPODYSTROPHY (BERARDINELLI-SEIP SYNDROME): Consanguinity of parents common; autosomal recessive; sexes equally affected; loss of subcutaneous fat within the first 2 years of life.

(D) **Acquired Lipoatrophic Diabetes:** Sporadic; predominantly in females.

Clinical Manifestations

(A) **Progressive Partial Lipodystrophy (Barraquer-Simons Syndrome):** Onset of symptoms usually between 5 and 15 years of age: fat loss from the face, arms, and trunk; normal or excessive fat deposition on the pelvic girdle and lower limbs; glomerulonephritis; hepatomegaly; diabetes; hyperlipidemia; mental retardation.

(B) **Familial Partial Lipodystrophy (Köbberling-Dunnigan Syndrome):** Two types: (1) limb lipodystrophy: loss of subcutaneous fat confined to the limbs, sparing the face and trunk; (2) limb and trunk lipodystrophy: the trunk affected, with the exception of the vulva (pseudolabial hypertrophy); diabetes mellitus; hyperlipoproteinemia; acanthosis nigricans present in some patients.

(C) **Congenital Total Lipodystrophy (Berardinelli-Seip Syndrome; Lipoatrophic Diabetes):** (a) *hirsutism; acanthosis nigricans; generalized absence of adipose tissue;* large hands and feet; large penis or clitoris in infancy; *accelerated growth and maturation;* prominent musculature; phlebomegaly; hepatosplenomegaly with cirrhosis; (b) mental retardation; (c) *insulin-resistant diabetes mellitus* not associated with ketosis; hypertriglyceridemia; elevated basal metabolic rate; decreased binding of insulin to its receptor; (d) oligomenorrhea; polycystic ovarian disease; (e) functional and morphologic abnormalities of the heart muscle and chambers: muscular hypertrophy; increased chamber size and myocardial indentation; systolic anterior movement of the mitral valve; wall motion abnormalities.

(D) **Acquired Lipoatrophic Diabetes:** Associated in some cases with infective processes (mumps; pertussis); difficult labor and delivery; etc.

Radiologic Manifestations of Congenital Total Lipodystrophy: (a) *absence of fat in soft tissues;* difficulty in abdominal organ delineation by computed tomography because of a paucity of fat; fatty liver (low computed tomographic attenuation; hyperechoic pattern on sonography); abnormally low or absent signal on magnetic resonance imaging evaluation of the bone marrow (atrophy of fatty tissue); peculiar distribution of adipose tissue: (1) absence of fat in the following sites: subcutaneous areas, intraabdominal and intrathoracic regions, bone marrow; (2) presence of fat at the following sites: orbits, palms and soles, periarticular, epidural, tongue, breasts, vulva, and buccal area; (b) *increased bone density; thickened cortex of tubular bones; prominent and hypertrophic epiphyses;* scattered areas of radiodensity and cystic changes in periarticular regions; magnetic resonance imaging: prolonged T_1 and T_2 times and marked gadolinium enhancement in radiographically normal–appearing long bones; fluid-fluid levels in the lytic lesions of the bones with peripheral enhancement after gadolinium infusion; (c) *advanced skeletal maturation;* (d) *thick calvaria;* calcification of the falx cerebri; excessive pneumatization of sinuses and mastoids; (e) *dense transverse bands in the vertebrae;* (f) *nephromegaly* with splaying of calices and infundibula; (g) hepatosplenomegaly; (h) *advanced dentition;* (i) miscellaneous abnormalities: enlargement of basal cisterns and the third ventricle with or without enlargement of the lateral ventricles, narrowing of interpediculate distances; polycystic ovarian disease.

Syndromes Associated with Lipodystrophy: (1) AREDYLD syndrome: Acro*R*enal–*E*ctodermal *DY*splasia–*L*ipoatrophic *D*iabetes; (2) SHORT syndrome: *S*hort stature; *H*yperextensibility of joint; *O*cular "depression"; *R*ieger anomaly; delayed *T*eething; other manifestations: distinct facial features; partial lipodystrophy; nonketotic hyperglycemia; diabetes mellitus secondary to severe insulin resistance; intrauterine growth retardation; slow weight gain; etc.; (3) generalized lipodystrophy, severe myopia, marfanoid habitus, and normal intelligence, in a 10-year-old girl.

LIPOID PROTEINOSIS (LIPOGLYCOPROTEINOSIS; URBACH-WIETHE DISEASE)

Clinical Manifestations: Onset of symptoms often at birth: (a) *mucosal involvement* of the oropharynx, larynx, and nose: diminished gustation; cracked lips; pale irregular buccopharyngeal mucosa; infiltration of the gingiva; diminished gag reflex; tethering of the tongue; limited tongue motility (board-like tongue); dysphagia; *hoarseness with an onset as early as neonatal;* thickened epiglottis; thickened arytenoepiglottic folds; thickened irregular false vocal cords; swollen arytenoids; plaque-like excrescence of the laryngeal mucosa; (b) *skin infiltration:* yellow or brown papules on the face, giving the skin a waxy look; beaded papules along the eyelids; nodular lesions on the elbows and knees; nonscarring alopecia; (c) *neuropsychiatric disorders:* seizures; mental retardation; choreoathetosis; paresthesia of the fingers; indifference to pain; behavioral problems; (d) *retinal degeneration;* (e) *elevated lipid levels in the blood;* (f) miscellaneous abnormalities: abnormal dentition; conduction type of hearing loss; intestinal bleeding secondary to massive submucosal deposits of hyaline material in the small bowel; (g) autosomal recessive inheritance.

Pathology: Infiltration of various tissues (skin, mucosa, central nervous system, respiratory system, gastrointestinal tract, lymph nodes, and striated muscles) by a complex glycolipoprotein.

Radiologic Manifestations: *Intracranial calcifications in the medial temporal region* that are located superolateral to dorsum sella and project over the medial aspect of the orbits in the frontal view (bean-shaped; inverted commas); areas of lucency within the calcification; *vocal cord thickening* (diffuse or nodular); reticular and nodular densities in the lung.

LOWE SYNDROME (Oculo-Cerebro-Renal Syndrome)

Clinical Manifestations: Onset of symptoms in early infancy: (a) *hypotonia at birth; physical and mental retardation* (near-normal intelligence in some cases); *maladaptive behaviors* (stubbornness; temper tantrums; stereotypic behaviors); (b) *cataract; glaucoma;* buphthalmos; corneal scarring; superficial granulations of the eyes; nystagmus; lenticular opacities in females heterozygous for this X-linked condition; (c) *progressive renal tubular dysfunction* (decreased ability to secrete hydrogen ions and to produce ammonia; hyperaminoaciduria; proteinuria; hyperchloremic acidosis; phosphaturia; hypophosphatemia); hematuria; granular casts; Fanconi syndrome; acute tubular necrosis; congenital nephrotic syndrome; (d) *hypophosphatemic rickets;* (e) joint hypermobility; tenosynovitis; joint effusion; (f) miscellaneous abnormalities: seizures; diminished or absent deep tendon reflexes; muscular hypoplasia; elevated serum concentrations of muscle enzymes; anemia; hyperhemolysis; episodes of fever; hyperactivity; high-pitched cry; fetal Lowe syndrome associated with elevated maternal serum and amniotic fluid α-fetoprotein; cryptorchidism; (g) X-linked recessive inheritance; possible genetic heterogeneity.

Radiologic Manifestations: (a) *rickets and/or osteoporosis;* (b) *pathologic fracture* through the shafts of long bones; healing with large callus formation; (c) frontal bossing; scoliosis; kyphosis; platyspondyly; cervical spine anomalies (increased motion at the C1-C2 level; fusion of C1 and the occiput; basilar impression); hip dislocation or subluxation; (d) central nervous system: (1) computed tomography: diffuse scalloping of the calvarial bones; ventricular dilatation; periventricular decrease in density; diffuse low-absorption areas in the cortical white matter; brain atrophy; (2) magnetic resonance imaging: nonhomogeneous areas of increased T_2-weighted signal intensity in the centrum semiovale; abnormal areas of high signal intensity in the periventricular white matter; periventricular white matter cystic lesions.

LYSINURIC PROTEIN INTOLERANCE

Etiology: Defective transport of the cationic amino acids lysine, arginine, and ornithine at the cell membrane.

Clinical Manifestations: Onset of symptoms in early childhood: (a) *failure to thrive; growth retardation; hypotonia; and episodes of stupor after eating protein-rich foods;* (b) predisposition in pediatric patients to develop pulmonary alveolar proteinosis, pulmonary hemorrhage, and glomerulonephritis; (c) very few adults with the clinical manifestations of pulmonary disease, but some asymptomatic individuals with radiologic signs of interstitial lung disease; (d) miscellaneous abnormalities: renal glomerulosclerosis; hemolytic anemia; bone marrow erythroblastophagocytosis; leukocytopenia; high serum IgG levels; pulmonary alveolar proteinosis; etc.; (e) autosomal recessive inheritance; genetic heterogeneity.

Radiologic Manifestations: (a) *osteoporosis;* fractures with minor trauma; metacarpal cortex thickening in some; rickets-like metaphyseal changes; end-plate impression of vertebrae; scoliosis; *skeletal maturation retardation;* (b) interstitial lung disease; high-resolution computed tomography of the lungs in asymptomatic patients demonstrating acinar nodules, inter- and/or intralobular thickening of the interstitial septa, and subpleural cysts; (c) nuclear studies: uneven distribution of perfusion and ventilation.

M

MADELUNG DISEASE (Launois-Bensaude Disease; Buschke Disease; Cervical Lipomatosis)

Clinical Manifestations: Onset in adulthood: (a) *massive lipomatosis:* normal fat that often begins on the back of the neck and extends symmetrically anteriorly to the submental region and to the thorax; may spread to the scrotal region; (b) respiratory system symptoms related to tracheal compression and recurrent palsy; (c) venous stasis of the chest wall in association with mediastinal involvement; (d) *neuromuscular abnormalities:* neuropathy; muscular weakness; tendon areflexia; muscle atrophy; tremor; cramps; etc.; (e) muscle biopsy and biochemical studies indicating mitochondrial dysfunction: ragged red fibers; reduced cytochrome *c* oxidase activity; (f) metabolic abnormalities: marked increase in adipose tissue lipoprotein lipase activity; plasma hyperalphalipoproteinemia; defect in the adrenergic-stimulated lipolysis in lipomatous tissue; hyperuricemia; reduced glucose tolerance; renal tubular acidosis; (g) red blood cell macrocytosis; macrocytic anemia; etc.; (h) most commonly noted in the countries around the Mediterranean Sea; male predominance; familial occurrence, autosomal dominant mode of inheritance has been postulated.

Radiologic Manifestations: *Lipomatosis (neck; mediastinum; below the trapezius muscle);* calcification/ossification within the lipomatous masses; tracheal narrowing and deformity; venous stasis; absence of pericardial, intraabdominal, retroperitoneal, and pelvic lipomatosis.

MANNOSIDOSES

I. α-MANNOSIDOSIS

Classification: Glycoprotein accumulation in tissues and organs, and excretion of oligosaccharides in urine: (1) type I homozygotes with severe disease, gross psychomotor retardation, hepatosplenomegaly, recurrent infections, short stature, dysostosis multiplex, and early death; (2) type II homozygotes with moderate retardation, deafness, near-normal stature, milder dysostosis multiplex, and survival to adult life.

Enzyme Deficiency: Deficiency of α-mannosidase leading to accumulation of mannose-rich glycoproteins in tissues.

Clinical Manifestations: Clinical features become apparent at about 1 to 3 years of age: (a) *craniofacial dysmorphism:* macrocephaly; coarse and puffy facial features; high frontal region; slight flattening of the nasal root; flat face; prominent mandible; macroglossia; large ears; widely spaced teeth; (b) *psychomotor retardation;* normal or accelerated early growth followed by *growth arrest; hypotonia; hyperreflexia;* (c) *corneal clouding; cataracts; ptosis;* wheel-like or spoke-shaped opacities in the lens; (d) *high-frequency mixed hearing loss* (common); (e) gingival and oral mucosal hyperplasia (histiocytic cells containing storage vacuoles and reticulogranular material); (f) excretion of glycoproteins in urine; abnormal α-mannosidase activity, demonstrable in cultured skin fibroblasts; hypogammaglobulinemia; vacuolized peripheral lymphocytes; coarse and dark granules in neutrophils; reduced α-mannosidase in cultured amniotic fluid cells; (g) autosomal recessive inheritance with considerable variation in clinical manifestations within the family.

Radiologic Manifestations: (a) *dysostosis multiplex of varying severity:* thick calvaria; dolichocephaly or brachycephaly; partial craniosynostosis; poor pneumatization of paranasal sinuses; widening of the ribs; mild flattening of the vertebrae; trapezoid-shaped vertebrae with anterior wedging or anterior beaking at the thoracolumbar junction; expansion of the diaphyses of tubular bones; mild bowing of long bones; slight irregularity of metaphyses; narrow basilar segment of the iliac wings, coxa valga; (b) osteoporosis; coarse bone trabeculae; (c) central nervous system: high signal intensity on T_2-weighted images involving parietooccipital white matter; cerebellar atrophy; communicating hydrocephalus; partial empty sella turcica.

II. ß-MANNOSIDOSIS

The major storage material is a disaccharide; autosomal recessive transmission; deficiency of ß-mannosidase; elevated urinary disaccharide levels; variable clinical manifestations (dysmorphic features; various degrees of neurologic deterioration; peripheral neuropathy; amyotrophy; deafness; mental retardation; angiokeratoma); cytoplasmic vacuolation of skin fibroblasts and lymphoid cells; prenatal diagnosis in the first trimester (ß-mannosidase activity analysis in the chorionic villi).

MAPLE SYRUP URINE DISEASE

Enzyme Deficiency: Deficiency of any of the subunits E1α, E1ß, or E2 of the branched-chain α-ketoacid dehydrogenase complex leading to elevation of branched-chain amino acid or ketoacid levels in blood and excretion of same in urine.

Classification: Various phenotypes: classical type (75% of the cases); intermittent; intermediate; thiamin-responsive.

Clinical Manifestations: Symptoms often occurring in the first postnatal days: (a) *vomiting; feeding difficulty; neurologic manifestations* (lethargy; shrill cry; hypotonicity; opisthotonos; convulsions; pseudotumor cerebri; respiratory difficulties; coma); mental retardation in surviving children; (b) *urine with characteristic odor (sweet, malty, or caramel-like);* (c) hypoglycemia (in some in the acute phase); (d) prenatal diagnosis with evaluation of the enzyme activity in cultured amniotic fluid cells; (e) postnatal diagnostic tests: plasma and urine assays for increased amino acids (leucine; isoleucine; valine); ferric chloride test (gray-blue color); 2,4-dinitrophenylhydrazine test (heavy yellow precipitate); (f) acrodermatitis enteropathica–like syndrome secondary to isoleucine deficiency during treatment of maple syrup urine disease; (g) cerebral edema causing death in infants and children; (h) autosomal recessive inheritance; genetic heterogeneity.

Pathology: (a) generalized status spongiosis of the white matter, reduced number of the myelin sheaths; increased cerebral water content, reduction in total brain lipid content, and aberrant dendritic development; (b) hair: structural defect in the fiber shaft.

Radiologic Manifestations: (a) *generalized brain edema plus a localized, more severe edema (the maple syrup urine disease edema) involving the deep cerebellar white matter, the dorsal part of the brain stem, the cerebral peduncles, and the dorsal limb of the internal capsule; improvement in response to treatment with total clearing or presence of residual changes (low-density zone around the lateral ventricles and small, low-attenuation lesions within the brain stem);* detection of cerebral accumulation of branched-chain amino acids by proton spectroscopy; progressive global (end-stage) brain atrophy over a period of several years in a missed or delayed diagnosis; (b) scoliosis.

MAURIAC SYNDROME

Clinical Manifestations: (a) *triad of poorly controlled diabetes, profound growth retardation, and hepatomegaly;* (b) miscellaneous abnormalities: protuberant abdomen; moon-shaped face; cushingoid fat deposition; retarded sexual maturation; malnutrition; edema; transient false sweat test (elevated sweat chloride level); glycogen infiltration of the liver; subtotal villous atrophy of the jejunum.

Radiologic Manifestations: *Retarded skeletal maturation;* osteoporosis.

MELAS SYNDROME (MITOCHONDRIAL MYOPATHY– ENCEPHALOPATHY–LACTIC ACIDOSIS–STROKELIKE EPISODES)

Clinical Manifestations: Variability in expression; onset in childhood or adulthood: (a) *encephalopathy: strokelike episodes;* fluctuating motor and visual symptoms; recurrent focal neurologic dysfunction (hemiparesis; hemianopsia; cortical blindness; etc.); episodic vomiting; episodic headache; sensorineural hearing loss; optic atrophy; seizures; ataxia; (b) *lactic acidosis* (raised blood and cerebrospinal fluid lactate); (c) *myopathy:* muscle weakness; exercise intolerance; (d) bilateral ptosis; external ophthalmoplegia; pigmentary retinopathy with macular involvement; (e) reduction in cytochrome *c* oxidase activity; a defect in NADH-coenzyme Q reductase; respiratory chain defects; ultrastructurally abnormal mitochondria; (f) very few familial cases have been reported (siblings; mother/child pairs).

Pathology: (a) *myopathy: ragged red fibers;* (b) *encephalopathy:* neuronal loss in the cerebral cortex; localized softening in the cerebral cortex; loss of myelin and fibrous gliosis in the subcortical and deep white matter; cerebral and cerebellar atrophy; ferrocalcific deposits in the capillary walls of the basal ganglia.

Radiologic Manifestations: (a) computed tomography: focal low-attenuation areas in the temporal and occipital regions; ventricular dilatation; basal ganglia calcification; cortical enhancement on post-contrast scans; development of brain atrophy in the low-attenuation regions; (b) magnetic resonance imaging: *transitory abnormalities ("migrating" infarcts) in association with strokelike episodes; multifocal hyperintense signal on T_2-weighted images in the cortex of the cerebrum, cerebellum, and immediately adjacent white matter);* (c) cerebral perfusion study using single photon emission computed tomography showing various patterns: decreased accumulation of the tracer at various sites after strokelike episodes; hyperemia persisting after strokelike episode.

Note: (a) *MELAS* is an acronym: *M*itochondrial myopathy–*E*ncephalopathy–*L*actic *A*cidosis–*S*trokelike episodes; (b) multiple migratory infarctlike lesions that are not limited to a particular vascular territory, particularly in the posterior part of cerebral hemisphere and basal ganglia in children, are considered to be diagnostic of MELAS syndrome.

MEMBRANOUS LIPODYSTROPHY (Nasu-Hakola Disease)

Clinical Manifestations: Onset of symptoms often in adolescence or young adult life: (a) *swelling and pain in joints;* fractures with minor trauma; (b) *neuropsychiatric symptoms* with onset in middle age (impairment of memory; euphoria; indifference; impotence or frigidity; ataxia; tremor; urinary incontinence; exaggerated deep tendon reflexes; pathologic reflexes; frontal syndrome; epileptic convulsions; peripheral motorsensory neuropathy); (c) abnormal electroencephalographic findings: slow activity; spike and wave complexes; spike discharges; (d) miscellaneous abnormalities: leukemia; disorder of intestinal motility; (e) autosomal recessive inheritance.

Pathology: (a) convoluted membranes interlaced with lipoid structures; leukodystrophy, general diffuse atrophy, and sclerosis of the white matter, especially in the frontal lobes; (b) secondary membranous lipodystrophy: local subcutaneous membranous lipodystrophy that occurs as a result of other skin diseases.

Radiologic Manifestations: (a) *osteopenia; thin cortices; pathologic fractures; radiolucent cystic areas with irregular borders involving the ends of the carpal and tarsal bones and the shafts, metaphyses, and epiphyses of tubular bones symmetrically;* Erlenmeyer deformity of the long bones with scalloping of the endosteal aspect of the cortex; skull and vertebrae not involved; (b) *white-matter atrophy* associated with ventricular dilatation; increased signal intensity of the white matter on T_2-weighted images and decreased signal intensity of thalamus, putamen, caudate nucleus, and cerebral cortex; (c) basal ganglia calcification.

MENKES DISEASE (Kinky-Hair Syndrome)

Clinical Manifestations: The disease is usually recognizable in the first 3 months of life: (a) *sparse, stubby, twisted, and fractured hairs; variation in diameter of the hair shafts;* (b) *developmental regression; mental retardation; seizures; ataxia; irritability; hypothermia;* intracranial hemorrhage; (c) laboratory findings: *low level of copper in plasma, urine, and hair; low level of plasma ceruloplasmin;* an increased number of free sulfhydryl groups and decreased number of disulfide bonds in hairs; cultured fibroblasts containing 4 to 6 times higher concentrations of copper than control cells; postmortem diagnosis by copper measurement in the muscle tissue (high); very high copper uptake (^{64}Cu) in cultured muscle cells; (d) copper measurement in the chorionic villi of the affected fetus in the first trimester (high); first-trimester prenatal diagnosis by deoxyribonucleic acid analysis; (e) *malabsorption and maldistribution of copper* *in body organs;* (f) miscellaneous abnormalities: cryptorchidism; cataracts; atypical form (hypotonicity; fine myoclonic movements; ataxia; delayed psychomotor development; pili torti); a female patient with 45X/46XX mosaicism; variability in clinical expression (the group of severely affected patients with long survival and the group of very mildly affected patients with late onset of symptoms); bleeding from gastric polyp; electroencephalographic abnormalities; clinical features resembling those of Menkes disease in infancy, but with occipital exostoses developing in adolescence; bladder rupture; (g) X-linked recessive inheritance; rare occurrence in females; prenatal diagnosis by mutation analysis.

Pathology and Pathophysiology: (a) copper absorption disrupted by the epithelial cells in the intestine; (b) progressive brain atrophy with diffuse neuronal loss and gliosis; myelin deficiency in the centrum semiovale and long tracts through the brain stem; cerebellar atrophy; microcephaly; subdural hygroma; subdural hematoma; cortical heterotopia; (c) accumulation of excessive amount of copper as copper-metallothionein in various organs and in the blood vessels; accumulation of large amount of copper in organelle-free cytoplasm; copper deficiency of the mitochondria; low serum, hepatic, and brain copper levels; decreased activity of copper-dependent enzymes, cytochrome oxidase A1 and A3 in liver, brain, and white cells; deficiency of dopamine ß-hydroxylase, with abnormal catecholamine levels in blood and cerebrospinal fluid; (d) hair pathology: twisting of the hair shaft (pili torti), periodic narrowing, and fragmentation.

Radiologic Manifestations: (a) bilateral symmetric *metaphyseal spurring* of long bones in infancy; flaring of ribs; osteoporosis; fracture(s); *diaphyseal periosteal reaction of long bones;* thickening of scapulae and clavicles; (b) *microcephaly;* excessive wormian bones in the posterior fontanelle region; (c) central nervous system abnormalities demonstrable by ultrasonography, computed tomography, magnetic resonance imaging, magnetic resonance angiography, and angiography: *delayed myelination or dysmyelination; progressive development of diffuse brain atrophy; ventricular dilatation; ischemic infarctions; extraaxial accumulation of fluid; low-density cortical areas on computed tomography; hypointense signals on T_1-weighted images; hyperintense signals on T_2-weighted images; widespread arterial changes* (narrowing; dilatation; tortuosity; elongation; supernumerary branches); *increased cerebral echoes;* "cystic" lesion in temporal lobes; (d) urinary tract abnormalities: bladder diverticula; hydronephrosis; ureteropelvic junction obstruction; hydroureter; vesicoureteral reflux; urinary tract infection; (e) miscellaneous abnormalities: intracranial vascular abnormalities in female carriers closely resemble those encountered in males with the disease; polypoid gastric mass; emphysema; round lumbar and thoracic vertebral bodies; tortuosity and elongation of intracranial arteries without evidence of cerebral atrophy, demyelination, or subdural hygroma in a patient treated with copper histidinate; one-sided magnetic resonance imaging findings in a patient suggesting ischemic lesions.

METACHROMATIC LEUKODYSTROPHIES

Enzyme Deficiency: A lysosomal storage disorder: (a) type A arylsulfatase deficiency in most patients; (b) metachromatic leukodystrophy due to the deficiency of an arylsulfatase A activator protein (sphingolipid activator protein B); (c) deficiency of arylsulfatase A in healthy individuals (pseudodeficiency).

Clinical Manifestations: Depend on the age of onset (autosomal recessive; genetic heterogeneity).

(A) LATE INFANTILE FORM: (a) *difficulty in walking; ataxia; defect in coordinating movement of the limbs; difficulty in swallowing; physical and mental deterioration; decerebrate posture;* abnormalities on evoked potential studies (somatosensory; visual; brain-stem auditory); (b) *severe constipation;* (c) *ichthyosis;* (d) *metachromatic granules in the urine; demonstration of various forms of arylsulfatase deficiency in leukocytes by electrophoretic techniques and cultured skin fibroblasts;* absence of arylsulfatase in amniotic fluid (chromatography); assay of chorionic villi for enzyme deficiency.

(B) JUVENILE FORM: Often seen initially with ataxia; progression slower than in the late infantile form.

(C) ADULT FORM: Often seen initially with progressive dementia and behavioral disorders (particularly schizophrenia-like psychosis); ataxia; spasticity; isolated peripheral neuropathy in some.

Pathology: Accumulation of metachromatically staining granules due to the presence of cerebroside sulfate (sulfatide) in the central nervous system and peripheral nerves (symmetric demyelination in the cerebral and cerebellar hemispheres, basal ganglia, brain stem, and long tracts of the spinal cord), bile duct epithelium, gallbladder wall, epithelial cells of the renal tubules, and other sites.

Radiologic Manifestations: (a) biliary tract: progressive inability of the gallbladder to concentrate bile, resulting in poor or nonvisualization of the gallbladder in roentgenologic studies; a thick gallbladder wall due to sulfatide deposition; intraluminal filling defects (globules of sulfatide or papillomatosis; "polyposis"); very echogenic gallbladder wall; very echogenic material within the gallbladder and common bile duct may be present before neurologic symptoms are detected; (b) megacolon; (c) central nervous system: computed tomographic demonstration of *degenerative disease with diminished attenuation in the brain tissue and progressive increased difference in attenuation values between the white and gray mat-*

ter, with changes most marked in the white matter; ventricular dilatation; brain atrophy; demyelination more accurately evaluated by magnetic resonance imaging; (d) miscellaneous abnormalities: lumbar kyphosis; wide ribs; irregular metaphyses; epiphyseal dysgenesis; narrowing of the base of the iliac wings; wide acetabular angles; osteopenia; epiphyseal dysgenesis/chondrodystrophia punctata; hypoplastic vertebral bodies; spondylolisthesis of T12 on L1; butterfly vertebral deformity.

METHYLMALONIC ACIDEMIA

Enzyme Deficiency: Methylmalonyl CoA mutase, with mutations occurring at different genetic sites; partial defects in enzyme activity.

Clinical Manifestations: A disorder of organic acid metabolism with onset of symptoms in neonates or in the first year of life: (a) *accumulation of methylmalonate in blood and urine; hyperammonemia; severe ketoacidosis;* (b) poor feeding; vomiting; lethargy; apneic episodes; (c) *progressive neurologic deterioration,* most commonly extrapyramidal; (d) miscellaneous abnormalities: renal tubular and glomerular dysfunction; tubulointerstitial nephritis; recurrent pancreatitis; cardiomyopathy; pancytopenia; recurrent infections; glutathione deficiency as a complication of methylmalonic acidemia; (e) autosomal recessive inheritance.

Radiologic Manifestations: Severe involvement of the globus pallidus: hypodensity (computed tomography) affecting the pallidal nuclei (nonenhancing in the acute phase after injection of contrast medium, but enhancing in the subacute phase); low signal intensity on T_1-weighted images and high signal intensity on T_2-weighted images in the early phase (edema of pallidal nuclei); progressive pallidal necrosis; diffuse low density of white matter in some cases; delay in myelination; widening of cerebrospinal fluid space.

MEVALONIC ACIDURIA

Enzyme Deficiency: Mevalonate kinase.

Clinical Manifestations: (a) *failure to thrive*; (b) *psychomotor retardation;* hypotonia; seizures; cerebellar signs (tremor, ataxia, and nystagmus); (c) recurrent diarrhea; (d) hepatosplenomegaly; lymphadenopathy; (e) *craniofacial dysmorphism:* microcephaly; dolichocephaly; wide fontanelles; triangular face; blue sclera; central cataracts; down-slanted eyes; large, low-set, and posteriorly rotated ears; (f) anemia; thrombocytopenia; leukocytosis; (g) *high concentration of mevalonic acid in plasma, urine, and amniotic fluid; severe deficiency of mevalonate kinase activity in fibroblasts, lymphocytes, and lymphoblasts; elevated creatine kinase;* (h) autosomal recessive inheritance.

Radiologic Manifestation: Metabolic encephalopathy: *microcephaly; cerebral atrophy; cerebellar atrophy; agenesis of vermis cerebelli.*

MILK-ALKALI SYNDROME

Clinical Manifestations: Hypercalcemia secondary to high calcium intake and excessive gastrointestinal calcium absorption: nausea; vomiting; weakness; headache; dizziness; ataxia; mental confusion; toxic psychosis; pancreatitis; etc.

Radiologic Manifestations: *Deposits of calcium in different body tissues* (nephrocalcinosis; soft-tissue calcification; corneal calcification); ^{99m}Tc uptake in nonosseous lesions; increased skeletal uptake of Tc-99m methylene diphosphonate.

Note: The classic triad: *metabolic alkalosis, hypercalcemia, and renal failure.*

MUCOLIPIDOSIS II (I-CELL DISEASE; LEROY I-CELL DISEASE)

Enzyme Deficiency: *N*-Acetylglucosamine-1-phosphotransferase.

Clinical Manifestations: Onset of symptoms in the first few months of life—may be evident from birth; inter- and intrafamilial variability: (a) *facial dysmorphism:* high forehead, flat bridge of the nose, anteverted nostrils, increased distance between the upper lip and nares, puffy eyelids, prominent epicanthal folds, and increased length of the philtrum; (b) fine granularity on slit-lamp examination; corneal opacity; increased corneal diameter; (c) *Hurler-like body configuration; marked psychomotor and growth retardation; thickened skin,* especially over the joints; thick and firm earlobes; *restricted motion of joints;* hypertrophied gingiva; widely spaced nipples; hepatomegaly; (d) miscellaneous abnormalities: recurrent respiratory infections; hoarse voice; hypertrophic cardiomyopathy; low levels of 1,25-(OH)2-D3, signs of hyperparathyroidism, and histologic findings of rickets in neonatal mucolipidosis; etc.; (e) autosomal recessive inheritance; genetic heterogeneity.

Laboratory Tests: *Markedly elevated serum β-hexosaminidase, iduronate sulfatase and arylsulfatase A activities; low acid hydrolase activity in fibroblast culture;* first-trimester prenatal evaluation by (1) *N*-acetylglucosamine-1-phosphotransferase assay (in chorionic villi and cultured trophoblasts); (2) amniotic fluid and maternal serum: increased levels of lysosomal enzymes.

Radiologic Manifestations

(A) EARLY INFANCY: (a) *osteopenia; subperiosteal diaphyseal bone deficiency; multiple areas of bone destruction, especially in the metaphyses of long bones; cortical bone erosion, particularly in the medial* *aspects of the proximal parts of the femora; pathologic fractures; congenital angulated fracture; modeling abnormalities of metacarpals and metatarsals; brachyphalangia; stippled calcification of the calcaneus;* (b) *ovoid vertebral bodies; narrowness of interpediculate distances in the lower thoracic regions;* intervertebral disc calcification; (c) pelvis: *flared iliac wings; horizontal acetabular roofs; supraacetabular constriction;* (d) rickets-like changes (a defect in calcium metabolism, related to the specific enzyme defect of mucolipidosis II, may be responsible for rickets-like changes).

(B) EARLY CHILDHOOD: (a) craniomegaly; thickened cranium (in some); normal or enlarged sella turcica; (b) *shortness of the long bones with abnormal tubulation; irregularity in ossification and widening of the metaphyses; varus deformity of the humeral neck; tilted distal ends of the radius and ulna;* (c) extreme hypoplasia of carpal bones; short metacarpals with rudimentary distal epiphyses and conical tapering to the base of the second through fifth metacarpals; *hypoplasia of the epiphyses of the phalanges at the base and conical bullet-shaped distal ends;* relatively normal-appearing tarsals, metatarsals, and phalanges of the feet; (d) short anteroposterior diameter of the thoracolumbar vertebrae; inferior *beaking of the vertebral bodies at T12 through L3;* hypoplastic odontoid process; atlantoaxial dislocation; spinal cord compression; (e) broad and spatulate-appearing ribs; (f) hypoplasia of the scapula; (g) *wide iliac flare with hypoplasia of the base; irregular contours of the pubis and ischium; hip dislocation;* (h) narrow trachea (storage material accumulation).

MUCOLIPIDOSIS III (PSEUDO-HURLER POLYDYSTROPHY)

Enzyme Deficiency: *N*-Acetylglucosamine-1-phosphotransferase; closely related to mucolipidosis II; abnormal storage of glycoproteins and glycolipids.

Clinical Manifestations: Onset of clinical manifestations usually in late infancy; clinical variability: (a) *short stature; coarse facies; progressive joint stiffness and flexion contractures; mild corneal clouding;* (b) miscellaneous abnormalities: mild mental retardation; valvular heart disease; self-mutilation; clinical presentation as rheumatologic disorder; presentation as transient tubular dysfunction; etc.; (c) autosomal recessive inheritance.

Laboratory Tests: Normal levels of urinary acid mucopolysaccharides; marked decrease in activities of several lysosomal hydrolases in cultured fibroblasts, with concomitant elevated activity of these hydrolases in serum and elevated activities in urine; coarse perinuclear refractile inclusions in cultured fibroblasts.

Radiologic Manifestations: Changes similar to those of Hurler and Hunter syndromes: (a) head and neck: *premature closure of the cranial sutures (in older cases); J-shaped sella turcica; mandibular prognathism; absence of dens;* (b) trunk: *short and thick clavicles; wide and slightly short ribs; beaking of some vertebrae (upper lumbar); flaring of the iliac wings; constriction of the iliac bodies; shallow acetabular fossae;* (c) limbs: *shortening and poor tubulation of long bones; broad metaphyses and small and flat epiphyses; proximal pointing of metacarpals; clawhand deformity; soft-tissue swelling around the interphalangeal joints; smallness and irregularity of carpal bones;* (d) mild to moderate delay in skeletal maturation.

MUCOLIPIDOSIS IV

Clinical Manifestations: Onset of symptoms in infancy; some variability in manifestations: (a) *low birth weight;* (b) *craniofacial features:* small head size, myopathic face, puffy eyelids, short forehead, prominent supraorbital ridges, hypoplastic malar areas, downturned corners of mouth, and broad palatine ridges; (c) ptosis; convergent strabismus; *pigmentary retinopathy; early or congenital corneal cloudiness;* (d) *mild to severe psychomotor retardation; hypotonia;* (e) autosomal recessive inheritance; submicroscopic deletion of 16q24.3; most diagnosed cases are among Ashkenazi Jews.

Laboratory Tests: (a) corneal and conjunctival biopsy specimens, cultured amniotic fluid cells, and fibroblast culture: *lysosomal inclusions;* (b) *lysosomal accumulation of lipid and water-soluble substances:* mono- and polysialogangliosides; lyso-bis-phosphatidic acid; lysophosphatidylcholine; phosphatidylethanolamine; (c) electron microscopy: typical abnormal inclusion bodies in various organ tissues (corneal and conjunctival biopsy material, chorionic cells, cultured amniotic fluid cells, and cultured fetal skin fibroblasts).

Radiologic Manifestations: No skeletal changes; no organomegaly; nonspecific brain abnormalities: hypodensity of white matter (computed tomography); partial agenesis of the corpus callosum; possible delayed myelination.

MUCOPOLYSACCHARIDOSES

Classification: Table ME-M-1.

Table ME-M-1 Classification of the Mucopolysaccharidoses

Type	Eponym	MPS Stored	Enzyme Deficiency	Clinical Manifestations
IH	Hurler	DS, HS	α-L-iduronidase	Dysostosis multiplex, organomegaly, mental retardation, corneal clouding
IS	Scheie	DS, HS	α-L-iduronidase	Stiff joints, normal intelligence, corneal clouding
II	Hunter	DS, HS	Iduronate sulfatase	Dysostosis multiplex, organomegaly, mental retardation, flesh-colored papules, no corneal clouding
IIIA	Sanfilippo	HS	Heparan sulfate sulfaminidase	Severe neurologic degeneration, no coarse features, behavior changes
IIIB	Sanfilippo	HS	α-N-acetyl-D glucosaminidase	Same as IIIA
IIIC	Sanfilippo	HS	Glucosamine-N-acetyl transferase	Same as IIIA
IIID	Sanfilippo	HS	N-acetyl glucosamine-6-sulfatase	Same as IIIA
IVA	Morquio	KS	N-acetyl galactosamine-6-sulfatase	Skeletal abnormalities, corneal clouding, odontoid hypoplasia
IVB	Morquio	KS	Keratan sulfate galactosidase	Same as IVA
VI	Maroteaux-Lamy	DS	N-acetyl galactosamine-4-sulfatase	Dysostosis multiplex, normal intelligence, corneal clouding, hepatosplenomegaly
VII	Sly	CS, DS, HS	ß-glucuronidase	Dysostosis multiplex, hepatosplenomegaly

From Finlayson LA: Hunter syndrome (mucopolysaccharidosis II). *Pediatr Dermatol* 7:150, 1990. Reprinted by permission of Blackwell Scientific Publishers.

MPS, Mucopolysaccharides; *DS*, dermatan sulfate; *KS*, keratan sulfate; *HS*, heparan sulfate; *CS*, chondroitin sulfate.

MUCOPOLYSACCHARIDOSIS I-H (Hurler Syndrome)

Enzyme Deficiency: α-L-Iduronidase.

Clinical Manifestations: Onset of detectable clinical findings by 1 to 2 years of age; fully developed picture: (a) *grotesque facial features:* scaphocephalic large head, protruding eyes, patulous lips, thick cheeks and jaw, low nasal bridge, flared nostrils, enlarged protruding tongue, and small malaligned teeth; (b) *severe mental retardation* (early bone marrow transplantation beneficial); no correlation between magnetic resonance imaging findings and the mental retardation; (c) coarse hair; hirsutism; (d) *corneal opacification;* glaucoma; (e) *dwarfism;* (f) *thoracolumbar gibbus;* (g) *protuberant abdomen; hernias;* (h) *flexion contracture* of all joints; clawhand deformity; (i) *aerodigestive tract obstruction* with the clinical manifestations of rhinitis; adenotonsillar enlargement; recurrent otitis media; harsh voice; stridor; dyspnea; cough; retraction; feeding difficulties; etc.; (j) *deafness;* (k) *hepatosplenomegaly;* (l) *cardiomyopathy; asymmetric septal hypertrophy; cardiac failure;* endocardial fibroelastosis of infancy; reduced QRS voltage; systemic hypertension associated with arterial narrowing at various sites; regression of cardiomyopathy after bone marrow transplantation; (m) autosomal recessive inheritance; mutational heterogeneity.

Laboratory Tests: *Excess storage of acid mucopolysaccharides in tissues and excess excretion in urine (dermatan sulfate and heparan sulfate);* prenatal diagnosis by analysis of α-L-iduronidase in chorionic villi.

Radiologic Manifestations

(A) Skeletal System: (a) craniofacial abnormalities: *large neurocranium; premature closure of the sagittal and lambdoid sutures; thick calvaria (particularly at the base); shallow orbits with vertically oriented roofs; enlarged J-shaped sella turcica; calcified stylohyoid ligament; thicker than normal, short and wide mandible with obtuse angle, short rami, and flat or concave condyle; abnormally directed molar teeth; dentigerous cysts and hyperplasia of dental follicles;* (b) vertebrae: *moderate dorsolumbar gibbus, hooklike dysplasia of the vertebrae at the apex of the gibbus,* decreased anteroposterior diameters of vertebral bodies, biconvex vertebral bodies, relatively long pedicles, and failure of development of the dens with resultant subluxation of C1 on C2; subluxation of C3 on C4; (c) thorax: *wide oar-shaped ribs; short and thick clavicles; thick elevated scapulae with poorly formed glenoid fossae;* (d) long bones: *widening of the midshaft* (particularly that of humerus); varus deformity of the humeral neck; tilt of the distal parts of the radius and ulna toward each other; (e) pelvis and hips: *flared small iliac wings; steep acetabular roofs; poorly formed and thickened ischial and pubic bones;* coxa valga; subluxation of the femoral heads; (f) hands: *widening of the diaphyses of metacarpals and the proximal and mid-*

dle phalanges ("sugarloaf" metacarpals); short phalanges; smallness and irregularity of the carpal bones; pointed proximal end of the second to fifth metacarpals; (g) feet: less severe deformities of the tarsals, metatarsals, and phalanges compared with the hands and wrists.

(B) CARDIOVASCULAR SYSTEM: (a) *cardiomyopathy* with thickening of the interventricular septum and left ventricular posterior wall; thickening of the valves; calcification of the mitral annulus; mitral stenosis; regression of cardiomyopathy after bone marrow transplantation; (b) arteriopathy: aortic narrowing (thoracic, abdominal); arterial narrowing (coronary, renal, mesenteric, vertebral, axillary, intercostal, lumbar, iliac).

(C) RESPIRATORY MANIFESTATIONS: (a) upper airway obstruction: hypoplastic mandible; macroglossia; temporomandibular joint ankylosis; short neck; abnormal cervical vertebrae; high epiglottis; mucopolysaccharide infiltration of the nasopharyngeal, oropharyngeal, hypopharyngeal, and laryngeal tissues; (b) narrow trachea; recurrent pneumonia and atelectasis.

(D) NERVOUS SYSTEM: (a) computed tomography: *low attenuation areas in the white matter;* (b) magnetic resonance imaging: *delayed myelination; high signal white-matter intensity on T_2-weighted images; cystic areas* (cribriform; sievelike; multicystic) involving centrum semiovale, peritrigonal white matter, corpus callosum, pericallosal region, and basal ganglia; (c) ventriculomegaly; (d) *expansion of subarachnoid space* (enlarged interhemispheric space; enlarged cortical sulci); *thickening of dura matter at the craniocervical junction, causing narrowing of the subarachnoid space and spinal cord compression;* (e) improved magnetic resonance imaging findings after bone marrow transplant (gray-white matter contrast; myelination; etc.).

MUCOPOLYSACCHARIDOSIS I-H/S (HURLER-SCHEIE COMPOUND)

Enzyme Deficiency: α-L-Iduronidase.

Clinical Manifestations: A phenotype intermediate between that of Hurler and Scheie compound; clinical signs appear between 1 and 2 years of age: (a) excessive birth weight and infantile growth; ultimate short height; (b) normal to mild retardation of intelligence; (c) *moderate joint stiffness and limitation of motion;* (d) *hepatosplenomegaly;* (e) *neurologic symptoms related to spinal cord compression;* (f) *corneal clouding;* (g) *thickened skin; hirsutism;* (h) psychosis; (i) *urinary excretion of dermatan sulfate and heparan sulfate;* (j) *impaired mucopolysaccharide degradation and correction by Hurler factor;* (k) miscellaneous abnormalities: hernias; nasal mucosal and sinus involvement with osteal obstruction; nasal polypoid formation; (l) autosomal recessive inheritance; one Hurler gene and one Scheie gene present at the affected gene locus.

Radiologic Manifestations: *Mild to moderate dysostosis multiplex* (refer to Hurler syndrome); cardiomegaly; myocardial dysfunction; mitral valvular disease; calcific mitral stenosis; concentric impingement on the subarachnoid space; cord compression; hydrocephalus; low white-matter density (computed tomography); dentigerous cysts.

MUCOPOLYSACCHARIDOSIS I-S (Scheie Disease)

Enzyme Deficiency: α-ʟ-Iduronidase.

Clinical Manifestations: Abnormalities usually appear in childhood: (a) *gargoylism;* (b) *corneal clouding;* retinitis pigmentosa; (c) *hepatosplenomegaly;* (d) *cardiac involvement;* hypertension; claudication; (e) *joint stiffness;* clawhand; genu valgum; carpal tunnel syndrome; (f) hearing loss; (g) normal intelligence or mild mental retardation; psychotic episodes; (h) excessive dermatan sulfate and heparan sulfate excretion in urine; impaired mucopolysaccharide degradation and correction by Hurler factor; (i) autosomal recessive inheritance.

Radiologic Manifestations: (a) *dysostosis multiplex* (refer to Hurler syndrome); (b) *cardiovascular disease:* valvular stenosis (aortic; mitral); coarctation of aorta; arterial narrowing at various sites; (c) miscellaneous abnormalities: deformities and cystic changes in the carpals, metacarpals, tarsals, metatarsals, and some other bones; femoral head dysplasia; widening of the clavicles and ribs.

MUCOPOLYSACCHARIDOSIS II (Hunter Disease)

Enzyme Deficiency: Defect of catabolism of acid glycosaminoglycans caused by deficiency of the lysosomal enzyme α-iduronate sulfate sulfatase.

Clinical Manifestations: Wide clinical spectrum ranging from normal intelligence to marked mental retardation; onset of clinically detectable findings between the ages of 2 and 4 years; physical features similar to but usually milder than those of Hurler disease: (a) *coarse facies, large nose with flattened bridge and flared nostrils, prominent lips, protruding tongue, large scaphoid head, and widely spaced teeth; short neck;* (b) *progressive neurologic deterioration; mental retardation;* destructive behavior; seizures; (c) *hepatosplenomegaly;* (d) hirsutism; coarse scalp hair; *thick skin; firm ivory-white papules and nodules that may coalesce to form ridges or a reticular pattern* (the skin lesions most common on the scapular areas; also occurring on the shoulders, upper arms, upper chest, and lateral thighs); (e) clear or cloudy cornea; papilledema; retinal degeneration; (f) mild dwarfism; (g) *flexion contractures* (flexed knees and elbows; prominent buttocks; clawhand); (h) *dorsolumbar kyphosis;* (i) upper respiratory infections; recurrent otitis media; progressive deafness; symptoms related to airway obstruction (pharynx; larynx; trachea); sleep apnea; tracheobronchomalacia; (j) protuberant abdomen; hernias; mucoid diarrhea; (k) *cardiac involvement* with valvular thickening due to accumulated mucopolysaccharides; valvular insufficiency; congestive heart failure; (l) X-linked recessive inheritance; identification of the carriers by means of mutation analysis.

Laboratory Tests: Urinary screening for mucopolysaccharides (dermatan sulfate; heparan sulfate); hair root and serum enzyme studies; testing for enzyme activity in white blood cells and skin fibroblasts; prenatal testing for enzyme activity in cells obtained by chorionic villus sampling or amniocentesis; enzyme determination in the serum of pregnant heterozygote women.

Radiologic Manifestations: (a) dysostosis multiplex *similar to Hurler syndrome, with findings being less severe* and progressing more slowly; (b) aerodigestive tract (mouth; pharynx; epiglottis; larynx; trachea): *obstruction due to soft-tissue infiltration;* heterogeneous signal intensity of the soft tissues on T_1-weighted magnetic resonance images and increased signal intensity on T_2-weighted images; (c) central nervous system: (1) computed tomography: low density in the white matter, the thalamus, and the basal ganglia; (2) magnetic resonance imaging: high signals in T_2-weighted images in the deep white matter, and areas of increased and decreased signals in T_1- and T_2-weighted images in the thalamus and the basal ganglia (honeycomb-like appearance; cribriform); reduced contrast of gray and white matter on T_2-weighted images; (3) age-dependent ventriculomegaly and brain atrophy; (4) cervical myelopathy; neurogenic bladder; (d) heart: valvular thickening; valvular insufficiency; cardiac failure.

MUCOPOLYSACCHARIDOSIS III (Sanfilippo Disease)

Enzyme Deficiency: Defective degradation of heparan sulfate caused by four lysosomal enzyme deficiencies with heparan sulfate accumulation in tissues and excretion in urine:

- Type A: heparan sulfate sulfamidase
- Type B: *N*-acetyl-α-D-glucosaminidase
- Type C: acetyl-CoA: α-glucosaminide *N*-acetyltransferase
- Type D: *N*-acetylglucosamine-6-sulfate sulfatase

Clinical Manifestations: Onset of detectable abnormalities in early childhood: (a) *mild coarsening of facial features;* normal height or mild dwarfism; (b) *minimal corneal clouding;* (c) *mild joint stiffness and claw-hand deformity;* (d) *mental and motor deterioration;* behavioral disorders; sleep disturbances; hyperactivity; insomnia; aggressive reactions to fear; dementia; (e) *hepatosplenomegaly;* (f) *cardiopathy;* (g) autosomal recessive inheritance; genetic heterogeneity.

Laboratory Tests: *Heparan sulfate accumulation in tissues and excretion in urine; prenatal diagnosis:* chorionic biopsy and enzyme assay; cultured amniotic fluid cell test; increased level of heparan sulfate in amniotic fluid.

Radiologic Manifestations: Much milder skeletal deformities than Hurler syndrome: (a) skeletal system: *marked thickening of the posterior aspect of the calvaria* in association with mild thickening of the base; underdevelopment of mastoid cells; *ovoid or rectangular appearance of the thoracic and lumbar vertebrae; thickened ribs;* broad iliac wings; steep acetabular roofs; small femoral heads; poor modeling of the tubular bones of the hand; tilt of the distal part of the radius toward the ulna; thick cortex of long bones and coarse trabeculae; (b) central nervous system: *cribriform changes* (peri- and supraventricular, parietal, white matter, corpus callosum, and basal ganglia); *low density of white matter and the thalamus (computed tomography); reduced contrast of gray and white matter on T_2-weighted images; prolonged T_1 and T_2 in the thalamus; cerebral atrophy; ventricular dilatation;* (c) *cardiopathy:* asymmetric septal hypertrophy; mitral regurgitation (valvuloplasty reported); mitral valve prolapse; aortic regurgitation; etc.

MUCOPOLYSACCHARIDOSIS IVA (MORQUIO DISEASE TYPE A; BRAILSFORD-MORQUIO SYNDROME)

Enzyme Deficiency: *N*-Acetylgalactosamine-6-sulfatase.

Classification: Clinical heterogeneity: (a) Morquio A, severe ("classic type"); (b) Morquio A, intermediate; (c) Morquio A, mild.

Clinical Manifestations: The disease usually becomes detectable between the first and third years of life; fully developed clinical picture: (a) *short-trunk dwarfism;* (b) mildly coarse facial features, broad mouth, and short nose; (c) *abnormal posture* (kyphosis at the thoracolumbar junction, prominent buttocks, pectus carinatum, and severe knock-knee); (d) *misshapen hands and feet;* (e) *hyperextensible joints;* (f) spinal cord compression due to atlantoaxial dislocation; chronic myelopathy with a slow or rapid rate of progression; quadriparesis; sudden death by respiratory arrest; (g) minimal corneal clouding; cataracts; (h) *normal intelligence;* (i) progressive deafness; (j) recurrent or chronic pneumonia; cardiac failure secondary to thoracic cage deformities; restricted pattern on ventilatory studies; hypoxemia due to right-to-left shunting (probably caused by microatelectasis); (k) valvular disease; cardiomyopathy; (l) dental abnormalities: thin enamel layers; smallness; more opaque than normal; pointed cusps of the permanent posterior teeth (concave and saucer-shaped biting surface; concave buccal surface); pitting of the buccal surfaces of the permanent posterior teeth; spade-shaped and spaced permanent maxillary incisors and deciduous teeth; (m) autosomal recessive inheritance.

Laboratory Tests: *Excess keratan sulfate excretion in the urine,* most marked in childhood; decreasing and becoming normal in adults; absence of keratosulfaturia in some cases in childhood; two-dimensional electrophoresis of urine glycosaminoglycans; enzyme deficiency in fibroblasts.

Radiologic Manifestations

(A) SKELETAL SYSTEM: (a) skull: mildly dolichocephalic skull; underdevelopment of mastoid cells; flat or concave mandibular condyles; (b) spine: *universal platyspondyly; small or disappearing odontoid process* of the axis; *atlantoaxial subluxation* resulting in narrowing of the spinal canal; irregular margins of the vertebral bodies; (c) thorax: *flaring of ribs; pectus carinatum;* short superoinferior height and increased anteroposterior diameter of the thorax; premature fusion of ossification centers of the sternum; (d) pelvis and hips: *constricted iliac wings; steeply oblique acetabular roofs; coxa valga; gradual disappearance of the ossified femoral head (aseptic necrosis);* (e) long bones: slight to moderate widening of the diaphyses and irregularity of the epiphyses and metaphyses of long bones in the advanced stage of the disease; (f) hands: *small and irregular carpal bones; pointed proximal end of the second through fifth metacarpals;* relatively wide first and fifth metacarpals and phalanges; (g) feet: irregular contour and delayed ossification of the tarsal bones; central constriction and shortness of the metatarsals and phalanges.

(B) DENTAL ABNORMALITIES: Thin enamel that does not extend as far down the neck of the tooth (thin enamel cap); widely spaced teeth; dental caries.

(C) CENTRAL NERVOUS SYSTEM: (a) *low density white matter (computed tomography); prolonged T_1 and T_2 in the white matter; ventriculomegaly; dilatation of the basal cisterns and subarachnoid space;* (b) *craniovertebral junction narrowing (dura matter thickening; atlantoaxial subluxation); spinal cord compression (thoracolumbar, less commonly cervicothoracic).*

(D) AIRWAY OBSTRUCTION: Narrow trachea; collapse of trachea during head flexion.

(E) CARDIAC ABNORMALITIES: Predominantly left-sided: valvular disease (thickening; stenosis; insufficiency); ventricular wall hypertrophy.

MUCOPOLYSACCHARIDOSIS IVB (MORQUIO DISEASE TYPE B)

Enzyme Deficiency: ß-Galactosidase.

Clinical Manifestations: Similar to Morquio disease: (a) *short stature; corneal clouding; chest deformity;* normal intelligence; normal enamel; *excess keratan sulfate excretion in the urine; oligosacchariduria;*

other reported abnormalities: cervical myelopathy; progressive mental handicap; (b) autosomal recessive inheritance.

Radiologic Manifestations: Skeletal abnormalities similar to Morquio disease, but with milder deformities (progressive spondyloepiphyseal dysplasia).

MUCOPOLYSACCHARIDOSIS VI (MAROTEAUX-LAMY SYNDROME)

Enzyme Deficiency: Arylsulfatase B (*N*-acetylgalactosamine-4-sulfatase) leading to the accumulation of the glycosaminoglycan substrate and dermatan sulfate, primarily in connective tissue and reticuloendothelial cell lysosomes.

Clinical Manifestations: Phenotypic variability related to broad molecular heterogeneity: (a) prominent forehead, sternal protrusion, and joint stiffness may be present at birth; (b) *growth arrest* at about 2 to 4 years of age; (c) *coarse facies,* usually less grotesque than those in Hurler syndrome; (d) *corneal opacity;* (e) normal mental development; (f) progressive hearing loss; (g) hepatosplenomegaly; (h) hernias; (i) hydrocephalus; optic atrophy; myelopathy (gait disturbances; pain; paresthesia; urinary and fecal incontinence); (j) aortic and mitral valve involvement; cardiac and respiratory failure; endocardial fibroelastosis; (k) *excess excretion of dermatan sulfate in the urine;* (l) autosomal recessive inheritance; genetic heterogeneity (severe, mild, and intermediate phenotypes).

Radiologic Manifestations

(A) SKELETAL SYSTEM ABNORMALITIES: Quite variable in severity and extent: (a) skull: *large dolichocephalic skull; large omega-shaped sella turcica; thick calvaria; premature closure of cranial sutures; large foramina of the emissary veins; short mandibular rami;* (b) spine: *oval or bullet-shaped vertebral bodies; kyphosis at the lower thoracic or upper lumbar regions with a wedge-shaped vertebra at the center of the curve; hypoplasia of the odontoid;* (c) thorax: *canoe-paddle appearance of the ribs; small and highly located scapulae; hypoplastic glenoid fossae; widening of the medial aspect of the clavicles;* (d) pelvis and hips: *irregularity and underdevelopment of the acetabular roofs; fragmentation of the femoral head (aseptic necrosis);* (e) limbs: *widening of the diaphyses of long bones and constriction of metaphyseal regions; hatchet-shaped proximal portions of the humeri; bowed radii and ulnae; irregularity of metaphyses and deformity of epiphyses; pointed base of metacarpals and widening of the shafts of short tubular bones.*

(B) CENTRAL NERVOUS SYSTEM: (a) prolonged T_1 and T_2 in various areas of the cerebral white matter; symmetrically low attenuation in the white matter on computed tomographic examination; hydrocephalus internus; brain atrophy; empty sella; (b) *ligamentous thickening and weakening causing* *vertebral subluxation and spinal cord compression, particularly at the atlantoaxial level; thickening of dura mater at the craniocervical junction.*

(C) AIRWAYS: Retropharyngeal and retrotracheal swelling; narrowing of the upper airways; narrow trachea.

(D) CARDIOVASCULAR SYSTEM: Valvular lesions; cardiomyopathy.

MUCOPOLYSACCHARIDOSIS VII (SLY DISEASE)

Enzyme Deficiency: ß-Glucuronidase.

Clinical Manifestations: Considerable phenotypic variation with minimal to marked clinical abnormalities (mild, moderate, and severe forms); onset of symptoms in early infancy and childhood: (a) *craniofacial dysmorphism:* large skull, coarse facies, hypertelorism, and gingivitis; (b) short neck; (c) *corneal clouding;* (d) *short stature;* protruding sternum; kyphosis; kyphoscoliosis; (e) *hepatosplenomegaly;* (f) *subnormal intelligence;* degeneration of speech, language, and hearing; (g) cardiovascular lesions: arterial fibromuscular dysplasia; arterial stenosis; aortic regurgitation; left-sided heart failure; (h) autosomal recessive inheritance.

Laboratory Tests: *Excessive excretion of dermatan sulfate and heparan sulfate; enzyme deficiency* in tissues, fibroblasts, leukocytes, and serum; enzyme deficiency evaluation of the amniotic fluid; first-trimester evaluation by chorionic villi sampling; glycosaminoglycan accumulation.

Radiologic Manifestations: Variable (patients with early onset of symptoms developing more severe manifestations): *dysostosis multiplex with various degrees of bone deformities* (J-shaped sella; platyspondyly; vertebral beaking; broadening of tubular bones; defective ossification of carpal and tarsal bones; hip dislocation; metatarsus adductus; etc.); atlantoaxial instability.

MULTIPLE SULFATASE DEFICIENCY (AUSTIN DISEASE)

Enzyme Deficiency: (a) Arylsulfatases A, B, and C; (b) iduronate-2-sulfate sulfatase; (c) *N*-acetylgalactosamine-6-sulfatase; (d) heparan *N*-sulfatase.

Clinical Manifestations: Classic clinical presentation in the first 2 years of life: (a) *developmental arrest followed by regression;* (b) *coarse facial features,* especially when onset of symptoms occurs in the first year of life (similar to Hunter syndrome); microcephaly; (c) *ichthyosis;* (d) *pigmentary retinopathy; corneal clouding; lens opacification; cherry-red spot; optic atrophy;* (e) *hepatosplenomegaly;* (f) *deafness; severe progressive dementia; pyramidal tract signs;* (g) miscellaneous abnormalities: gibbus; cardiac involvement; neonatal form; juvenile form; etc.; (h) autosomal recessive inheritance.

Radiologic Manifestations: Combined features of metachromatic leukodystrophy, Maroteaux-Lamy, Morquio, Sanfilippo type A, and Hunter diseases: *dysostosis multiplex* (refer to Hurler syndrome); *cerebral leukodystrophy; brain atrophy; hydrocephalus;* cervical cord compression (thickened posterior arch of C1, narrow foramen magnum, and meningeal thickening).

N

NAVAJO NEUROPATHY

Clinical Manifestations: (a) *sensorimotor neuropathy:* weakness; acral mutilation; corneal insensitivity; ulceration and scarring; autonomic dysfunction; slow nerve conduction velocities; *failure to thrive; short stature;* scoliosis; sural nerve biopsy: *almost total loss of myelinated fibers;* (b) autosomal recessive inheritance.

Radiologic Manifestations: Cerebral and cerebellar white matter disease: decreased signal intensity on T_1-weighted images and increased signal intensity on T_2-weighted images.

Note: The preceding clinical manifestations are those of type A Navajo neuropathy. Autonomic disturbances and severe neuropathic arthropathy are the major manifestations of type B disease.

NELSON SYNDROME

Definition: Development of an adrenocorticotropic hormone–secreting pituitary tumor following total adrenalectomy for Cushing syndrome associated with adrenal hyperplasia (pituitary-dependent Cushing syndrome).

Clinical Manifestations: Development or worsening of skin and mucosal hyperpigmentation after adrenalectomy for Cushing syndrome; clinical manifestation of pituitary tumor (particularly important in microadenomas); headaches; bitemporal hemianopia; etc.

Radiologic Manifestations: Sellar enlargement and deformity; pituitary tumor (magnetic resonance imaging better than computed tomography in demonstrating the tumor development): displacement of the infundibulum or optic chiasm; infiltration of the cavernous sinus.

NEUROACANTHOCYTOSIS (Levine-Critchley Syndrome)

Clinical Manifestations: Adult onset of symptoms: (a) *progressive orofacial dyskinesia and choreic movements of the limbs; tongue and/or* *lip biting; peripheral neuropathy; acanthocytosis in peripheral blood; normal plasma β-lipoprotein; increased level of serum creatine kinase;* cardiomyopathy; generalized seizures; cognitive deficits; parkinsonism; pes cavus; abnormal composition of tightly bound fatty acids of erythrocyte membrane proteins; (b) most likely autosomal recessive inheritance.

Pathology: *Atrophy and gliosis of the caudate, putamen, and globus pallidus;* ventriculomegaly (especially the anterior horns); other sites of atrophy: thalamus, substantia nigra, and anterior horns of the spinal cord.

Radiologic Manifestations: *Bilateral caudate and putamen atrophy;* glucose hypometabolism of the caudate and putamen (positron emission tomography); hypoperfusion of frontal lobes (cerebral blood flow tomography).

NEURONAL CEROID LIPOFUSCINOSIS (Batten Disease)

Classification and Clinical Manifestations: (a) accumulation of autofluorescent ceroid-lipofuscin pigment in the brain and other tissues (Table ME-N-1); (b) autosomal recessive inheritance.

Radiologic Manifestations: Rapid progression of cerebral abnormalities in the first four years of life: (a) *brain atrophy* (most severe in the cerebellum); magnetic resonance imaging: hyperintense periventricular white matter, especially around the bodies and atria of the lateral ventricles (periventricular rim); significant decrease in signal intensity in the thalami and/or putamina; (b) single photon emission computed tomography: hypoperfusion of the cerebellum; (c) positron emission tomography: reduced regional cerebral metabolic rate.

NIEMANN-PICK DISEASE (Sphingomyelin Lipidoses)

Enzyme Deficiency: Sphingomyelinase deficiency in types A and B; diagnosis by enzymatic assay of white blood cells or fibroblasts.

Clinical Classification and Manifestations

(A) Type A (Acute Neuronopathic Form): Onset of symptoms in infancy: (a) *feeding difficulties;* (b) *weight loss; cachexia;* (c) *regressive intellectual capabilities; hypotonia; flaccidity;* (d) *hepatosplenomegaly; protuberant abdomen;* (e) brownish yellow skin discoloration; (f) ocular manifestations: *cherry-red spots* (50% of patients); corneal opacification; retinal opacification; brownish discoloration of the anterior lens capsule; (g) *foamy histiocytes* in the bone marrow, spleen, lymph nodes, adrenal medulla, and the alveoli of the lungs.

(B) Type B (Chronic Form without Central Nervous System Involvement): Onset of symptoms in infancy: (a) *hepatosplenomegaly;* (b) recurrent pneumonias; (c) *delayed growth and height;* (d) anemia; (e)

Table ME-N-1   Diagnostic Criteria for Some Established Human Forms of Neuronal Ceroid Lipofuscinosis (NCL, Batten Disease)

Nosological Entity Eponyms and Other Designations	Infantile NCL (INCL) Santavuori-Haltia Disease; CLN1 MIM 256730	Late-Infantile NCL (LINCL) Jansky-Bielschowsky Disease; CLN2 MIM 204500	Early Juvenile NCL; Late Infantile NCL Variant	Juvenile NCL (JNCL) Spielmeyer-Vogt Disease; CLN3 MIM 204200	Adult NCL; Kufs Disease MIM 204300
Incidence per 100,000 live births	7.7 (Finland)	2.2 (British Columbia) 0.5 (Germany)		0.5-0.7 (British Columbia, Germany, Holland) 4.8 (Finland)	
Clinical leading symptoms					
Onset and progression of visual failure	12-22 months	2-3 years Progression to blindness slow	4-5 years	4-9 years Blind by age 6-14 years	—
Onset of seizures	14-24 months	2½-3½ years (severe)	5-6 years	8-16 years	
Onset of dementia	6-18 months	2½-3½ years	5-9 years	6-9 years	30 years
Inability to walk	12-18 months	3½-6 years	10-20 years	10->20 years	
Motor disorders	Stereotypic hand movements Choreoathetosis	Myoclonus	Myoclonus	Rigidity in some Myoclonus	Facial dyskinesia Myoclonus
Other findings				Slurred speech, echolalia (onset 10-14 years)	Psychotic symptoms
Death	<14 years	10-15 years	10-30 years	20-40 years	

From Kohlschütter A, Gardiner RM, Goebel HH: Human forms of neuronal ceroid-lipofuscinosis (Batten disease): consensus on diagnostic criteria, Hamburg 1992, *J Inherit Metab Dis* 16:241, 1993. Used by permission.

Continued

Table ME-N-1 Diagnostic Criteria for Some Established Human Forms of Neuronal Ceroid Lipofuscinosis (NCL, Batten Disease)—cont'd

Nosological Entity Eponyms and Other Designations	Infantile NCL (INCL) Santavuori-Haltia Disease; CLN1 MIM 256730	Late-Infantile NCL (LINCL) Jansky-Bielschowsky Disease; CLN2 MIM 204500	Early Juvenile NCL; Late Infantile NCL Variant	Juvenile NCL (JNCL) Spielmeyer-Vogt Disease; CLN3 MIM 204200	Adult NCL; Kufs Disease MIM 204300
Retinal pathology					
Macular degeneration	+	+	+	+	−
Pigment aggregation	−	+	+	+	−
ERG absent by age	12 months	3-4 years	4-5 years	5-7 years	−
Neurophysiology					
EEG: helpful findings	Flattening 18-24 months Isoelectric 3-4 years Photic response absent	Large polyspikes after single flashes (at early stage)			
Visual evoked potential	↓, Absent > 12 months	↑↑	↑↑	→	→
Somatosensory evoked potential	↓, Absent < 12 months	↑↑	↑↑	→	→
Neuroimaging					
CT/MRI—brain atrophy	++	+	+	+	+

Morphology

LM vacuolated lymphocytes	—	—	—	++	—
EM of predominant inclusions	Granular	Curvilinear	Curvilinear Fingerprint	Fingerprint Curvilinear (Granular)	Granular Fingerprint
Preferred tissue	Skin Rectal	Skin Rectal	Skin Rectal	Skin Lymphocyte Rectal	Skin Rectal Muscle Brain
Biochemistry					
Subunit c* accumulated	—	++		+	+
Genetics					
Inheritance	AR	AR	AR	AR	AR,AD
Chromosomal location	1p	≠ locus for CLN1 ≠ locus for CLN 3		16p	
Prenatal diagnosis	Established (DNA linkage; EM of CV, AFC	Possible (EM of CV, AFC; subunit c* in CV)		Possible (DNA linkage; EM of CV, AFC, fetal skin, lymphocytes; subunit c* in CV)	
Carrier testing	Possible in selected cases				

From Kohlschütter A, Gardiner RM, Goebel HH: Human forms of neuronal ceroid-lipofuscinosis (Batten disease): consensus on diagnostic criteria, Hamburg 1992, *J Inherit Metab Dis* 16:241, 1993. Used by permission.

AD, Autosomal dominant; *AFC,* amniotic fluid cells; *AR,* autosomal recessive; *CV,* chorionic villi; *EM,* electron microscopy; *LM,* light microscopy; +, present; −, absent; ↑, elevated;↓, decreased.

*Subunit c of mitochondrial ATP synthase.

foam cells in the bone marrow; visceral infiltration with lipid-laden histio-cytes; accumulation of sphingomyelin in multiple tissues; (f) first-trimester prenatal diagnosis: chorionic villi and chemical study; (g) miscellaneous abnormalities: polyglandular involvement; liver cirrhosis; lung involve-ment; fatal liver failure; increased alkaline phosphatase levels (may be asymptomatic); increased serum transaminase concentration; hyperlipi-demia; association with familial Mediterranean fever; presentation as recurrent episodes of osteomyelitis.

(C) TYPE C (CHRONIC NEURONOPATHIC FORM; JUVENILE FORM): An entity distinct from types A and B, characterized by deficient intracellular transport of exogenously derived cholesterol, and accumulation of choles-terol in lysosomes; onset of symptoms from infancy through adulthood: (a) *hepatosplenomegaly;* (b) *progressive neurologic manifestations:* regres-sive intellectual capabilities; ataxia; seizures; loss of coordination; hyper-tonia; hyperactive reflexes; (c) *cholestasis;* (d) *foamy macrophages in the bone marrow; defect of cholesterol esterification in cultured fibroblasts;* ultrastructural examination of skin biopsy showing lysosomes containing loosely arrayed dark lamellated structures within a clear matrix; prenatal diagnosis in families with the classic biochemical phenotype (cultured amniotic fluid cells; cultured chorionic villus cells); (e) death in childhood or adolescence; (f) miscellaneous abnormalities: biliary atresia and meco-nium ileus; presentation as "neonatal hepatitis"; clinical heterogeneity in a sibship; cataplexy (abrupt loss of muscle tone, reversible); fetal ascites; fatal pulmonary form; higher mortality in patients with preschool onset than in patients with school-age onset of the disease; psychosis as the ini-tial manifestation of adult-onset Niemann-Pick disease, type C.

(D) TYPE D (NOVA SCOTIA VARIANT): A neurovisceral disease with onset of symptoms in early childhood and a clinical picture similar to that of type C; patients with a common ancestry from the coastal area in west-ern Nova Scotia; abnormal intracellular cholesterol metabolism.

(E) TYPE E (ADULT, NONNEURONOPATHIC FORM): (a) *moderate hep-atosplenomegaly;* (b) *foam cells in the bone marrow;* (c) biochemically closely related to type C.

(F) Autosomal recessive inheritance; genetic heterogeneity of type C.

Pathology: A heterogeneous group of metabolic disorders with the common feature of variable degree of sphingomyelin accumulation in dif-ferent tissues (liver; spleen; lungs; thymus; etc.); foam cells in the bone marrow; storage within neurons and phagocytic cells in the white matter (Niemann-Pick cells), and in the leptomeninges and choroid plexuses; demyelination; gliosis.

Radiologic Manifestations: (a) skeletal system: *widening of the medullary cavities of the ribs and long bones; thinning of the cortices and expansion of the shafts of tubular bones;* Erlenmeyer-flask deformity of distal portions of the femora; anterior notching of the vertebrae at the thoracolumbar junction; *osteoporosis;* spontaneous fractures; coxa valga; notch defects in the proximal humeral diaphysis and metaphysis of older children (also noted in normal children); punctate calcific deposits inferior to the sacrum and coccyx, in the hips and feet (in two infants); (b) visceral involvement: *hepatosplenomegaly;* diffuse liver calcification; renomegaly; miliary, nodular, or reticular infiltration of the lungs; diffuse lung calcification; (c) central nervous system (types A and C): *demyelination, gliosis;* (d) miscellaneous abnormalities: echogenic splenic tumors in types B and C; hypoplasia of the corpus callosum in type C; abnormal lipid signals in the brain of a case of type C Niemann-Pick disease (shown by magnetic resonance spectroscopy); liver lesions in a case of type B Niemann-Pick disease (related to sea-blue histiocyte syndrome).

O

OCCIPITAL HORN SYNDROME (X-Linked Cutis Laxa)

Enzyme Deficiency: Lysyl oxidase.

Clinical Manifestations: A disorder of copper transport: (a) *long, thin face; high forehead; highly arched palate; occipital bony protuberances;* (b) *soft and lax skin; mildly hyperextensible skin; easily bruised; atrophic scars; digital hypermobility; limited extension at the elbows and knees;* (c) coarse and abundant hair; (d) chronic diarrhea and malabsorption; (e) low-normal intelligence; (f) miscellaneous abnormalities: persistent open anterior fontanelle; hooked nose; long philtrum; long neck; narrow shoulders; narrow rib cage; pectus excavatum; pectus carinatum, cardiac murmur; syncopal episodes; respiratory and urinary tract infections; micturition disturbances; inguinal hernia; seizures; generalized muscular atrophy; (g) X-linked inheritance.

Laboratory Tests: *Low copper concentration (serum; hair); low serum ceruloplasmin; abnormalities in cultured fibroblasts* (low lysyl oxidase activity; increased copper content; increased ^{64}Cu incorporation; accumulation of metallothionein or metallothionein-like protein; increased extractability of newly synthesized collagen; reduced conversion of newly synthesized collagen into insoluble form).

Radiologic Manifestations: (a) *bilateral, parasagittal, and symmetric occipital bony protuberances ("occipital horns");* (b) osteopenia; (c) limb: widening and bowing of multiple long bones at tendinous and ligamentous insertion sites; wavy appearance of the cortices of the tubular bones; capitate-hamate fusion; dislocated radial head; bulbous ulnar coronoids; flattened glenoid fossa; broad scapular neck; expanded distal digital tufts; coxa valga; genu valgum; fibular shortening; tarsal abnormalities; pes planus; (d) trunk: pectus excavatum; pectus carinatum; deformed clavicles (hammer-shaped); rib irregularity; mild platyspondyly; broad, round iliac wings; expanded ischial and pubic bones; flattened acetabular roofs; (e) *bladder diverticula* with tendency to recur postoperatively; bladder rupture; obstructive uropathy; (f) miscellaneous abnormalities: intracranial arterial narrowing; ectatic carotid arteries; hiatal hernia.

Note: This syndrome was formerly known as occipital horn–type Ehlers-Danlos syndrome (Ehlers-Danlos type IX).

ORNITHINE TRANSCARBAMYLASE DEFICIENCY

Enzyme Deficiency: Ornithine carbamoyl transferase.

Clinical Manifestations: An inborn error of the urea cycle with a postnatal onset of symptoms and fluctuating course: (a) *vomiting; lethargy; feeding difficulties; grunting; tachypnea; respiratory alkalosis;* (b) *seizures; hypertonicity or hypotonicity; abnormal electroencephalographic findings; coma;* (c) *hyperammonemia; elevated levels of glutamine and alanine; orotic aciduria after a standard protein load;* (d) miscellaneous abnormalities: often fatal hyperammonemic encephalopathy in affected males; carrier females usually asymptomatic; hemorrhagic diathesis (pulmonary; intracranial; gastrointestinal); recurrent episodes of bizarre behavior; neuropathologic changes acquired in utero; strokelike episodes; sudden onset of clinical manifestations after aspirin ingestion; spongiform and cystic degeneration of the brain substance and gliosis of the white matter in advanced cases; (e) X-linked inheritance; a heterogeneous metabolic disorder caused by a variety of defects in the ornithine transcarbamylase gene (mapped to Xp21.1); variable expression in females; frequent new mutations.

Radiologic Manifestations: *Cerebral swelling, diffuse low attenuation changes in the cerebral white and gray matter on computed tomography; high signals on the T_2-weighted magnetic resonance images* (the changes may be partially reversible); changes in gray and white matter resembling infarcts on computed tomography and magnetic resonance imaging in patients with the clinical manifestations of strokelike episodes; cavitation at the base of the sulci; *brain atrophy in advanced cases.*

OVARIAN HYPERSTIMULATION SYNDROME

Clinical Manifestations: Onset of symptoms usually 5 to 7 days after ovulation; mild to severe manifestations: (a) mild form: lower abdominal discomfort, no significant weight gain, and *enlarged ovaries* (less than 5 cm in average diameter); (b) severe form: *ovarian enlargement more than 10 cm* *in average diameter, hemoconcentration, hypotension, oliguria, and electrolyte imbalance;* (c) side effect of treatment with fertility drugs; occurrence after follicular aspiration; occurrence in premature infants (estradiol-producing ovarian cysts); (d) miscellaneous abnormalities: arterial and venous thromboses; prerenal azotemia; edema; adult respiratory syndrome; high concentrations of the renin-angiotensin-aldosterone system.

Radiologic Manifestations: *Enlarged ovaries mainly due to the presence of multiple thin-walled cysts,* often located in the periphery; *ascites; pleural effusion;* pericardial effusion; complication (ovarian rupture; ovarian torsion).

OXALOSIS (HYPEROXALURIA)

Classification

(A) PRIMARY OXALOSIS: A defect in glyoxylate metabolism resulting in an increased synthesis of oxalic acid: (a) type I: excessive urinary excretion of oxalic, glyoxylic, and glycolic acids due to a deficiency of the peroxisomal enzyme alanine-glyoxylate aminotransferase; genotypic and phenotypic heterogeneity; (b) type II: excessive urinary excretion of L-glyceric acid and oxalic acid due to combined deficiencies of D-glyceric dehydrogenase and glyoxylate reductase.

(B) SECONDARY OXALOSIS: Ethylene glycol ingestion; pyridoxine deficiency; ileal resection; excess ingestion of oxalate or its precursors; methoxyflurane anesthesia; liver cirrhosis; renal failure; renal tubular acidosis; sarcoidosis; long-term hemodialysis (hemodialysis oxalosis synovitis); intravenous xylitol treatment (renocerebral oxalosis); small-bowel bypass for morbid obesity; steatorrhea; diabetes mellitus; excessive vitamin C ingestion; sarcoidosis; Shwachman syndrome; cystic fibrosis; long-term hemodialysis (cutaneous oxalosis).

Clinical Manifestations: Heterogeneous presentation and clinical course, ranging from the malignant neonatal form causing death in infancy to the milder form in which the patient may not become symptomatic until adulthood: (a) *urinary calculi;* urinary tract infections; *renal failure;* (b) *growth delay;* (c) miscellaneous abnormalities: acute arthritis; cardiac arrhythmias; secondary cutaneous oxalosis; bulbous enlargement of the tips of the fingers and extrusion of calcium oxalate from nail beds; pancytopenia (related to bone marrow obliteration by calcium oxalate crystals); hepatosplenomegaly; hematuria in acquired hyperoxaluria; secondary oxalosis and sperm granuloma of the epididymis; oxalosis associated with aluminum bone disease; progressive hand gangrene; (d) autosomal recessive inheritance; heterozygous carriers; genetic heterogeneity.

Laboratory Tests: (a) type I primary: *excessive urinary excretion of oxalic, glyoxylic, and glycolic acids; determination of enzyme activity in* *liver tissue;* (b) type II primary: *excessive urinary excretion of oxalate and L-glycerate; determination of enzyme deficiency in leukocytes and liver tissue; hyperoxalemia;* hypercalcemia; high levels of serum parathyroid hormone (secondary hyperparathyroidism).

Pathology: (a) deposition of the calcium salt of oxalate: kidneys; bones; soft tissues; vessels; the conduction system of the heart; central nervous system; eyes; rete testis; etc.; (b) nephrocalcinosis; renal calculi; pyelonephritis; progressive renal destruction and atrophy.

Radiologic Manifestations: (a) urinary system: (1) *increased kidney radiopacity;* (2) *closely packed, marked increased echogenicity of the renal parenchyma as compared with renal sinus fat;* (3) computed tomography: *uniformly dense cortex and medulla; parenchymal loss in the later stage of the disease;* (4) *renal scintigram: poor perfusion and function;* (5) *radiopaque renal calculi;* (6) *nephrocalcinosis;* (b) *skeletal system changes in primary types related to oxalosis and renal osteodystrophy:* narrow transversal radiolucent band adjacent to physis; irregular transverse sclerotic metaphyseal band; subchondral areas of sclerosis in the long bones; intraosseous and periosteal tophi (calcium oxalate); "rugger-jersey" vertebrae; pathologic fractures; slow healing at the fracture sites; extrusion of crystalline material from bone; epiphyseal displacement; osteoporosis in the early phase of the disease; diffuse bone sclerosis in the advanced stage; diffuse increased uptake on nuclear bone scan (with reversal in response to treatment); (c) vascular and soft tissue calcification; (d) retarded skeletal maturation; (e) extraosseous uptake on bone scintigraphy: heart; kidneys (with reversal in response to treatment).

Note: (a) type I primary oxalosis is more common than type II; (b) in secondary oxalosis, the skeletal and soft-tissue manifestations related to oxalosis and renal osteodystrophy are generally much less prominent; (c) the extent of bone disease is related to the severity of hyperoxaluria.

P

PARANEOPLASTIC SYNDROMES

Definition: Remote effect of neoplasia due to known hormone production in some cases and unknown mechanism in others.

Clinical and Radiologic Manifestations

(A) ENDOCRINE DISORDERS

1. *Cushing syndrome* (production of adrenocorticotropic hormone by neoplasm): carcinoma of the lung; malignant epithelial thymoma; islet cell carcinoma; small cell carcinoma; carcinoids; car-

cinomas of the larynx and salivary glands; medullary thyroid carcinoma; ovarian carcinoma; pheochromocytoma; most of amine precursor uptake and decarboxylation (APUD) series origin; Ewing sarcoma.

2. *Hypoglycemia* (associated with non–islet cell neoplasms): fibrosarcomas; other sarcomas; benign fibromas; mesotheliomas; adrenal cortical carcinoma; lymphomas; gastrointestinal carcinomas.

3. *Hyperglycemia:* glucagon-producing islet cell neoplasms; enteroglucagon-producing renal carcinoma; somatostatin-containing islet cell neoplasm.

4. *Hypercalcemia:* osseous metastases; elevated levels of parathormone and hypercalcemia (carcinomas of the lung; esophageal neoplasms with ectopic hyperparathyroidism; squamous carcinomas of the head and neck region; carcinomas in other locations; lymphomas; leukemias).

5. *Hypocalcemia and osteomalacia:* hypocalcemia very rarely associated with neoplasia; rickets and osteomalacia have been reported with various "tumors" (hemangiomas of bones or soft tissues; hemangiopericytoma; giant cell tumor; osteoblastoma; fibrous dysplasia; malignant neurinoma; sarcoma; epidermal nevus syndrome; nonosteogenic fibroma; etc.).

6. *Inappropriate secretion of antidiuretic hormone:* lung cancer; digestive system cancer; lymphoma.

7. *Carcinoid syndrome* associated with noncarcinoid neoplasms: adenocarcinoma of the pancreas; islet cell neoplasms; small cell carcinoma of the lung; medullary carcinoma of the thyroid; most of APUD series origin.

8. *Gynecomastia:* nonseminomatous carcinomas of the testis; liver cell and renal carcinomas; lung carcinomas; etc.

9. *Hyperthyroidism:* hydatidiform mole or choriocarcinoma; nonseminomatous testicular carcinoma.

10. *Hypertension:* pheochromocytoma; neuroblastoma; aldosteronoma; renal tumors (Wilms; renal cell carcinoma; hemangiopericytoma; etc.).

(B) HEMATOLOGIC DISORDERS

1. *Polycythemia:* renal tumors (Wilms; renal cell carcinoma); liver cell carcinoma; cerebellar hemangioblastoma; leiomyomas of the uterus; renal cystic disease; hydronephrosis; etc.

2. *Erythroid aplasia:* thymoma; cancer of the lung, stomach, or thyroid; lymphoid neoplasia.

3. *Hemolytic anemia:* lymphoid malignancies; carcinomas of the ovary, stomach, colon, lung, cervix, or breast.

4. *Thrombocytosis and leukocytosis:* metastatic lesions, especially with marrow involvement.

(C) Coagulopathies

1. *Intravascular coagulation:* acute progranulocytic leukemia; carcinoma of the prostate; mucin-producing adenocarcinomas.
2. *Venous thrombosis:* neoplasms of the stomach, pancreas, ovary, lung, colon, etc.
3. *Dysfibrinogenemia:* liver cell carcinoma; metastatic liver tumors; etc.

(D) Protein Disorders

1. *Amyloidosis:* myeloma; macroglobulinemia; lymphomas; renal cell carcinoma; gastric carcinoma.
2. *Paraproteinemia* (monoclonal gammopathy): plasmacytic neoplasms; carcinomas; sarcomas; lymphomas; leukemias.

(E) Digestive Disorders

1. *Zollinger-Ellison syndrome:* non–beta cell adenomas or carcinomas of the pancreas or duodenum; mucinous adenocarcinoma of the ovary; ductal adenocarcinoma of the pancreas.
2. *Multiple endocrine neoplasia* (MEN):
   a. MEN-I: gastrinomas or insulinomas; parathyroid and pituitary neoplasms.
   b. MEN-IIA: medullary carcinoma of the thyroid, pheochromocytoma, and parathyroid neoplasm.
   c. MEN-IIB: medullary carcinoma of the thyroid, pheochromocytoma, and dermal or mucosal neuromas.
3. *Diarrhea and tumors:* Zollinger-Ellison syndrome; carcinoid syndrome; "pancreatic cholera" (non–beta islet cell neoplasm; vasoactive intestinal polypeptide production).

(F) Nephrogenic Hepatic Dysfunction Syndrome: Liver dysfunction associated with renal cell carcinoma.

(G) Renal Dysfunction

1. *Nephrotic syndrome:* lymphomas; carcinomas of the lung, stomach, colon, or ovary.
2. *Tubular dysfunction:* multiple myeloma; idiopathic light-chain proteinuria; acute nonlymphocytic leukemia.

(H) Musculoskeletal Disorders

1. *Hypertrophic osteoarthropathy:* malignant (primary or secondary) or benign lung tumors; intraabdominal cancers.
2. *Dermatomyositis:* carcinoma of the breast, lung, ovary, or stomach; leukemias; lymphomas; sarcomas.
3. *Childhood polymyositis:* immunoblastic sarcoma.
4. *Polymyopathy* (types I and II atrophy; necrosis): small cell lung carcinoma.

(I) Skin Disorders

1. *Acanthosis nigricans:* adenocarcinomas (stomach; etc.).

2. *Miscellaneous dermatoses:* pellagra-like lesions (carcinoid syndrome); porphyria cutanea tarda (liver cell carcinoma or adenoma); pemphigus vulgaris or bullous pemphigoid; nodular panniculitis (adenocarcinoma of the pancreas); acquired hypertrichosis; erythema gyratum repens; acquired ichthyosis; hyperkeratosis of the palms and soles; sebaceous adenomas; cutaneous angiitis and arthritis associated with myeloproliferative disorders (myelofibrosis; myelogenous leukemia).

(J) NEUROLOGIC DISORDERS

1. *Central nervous system*
   a. *Progressive multifocal leukoencephalopathy:* leukemia; lymphoma; myeloma; carcinoma; polycythemia vera.
   b. *Limbic encephalopathy:* carcinomas of the lung, uterus, breast, etc.; magnetic resonance imaging is the method of choice for central nervous system evaluation (signal abnormalities in the involved gray and white matter, particularly the hippocampus and amygdala).
   c. *Pontine lesions* (central pontine myelinolysis): leukemia; etc.
   d. *Cerebellar atrophy:* carcinomas of the lung, breast, ovary, or kidney; lymphomas.
   e. *Opsoclonus-myoclonus:* neuroblastoma; ganglioneuroma; ganglioneuroblastoma.
   f. *Opsoclonus:* breast neoplasm.
   g. *Myelopathy:* visceral carcinoma; retroperitoneal lymphoma.
2. *Peripheral nervous system*
   a. *Subacute sensory neuropathy:* small cell lung carcinoma; epithelial ovarian cancer.
   b. *Peripheral neuropathies:* lymphomas; plasma cell dyscrasias.
3. *Neuromuscular junction*
   a. *Myasthenia gravis:* thymoma; thymic hyperplasia.
   b. *Myasthenic syndromes:* nonthymic neoplasms; especially small cell carcinoma of the lung (Lambert-Eaton syndrome).

(K) EYES: *Retinopathy:* small cell lung carcinoma.

PATTERSON SYNDROME

Clinical Manifestations: (a) normal birth weight; body disproportion noted at birth with *large hands, feet, nose, and ears;* (b) *cutis laxa* (present from birth); *generalized bronzed hyperpigmentation* (present from birth); *hirsutism;* (c) *mental retardation;* epilepsy; (d) kyphoscoliosis; deformities of the extremities with *swelling in joint regions* related to bone deformities; (e) *endocrine disorders:* hyperadrenocorticism; cushioned features; diabetes mellitus; premature adrenarche with elevated dehydroepiandrosterone and androstenedione levels; (f) survival beyond infancy.

Radiologic Manifestations: (a) *thickening of the cranial vault and base of the skull; thickening and deformity of facial bones; deformed vertebral bodies* with irregular and dense end-plates; platyspondyly of the cervical vertebrae; hypoplasia of the odontoid process; anterior displacement of the atlas; ovoid configuration of the thoracic and lumbar vertebrae; marked deformity of ribs, clavicles, and scapulae; progressive deformity and failure of ossification of the pubic bones, ischii, triradiate cartilages, and margins of the sacroiliac joints; flattening and irregularity of the acetabular roofs; *short, deformed tubular bones with poor enchondral bone formation; irregular metaphyseal ossification, and sclerotic metaphyseal changes;* (b) *severe retarded skeletal maturation.*

PEARSON SYNDROME

Clinical Manifestations: A multisystem disease due to abnormal mitochondrial deoxyribonucleic acid; onset of symptoms in infancy: (a) *refractory sideroblastic anemia (transfusion-dependent macrocytic anemia), vacuolization of marrow precursors;* neutropenia; thrombocytopenia; mitochondrial deoxyribonucleic acid rearrangement; (b) *pancreatic exocrine dysfunction;* pancreatic fibrosis; (c) lactic acidosis resulting from defective oxidative phosphorylation; deletions in the mitochondrial genome; 3-methylglutaconic aciduria; (d) miscellaneous abnormalities: liver failure; renal tubular dysfunction; renal failure; adrenal insufficiency; growth hormone deficiency; insulin-dependent diabetes; sepsis; corneal opacities; etc.

Radiologic Manifestations: *Encephalopathy:* increased signal intensity (T_2-weighted images) in the white matter of cerebral hemispheres and also in the globus pallidus, periaqueductal area, cerebral peduncles, and the pons; brain atrophy.

PELIZAEUS-MERZBACHER DISEASE

Classification: (a) type I (classic): X-linked; the gene for proteolipid protein mapped to Xq–22 position; (b) type II: either X-linked recessive or autosomal recessive inheritance; (c) type III: transitional form, with manifestations similar to those of type II, but slower progression of the disease; sporadic or possible autosomal transmission; (d) type IV: autosomal dominant inheritance, adult onset of symptoms; (e) type V: a variant form with patchy demyelination; autosomal recessive inheritance; (f) type VI: a demyelination variant of Cockayne syndrome; autosomal recessive inheritance.

Clinical Manifestations

(A) TYPE I (CLASSIC): Onset of symptoms during infancy: (a) *nystagmus; intermittent tremor and shaking movements of the head; choreoathetoid movements; ataxia; progressive pyramidal, dystonic, and cerebellar signs; spastic quadriparesis; psychomotor deterioration; optic atrophy;* abnormal brain-stem, auditory, and visual somatosensory evoked potentials; (b) miscellaneous abnormalities: microcephaly; laryngeal stridor; feeding problems; seizures; chronic course with slow progression of the neurologic manifestations after 5 or 6 years of age; death in adolescence or early adulthood.

(B) TYPE II: More severe disease than type I with earlier onset of symptoms and more pronounced neurologic manifestation; death often in early childhood.

Pathology: (a) dysmyelination/demyelination with islands of preserved myelin around blood vessels ("tigroid" or "leopard-skin" pattern); cerebral and cerebellar atrophy; ventriculomegaly; variable astrogliosis; accumulation of lipid-laden macrophages; nearly intact neurons and axons; (b) severe deficiency of myelin lipids; absence of proteolipid apoprotein (lipophilin); (c) prenatal diagnosis by deoxyribonucleic acid analysis on chorionic villus specimen.

Radiologic Manifestations: (a) computed tomography: usually normal in the early course of the disease; *decreased attenuation of white matter; brain atrophy;* (b) magnetic resonance imaging: *symmetric increased signals in the white matter (T_2-weighted images) compared with gray matter (reversal of the normal gray/white matter signal relationship);* foci of normal intensity scattered within the abnormal white matter (possibly corresponding to the "tigroid" pathologic pattern); *decreased basal ganglia and thalamic signals on T_2-weighted images; brain atrophy;* detection of carrier state.

PEROXISOMAL DISORDERS

Classification and Mode of Inheritance

1. Acatalasemia: catalase deficiency; autosomal recessive.
2. Hyperoxaluria type I: deficiency of alanine-glyoxylate aminotransferase; autosomal recessive.
3. Hyperpipecolic acidemia: generalized loss of peroxisomal functions.
4. Infantile Refsum disease: generalized loss of peroxisomal functions; autosomal recessive.
5. Neonatal adrenoleukodystrophy: generalized loss of peroxisomal functions; autosomal recessive.
6. Pseudoneonatal adrenoleukodystrophy: deficiency of fatty acyl-CoA oxidase; autosomal recessive.

7. Pseudo-Zellweger syndrome: thiolase deficiency; autosomal recessive.
8. Refsum disease (adult): deficiency of phytanic acid oxidase; autosomal recessive.
9. Rhizomelic chondrodysplasia punctata: deficiency of dihydroxyacetone phosphate acyltransferase, alkyl dihydroxyacetone phosphate synthase, and phytanic acid oxidase; autosomal recessive.
10. X-linked adrenoleukodystrophy and adrenomyeloneuropathy: deficiency of very long chain fatty acyl CoA synthetase; childhood, adolescent, and adult forms.
11. Zellweger syndrome: generalized loss of peroxisomal functions; autosomal recessive.
12. Zellweger-like syndrome: deficiency of multiple peroxisomal ß-oxidation enzymes.

Radiologic Manifestations: Neuronal migrational disorders; dysmyelination; hypomyelination; demyelination; etc.

PHENYLKETONURIA (PKU; Hyperphenylalaninemia)

Enzyme Deficiency: Deficiency of hepatic phenylalanine hydroxylase (faulty conversion of phenylalanine to tyrosine).

Clinical Manifestations

(A) Classic Phenylketonuria: (a) *usually fair-skinned child with blond hair and blue eyes;* (b) *neurologic symptoms:* poor coordination; tremor; dystonia; athetoid movements; hyperactivity; progressive loss of motor function; seizures; mental retardation; (c) *abnormal electroencephalographic findings:* single repetitive or multiple spikes and/or sharp waves; focal or scattered; (d) *eczema;* scleroderma-like skin lesions; (e) miscellaneous abnormalities: vomiting in infancy; unusual odor; impaired sensitivity to visual contrast in children treated for PKU; association with myotonic dystrophy in an infant; occurrence of phenylketonuria and galactosemia within the same family; autistic syndrome; agoraphobia; congenital heart disease; vitamin B_{12} deficiency.

(B) Phenylketonuria Variants: (a) *dihydropteridine reductase deficiency* (malignant phenylketonuria); *biopterin synthesis deficiency:* (1) hyperphenylalaninemia; (2) *progressive cerebral deterioration and seizures despite adequate dietary control of phenylalanine blood concentrations;* (3) association with neuroblastoma; (b) deficiencies of two enzymes, GTP-cyclohydrolase and 6-pyruvoyl tetrahydropterin synthase, resulting in defective tetrahydrobiopterin biosynthesis (1% to 3% of all reported forms of hyperphenylalaninemia).

(C) Maternal Phenylketonuria Syndrome (Abnormalities in Nonphenylketonuric Offspring of Mothers with Phenylketonuria): Low birth weight; microcephaly; developmental delay; mental retardation;

heart defects; facial dysmorphism; premature closure of cranial sutures in some of these children; miscarriages.

(D) Autosomal recessive inheritance; heterogeneity at the clinical, protein, and deoxyribonucleic acid levels.

Laboratory Tests: *Urinary excretion of phenylpyruvic acid; persistent blood phenylalanine levels above 6 mg/100 ml;* possibility of detecting disease in the first few hours of life by testing blood for phenylalanine (over 2 mg/dl necessitates reevaluation); prenatal diagnosis by means of a cloned human phenylalanine hydroxylase gene probe (analysis of deoxyribonucleic acid isolated from cultured amniotic fluid cells).

Radiologic Manifestations

(A) SKELETAL SYSTEM: osteopenia (diet-related); widening and cupping of the metaphysis (wrist); calcified spicules of cartilage projecting into the growth cartilage from the metaphyses of growing bones in infants; incorporation of calcified cartilage into the metaphysis with progression of bone growth; growth arrest lines; retarded skeletal maturation.

(B) CENTRAL NERVOUS SYSTEM: (a) classic PKU: (1) *demyelination/ dysmyelination* of varying degrees presenting as bandlike and/or confluent patchy areas of increased signal intensity on T_2-weighted sequences, most marked in the periventricular deep cerebral white matter; subcortical white matter involvement in some; less severe white matter abnormalities in patients with adequately controlled blood phenylalanine levels; cortical atrophy; (2) proton in vivo spectroscopy: abnormalities shown in the periventricular, basal ganglia, and cerebellum, with good correlation between an increased signal on T_2-weighted images and clinical findings; (b) PKU variants: *demyelination/dysmyelination* with hyperintense areas in the white matter on T_2-weighted magnetic resonance images; cavitary lesions in the white matter; basal ganglia calcification; diffuse cerebral atrophy; (c) magnetic resonance imaging of maternal PKU offspring: hypoplasia of the corpus callosum; delayed myelination.

POLYCYSTIC OVARY SYNDROME (STEIN-LEVENTHAL SYNDROME)

Clinical Manifestations: Defined as *functional, gonadotropin-dependent ovarian hyperandrogenism;* disturbance of the hypothalamic-pituitary-adrenal axis; lack of clinical uniformity: (a) *ovulatory dysfunction:* oligomenorrhea or amenorrhea, infertility, and dysfunctional uterine bleeding; (b) *excessive androgen production: hirsutism, acne, and excessive sebaceous gland secretions;* (c) *anabolic state:* obesity and difficulty in losing weight; (d) miscellaneous abnormalities: association with insulin insensitivity and oligo/amenorrhea; occurrence in several members of some families; an increased occurrence of tetraploidy in two sisters and their mother; endometrial carcinoma; increased risk of developing coronary artery disease.

Radiologic Manifestations: (a) *enlarged ovaries* (in 70% of cases); (b) ultrasonography: *ovarian cysts;* large follicular size and ovarian volume compared with normal controls; increased ovarian stroma echogenicity; (c) magnetic resonance imaging: more accurate than ultrasonography in demonstrating the characteristic small peripheral ovarian cysts; (d) mammography: decrease in glandular parenchyma; (e) scintigraphic evidence of adrenal cortical dysfunction.

Note: Other diseases associated with polycystic ovaries are congenital adrenal hyperplasia, Cushing syndrome, hyperinsulinemia, hyperprolactinemia, and hypothyroidism.

POLYGLANDULAR AUTOIMMUNE DISEASE

Classification

(A) TYPE I (POLYENDOCRINOPATHY–CANDIDIASIS–ECTODERMAL DYSTROPHY; WHITAKER SYNDROME): At least two of the three conditions (the triad) must be present: *Addison disease, hypoparathyroidism, and chronic mucocutaneous moniliasis;* autosomal recessive transmission; associated immune disorders may be present.

(B) TYPE II (SCHMIDT SYNDROME): Addison disease plus one or both of the following two conditions: autoimmune thyroid disease (chronic lymphocytic thyroiditis, Graves disease, or spontaneous myxedema) and insulin-requiring diabetes; autosomal dominant trait with variable expressivity has been reported; associated immune disorders may be present.

(C) TYPE III: Co-occurrence of autoimmune thyroid disease and another associated autoimmune disease, but without adrenal insufficiency: III-A: diabetes mellitus; III-B: pernicious anemia; III-C: another organ-specific autoimmune disorder.

Clinical and Radiologic Manifestations: (a) *mucocutaneous:* alopecia; dry skin; brittle and rigid nails; *chronic moniliasis;* vitiligo; (b) *polyendocrinopathy:* acquired primary hypogonadism; chronic lymphocytic thyroiditis; Graves disease; hypophysitis; insulin-requiring diabetes; myasthenia gravis; nontuberculous Addison disease; spontaneous acquired hypoparathyroidism; (c) malabsorption syndrome; atrophic gastritis; (d) chronic active hepatitis; primary biliary cirrhosis; (e) pernicious anemia; iron deficiency anemia; (f) quantitative immunoglobulin abnormalities; antisperm antibodies; (g) miscellaneous abnormalities: (1) type I: keratoconjunctivitis; Sjögren syndrome; exophthalmos; dental abnormalities (chalky teeth; pitted crowns; transverse grooves); acquired hyposplenism; chronic hoarseness due to candidal laryngitis; thymoma; thymic dysplasia; (2) type II: metaphyseal osteopenia; coexisting hypothyroidism and sarcoidosis; arterial (aorta; iliofemoral artery) calcification; basal ganglia calcification; (3) type III: diffuse alveolar hemorrhage due to anti–basement membrane antibody disease; association with celiac disease and sarcoidosis in a female patient.

Note: In most patients, candidiasis develops in childhood; the other components of type I may develop as late as the fifth decade.

PORPHYRIAS

Classification and Clinical Manifestations
(A) ERYTHROPOIETIC PORPHYRIA

1. Congenital erythropoietic porphyria (Gunther disease): Autosomal recessive inheritance (several mutations have been described); photosensitivity; cutaneous hyperfragility; burning sensation; vesicle and blister formation; superficial erosions on hands and face; dark reddish discoloration of deciduous teeth; mutilating tendency of the scars; loss of eyelids; ectropion; scleromalacia perforans; hypertrichosis; progressive sclerodermatous lesions; mutilation of the nose, ears, mouth, and fingers; transformation of the hands into stumps; *uroporphyrinogen III cosynthase deficiency;* high amounts of porphyrins in urine and feces; large amount of porphyrins in red blood cells and bone marrow erythroblasts.

2. Erythropoietic protoporphyria: Autosomal dominant inheritance with variable penetrance or autosomal recessive (less common); onset of symptoms usually in childhood; photosensitivity; burning sensation; erythema; edema; vesicle and blister formation; fever in some cases; thickening and yellowish discoloration of skin; varioliform scars; liver involvement (cirrhosis; hepatic failure); *ferrochelatase deficiency;* increased protoporphyrin in red blood cells.

3. Hepatoerythropoietic porphyria: Autosomal recessive inheritance; considered to be due to a homozygous *defect in uroporphyrinogen decarboxylase activity;* extremely rare; onset usually in infancy; photosensitivity; red urine; hyperfragility; hypertrichosis; scleroderma-like skin lesions; mutilation at various sites (face; fingers); no hemolytic anemia; no splenomegaly; no erythrodontia; hemiplegia (a lesion in the pons; case report).

(B) HEPATIC PORPHYRIA

1. Acute intermittent porphyria: Autosomal dominant inheritance; *uroporphyrinogen I synthase deficiency;* drug-induced visceral pain; muscle group or respiratory paralysis; behavioral problems ("peculiar"; depressed; hysterical; etc.).

2. Hereditary coproporphyria: Autosomal dominant inheritance; *coproporphyrinogen oxidase deficiency;* photosensitivity (rare); drug-induced visceral pain; paralysis; etc.

3. Variegata porphyria: Autosomal dominant inheritance; *protopor-phyrinogen oxidase or ferrochelatase deficiency;* light-induced blisters; hyperpigmentation; hirsutism; neuropathy; etc.
4. Porphyria cutanea tarda: Autosomal dominant inheritance (in some families); *uroporphyrinogen decarboxylase deficiency;* light-induced blisters; hyperpigmentation; hirsutism; epidermal inclusion cysts; diabetes; liver tumor (rare).

Radiologic Manifestations: (a) congenital erythropoietic porphyria: (1) atrophy of soft tissues; scleroderma-like cutaneous and subcutaneous calcifications; (2) skull: sun-ray spiculation and diploic widening; round sclerotic skull lesions (with progressive enlargement); "salt and pepper" skull; dura mater calcification; (3) osteopenia; fractures related to osteopenia; vertebral compression fractures; thoracic kyphosis; imperfect modeling of the bones; delayed epiphysiometaphyseal fusion; multiple osteolytic and sclerotic lesions; acro-osteolysis; shortening of fingers; mutilation of distal fingers; (b) acute intermittent porphyria: pseudoobstruction of the alimentary tract (autonomic dysfunction); (c) nodular focal fatty infiltration of liver in acquired porphyria cutanea tarda; (d) porphyric encephalopathy: ischemic brain changes (magnetic resonance imaging: diffuse, predominantly gyriform cortical contrast–enhanced cerebral hemispheres).

PRASAD SYNDROME (Geophagia Syndrome)

Clinical Manifestations: *Geophagia; iron deficiency with microcytic anemia and iron malabsorption; hepatosplenomegaly; short stature; hypogonadism; delay in puberty; zinc deficiency;* shortening and blunting of the small intestinal villi; alterations in the ultrastructure of intestinal mucosa, especially in Paneth cells.

Radiologic Manifestations: *Retarded skeletal maturation; radiopaque materials within the digestive tract; hepatosplenomegaly;* cardiomegaly; thick calvaria due to anemia.

PROTEIN S DEFICIENCY

Clinical and Radiologic Manifestations: Protein S produced by liver and acts as a cofactor for protein C: (a) *thrombosis:* spontaneous or in association with known factors (pregnancy; trauma; contraceptive use; immobilization; surgery; infection): deep veins; splanchnic veins; cerebral vessels; peripheral arteries; placenta; vessels supplying the femoral heads; etc.; (b) pulmonary embolism; (c) autosomal dominant inheritance, limited penetrance, and variable expression.

Note: (a) the risk of thromboembolism is high among the asymptomatic deficient relatives of symptomatic patients with protein C or protein S deficiency; (b) stroke in young adults associated with protein S deficiency is uncommon.

PSEUDOHYPOPARATHYROIDISM (ALBRIGHT HEREDITARY OSTEODYSTROPHY; PHP; PPHP)

Classification: Variable pattern of inheritance: autosomal dominant, autosomal recessive, and X-linked dominant forms; phenotypic variability; genetic heterogeneity; marked excess of maternal transmission; different subtypes of PHP in the same family:

(A) PSEUDOHYPOPARATHYROIDISM (PHP): Hypocalcemia and hyperphosphatemia that do not respond adequately to parathormone.

1. Type I a (classic form): Albright hereditary osteodystrophy somatotype present in most cases; low serum calcium; high serum phosphate; high immunoreactive parathyroid hormone (PTH); lack of normal increase in urinary excretion of cyclic adenosine monophosphate (cAMP) and phosphate in response to PTH; decreased Gs protein function; decreased synthesis of 1,25(OH)2D3.

2. Type I b: presence of the preceding biochemical abnormalities with normal Gs protein activity.

3. Type II: Albright hereditary osteodystrophy somatotype usually absent; low serum calcium; normal or high serum phosphate; high immunoreactive PTH; decreased phosphate excretion in response to PTH challenge; normal cAMP excretion in response to PTH challenge; normal Gs protein activity.

(B) PSEUDOPSEUDOHYPOPARATHYROIDISM (PPHP; NORMOCALCEMIC PHP): Albright hereditary osteodystrophy somatotype and normocalcemia.

Clinical Manifestations: Characterized by *end organ resistance to the action of PTH:* (a) *short stature;* (b) *round face and depressed nasal bridge;* (c) *obesity;* (d) seizures; *mental retardation;* (e) short fingers and/or toes; positive "knuckle sign"; (f) cataract; retinopathy involving mostly rods; (g) *abnormal dentition:* hypodontia; enamel hypoplasia; small crowns; enlarged pulp chambers; pulp stones; root canals with open apices; blunted roots; delayed eruption of deciduous and permanent teeth; thickening of the lamina dura; extensive caries; early tooth loss; (h) *hypocalcemia and hyperphosphatemia that do not respond adequately to PTH in pseudohypoparathyroidism; normal calcium and phosphorus in pseudopseudohypoparathyroidism;* no increase in urinary excretion of cAMP in response to PTH injections; increased serum PTH levels; (i) other associated endocrine abnormalities: hypothyroidism due to thyroid-stimulating hormone deficiency; gonadotropin deficiency; growth hormone releasing factor deficiency; decreased cAMP response to glucagon and isoproterenol; abnormal prolactin response to thyrotropin; (j) miscellaneous abnormalities: cardiac failure; various unusual dermatoglyphic patterns; association with rickets; progressive paraparesis with ossification of the posterior longitudinal ligament (C4 to C5); defective membrane-bound receptor–adenylate cyclase complex; platelet aggregation abnormalities; proximal 15q chromosomal deletion (resembling that found in Prader-Willi syndrome) in a mother and her daughter with Albright hereditary osteodystrophy; coexistence with D brachydactyly in a family; defective G proteins; postinfancy change in PTH responsiveness in the child of a woman with PHP; presentation with hysterical paralysis and subsequent rapid-cycling bipolar mood disorder; transient PHP of the neonates (transient hypoparathyroidism associated with elevated PTH levels).

Radiologic Manifestations: (a) thick calvaria (in about one third of cases); (b) central nervous system: *extensive bilateral symmetric cerebral and cerebellar dentate nucleus calcifications;* high signal intensities in putamina, pulvinars, and dentate nuclei on T_1-weighted magnetic resonance images; spinal stenosis; spinal cord compression (osseous tubercle on the anterolateral margin of the foramen magnum; ossification of the posterior longitudinal ligament); (c) *soft-tissue calcification/ossification;* (d) *disproportionate shortness and/or deformity of the metacarpals, metatarsals, and phalanges;* premature fusion of the epiphyses of the hands; cone-shaped epiphyses of the hands; a typical pattern profile (similar to acrodysostosis); (e) other reported skeletal abnormalities: bowing of long bones; coxa vara or valga; syndactyly; osteochondromas; subperiosteal bone resorption; radiolucent lesions caused by either brown tumors or bone cysts; slipped capital femoral epiphyses; focal areas of osteosclerosis; periosteal neoostosis; osteopenia; (f) miscellaneous abnormalities: association with hyperparathyroid bone disease; osteitis fibrosa cystica; intracardiac (within ventricular septum) calcification.

PYRUVATE DEHYDROGENASE COMPLEX DEFICIENCY

Clinical Manifestations: Variable presentations and clinical diversity: (a) *severe lactic acidosis in the neonatal period; recurrent episodes of lactic acidosis and associated neurologic disorders; chronic acidosis throughout childhood;* (b) *neurologic manifestations:* slow mental and physical development; microcephaly; cerebellar ataxia; seizures; spasticity; Leigh encephalopathy; etc.; (c) *lactic acidemia* (most common defined cause of primary lactic acidosis in infancy and early childhood); (d) *deficient pyruvate dehydrogenase activity in cultured fibroblasts;* (e) *elevated levels of lactate and pyruvate in the cerebrospinal fluid and blood;* (f) miscellaneous abnormalities: subacute/chronic neurodegenerative disease without significant metabolic acidosis; (g) X-linked inheritance; intrafamilial heterogeneity; most of the mutations are in the X-linked $E_{1\alpha}$ gene.

Radiologic Manifestations: (a) magnetic resonance imaging: *brain dysgenesis/atrophy* (cerebrum, cerebellum, and brain stem) with grossly dilated ventricles; corpus callosum agenesis; leukodystrophy; abnormal signals in the basal ganglia; (b) proton magnetic resonance spectroscopy: abnormal brain lactate metabolism.

PYRUVATE KINASE DEFICIENCY ANEMIA

Clinical Manifestations: Onset usually in infancy; very variable expression: (a) *hemolytic anemia; jaundice;* (b) low hemoglobin levels; macrocytosis; normochromic erythrocytes; slight anisocytosis and poikilocytosis; *deficiency of glycolytic enzyme pyruvate kinase;* (c) *splenomegaly; hepatomegaly;* (d) miscellaneous abnormalities: fetal anemia; hydrops fetalis; frontal bossing; chronic leg ulcer; hemolytic anemia and functional abnormality of pyruvate kinase in the presence of elevated red blood cell enzyme activity; hemochromatosis; (e) autosomal recessive inheritance.

Radiologic Manifestations: *Widened diploic space; vertical calvarial striations; atrophy of the outer table of skull;* mild demineralization of long bones; thinning of cortices; failure of tubulation; cardiomegaly; cholelithiasis; hepatosplenomegaly detectable on antenatal ultrasound study; hydrops fetalis.

R

REFSUM DISEASE

I. CLASSIC REFSUM DISEASE (PHYTANIC ACID STORAGE DISEASE)

Enzyme Deficiency: A defect in the α-oxidation of phytanic acid due to phytanic acid α-oxidase deficiency, resulting in an accumulation of C20 branched fatty acid (phytanic acid) in various tissues.

Clinical Manifestations: Onset of symptoms in childhood or early adulthood: (a) *cerebellar ataxia; polyneuropathy; enlargement of peripheral nerves; hyposmia; nerve deafness;* (b) *progressive visual deterioration; night blindness; optic atrophy; pigmentary retinal degeneration;* (c) *ichthyosis;* (d) *raised phytanic acid value in plasma;* in utero diagnosis by a determination of phytanic acid oxidase activity and very long chain fatty acids in cultured amniotic cells; (e) impaired renal hemodynamic and tubular function, etc.; (f) autosomal recessive inheritance.

Radiologic Manifestations: (a) symmetric epiphyseal dysplasia, particularly at the knees (flattening and irregularity of the subchondral bone); marginal osteophytes; "inverted V" appearance of intercondylar femoral notch; (b) shortening and deformity of the tubular bones in the hands and feet; short conical terminal phalanx of the thumbs.

II. GENERALIZED PEROXISOMAL DISORDER (INFANTILE REFSUM DISEASE)

Clinical Manifestations: Onset of symptoms in newborn period: (a) *hypotonia; craniofacial dysmorphism; transient jaundice; gastrointestinal illness (diarrhea; vomiting; malabsorption); hepatomegaly; seizures; growth retardation; psychomotor retardation;* (b) *biochemical changes:* elevated phytanic acid concentrations in plasma combined with tissue phytanic acid oxidase deficiency; elevated levels of plasma and skin fibroblast C24 and C26 fatty acids; abnormal bile acid metabolites; increased plasma pipecolic acid levels; etc.; (c) consistent with autosomal recessive transmission.

Radiologic Manifestations: Osteopenia; magnetic resonance imaging: decreased signal intensity on T_1-weighted images and increased signal intensity on T_2-weighted images in the dentate nuclei.

RENAL TUBULAR ACIDOSIS (RTA)

Pathophysiology: Disorder of renal acidification leading to metabolic acidosis, often without reduced renal mass.

Classification

(A) TYPE 1 (DISTAL) RTA: Inappropriately high pH of urine in association with persistent hyperchloremic acidosis, absence of glycosuria, hyperphosphaturia, or excessive bicarbonate excretion; autosomal dominant inheritance in some cases; occurrence with the use of certain drugs and in various autoimmune disorders.

(B) TYPE 2 (PROXIMAL) RTA (BUTLER-ALBRIGHT DISTAL TUBULAR ACIDOSIS): Defect in acidification in the proximal tubule leading to alkali loss, high pH of urine, and heavy bicarbonaturia; occurrence in association with various drugs, amyloidosis, multiple myeloma, Sjögren syndrome, medullary cystic disease, vitamin D deficiency, and genetic disorders (cystinosis; Wilson disease; fructose intolerance; Lowe syndrome; tyrosinemia; etc.); autosomal recessive inheritance or sporadic in the primary form of type 2 RTA.

(C) TYPE 3 (HYBRID) RTA: Formerly used in reference to infants with renal bicarbonate wasting associated with a distal acidification disorder and inappropriately high urinary pH; it is considered to be a variant of type 1.

(D) TYPE 4 RTA: Metabolic acidosis, hyperkalemia, and decreased glomerular filtration rate.

Clinical Manifestations: (a) *arthralgia; myalgia;* low back pain; *muscle weakness; growth retardation;* recurrent nephrolithiasis; (b) other reported abnormalities: distal RTA in polyarteritis nodosa; medullary sponge kidney.

Radiologic Manifestations: *Nephrocalcinosis; nephrolithiasis;* generalized *skeletal demineralization* of mild to marked severity; pathologic fractures; retarded skeletal maturation.

Association with Syndromes/Metabolic Disorders

1. RTA type 1 in association with Shwachman syndrome.
2. RTA type 4 in association with diabetes mellitus (diabetic nephropathy), chronic renal parenchymal damage, and interstitial nephritis.
3. Association of proximal RTA and glycogen storage diseases.
4. The syndrome of RTA and nerve deafness.
5. Carnitine palmitoyltransferase type 1 deficiency associated with RTA.
6. Cytochrome *c* oxidase deficiency in muscle with dicarboxylic aciduria and RTA.
7. Neuroaxonal dystrophy, RTA, and hyperdense lesions (computed tomography) in the thalamus and basal ganglia in a sibship.

Note: (a) skeletal abnormalities in RTA are often limited to patients with type 2 disease or azotemic individuals; (b) nephrocalcinosis is common in distal RTA, rare in proximal RTA, and usually absent in type 4 disease; (c) RTA associated with vesicoureteral reflux and growth failure has been reported in several children.

RICKETS/OSTEOMALACIA

Classification

(A) ABNORMAL VITAMIN D METABOLISM

1. Vitamin D deficiency: Inadequate exposure to sunlight; deficient intake of vitamin D; malabsorption.
2. Hepatic origin: Anticonvulsant therapy (increased hepatic metabolism); liver disease (failure of 25-hydroxylation).
3. Renal origin: Renal osteodystrophy; vitamin D–dependent rickets; parathyroid disorders (hypoparathyroidism; hyperparathyroidism; pseudohypoparathyroidism); maternal renal insufficiency as a cause of congenital rickets and secondary hyperparathyroidism.

(B) PHOSPHATE LOSS DUE TO RENAL TUBULAR DISORDERS

1. Vitamin D–resistant rickets (X-linked hypophosphatemia).
2. Fanconi syndrome.
3. Renal tubular acidosis.

(C) TUMOR-RELATED (ONCOGENIC RICKETS/OSTEOMALACIA): Hemangiomas of bone or soft tissues; hemangiopericytoma; giant cell tumor;

osteoblastoma; nonossifying fibroma; metastatic neuroblastoma; epidermal nevus syndrome; giant nevocellular nevi.

(D) SKELETAL DYSPLASIAS: Fibrous dysplasia; melorheostosis.

(E) CALCIUM DEFICIENCY: Dietary.

Clinical Manifestations

(A) VITAMIN D DEFICIENCY RICKETS: (a) muscle weakness; waddling gait; bone pain; growth failure; irritability; sweating; respiratory distress in small preterm infants; frontal and parietal bossing; pigeon breast; Harrison groove; rachitic rosaries; enlarged costochondral junctions; kyphoscoliosis; pelvic deformity; knobby joints, particularly in the wrist and ankle regions; abnormal limb curvatures; etc.; (b) normal or decreased serum calcium levels; decreased serum phosphate levels; increased alkaline phosphatase levels; increased aminoaciduria; (c) miscellaneous abnormalities: osteomalacia of the mother/rickets of the newborn; pseudotumor cerebri; congenital rickets associated with magnesium sulfate infusions for tocolysis.

(B) VITAMIN D–DEPENDENT RICKETS: (a) deficiency of the renal enzyme 1 α-hydroxylase, which converts 25-OH-D to 1,25(OH)2D in type 1; target organ resistance to 1,25(OH)2D in type 2; (b) clinical and biochemical manifestations similar to vitamin D–deficiency rickets; onset in early infancy in most cases (earlier than in nutritional deficiency type of rickets); hypocalcemia resulting from poor intestinal absorption; secondary hyperparathyroidism; hair abnormalities (generalized alopecia or sparse hair); (c) autosomal recessive inheritance.

(C) X-LINKED HYPOPHOSPHATEMIA: (a) dwarfism; growth retardation; bowleg; waddling gait; protuberant abdomen; rachitic rosaries; etc.; (b) hypophosphatemia (diminished tubular resorption of inorganic phosphate); elevated serum alkaline phosphatase levels; (c) rickets unresponsive to usual amounts of vitamin D; (d) miscellaneous abnormalities: nephrocalcinosis; tertiary hyperparathyroidism during high phosphate therapy; nocturnal hyperparathyroidism; (e) X-linked dominant inheritance (Xp22.1); sporadically occurring cases.

(D) TUMOR-RELATED RICKETS/OSTEOMALACIA: Weakness; proximal myopathy; hypophosphatemia; normal serum calcium levels; reduced 1,25(OH)2D levels; aminoaciduria, particularly glycinuria; rapid response to tumor removal.

Radiologic Manifestations

(A) OSTEOMALACIA

1. Vitamin D–deficiency osteomalacia: Skeletal deformities (limbs, spine, thorax, and pelvis); diminished bone density; coarsened trabeculae; mottled bone texture; cortical thinning; intercortical striations; pseudofractures (Looser lines); sclerosis at the sites of pseudofractures; spinal stenosis.

2. X-linked hypophosphatemia: Bowing of the tubular bones; osteo-arthritis (ankles, knees, feet, sacroiliac joints, and wrists); flaring of the iliac wings; trapezoidal distal femoral condyles; shortening of the talar neck; flattening of the talar dome; enthesopathic changes (bone proliferation at the sites of ligament, tendon, joint capsule, and interosseous membrane attachment); spinal stenosis (new bone formation in the ligamentum flavum; facet joint hyper-trophy; etc.); abnormal Tc-99m methylene diphosphonate scinti-grams (focal tracer accumulation in diaphyseal cortices and peri-articular and extraarticular regions).

(B) RICKETS
1. Vitamin D–deficiency: (a) demineralization; widening of the epi-physeal plates; metaphyseal cupping; irregularity and indistinct-ness of the provisional zone of calcification; poorly ossified epi-physes with indistinct borders; coarsened trabeculae; unsharp border of the inferior scapular angle and iliac crest; poor sub-periosteal new bone formation of mandible; pathologic fractures; skeletal deformities; (b) miscellaneous abnormalities: seizures and demineralization of the skull as presenting manifestations; prema-ture closure of cranial sutures; fractures in preterm infants.
2. Vitamin D–dependent: Rachitic changes with onset in early infancy, often severe, and rapidly progressive; pathologic fractures.
3. X-linked hypophosphatemic rickets: (a) mild to moderate rachitic changes in childhood; bowing of long bones, particularly in the lower limbs; coarse trabecular pattern; Looser zones and fractures in older individuals; mild osteopenia in childhood; generalized osteosclerosis in adulthood; (b) miscellaneous abnormalities: par-tial premature epiphyseal closure; premature cranial synostosis; absence of rachitic abnormalities in some patients; thoracic spinal stenosis; nephrocalcinosis (treatment-related).

ROTOR SYNDROME

Clinical Manifestations: (a) chronic, predominantly conjugated hyper-bilirubinemia without evidence of hemolysis; (b) plasma retention of sulfo-bromophthalein 45 minutes after the intravenous injection of a 5 mg/kg dose exceeds 25%; (c) normal liver histology (no excess pigmentation); defective hepatic glutathione S-transferase; (d) marked increase in the total coproporphyrin excretion in the urine; (e) autosomal recessive inheritance.

Radiologic Manifestations: ^{99m}Tc HIDA cholescintigraphy: nonvisu-alization of the bile ducts, nonvisualization or very faint visualization of liver with slow uptake, persistent visualization of the cardiac blood pool, and prominent kidney excretion.

S

SALLA DISEASE (Sialuria, Finnish Type)

Clinical Manifestations: Onset in infancy or early childhood; wide phenotypic variation: (a) *mental and physical retardation;* (b) *ataxia, athetosis, abnormal deep tendon reflexes, inability to walk, impaired speech, and epileptic fits;* (c) *moderate to marked increase in the excretion of free N-acetylneuraminic acid (sialic acid) in urine;* prenatal detection (increased free sialic acid in amniocytes); (d) miscellaneous abnormalities: slight corneal opacities; pale optic disc; hypertelorism; inguinal hernia; abnormal electroencephalographic findings; congenital ascites; (e) autosomal recessive inheritance; locus on the long arm of chromosome 6.

Radiologic Manifestation: (a) thick calvarium in adult patients; (b) magnetic resonance imaging appearance of cessation of myelination in infancy; brain atrophy in some.

Note: The eponym *Salla disease* refers to the geographic area in northern Finland from which the patients originated.

SCURVY (Vitamin C Deficiency)

Clinical Manifestations

(A) Children: Onset of symptoms usually between 3 months and 2 years of age: (a) irritability; pain, swelling, tenderness, pseudoparalysis of the legs, frog-leg position, and external hemorrhage (skin; mucous membranes); anemia; swelling of the gums; (b) costal rosaries; limb deformities.

(B) Adults: Muscle fatigue; petechiae, purpura, ecchymoses, and subcutaneous and mucosal bleeding; swelling, pain, and discoloration of the lower limbs; decreased range of motion of the ankle and knee joints; enlargement and hyperkeratosis of the hair follicles with a red hemorrhagic halo; corkscrew deformity and swan neck deformity of hair; anemia.

(C) Miscellaneous Abnormalities: association with panniculitis; association with wet beriberi; etc.

Pathology: Vitamin C deficiency results in reversible atherosclerosis in latent scurvy and microvascular complications such as widespread capillary hemorrhage in acute scurvy (vitamin C being essential element in the synthesis of collagen, the protein most needed for the maintenance of vascular integrity).

Radiologic Manifestations: Generalized osteoporosis; ground-glass appearance; thickening of the provisional zone of calcification (Fränkel sign); white rim about the epiphyseal center (Wimberger sign); metaphyseal zone of demineralization; "corner sign" (subepiphyseal infraction); fracture with epiphyseal slipping; subperiosteal hemorrhage; subperiosteal calcifying hematoma; metaphyseal cupping; ball-in-socket deformity of the epiphyseal-metaphyseal junction; improvement of the deformity in a long range follow-up; premature closure of central epiphyseal growth plate.

SHEEHAN SYNDROME

Clinical Manifestations: *Necrosis of the pituitary during the postpartum period;* secondary atrophy of thyroid, adrenal cortex, and ovaries: (a) *acute postpartum shock followed by asthenia; failure of lactation; amenorrhea or menstrual irregularity;* pallor; anorexia; brachycardia; hypotension; weight loss; cachexia; clinical manifestations of hypothyroidism, adrenal insufficiency, and gonadal insufficiency; (b) lower than normal response to provoked combined pituitary stimulation; (c) miscellaneous abnormalities: acute hypoglycemic coma; thrombasthenia as a cause of the syndrome; Sheehan syndrome presenting as a psychosis; pericardial effusion and hyponatremia as a clinical presentation of the syndrome; hypercalcemia associated with secondary Sheehan syndrome; etc.

Radiologic Manifestations: (a) *small sella turcica;* (b) *empty sella turcica* (partial or complete); *visible pituitary stalk; pituitary residue usually less than third of normal size;* hypodense (computed tomography) residual pituitary gland; (c) magnetic resonance imaging in pituitary apoplexy (sudden degeneration of pituitary gland): enhancement of adjacent dura after injection of contrast medium has been observed.

SHWACHMAN SYNDROME (SHWACHMAN-DIAMOND SYNDROME)

Clinical Manifestations: Onset of symptoms in infancy: (A) *growth retardation; low birth weight; short-limbed dwarfism;* (b) *exocrine pancreatic insufficiency associated with malabsorption syndrome;* (c) *recurrent infections;* (d) *leukopenia and/or neutropenia; defective neutrophil chemotaxis; thrombocytopenia; anemia;* (e) miscellaneous abnormalities: myocardial necrosis; respiratory distress in neonatal period; eczema; hepatic dysfunction; liver cirrhosis; dysgammaglobulinemia; renal dysfunction; dental decay and enamel hypoplasia; spontaneous chromosomal breakage; leukemia; etc. (f) autosomal recessive inheritance.

Radiologic Manifestations: (a) *Metaphyseal dysplasia* (small lucent patches and sclerotic serrations at or adjacent to provisional zone of calcification); *irregular ossification of the anterior rib ends;* (b) *lipomatosis of the pancreas* (computed tomography and ultrasonography); (c) miscellaneous abnormalities: coxa vara, slipping of capital femoral epiphysis; abnormal tubulation of long bones; clinodactyly; phalangeal hypoplasia; narrowing of sacrosciatic notches; skeletal maturation retardation.

SIALIC ACID STORAGE DISEASES

Classification and Manifestations
1. Sialidosis (neuraminidase deficiency).
2. Salla disease.
3. Sialuria: Hepatosplenomegaly, developmental delay, difficulty with fine motor skills, etc.; urinary excretion of free sialic acid.
4. Infantile sialic acid storage disease: A rapidly progressive neurovisceral storage disorder with onset of symptoms in early infancy: unusually fair complexion, coarse facial features, severe mental and motor retardation, dystonia, hepatosplenomegaly, nephrosis, vacuolization of peripheral lymphocytes, and short life span.

SIALIDOSIS

Definition: A group of inborn errors of metabolism caused by the intracellular accumulation of sialic acid–containing oligosaccharides.
Enzyme Deficiency: Glycoprotein-specific *N*-acetylneuraminidase.
Clinical Manifestations
(A) EARLY INFANTILE FORM SIALIDOSIS (CONGENITAL SIALIDOSIS): *Nonimmune hydrops fetalis, ascites, hepatosplenomegaly, failure to thrive, and recurrent infections; death usually occurs within the first year of life;* prenatal diagnosis (cultured amniotic cells).

(B) LATE INFANTILE FORM SIALIDOSIS: *Motor retardation, progressive neurologic deterioration, axial hypotonia, limb hypertonicity, hepatosplenomegaly, coarse facial features, and recurrent infections;* death in early childhood.

(C) JUVENILE FORM SIALIDOSIS (PREVIOUSLY KNOWN AS MUCOLIPIDOSIS I): *Progressive neurologic deterioration, impaired hearing, impaired speech, Hurler-like appearance in early childhood, hernias, myoclonus, ataxia, cherry-red macular spot, mental retardation, and hepatosplenomegaly;* survival into early adulthood.

(D) ADULT FORM SIALIDOSIS (CHERRY-RED SPOT–MYOCLONUS SYNDROME): Onset in adolescence, *progressive myoclonus, bilateral macular cherry-red spots, gradual visual loss, and normal or near-normal intelligence;* death in the fourth decade of life.

(E) Autosomal recessive inheritance.
Radiologic Manifestations
(A) INFANTILE FORM SIALIDOSIS: Coarsened bony trabecular pattern mainly in the long bones; metaphyseal irregularity and increased density; stripelike intracranial echogenicities in the region of the basal ganglia with color Doppler demonstrating blood flow within the echogenicities (vasculopathy).

(B) JUVENILE FORM SIALIDOSIS: *Mild to moderate dysostosis multiplex:* flat vertebral bodies; beaking of vertebral bodies; irregular vertebral end-plates; small and flared iliac wings; shallow acetabular roofs; flat capital femoral epiphyses; coxa valga; thickened calvaria; mandibular prognathism; osteopenia; thin cortex of the tubular bones; cystic type of changes of the phalanges; bifid ossification of the calcaneus; skeletal maturation retardation; cardiomegaly; persistent pulmonary infiltrates.

SICKLE CELL ANEMIA

Etiology: (a) the presence of abnormal ß-chain in hemoglobin S (valine substituted for glutamic acid) results in erythrocyte sickling at a reduced oxygen tension; the deformed and fragmented erythrocyte associated with an increase in blood viscosity leads to occlusion of small blood vessels and infarct; (b) autosomal recessive inheritance.

Classification: (a) homozygous sickle cell disease (SS disease), severe anemia; (b) sickle cell–hemoglobin C disease (SC disease), mild anemia; (c) sickle cell–α-thalassemia (SS–α-thalassemia), severe anemia; (d) sickle cell–ß-thalassemia, mild to severe anemia.

Clinical Manifestations

(A) GENERAL MANIFESTATIONS: Anemia; jaundice; liver and biliary tract dysfunction; hepatomegaly; splenomegaly in the early stage; splenic fibrosis in a later stage; abdominal crisis (intravascular thrombosis; infarcts; pain; vomiting; distension); splenic sequestration crises; chronic leg ulcer; "ulcer osteoma."

(B) SKELETAL SYSTEM: Painful limbs: bone infarcts; hand-foot syndrome (swelling; tenderness; fever; leukocytosis); osteomyelitis (*Salmonella* or *Staphylococcus* infections); arthralgia; arthritis; hemarthrosis.

(C) RESPIRATORY SYSTEM: Pulmonary infarcts; recurrent pneumonias; reduced peak expiratory flow rate in children with multiple episodes of acute chest syndrome; restrictive ventilatory defect characterized by low vital capacity and total lung capacity; sleep-related upper airway obstruction and baseline hypoxemia; abnormally small lungs (particularly in those with SS hemoglobin); diffuse lung fibrosis and cor pulmonale (rare).

(D) CARDIOVASCULAR SYSTEM: Cardiomegaly; congestive heart failure; abnormal septal Q waves; ventricular dysfunction; pulmonary hypertension; cor pulmonale; postmortem evidence of myocardial infarction.

(E) NERVOUS SYSTEM: Stroke in 6% to 16% of children with sickle cell anemia; seizures; hemiplegia; stupor; coma; cerebral infarction; intracranial hemorrhage; spinal cord infarction; isolated neuropathies due to anatomic proximity to infarcted bones; ocular manifestations; recurrent cerebral ischemia during hypertransfusion therapy; neuropsychologic impairment in school-age children; sensorineural hearing loss in sickle cell crisis; high leukocyte count and an acute decrease of hemoglobin reported as risk factors for stroke in patients with homozygous sickle cell disease; severe hypoxemia secondary to acute sternal infarction.

(F) URINARY SYSTEM: Focal glomerular sclerosis; urinary concentration defect; impaired renal acidification and potassium excretion; proteinuria; supranormal proximal tubular function (increased reabsorption of phosphate and increased secretion of creatinine); hematuria; papillary necrosis; renal failure.

(G) PRENATAL DIAGNOSIS: First-trimester diagnosis with chorionic villus sampling (enzymatic deoxyribonucleic acid test); amniocentesis in the second trimester.

(H) MISCELLANEOUS ABNORMALITIES: (a) painful crises (acute chest syndrome, abdominal crises); (b) growth disturbances; abnormal body shape: reduction in weight, height, sitting height, limb length, and skinfold thickness; increased anteroposterior chest diameter; (c) retinopathy; exophthalmos associated with bone infarction; (d) fat embolism (bone marrow necrosis); ischemic colitis; myonecrosis secondary to muscle infarction; myofibrosis; (e) priapism (indication of severe disease in adults); (f) bacteremia; liver abscess; (g) others: lymphadenopathy; mitral valve prolapse; vitamin C deficiency; hypothyroidism in adults receiving multiple blood transfusions (iron overload); association with sarcoidosis.

Radiologic Manifestations

(A) SKELETAL SYSTEM

1. Skull: Granular pattern; widening of diploic space; decreased width of the outer table; hair-on-end appearance; decreased calvarial density; focal radiolucent areas; focal or diffuse osteosclerosis; radiolucency and coarsening of the bony trabeculae of the mandible; prominent lamina dura; orbital bone infarction; calvarial infarction; iron deposition in cranial bone marrow (transfusion therapy).

2. Spine and pelvis: Osteoporosis; depression of end-plates with a squared-off appearance of the indentation; prominent vertical bony trabeculae; increased thoracic kyphosis and lumbar lordosis; prominence and persistence of anterior vascular foramina of the thoracic vertebral bodies in children; pelvic osteomyelitis; osteitis pubis; protrusio acetabuli; infarction of the ilia.

3. Thorax: Sternal infarction; sternal cupping; patchy areas of rarefaction and/or sclerosis of the ribs; rib infarction (demonstrated by ^{99m}Tc diphosphonate bone scan) in patient with acute chest syndrome.

4. Long bones: (a) diaphyseal infarction (mottled and strandy medullary sclerotic densities; cortex-within-cortex pattern; cortical fissuring; massive infarct of the entire shaft in children; scinti-

graphic demonstration of infarcted segment); (b) epiphyseal infarction (proximal humeral and femoral epiphyses most common sites; osteonecrosis; collapse and disintegration; osteosclerosis); (c) osteomyelitis (*Salmonella; Staphylococcus aureus;* etc.); (d) miscellaneous abnormalities: pathologic fractures; "ulcer osteoma" (chronic ulcer in the superficial tissues adjacent to the involved bone); tibiotalar slant.

5. Hands and feet: Hand-foot syndrome in children (most frequent between 6 months and 2 years of age; "dactylitis"; soft-tissue swelling; bone resorption in infarcted or infected areas; periosteal elevation and subperiosteal new bone formation); slender marfanoid fingers or brachydactyly associated with cone-shaped epiphyses and concave metaphyses of the metacarpal bones and phalanges; terminal phalangeal sclerosis; erosive disease of the calcaneus (loss of definition of the cortical margin in the superior aspect of the bone).

6. Retarded skeletal maturation.

7. Arthropathy: Joint effusion (noninflammatory); septic arthritis; hemarthrosis.

8. Bone infarction: (a) radionuclide scintigraphy: photopenic defect in the femoral or humeral head as an earliest manifestation of avascular necrosis; cortical bone–seeking radiopharmaceuticals (Tc-99m phosphate compounds) may show a similar picture to that of osteomyelitis in cases with medullary osteonecrosis; bone marrow scanning with ^{99m}Tc sulfur colloid demonstrating decreased marrow activity in bone infarction; Ga citrate imaging very useful in differentiating bone marrow infarction and osteomyelitis; (b) magnetic resonance imaging: various patterns in avascular necrosis: T_1-weighted images: low signal intensity (homogeneous, heterogeneous, or ringlike pattern of decreased signal surrounding the high signal intensity of fatty marrow); T_2-weighted images: double-line ring (high signal bordering the ring); edema in acute infarction; cystic lesions; magnetic resonance imaging helpful in differentiating between acute and chronic marrow infarcts; significant inhomogeneity of bone marrow in asymptomatic patients; magnetic resonance imaging not helpful in differentiating between acute infarct and acute osteomyelitis; (c) computed tomography: "asterisk sign" of femoral head (normal central density with star-shaped appearance): loss of rays of asterisk, increased peripheral density, sclerosis, deformity, and intraosseous cyst; computed tomography not useful for early detection of avascular necrosis of epiphyses.

(B) CHEST: (a) acute chest syndrome due to pneumonia or infarction (chest radiography and ventilation-perfusion scintigraphy are not diagnostic in differentiating between pneumonia and pulmonary infarct); 3-mm chest computed tomography helpful in differential diagnosis by demonstrating a ground-glass attenuation in microvascular occlusion; pleural effusion; rib infarction; (b) pulmonary hypertension and cor pulmonale following repeated episodes of pulmonary vascular occlusion; cardiomegaly; congestive heart failure; increased left atrial, left ventricular, and aortic root dimensions; increased left ventricular wall thickness; (c) extramedullary hematopoiesis (masses in the paravertebral region).

(C) URINARY SYSTEM: (a) renal enlargement; thickening of the renal medulla; focal cortical hypertrophy; caliceal clubbing; papillary necrosis; (b) pyelonephritis; (c) perirenal hematoma; (d) renal arteriography: focal cortical hypertrophy; "pseudobrain" nephrogram due to a mixture of hypertrophy and scar formation; thinning of the cortex; medullary hypertrophy; pruning of the arterial tree; (e) magnetic resonance imaging of sickle-cell nephropathy: decreased relative cortical signals, most evident on T_2-weighted images; (f) renal vein thrombosis; (g) unusual renal accumulation of Tc-99m phytate and Tc-99m HMDP; (h) focal and diffuse increased echogenicity in the renal parenchyma.

(D) CENTRAL NERVOUS SYSTEM
1. Vascular occlusion of major arteries or distal branches (partial or complete): (a) magnetic resonance imaging: cerebrovascular disease; (b) ultrasonography: cerebral vascular stenosis resulting in elevated flow velocity shown by transcranial and extracranial Doppler ultrasonography; increased velocity in ophthalmic artery and middle cerebral artery; decreased resistive index secondary to increased diastolic flow; reversal of flow especially in ophthalmic artery; absence of detectable flow in the middle cerebral artery or anterior cerebral artery when good flow is detected in posterior cerebral artery; increased velocity in posterior cerebral and/or increased velocity in vertebral and basilar circulation; decreased velocity in vessel supplying infarcted area; (c) abnormalities on localized proton resonance spectroscopy in stroke; (d) stable Xenon-enhanced computed tomography: decreased cerebral blood flow (total, hemispheral, or regional); (e) central nervous system parenchymal changes, particularly in the general regions of arterial border zones between the major cerebral arteries and adjacent deep white matter (distal small-vessel disease); (f) magnetic resonance imaging: evidence of infarction/ischemia in the absence of a recognized cerebrovascular accident.
2. Extramedullary hemopoiesis: Extradural mass within the spinal canal, displacing the cord.
3. Miscellaneous abnormalities: Intracranial hemorrhage (intracerebral; subarachnoid); intracranial aneurysm(s); retroorbital and

epidural hematoma (associated with bone infarct); postangiographic blindness; vein of Galen and straight sinus thrombosis.

(E) ABDOMEN: (a) spleen: infarcts; rupture; hemorrhage; calcification; acute splenic sequestration crisis (patent splenic vein; enlarged spleen; hypoechoic lesions; low attenuation on computed tomography; hyperintense lesions on both T_1- and T_2-weighted magnetic resonance images suggestive of subacute hemorrhage); (b) liver: infarcts; hepatic vein thrombosis; abscess; (c) biliary tract: cholelithiasis (calcium bicarbonate); biliary sludge; gallbladder wall thickening; abnormal biliary scintigraphy (delayed gallbladder visualization consistent with chronic cholecystitis); (d) bowel distension (related to vascular occlusion); (e) miscellaneous abnormalities: appendicitis; focal hepatic nodular hyperplasia; focal echogenic lesions in the spleen in patients with no symptoms related to the spleen; transfusional hemosiderosis of liver and pancreas (shown by ultrasonography and magnetic resonance imaging); retroperitoneal fibrosis (in sickle cell trait).

(F) SOFT TISSUES: Soft-tissue changes (edema; inflammation; and ischemia) with or without adjacent bone marrow abnormalities; myonecrosis; altered muscle metabolism shown by magnetic resonance spectroscopy in patients with leg ulcers.

SJÖGREN-LARSSON SYNDROME

Enzyme Deficiency: Fatty alcohol: NAD+ oxidoreductase.

Clinical Manifestations: (a) *congenital ichthyosis;* (b) *spastic diplegia or tetraplegia;* (c) *mental retardation; speech defects;* (d) *retinopathy* (retinal "glistening dots"); superficial punctate epithelial erosions of the cornea; conjunctivitis; blepharitis; photophobia; (e) short stature; (f) *reduced activity of the fatty alcohol: NAD+ oxidoreductase activity in cultured skin fibroblasts and peripheral leukocytes;* carrier detection by measurement of fatty alcohol: NAD+ oxidoreductase (FAO) complex and fatty aldehyde dehydrogenase component of FAO in cultured skin fibroblasts; (g) prenatal diagnosis: skin biopsy (hyperkeratosis); (h) miscellaneous abnormalities: seizures; joint hyperextensibility; increased muscle tone; increased deep tendon reflexes; kyphoscoliosis; defective sweating; enamel hypoplasia; dermatoglyphic anomalies; (i) autosomal recessive inheritance; variable expressivity; fatty aldehyde dehydrogenase maps to chromosome 17p11.2.

Radiologic Manifestations: (a) *demyelination in the cerebral white matter, corticospinal and vestibulospinal tracts;* internal hydrocephalus; (b) short metacarpals and metatarsals; epiphyseal-metaphyseal dysplasia; foot deformities and flexion contractures; widening of the symphysis pubis; nonossified pubis; hypoplasia of the femoral head; retarded skeletal maturation; (c) miscellaneous abnormalities: dental dysplasia; hypertelorism; basilar impression; Dandy-Walker malformation.

SMITH-LEMLI-OPITZ SYNDROME TYPE I

Clinical Manifestations: A metabolic–multiple congenital anomalies–mental retardation syndrome: (a) *low birth weight; failure to thrive;* (b) *hypotonia at birth; progressive spasticity in childhood;* (c) moderate to severe *mental retardation;* (d) *typical facies:* microcephaly, blepharoptosis, inner epicanthal folds, strabismus, short nose with a broad bridge, anteverted nostrils, broad maxillary anterior alveolar ridge, micrognathia, and slanted auricles or low-set ears; (e) short neck; (f) short and narrow shoulders; syndactyly of the second and third toes; (g) *urogenital anomalies:* hypospadias; cryptorchidism; cleft scrotum; pseudohermaphroditism; micropenis; microurethra; hypoplastic scrotum; 46,XY with female external genitalia; (h) ocular abnormalities: cataracts; absence of lacrimal punctae; posterior synechiae; ptosis; epicanthal folds; choroidal hemangioma; pale discs; neuronal atrophy; (i) hepatomegaly; pancreatic anomalies; adrenal enlargement; (j) miscellaneous abnormalities: highly arched or cleft palate; long tapered fingers; sacral dimple; abnormal electroencephalographic and electrocardiographic findings; acrocyanosis of the hands and feet; hypoplasia of the thymus; irritability; typical shrill screaming; frequent vomiting and regurgitation; abnormal dermatoglyphics; Hirschsprung disease; prematurity; few cases reported in adults; early death; (k) autosomal recessive inheritance.

Laboratory Findings: (a) *defect in biosynthesis of cholesterol* due to a block in the pathway for synthesis of cholesterol via 7-dehydrocholesterol; *low level of blood cholesterol; very high concentration of 7-dehydrocholesterol* (cholesterol precursor); deficiency in normal bile acids in urine; detection of defective 3 beta-hydroxysterol delta 7-reductase activity in cultured fibroblasts; (b) prenatal diagnosis: analysis of 7-dehydrocholesterol in amniotic fluid; chorionic villi biopsy.

Radiologic Manifestations: (a) *microcephaly;* scaphocephaly; micrognathia; (b) mild to moderate hydrocephalus involving one or more ventricles; hypoplasia of the frontal lobes, the corpus callosum, the cerebellum, and the brain stem; paucity of white matter in cerebellum; periventricular gray matter heterotopias; irregular frontal gyri; pachygyria; (c) *soft-tissue syndactyly of the second and third toes;* (d) swallowing mechanism dysfunction in early infancy; gastroesophageal regurgitation and recurrent pneumonia; (e) urinary tract anomalies: ureteropelvic junction obstruction; vesicoureteral reflux; hydronephrosis; collecting system duplication; positional renal abnormalities; renal cystic dysplasia; renal agenesis; etc.; (f) prenatal ultrasonography: increased first-trimester nuchal translucency (fluid accumulation) with subsequent subsidence of the nuchal fluid; (g) miscellaneous abnormalities: congenital heart disease; pyloric stenosis; polydactyly; brachydactyly; clinodactyly; hypoplasia of the thumbs, which are low-set on the hands; clubfoot; stippled epiphyses.

SMITH-LEMLI-OPITZ SYNDROME TYPE II

Clinical Manifestations: (a) *intrauterine growth retardation;* oligohydramnios; birth asphyxia; (b) *distinctive face* (round face, ptosis, epicanthal folds, broad nasal bridge, and anteverted nares); facial hemangiomas; *microcephaly; micrognathia; cleft palate;* small tongue; tongue cysts; redundant sublingual tissues; (c) short neck with redundant skin folds; (d) *postaxial polydactyly* (hands and/or feet); soft-tissue syndactyly of second and third toes; (e) *genital ambiguity or pseudohermaphroditism in XY males;* (f) *congenital heart defects;* (g) internal organ abnormalities: pulmonary hypoplasia; unilobated lungs; large adrenals; pancreatic islet cell hyperplasia; Hirschsprung disease; pyloric stenosis; renal agenesis; renal cystic dysplasia; (h) miscellaneous abnormalities: cataracts; developmental delay; maternal estriol levels unrecordable during the late stage of pregnancy and suppression of maternal adrenal function; poor suck and feeding; vomiting, abdominal distension; recurrent respiratory infections; short limbs; joint contractures; de novo balanced translocation involving 7q32; abnormalities of cholesterol and bile acid biosynthesis; (i) autosomal recessive inheritance.

Radiologic Manifestations: (a) prenatal ultrasonographic findings: growth retardation; heart defect; limb shortening; finger anomalies; renal anomaly; breech presentation; decreased fetal movement; nuchal membrane; etc.; (b) central nervous system: microcephaly; hydrocephaly; absent corpus callosum; polymicrogyria; cerebellar hypoplasia; holoprosencephaly; cerebral atrophy; lipoma of the sella turcica; lumbar meningomyelocele; (c) miscellaneous abnormalities: persistent open posterolateral fontanelle; thin ribs; hypoplastic thumb metacarpals; high ovoid lumbar bodies; increased number of sternal ossification centers.

SOMATOSTATINOMA SYNDROME

Etiology: Pancreatic tumor producing somatostatin-like immunoreactivity and bioactivity.

Clinical and Radiologic Manifestations: (a) *dry mouth, dyspepsia, postprandial fullness, steatorrhea, and diabetes mellitus;* (b) *normocytic, normochromic anemia;* (c) *pancreatic tumor or extrapancreatic tumor* (duodenum or papilla of Vater, resulting in chronic pancreatitis); (d) miscellaneous abnormalities: association of duodenal somatostatinoma with neurofibromatosis; hypercalcemia; congenital pseudoarthrosis; cholelithiasis.

SPHEROCYTOSIS (MINKOWSKI-CHAUFFARD DISEASE)

Pathophysiology: Deficiency of spectrin (a protein of the erythrocyte membrane skeleton) resulting in the formation of spherocytes that lack normal strength; the spherocytes trapped in the splenic red pulp have a short survival period and are destroyed.

Clinical Manifestations: Variable clinical severity: (a) *jaundice;* (b) *splenomegaly;* (c) *chronic hemolytic anemia* with an onset in childhood or adolescence; *spherocytes in the peripheral blood; increased osmotic fragility of erythrocytes; shortened life span of erythrocytes* from an affected person in a normal recipient; rapid hemolysis of spherocytes in the spleen; (d) diagnosis in newborn infants: increased osmotic fragility of fresh and incubated red blood cells, moderately increased autohemolysis, and partial reduction of autohemolysis by the addition of glucose; (e) miscellaneous abnormalities: atypical hyperbilirubinemia in newborns; aplastic crisis; leg ulcerations; congestive heart failure; myeloproliferative disorders; myelolipoma of adrenal gland; acute lymphoblastic leukemia in a child; (f) autosomal dominant inheritance in about 75% of the cases; sporadic or autosomal recessive inheritance in other cases.

Radiologic Manifestations: (a) *bilirubin stones;* (b) *osteoporosis; widening of the medullary canal of tubular bone;* widening of the diploic space; hair-on-end appearance of the calvaria; (c) extramedullary hematopoiesis (paravertebral); (d) secondary hemochromatosis (related to repeated transfusions); (e) splenomegaly, usually with a homogeneous increased echogenicity; well-defined focal defects of high echogenicity relative to the normal spleen (soft areas composed of dilated sinuses and extramedullary hemopoiesis); splenic rupture; (f) ischemic cerebral accident.

SULFITE OXIDASE DEFICIENCY

Classification: (a) isolated enzyme deficiency (rare); (b) part of the group of enzymes sharing the common molybdenum-pterin cofactor.

Clinical Manifestation: Clinical manifestations related to endogenous sulfite intoxication (failure of oxidation of inorganic sulfite to sulfate): (a) *degenerative brain changes:* seizures; spastic quadriparesis; blindness; lens dislocation; mental retardation; microcephaly; etc.; (b) *abnormal metabolites* in urine, plasma, and cerebrospinal fluid (sulfite and others); (c) miscellaneous abnormalities: presentation as Leigh disease.

Radiologic Manifestations: Cerebral edema in early infancy; brain atrophy, cystic changes, and cerebral calcification.

SYNDROME OF INAPPROPRIATE SECRETION OF ANTIDIURETIC HORMONE (INAPPROPRIATE SECRETION OF ANTIDIURETIC HORMONE SYNDROME)

Etiology: *Ectopic production of antidiuretic hormone induced by nonosmotic stimuli:* (1) neoplasia at various sites, particularly bronchogenic carcinoma; (2) infections in various organs; (3) central nervous system diseases including trauma, infection, vascular occlusion, neoplasm, vasculitis, multiple sclerosis, cerebral atrophy, hypoplastic corpus callosum, and surgery; (4) medications: antidepressants and antipsychotics, antineoplastics, contrast agents, hypoglycemics, nonsteroidal antiinflammatory agents, and thiazide diuretics; (5) others: acute asthma; acute bronchitis; chronic obstructive pulmonary disease; pneumothorax; cystic fibrosis; psychosis; spinal fusion; pregnancy; etc.

Types: (a) transient and self-limited; (b) chronic and persistent.

Clinical Manifestations: Normovolemic or near-normovolemic hyponatremia in a patient with unrestricted water intake; inappropriately high urine osmolarity; high urinary excretion of sodium; normal renal function; correction of the hyponatremia by fluid restriction.

Radiologic Manifestations: (a) those of the etiologic factors listed under Etiology; (b) magnetic resonance imaging: absence of normal high intensity signal of neurohypophysis.

T

TESTICULAR FEMINIZATION (ANDROGEN INSENSITIVITY SYNDROME)

Clinical Manifestations: (a) *XY karyotype; female phenotype; testes secrete androgens;* (b) *primary amenorrhea and sterility;* (c) *inguinal hernia;* (d) *intraabdominal, inguinal, or intralabial testicular location;* (e) *small or absent clitoris; blind-ending vaginal pouch; absent cervix on rectal examination;* (f) *lack of a cytosolic receptor for dihydrotestosterone* in androgen-dependent tissues; plasma testosterone levels in the male range; normal follicle-stimulating hormone concentration; elevated luteinizing hormone levels; (g) X-linked recessive or sex-modified autosomal dominant.

Radiologic Manifestations: Ultrasonography and magnetic resonance imaging: *absence of uterus and ovaries; presence of testes.*

Note: The syndrome may occur in complete form (phenotypically female) or incomplete form (variable appearance of the external genitalia depending on the degree of androgenic insensitivity).

THALASSEMIA

Biochemical Classification: (a) α-thalassemia: deficiency of α-globin chain synthesis; (b) ß-thalassemia: deficiency of ß-globin chain synthesis; (c) others: less common, hemoglobin polypeptide chains (∂; ∂ß).

Clinical Types: (a) thalassemia major (homozygote; Cooley anemia): two similar or identical genes for thalassemia; (b) thalassemia minor (heterozygote), mildly affected; (c) thalassemia intermedia (heterozygote), moderately affected.

Clinical Manifestations (Thalassemia Major)

(A) GENERAL MANIFESTATIONS: (a) severe anemia, jaundice; (b) hepatosplenomegaly; (c) cephalofacial deformities: prominent parietal and frontal bones; depressed nasal bridge; hypertelorism; prominent maxilla with an overbite on the mandible; retraction of the upper lip; protrusion of the incisors ("rodent facies"); (d) dwarfism; adult height deficiency.

(B) CARDIOVASCULAR SYSTEM: Cardiomegaly; pericardial effusion; pericarditis; disturbance of conductions and rhythm; right and left ventricular dysfunction (shown by radionuclide angiography) related to excessive iron deposition in the myocardium as a result of recurrent transfusions; congestive heart failure.

(C) ENDOCRINE DISORDERS: Hypogonadotropic hypogonadism (retarded sex characteristics); hypoparathyroidism; hypothyroidism; reduced growth hormone; reduced thyroid hormone reserve; diabetes mellitus.

(D) CENTRAL NERVOUS SYSTEM: Symptoms related to compression by extramedullary hematopoiesis (low back pain; paraplegia; generalized epileptiform seizures; etc.); intracranial hemorrhage and circulating coagulation inhibitor in ß-thalassemia major.

(E) SKELETAL SYSTEM: Gout; arthropathy (secondary to hemochromatosis); osteomyelitis; septic arthritis; association with pyknodysostosis (heterozygous ß-thalassemia).

(F) EAR, NOSE, AND THROAT: Enlargement of the adenoids and tonsils; hypertrophy of the nasal turbinates; conductive hearing loss; mixed-type hearing loss.

(G) MISCELLANEOUS ABNORMALITIES: Iron overload (liver cirrhosis; myocardial degeneration; endocrinopathies); bilirubin stones; scurvy despite a normal intake of vitamin C; mild to moderate small-airway obstruction and hyperinflation in homozygous ß-thalassemia; deletion of all four α-globin loci (Bart hemoglobin hydrops fetalis syndrome); hypersplenism in thalassemia major; renal cortical foci of extramedullary hematopoiesis.

Laboratory Tests (Thalassemia Major): (a) hypochromic microcytic anemia; poikilocytosis; polychromatophilia; target cells; nucleated erythroid precursors; decreased red cell survival; increased serum bilirubin and fecal urobilinogen; elevated serum iron level; excess hemoglobin A2 (over 3%) and hemoglobin F (50% to 90%); elevated serum iron level; (b) prenatal diagnosis by a method that allows determination of the mutations in both parental and fetal deoxyribonucleic acid on the same day.

Radiologic Manifestations

(A) SKELETAL SYSTEM

1. Skull: Osteoporosis with a granular pattern; expansion of the diploic space, most prominent in the frontal bone; thinning of the outer table; hair-on-end appearance; enlarged calvarial vascular markings; osseous lamellae parallel with the inner table; circumscribed lytic lesions; hypertelorism; hypoplasia of the paranasal sinuses due to osseous expansion of the facial bones (marrow hyperplasia); malocclusion of the jaws; dental displacement and deformities.

2. Trunk: Osteoporosis; coarse bony trabeculae; thinning of the cortex; rib-within-rib appearance; costal widening; rib notching; accentuation of vertical bone trabeculae of the vertebrae; biconcave vertebral configuration ("fish vertebrae"); scoliosis; medullary hyperplasia of the pelvic bones and clavicles.

3. Tubular bones: Widened medullary cavity; thinning of the cortex; underconstriction; premature closure of growth plates; pathologic fractures; perpendicular periosteal spiculation; enlarged phalangeal nutrient foramina; aseptic necrosis of the femoral head; computed tomography: cortical destruction and invasion of marrow tissue outside the medullary space.

4. Miscellaneous abnormalities: Skeletal maturation retardation; avidity of radiogallium for bone (marrow cavity hypertrophy); mild skeletal changes or "normal bones" (including craniofacial structures) in patients who had received adequate blood transfusions in early childhood.

(B) CHEST AND ABDOMEN: (a) extramedullary hematopoiesis: multiple lobular intrathoracic and intraabdominal masses adjacent to the ribs and thoracic vertebrae; pelvic masses; (b) transfusional hemochromatosis (liver; spleen; pancreas; lymph nodes); (c) hepatosplenomegaly; gallstones; gallbladder sludge; porcelain gallbladder; (d) renal enlargement.

(C) NERVOUS SYSTEM: (a) intracranial, paraspinal, and intraspinal extramedullary hematopoiesis (soft-tissue epidural masses having magnetic resonance signal of similar or slightly higher intensity compared with the adjacent bone marrow) causing compression symptoms (brain; spinal cord; cauda equina; nerve roots); spinal cord constriction and atrophy, with high signal intensity within the spinal cord suggestive of postcompressive myelomalacia or gliosis; intracranial hemorrhage; (b) gonadotropin insufficiency due to pituitary siderosis related to repeated blood transfusions: marked loss of signal intensity in the anterior lobe.

Treatment-Related Manifestations

(A) HEMOCHROMATOSIS DUE TO REPEATED BLOOD TRANSFUSIONS: Myocardial degeneration; gonadotropin insufficiency secondary to pituitary siderosis (loss of signal intensity in the anterior lobe on T_2-weighted magnetic resonance images); hepatosplenomegaly; increased density of the liver, spleen, and lymph nodes with magnetic resonance imaging showing hypointense hemosiderin deposits; liver cirrhosis; highly echogenic pancreas; etc.

(B) CHELATION THERAPY (DEFEROXAMINE INFUSIONS): (a) pulmonary syndrome of moderate to life-threatening severity characterized by tachypnea, hypoxemia, a diffuse interstitial pattern on chest roentgenogram, and restrictive dysfunction on pulmonary function studies; (b) deferoxamine-induced bone dysplasia: growth plate and metaphyseal irregularity (magnetic resonance imaging: signal characteristics consistent with hyaline cartilage); widened growth plates; decreased spinal height (platyspondyly); increased thoracic kyphosis; vertebral flattening and elongation anteriorly; intervertebral disc calcification; genu varum; etc.; (c) growth failure.

(C) GONADAL DAMAGE: Increased gonadotropin concentrations indicating gonadal damage after allogenic bone marrow transplantation in girls (probably related to the use of high doses of busulphan and cyclophosphamide).

Note: (a) ATR-X (*Alpha-Thalassemia/mental Retardation syndrome): X-linked inheritance* (Xq12–q21.31); short stature; craniofacial dysmorphism (microcephaly; midfacial hypoplasia; anteverted nares; wide mouth; prominent lower lip; large central incisors; etc.); hypogenitalism; (b) ATR-16: *Alpha-Thalassemia/mental Retardation,* and large deletion of the tip of chromosome 16p involving the α-globin locus.

3-HYDROXY-3-METHYLGLUTARYL-COENZYME A LYASE DEFICIENCY

Clinical Manifestations: A defect in amino acid and ketone metabolism: *seizures; hypoglycemia, acidosis, and absence of ketonuria; hepatomegaly; enzyme deficiency in cultured skin fibroblasts;* mental retardation.

Radiologic Manifestations: Macrocephaly; *leukodystrophy with preferential involvement of the deeper arcuate fibers:* hypodensity on computed tomography; white-matter cavitation; foci of hyperintensity on T_2-weighted images in the subcortical white matter; prominent sulci; mild to severe ventriculomegaly; brain atrophy.

TUMORAL CALCINOSIS

Clinical Manifestations: Onset of symptoms in the first or second decade of life: (a) *painless, hard, large, or small mass or masses over the extensor surface of joints;* (b) limited joint motion; inhibition of normal muscular function in association with large calcific masses; (c) slow growth of the masses over period of years; (d) biochemical features: hyperphosphatemia; elevated renal phosphate reabsorption; elevated serum 1,25-dihydroxyvitamin D levels; normal renal function; normocalcemia; normal alkaline phosphatase levels; (e) sinus formation associated with a whitish, chalky discharge to the skin (amorphic Ca apatite); (f) head and neck manifestations: involvement of the mucous membranes (gingivitis; perlèche; papillary hyperplasia of the lip vermilion and velvety red macules on the tongue, palate, and buccal mucosa; hoarseness) preceding the development of calcified nodules; retruded maxilla and relative mandibular prognathism; (g) miscellaneous abnormalities: tumoral calcinosis of the fingers; elevated sedimentation rate; erythematous rash; acrocyanosis; palmoplantar hyperhidrosis; hyperglobulinemia; onset in early infancy; pseudoxanthoma elasticum–like picture (retinal angioid streaks; skin calcifications; vascular calcifications; etc.); atypical presentation (absence of paraarticular masses); secondary infection and abscess formation; (h) approximately one third of reported cases are familial (mostly autosomal recessive inheritance); variability in expression; no sex predominance; more commonly reported in blacks.

Radiologic Manifestations: (a) *dense round or oval-shaped calcium deposits in the juxtaarticular regions* that measure from a few millimeters to several centimeters in diameter; may have a multinodular appearance; hip, elbow, shoulder, ankle, wrist, and foot the most common sites; sedimentation of calcified material within fluid-filled cysts; (b) periosteal reaction of tubular bones; smooth bony erosion adjacent to the mass; (c) bone scintigraphy: increased uptake of the calcified paraarticular masses and the involved bones; (d) computed tomography: (1) calcific paraarticular masses with varied appearance (from small solid to large cystic); (2) calcification of various tissues (skin; vessels; dura, articular cartilages, and articular capsules of hand); (3) marrow abnormalities (increased attenuation; spotty calcification in the marrow of the tubular bones and the diploic space of skull); (e) magnetic resonance imaging: high signal intensity on T_2-weighted images despite a large calcific component of the paraarticular masses; increased signal intensity of marrow on T_2-weighted images and also foci of decreased T_2 signal in the marrow corresponding to the small calcific deposits; (f) dental abnormalities: pulp stones with obliteration of the cavity; short and bulbous roots; (g) miscellaneous abnormalities: wrist arthropathy with the radiographic appearance of calcium pyrophosphate dihydrate crystal deposition disease; intervertebral disc calcification; paraspinal cervical soft-tissue mass with bony involvement.

Note: Tumoral calcinosis is classified into two types: idiopathic and secondary.

TYROSINEMIA TYPE I

Enzyme Deficiency: Fumarylacetoacetase hydrolase (FAH).

Clinical Manifestations

(A) ACUTE HEREDITARY TYROSINEMIA: Considerable clinical variations; occurrence of acute and chronic forms in the same family; the earlier the onset of symptoms, the poorer the prognosis: (a) onset in the first year of life, rapid lethal course; (b) *lethargy; irritability; failure to gain weight; fever; jaundice; diarrhea; ecchymosis; melena;* (c) *ascites; splenomegaly; hepatomegaly; liver failure; cardiomyopathy; proximal renal tubular defects;* renal acidosis; (d) elevated liver transaminases, γ-glutamyltranspeptidase, and bilirubin; depressed coagulation factors; *elevated blood tyrosine, methionine, and α-fetoprotein;* phosphaturia; glucosuria; hyperaminoaciduria; elevated excretion of ∂-aminolevulinic and phenolic acids.

(B) CHRONIC HEREDITARY TYROSINEMIA: (a) *hepatic cirrhosis;* (b) *generalized renal reabsorption defects* (Fanconi renotubular syndrome); reduced glomerular filtration; *hypophosphatemic rickets;* (c) neurologic crises: episodes of severe peripheral neuropathy (severe pain with extensor hypertonia; vomiting; paralytic ileus; muscle weakness; respiratory paralysis necessitating mechanical ventilation); self-mutilation; elevated urinary excretion of ∂-aminolevulinic acid (a neurotoxic intermediate of porphyrin biosynthesis); (d) *renal tubular defect* (absent in some cases); transaminases and methionine normal or elevated; depressed vitamin K–dependent coagulation factors; elevated excretion of phenolic acid; slightly elevated γ-glutamyltranspeptidase; *elevated plasma tyrosine;* (e) miscellaneous abnormalities: recurrent bleeding; hepatoma; porphyria-like syndrome with respiratory failure; mental retardation; chromosomal instability.

(C) Autosomal recessive inheritance.

Laboratory Tests: (a) acute and chronic forms: (1) increased levels of succinylacetone or the precursors; (2) fumarylacetoacetase deficiency (demonstrated in lymphocytes, fibroblasts, and possibly erythrocytes); (b) prenatal diagnosis: (1) determination of succinylacetone in amniotic fluid supernatant; (2) assay of FAH activity in cultured amniotic fluid cells; (3) determination of FAH in chorionic villus material; (4) mutation analysis on chorionic villi.

Radiologic Manifestations: (a) *vitamin D–resistant rickets;* (b) *nephromegaly; renal stones; nephrocalcinosis;* (c) liver: *cirrhosis* in early childhood; hepatocellular carcinoma; computed tomographic liver patterns: (1) normal liver attenuation or diffuse low attenuation; (2) mixed background liver attenuation with high-density nodules; (3) mixed background attenuation with high- and low-density nodules; (4) low-density nodules; magnetic resonance imaging: hepatic nodules of high signal intensity on both T_1- and T_2-weighted images; (d) miscellaneous abnormalities: dense bony spicules projecting from metaphysis into the epiphyseal growth plate associated with widening and cupping of the metaphysis; unusually intense skeletal uptake of gallium-67 citrate.

Note: Other disorders of tyrosine metabolism (hypertyrosinemia): (a) tyrosinemia type II (Richner-Hanhart syndrome): autosomal recessive inheritance; tyrosine transaminase deficiency; corneal erosions and plaques; palm and sole erosions and hyperkeratoses; mental retardation in some; the gene defect is localized to chromosome 16; intrafamilial variation in phenotype; (b) neonatal transitory tyrosinemia: *p*-OH-phenylpyruvic acid oxidase deficiency; infants may be lethargic, have difficulty in feeding, experience impaired motor activity, etc.; (c) the term tyrosinosis usually used in reference to the case reported by Medes in 1932; the enzyme defect not determined; (d) hypertyrosinemia in patients with liver disease; (e) tyrosinemia type III (4-hydroxyphenylpyruvic acid oxidase deficiency): mental deficiency.

V

VIPoma SYNDROME (WDHA Syndrome; Watery Diarrhea–Hypokalemia-Achlorhydria Syndrome; Verner-Morrison Syndrome)

Etiology: *Pancreatic non–beta islet cell tumor (VIPoma) or hyperplasia;* other less common causes: bronchogenic carcinoma; pheochromocytoma; ganglioneuroblastoma; ganglioneuroma; liver VIPoma; etc.

Clinical Manifestations: (a) *watery diarrhea* (tea-colored watery stools); (b) *hypokalemia; gastric hypochlorhydria* (more common) or achlorhydria; *elevated levels of plasma vasoactive intestinal polypeptide;* (c) miscellaneous abnormalities: significant weight loss; dehydration, and electrolyte depletion; tetany due to hypomagnesemia; increased tear secretion.

Radiologic Manifestations: (a) mass with compression of the stomach and/or duodenum; (b) bowel distension; multiple air-fluid levels in the bowel; (c) arteriography: *hypervascular mass with hypertrophied feeding vessels; persistent dense capillary stain;* (d) computed tomography: *pancreatic tumor demonstrable in about one third of WDHA cases;* (e) endoscopic retrograde cholangiopancreatography study showing pancreatic duct distortion by the mass; search for neural crest tumor.

Note: VIP (*V*asoactive *I*ntestinal *P*olypeptide) was originally isolated from porcine gut and given this name because it produces systemic vasodilatation in dogs.

VITAMIN A DEFICIENCY

Clinical and Radiologic Manifestations: Growth retardation; anemia; recurrent infections; immune abnormalities in T-cell subsets (reversible with vitamin A supplementation); increased intracranial pressure: bulging fontanelles; widening of sutures.

VITAMIN A INTOXICATION

Etiology: (a) acute poisoning due to a large single dose of 300,000 to 1,000,000 IU; ingestion of polar bear liver or shark liver; (b) chronic poisoning due to intake of 100,000 IU or more per day for 6 months or longer; daily ingestion of chicken liver in infancy; long-term parenteral hyperalimentation.

Clinical Manifestations

(A) ACUTE HYPERVITAMINOSIS A: Insomnia or irresistible desire to sleep, drowsiness, sluggishness, irritability, headaches, vomiting, peeling of skin, increased intracranial pressure, and acute hydrocephalus.

(B) CHRONIC HYPERVITAMINOSIS A

1. Fetal: Malformations of the central nervous system with exposure in early pregnancy.
2. Early infancy: Anorexia, hyperirritability, tenderness and swelling of the scalp, bulging fontanelles, and craniotabes.
3. Children: Anorexia, hyperesthesia, irritability, limb pain and swelling, loss of hair, pruritus, rhagades, impaired attention span, emotional instability, focal motor seizures, electroencephalographic abnormalities, pseudotumor cerebri, hepatosplenomegaly, and hepatic fibrosis.
4. Adolescents and adults: Skin dryness, maculopapular rash, fissures, desquamation, pigmentation, pruritus, loss of hair, brittle nails, yellow discoloration of the skin, gingivitis, generalized weakness, fatigue, pain in bones and joints, tenderness of limbs, anorexia, headaches, muscle stiffness, papilledema, diplopia, psychiatric symptoms, insomnia, somnolence, exophthalmos, hepatomegaly, liver cirrhosis, splenomegaly, absent or decreased menorrhea, weight loss, polyuria, polydipsia, edema of the lower limbs, epistaxis, lymphadenopathy, and hypercalcemia.

Radiologic Manifestations

(A) EARLY INFANCY: Thinness and poor mineralization of the skull; relative hyperostosis of the sutural margins; hydrocephalus; osteopenia; cup-shaped, sharply demarcated, and widened metaphyses.

(B) CHILDREN: Widening of cranial sutures; hyperostosis of the occipital and temporal bones; normal-appearing or enlarged cerebral ventricles and subarachnoid space; thickening of the mandible; cortical hyperostosis of the tubular bones; pleural effusion; ascites; increase in ^{99m}Tc pyrophosphate uptake in the diaphyses of long bones (present before the appearance of radiographic manifestations).

(C) ADOLESCENTS AND ADULTS: Demineralization of the floor of the sella turcica simulating an intrasellar tumor, with return to normal after vitamin A ingestion is discontinued; wavy and laminated periosteal calcification of the tubular bones; skeletal hyperostoses.

Note: Hyperostotic changes in the axial and appendicular skeleton have been reported in adults with the use of synthetic retinoids, including isotretinoin.

VITAMIN B$_1$ DEFICIENCY (BERIBERI; THIAMIN DEFICIENCY)

Clinical and Radiologic Manifestations: (a) *generalized weakness, anorexia, and failure to thrive;* (b) *cardiomyopathy:* tachycardia; arrhythmias; cardiomegaly; heart failure; increased QT interval, inversion of T waves, and low voltage; (c) psychiatric disorders; laryngeal nerve paralysis; pain; burning feet; tenderness of the nerve trunks; ataxia, loss of coordination; loss of deep sensation; optic nerve atrophy; increased intracranial pressure; meningism; coma; (d) *elevated levels of blood pyruvic acid and lactic acid; low levels of red cell transketolase and high blood and urinary levels of glyoxylate.*

Note: (a) cardiovascular beriberi has the following two forms of clinical presentations: (1) predominantly right-sided heart failure associated with a high cardiac output failure (due to peripheral vasodilatation); (2) Shoshin beriberi or acute pernicious beriberi: cardiovascular collapse; (b) thiamine-responsive anemia syndrome: anemia associated with diabetes mellitus and sensorineural deafness; (c) association of scurvy with wet berberi.

VITAMIN B$_{12}$ DEFICIENCY

Etiology: Strictly vegetarian diet; breast-fed infants with the mother on strictly vegetarian diet (vegan diet); malabsorption of B$_{12}$ vitamin; after gastric surgery for obesity.

Clinical Manifestations: Insidious onset of symptoms: (a) *progressive psychomotor regression;* confusion; depression; delusions; mental slowness; (b) *symptoms of subacute combined degeneration of the spinal cord:* weakness; unsteadiness of gait; paresthesias of the hands and feet; absent tendon reflexes in the legs; loss of joint position and vibration sense; positive Romberg sign; pseudoathetosis of the upper limbs due to severe loss of joint position sense; (c) *megaloblastic anemia;* (d) *diminished plasma level of vitamin B_{12};* (e) dramatic improvement of clinical manifestations with vitamin B_{12} therapy.

Radiologic Manifestations: Computed tomography: "brain atrophy" in infancy with improvement during B_{12} therapy; intrathoracic extramedullary hematopoiesis secondary to B_{12} and folate deficiency.

Note: (a) low serum vitamin B_{12} levels and abnormalities of vitamin B_{12} metabolism have been reported in patients with acquired immunodeficiency syndrome; (b) neuropsychiatric manifestations of vitamin B_{12} deficiency may be present with anemia.

VITAMIN D INTOXICATION

Clinical Manifestations: (a) history of excessive intake of vitamin D over a period of a few days to several years; drinking milk that is incorrectly or excessively fortified with vitamin D; (b) *loss of appetite, abdominal cramps, nausea, vomiting, polydipsia, polyuria, seizures, and coma;* (c) *renal insufficiency;* impaired ability to concentrate urine; (d) *generalized calcinosis;* (e) *hypercalcemia, hypercalciuria,* elevated blood urea nitrogen levels, elevated serum creatinine levels, and abnormal urine sediment.

Radiologic Manifestations: (a) *generalized calcinosis* (falx; tentorium; kidneys; myocardium; lung; gastric wall; adrenal; parathyroid and thyroid glands; pancreas; skin; arteries; joints; periarticular); (b) *dense transverse metaphyseal bands; cortical thickening of tubular bones; bone sclerosis; dense vertebral end plates; thickening of the calvaria;* osteoporosis in some adult patients.

VON WILLEBRAND DISEASE

Classification: Type I: mild reduction in the concentration of von Willebrand factor (vWF); type II: decreased proportion of high molecular weight multimers; type III: barely detectable concentration of vWF.

Clinical and Radiologic Manifestations: (a) *hemorrhagic disorder:* visceral bleeding (posttraumatic; postsurgical); external bleeding (easy bruising; epistaxis; gingival bleeding); rare occurrence of hemarthrosis; (b) *prolonged bleeding time;* reduced glass bead adherence; reduced factor VIII procoagulant activity (VIII:C); decreased ristocetin-induced platelet aggregation (VIII:RCOF); reduced factor VIII–related antigen (VIII:Ag); (c) high incidence of association with mitral valve prolapse; (d) association with hereditary hemorrhagic telangiectasia; gastrointestinal angiodysplasia; (e) acquired von Willebrand disease associated with angiodysplasia, hypothyroidism; (f) miscellaneous abnormalities: von Willebrand disease associated with thrombocytopenia, platelet function defect, and an abnormal factor VIII molecule; fetal periventricular hemorrhage; pseudoaneurysm; (g) autosomal dominant and autosomal recessive inheritance.

W

WILSON DISEASE (HEPATOLENTICULAR DEGENERATION)

Pathophysiology: A disorder of copper metabolism with impaired ability of the liver to handle copper and excrete it in the bile, resulting in the excessive accumulation of copper in various organs (central nervous system; kidneys; liver; cornea; etc.), a low serum ceruloplasmin level, and an increased rate of urinary copper excretion.

Clinical Manifestations: Onset in childhood: (a) *neurologic disorders* (variable in frequency and severity): lethargy; abdominal pain; malaise; poor coordination; tremor; psychologic disorders; drooling; dysphagia; dysarthria; masked face; disturbed locomotion; dystonia and hypertonia; choreoathetosis; blurred vision; headache; seizures; coma; (b) *Kayser-Fleischer ring at the limbus of the cornea;* (c) *jaundice; hepatomegaly; hepatocellular necrosis; liver cirrhosis; splenomegaly;* (d) *renal dysfunction:* Fanconi syndrome; renal tubular acidosis (proximal and distal tubular dysfunction); decreased renal plasma flow; decreased glomerular filtration rate; aminoaciduria; urolithiasis; (e) *cupriuria; elevated "free" copper and deficiency of ceruloplasmin; spectrometric demonstration of high corneal copper content;* (f) subclinical dysfunction in major sensory pathways: somatosensory; brain-stem auditory and pattern-reversal visual evoked potentials; (g) miscellaneous abnormalities: (1) blood: hemolytic anemia (which may be the presenting manifestation in response to the ingestion of food with a high copper content); bleeding tendency; persistent hypertransaminasemia; (2) cardiovascular: electrocardiographic abnormalities (left ventricular hypertrophy; biventricular hypertrophy; early repolarization; ST depression and T inversion; premature atrial or ventricular contractions; atrial fibrillation; sinoatrial block; Mobitz type 1 atrioventricular block; orthostatic hypotension; (3) skin/hair: keratitis; hyperpigmentation of the legs; "uncombable hair syndrome"; (4) other manifestations: edema; arthralgias; ascites; fever; pancreatitis; gigantism; cardiac death (h) autosomal recessive; chromosomal localization: 13q14–q21; deoxyribonucleic acid–based diagnosis: carrier detection, diagnosis in the presymptomatic phase of the disease, and transabdominal chorionic villi biopsy diagnosis; heterozygous carriers may develop mild abnormalities of copper metabolism.

Radiologic Manifestations: (a) skeletal system: (1) osteoporosis; osteomalacia or rickets; (2) arthropathy; osteochondritis dissecans; subarticular cysts; paraarticular calcific deposits; chondrocalcinosis; irregularity of vertebral body contour; "squaring" of vertebral bodies; Schmorl nodes; wedge-shaped vertebral bodies; juvenile kyphosis; disc space narrowing; (3) spontaneous fractures; (4) retarded skeletal maturation; (b) portal hypertension; increased computed tomographic density of the liver (case report); splenomegaly; pancreatic distortion due to splenomegaly; (c) renal stones; (d) cholelithiasis; (e) central nervous system: (1) computed tomography: low attenuation in the basal ganglia (reversible under treatment); cavitation of the basal ganglia; selective dilatation of the frontal horn secondary to atrophic changes in the caudate and anterior lenticular nuclei; red nucleus, dentate nucleus, brain stem, and frontal cortex occasionally involved; (2) magnetic resonance imaging: *lesion with decreased signal intensity on T_1-weighted images and increased signal intensity on T_2-weighted images measuring 3 to 15 mm in diameter located in lenticular, thalamic, caudate and dentate nuclei, as well as in the brain stem and white matter;* atypical decreased T_2 signal intensity in some cases; cavitations in basal ganglia and thalami; thickened and bright claustrum on long-TR magnetic resonance images; brain atrophy; contrast enhancement of cerebral lesions after penicillamine therapy; resolution of "magnetic resonance imaging lesions" following long-term zinc therapy; (3) positron emission tomography: diffusely reduced glucose metabolism.

WINCHESTER SYNDROME

Clinical Manifestations: (a) short stature; (b) polyarthralgia, progressive joint deformities, and flexion contractures of small and large joints; (c) coarse facial features; (d) skin thickening and hyperpigmentation; hypertrichosis; (e) skin biopsy: fibroblastic hyperplasia; abnormal collagen bundles in the deep dermis; characteristic ultrastructural dilatation of mitochondria in fibroblasts (electron microscopy); excessive collagen turnover; (f) gum hypertrophy; (g) peripheral corneal opacities; (h) miscellaneous abnormalities: intestinal lymphangiectasia and protein-losing enteropathy; excessive oligosaccharides in the urine; (i) autosomal recessive inheritance.

Radiologic Manifestations: Extensive progressive skeletal disease: (a) bone resorption, most marked in the carpals and metacarpal articular margin; (b) osteoporosis; (c) thinning of long bones; (d) resorption of the distal phalanges; (e) subluxation of C1 on C2; kyphoscoliosis; (f) misshapen pelvis; destruction of the femoral heads; (g) expanded clavicle; wide and thin ribs; (h) delayed closure of the anterior fontanelle; widely open sutures and prominent frontal region; flat mandibular condyles; delayed tooth eruption; (i) miscellaneous abnormalities: compression fracture of the vertebrae; protrusio acetabuli; ankylosis involving the small joints of the feet; radial and ulnar artery hypoplasia; hypervascularity in areas of apparent active bone resorption.

WOLMAN DISEASE

Enzyme Deficiency: Lysosomal acid lipase (acid cholesteryl ester hydrolase).

Clinical Manifestations: Onset in early infancy: (a) *failure to thrive;* (b) *diarrhea; steatorrhea;* (c) *protuberant abdomen;* (d) *hepatosplenomegaly;* jaundice; (e) *anemia;* (f) *storage of cholesteryl esters and triglycerides in various tissues* (liver; spleen; intestine; kidneys; thymus; adrenal glands; blood cells); (g) jejunal mucosal abnormalities: distorted and club-shaped intestinal villi as a result of infiltration of foam cells into the lamina propria of the mucosa; marked shortening and irregularity of the microvilli of the epithelial cells and severe impairment of disaccharidase activity on electron microscopy; loss of the sugar- and amino acid–evoked potential differences in the jejunum; (h) subarachnoid hemorrhage; (i) autosomal recessive inheritance.

Radiologic Manifestations: (a) *punctate calcific foci distributed throughout enlarged adrenal glands;* flattening of the superior pole of the kidneys without displacement of the kidneys or distortion of the pelvicaliceal system; marked echogenicity of the adrenals; cortical calcification and markedly enlarged adrenal glands (computed tomography); (b) *hepatosplenomegaly;* decreased attenuation value (computed tomography) of the liver, attenuation value that may be less than that of the spleen; (c) miscellaneous abnormalities: paucity of subcutaneous fat; generalized osteoporosis; multiple "growth lines" in bones; involution of the thymus; highly echogenic thickened bowel walls due to fat deposition within the lamina propria.

X

XANTHINE OXIDASE DEFICIENCY

Enzyme Deficiency: Xanthine oxidase, which catalyses the transformation of hypoxanthine to xanthine and xanthine to uric acid; enzyme deficiency demonstrable by evaluation of the liver or intestinal mucosa.

Clinical Manifestations: (a) *xanthinuria;* hypouricemia; hypouric aciduria; increased urinary excretion of oxypurines, hypoxanthine, and xanthine; *xanthine stones;* (b) muscle cramp; myopathy; polyarthritis; (c) autosomal recessive inheritance.

Radiologic Manifestations: *Nephrolithiasis.*

Note: (a) the disease may present as the classic form (isolated xanthine oxidase deficiency) or as a defect of a molybdenum-containing cofactor present in both xanthine oxidase and sulfite oxidase complexes; the second form is associated with severe neurologic manifestations and early death in infancy; (b) a high incidence of the classic form in individuals of Lebanese extraction has been reported.

Z

ZELLWEGER SYNDROME (Cerebro-Hepato-Renal Syndrome)

Biochemical Abnormalities: Absence of peroxisomes in hepatocytes and renal proximal tubule cells; marked deficiency of plasmalogens in the liver, kidney, brain, muscle, and heart; absence of histochemical staining for catalase in liver; deficiency of peroxisomal enzyme dihydroxyacetone phosphate acyltransferase (DHAPAT); accumulation of very long chain fatty acids; fibroblasts containing unprocessed thiolase and unprocessed acyl-CoA oxidase.

Clinical Manifestations: (a) *craniofacial dysmorphism:* macrocephaly; round flat face; high forehead; micrognathia; widely open suture and fontanelles; ocular hypertelorism; mongoloid slant of the orbital fissures; epicanthal folds; periorbital edema; external ear defect; highly arched palate; (b) *marked muscular hypotonia; decreased or absent reflexes; psychomotor retardation; seizures;* nystagmus; poor sucking; severe hearing impairment; marked abnormal neurophysiologic study (electroencephalography, brain stem auditory evoked potentials, and somatosensory evoked potentials); (c) cataract; prominent Y-suture; glaucoma; corneal clouding; Brushfield spots; pigmentary retinopathy; optic nerve dysplasia/hypoplasia; blindness; (d) *hepatomegaly;* proteinuria; hypoprothrombinemia; abnormal liver function values; elevated serum iron level and iron-binding capacity; hemosiderosis and iron deposition in macrophages of the bone marrow; (e) miscellaneous abnormalities: small for gestational age; jaundice of unusual degree and duration in newborn; congenital cardiovascular anomalies; camptodactyly; cubitus valgus; deep sacral dimple; hypospadias; cryptorchidism; hypertrophic pyloric stenosis; microdeletion of the proximal long arm of chromosome 7; mild variant without the characteristic facial features; (f) autosomal recessive inheritance; the human peroxisome assembly factor-1 gene responsible for Zellweger syndrome assigned to chromosome 8q21.1.

Laboratory Diagnostic Tests: (a) prenatal: demonstration of a deficiency of the enzyme DHAPAT in the amniotic fluid cells; absence of peroxisomes in cultured amniotic fluid cells; (b) postnatal: absence of peroxisome in the liver biopsy specimen; absence of DHAPAT activity; high levels of saturated very long chain fatty acids in cultured fibroblasts; analysis of very long chain fatty acids in the blood spots collected at neonatal screening.

Pathology: (a) brain dysgenesis: microgyria; pachygyria; agenesis or hypoplasia of the corpus callosum; cerebral/cerebellar heterotopias; enlarged lateral ventricles; ependymal abnormalities; cerebellar hypoplasia; olivary hypoplasia; sudanophilic leukoencephalomyelopathy; gliosis; glycogen storage; (b) renal cortical microcysts; tubular ectasia; hydronephrosis; (c) cirrhosis; biliary dysgenesis; siderosis; absent peroxisomes; abnormal mitochondria; diminished smooth endoplasmic reticulum; (d) congenital heart disease: ventricular septal defect; patent ductus arteriosus; (e) miscellaneous abnormalities: pancreatic islet cell hyperplasia; thymic hypoplasia; intestinal lymphangiectasia.

Radiologic Manifestations: (a) *chondral, articular, and periarticular soft-tissue calcifications,* especially in the patellae, acetabular regions, hyoid bone, and areas of the greater trochanters; (b) bell-shaped thorax; (c) limb anomalies: flexion deformities of the fingers; cubitus valgus; metatarsus adductus; talipes equinovarus; rocker-bottom feet; metatarsus varus; (d) retarded bone age; (e) dolichocephaly; wide-open sutures; large fontanelles; subependymal germinal cysts; ventricular dilatation; colpocephaly; hypogenesis of the corpus callosum; pachygyria in the perisylvian region; (f) renal cortical cysts; (g) proton nuclear magnetic resonance spectroscopy: marked decrease of N-acetylaspartate in white and gray matter, thalamus, and cerebellum.

ZOLLINGER-ELLISON SYNDROME

Clinical Manifestations: (a) *severe recurrent peptic ulcers;* (b) *watery diarrhea;* (c) *gastric hypersecretion hyperchlorhydria* (the secretin provocation test may be necessary to demonstrate gastric acid hypersecretion); (d) malabsorption syndrome; (e) radioimmunoassay of circulating serum gastrin; (f) miscellaneous abnormalities: endocrine abnormalities in about 30% of cases (pituitary tumor; hyperparathyroidism; insulinoma; multiple endocrine adenomatosis; duct adenocarcinoma of the pancreas; ovarian mucous cyst adenocarcinoma); osteoblastic bone metastasis; Cushing syndrome.

Pathology: (a) *gastrin-secreting lesions,* most commonly of pancreatic origin (adenocarcinoma; adenoma; hyperplasia), tumors less commonly located in duodenum or at other sites; (b) *peptic ulcer or ulcers.*

Radiologic Manifestations: (a) *peptic ulcer or ulcers of the stomach, duodenum, and jejunum in an atypical location; large mucosal folds of the stomach, duodenum, and jejunum; gastric hypersecretion; megaduodenum; small-bowel edema; increased intraluminal fluid; dilatation of the jejunum and ileum;* peptic esophagitis and esophageal ulceration; (b) ultrasonography of gastrinomas (low sensitivity; useful as the initial imaging modality and for intraoperative tumor localization): homogeneous area of low echogenicity in the pancreas; tumor calcification; (c) localization of gastrinoma by endoscopic ultrasonography (successful in 60% of case); (d) computed tomography for localization and staging of islet cell tumors: *calcification; tumor enhancement after contrast medium;* hepatic metastases; secondary abnormalities (thickening of the gastric, duodenal, or jejunal wall; increased fluid in the duodenum or small bowel); (e) magnetic resonance imaging of extrahepatic gastrinomas (low sensitivity, particularly for small tumors): increased relative signal intensity on the T_2-weighted images of primary lesion and metastatic lymph nodes; *variable signal intensity on the T_1-weighted image of the primary tumors* (magnetic resonance imaging very sensitive in detecting and assessing the extent of hepatic metastatic gastrinoma, but not as useful as arteriography in detecting primary tumor); (f) celiac arteriography: *tumor stain;* prominent gastric and intestinal venous opacification; selective arterial secretin injection test for localizing gastrinoma; (g) transhepatic selective catheterization of the pancreatic veins for venous sampling and reliable localization of gastrin-secreting islet cell tumors; (h) portal venous sampling (pancreaticoduodenal venous arcade): gastrin; (i) miscellaneous abnormalities: nephrocalcinosis; hypervascular liver metastases; bone metastases; Zollinger-Ellison syndrome as part of the multiple endocrine neoplasm I syndrome; kidney stones; esophageal involvement related to gastroesophageal reflux (esophagitis; stricture formation; Barrett esophagus); peptic ulcer perforation as the presenting manifestation; cholelithiasis following total gastrectomy.

Index-Gamuts

A

Acetabular angle: small; flared iliac wing
  Aminopterin fetopathy, 8
  Brachmann–de Lange syndrome, 22
  Caudal dysplasia sequence, 31
  Cephaloskeletal dysplasia, 32
  Chromosome 13 trisomy syndrome, 37
  Down syndrome, 57
  Hypothyroidism (cretinism), 300
  Mucolipidosis II, 323
  Mucolipidosis III, 324
  Mucopolysaccharidosis I-H, 327
  Mucopolysaccharidosis III, 330
  Mucopolysaccharidosis IVA, 331
  Nail-patella syndrome, 137
  Prune-belly syndrome, 170
  Pterygium syndromes, 171
  Rubinstein-Taybi syndrome, 182
  Shwachman syndrome, 363

Achalasia (esophagus)
  Achalasia-adrenal-alacrima syndrome, 2
  Amyloidosis, 245
  Down syndrome, 57
  Scleroderma, 186

Acro-osteolysis; distal phalangeal erosion
  Acrogeria, 4
  Diabetes mellitus, 262
  Ehlers-Danlos syndrome, 63
  Epidermolysis bullosa, 67
  Gout, 280
  Hajdu-Cheney syndrome, 87
  Hyperparathyroidism, 290
  Insensitivity to pain (congenital), 101
  Lesch-Nyhan syndrome, 310
  Lipoid dermatoarthritis, 115
  Mandibuloacral dysplasia, 120
  Mixed connective tissue disease, 131
  Osteomalacia, 360
  Pachydermoperiostosis, 155

  Papillon-Lefèvre syndrome, 157
  Porphyrias, 353
  Progeria, 168
  Raynaud syndrome, 173
  Reiter syndrome, 174
  Rothmund-Thompson syndrome, 181
  Satoyoshi syndrome, 184
  Scleroderma, 186
  Singleton-Merten syndrome, 191
  Sjögren syndrome, 192
  Thevenard syndrome, 208
  Werner syndrome, 224
  Winchester syndrome, 384

Adipose tissue: absent or deficient
  Cockayne syndrome, 40
  Diencephalic syndrome, 55
  Fetal alcohol syndrome, 71
  Leprechaunism, 310
  Lipodystrophy (lipoatrophic diabetes), 311
  Progeria, 168
  Rothmund-Thomson syndrome, 181
  SHORT syndrome, 265
  Werner syndrome, 224
  Wiedemann-Rautenstrauch syndrome, 226

Adrenal gland, large
  Addison disease, 237
  Adrenal hyperplasia (congenital), 238
  Amyloidosis, 245
  Cushing syndrome, 258

Adrenal insufficiency
  Achalasia-adrenal-alacrima syndrome, 2
  Addison disease, 237
  Addison–hypoparathyroidism–adrenogenital syndrome, 237
  Adrenoleukodystrophy, 239
  Amyloidosis, 245
  Deprivation dwarfism, 260
  Hemochromatosis, 281
  Pituitary diseases

389

POEMS syndrome, 161
Polyglandular autoimmune disease, 352
Sheehan syndrome, 363
Waterhouse-Friderichsen syndrome, 222
Alopecia; hypotrichosis
  Acrodermatitis enteropathica, 234
  Autosomal-recessive sparse hair
  Biotinidase deficiency, 248
  Cardio-facio-cutaneous syndrome, 26
  CHILD syndrome, 36
  Clouston syndrome, 39
  Cockayne syndrome, 40
  Coffin-Siris syndrome, 42
  Cranioectodermal dysplasia, 45
  Cronkhite-Canada syndrome, 47
  Down syndrome, 57
  Dubowitz syndrome, 59
  Dyskeratosis congenita, 60
  Ectodermal dysplasia (hypohidrotic), 61
  Encephalo-cranio-cutaneous lipomatosis,
    66
  Epidermal nevus syndrome, 66
  GAPO syndrome, 80
  Goltz syndrome, 83
  Hallermann-Streiff syndrome, 88
  Homocystinuria, 285
  Hypomelanosis of Ito, 98
  Hypoparathyroidism, 296
  Hypopituitarism (anterior lobe), 298
  Incontinentia pigmenti, 100
  Laron syndrome, 309
  Mandibuloacral dysplasia, 120
  Marinesco-Sjögren syndrome, 122
  Menkes disease, 319
  Neu-Laxova syndrome, 139
  Oculo-dento-osseous dysplasia, 147
  Odonto-tricho-melic syndrome, 148
  Oro-facio-digital syndrome I, 150
  Pallister-Killian syndrome, 156
  Polyglandular autoimmune disease, 352
  Progeria, 168
  Pterygium syndromes, 171
  Rothmund-Thomson syndrome, 181
  Seckel syndrome, 188
  Tricho-odonto-onychial dysplasia
  Vohwinkel syndrome, 219
  Werner syndrome, 224
Ambiguous genitalia
  Aniridia-Wilms tumor association, 10
  Meckel syndrome, 125
  Pterygium syndrome (popliteal web), 171

Amputation (congenital or acquired); reduc-
    tion defect
  Ainhum, 6
  Amniotic band sequence, 9
  Diabetes mellitus, 262
  Insensitivity to pain (congenital), 101
  Keratosis palmaris et plantaris familiaris
    (tylosis), 107
  Lesch-Nyhan syndrome, 310
  Scleroderma, 186
  Vohwinkel syndrome, 219
Anemia
  Aarskog syndrome, 2
  Aase syndrome, 2
  Aluminum intoxication, 245
  Banti syndrome, 15
  Blind loop syndrome, 20
  Celiac disease, 254
  Chédiak-Higashi syndrome, 35
  Copper deficiency, 258
  Cronkhite-Canada syndrome, 47
  Diamond-Blackfan syndrome, 54
  Dubowitz syndrome, 59
  Dyskeratosis congenita, 60
  Fabry disease, 266
  Fanconi anemia, 69
  Felty syndrome, 70
  Glucagonoma syndrome, 274
  Goodpasture syndrome, 84
  Hemolytic uremic syndrome, 90
  Hemosiderosis (idiopathic pulmonary),
    284
  Hereditary nonspherocytic anemia
  Holt-Oram syndrome, 94
  Hypereosinophilic syndrome (idiopathic),
    96
  Hyperostosis–hyperphosphatemia syn-
    drome, 97
  Hyperthyroidism, 294
  Hypophosphatasia, 297
  Hypothyroidism, 300
  Iron deficiency anemia, 305
  Kwashiorkor, 308
  Lead intoxication
  Lowe syndrome, 314
  Ménétrier syndrome, 127
  Mixed connective tissue disease, 131
  Nephronophthisis, 138
  Niemann-Pick disease, 336
  Paraneoplastic syndromes, 344
  Pearson syndrome, 348

Peutz-Jeghers syndrome, 159
Plummer-Vinson syndrome, 161
Polyglandular autoimmune disease, 352
Porphyrias, 353
Prasad syndrome, 354
Pyruvate kinase deficiency anemia, 357
Sea-blue histiocyte syndrome, 188
Shwachman syndrom, 363
Sickle cell anemia, 365
Somatostatinoma syndrome, 371
Spherocytosis, 372
Stagnant small-bowel syndrome, 198
TAR syndrome, 206
Thalassemia, 374
Tyrosinemia type I, 378
Vitamin A deficiency, 380
Vitamin B_{12} deficiency, 381
Weismann-Netter syndrome, 224
Wilson disease, 383
Wiskott-Aldrich syndrome, 228
Aneurysm (arterial)
Behçet syndrome, 18
Contractural arachnodactyly, 44
Ehlers-Danlos syndrome, 63
Hughes-Stovin syndrome, 95
Hyperimmunoglobulinemia E syndrome,
96
Hypothenar hammer syndrome, 99
Kawasaki syndrome, 106
Maffucci syndrome, 119
Marfan syndrome, 121
Anhidrosis; hypohidrosis
Cockayne syndrome, 40
Ectodermal dysplasia (hypohidrotic), 61
Menkes disease, 319
Shy-Drager syndrome, 190
Sjögren-Larsson syndrome, 369
Anophthalmia
Branchio-oculo-facial syndrome, 23
Chromosome 13 trisomy syndrome, 37
Lenz microphthalmia syndrome, 113
Oculo-auriculo-vertebral spectrum, 147
Waardenburg anophthalmia syndrome,
220
Anorectal anomaly
Apert syndrome, 11
Baller-Gerold syndrome, 14
Cat-eye syndrome, 30
Caudal dysplasia sequence, 31
CHARGE association, 34
Currarino triad, 49

DiGeorge syndrome, 55
Down syndrome, 57
Duane syndrome, 59
Dyskeratosis congenita, 60
Femoral hypoplasia–unusual facies syn-
drome, 70
Fetal hydantoin syndrome, 72
FG syndrome, 73
Fraser syndrome, 77
Johanson-Blizzard syndrome, 103
Kaufman-McKusick syndrome, 106
Meckel syndrome, 125
Opitz BBBG syndrome, 149
Pallister-Hall syndrome, 156
Potter sequence, 166
Sirenomelia, 192
Splenogonadal fusion/limb deformity, 196
Spondylocostal dysostoses (Jarcho-Levin
syndrome), 197
Townes-Brocks syndrome, 210
VATER association, 218
Aortic valvular disease
Alkaptonuria, 243
Chronic granulomatous disease of child-
hood, 256
Cogan syndrome, 43
Ehlers-Danlos syndrome, 63
Floppy valve syndrome, 75
Heyde syndrome, 93
Hyperlipoproteinemias, 287
Mannosidoses, 316
Marfan syndrome, 121
Marfanoid hypermobility syndrome, 122
Mucolipidosis III, 324
Mucopolysaccharidoses, 325
Reiter syndrome, 174
Relapsing polychondritis, 175
Turner syndrome, 214
Williams syndrome, 227
Arachnodactyly
Antley-Bixler syndrome, 11
Contractural arachnodactyly, 44
Ehlers-Danlos syndrome, 63
Gorlin syndrome, 85
Homocystinuria, 285
Marden-Walker syndrome, 121
Marfan syndrome, 121
Multiple endocrine neoplasia,type IIB, 135
Shprintzen-Goldberg syndrome, 189
Sotos syndrome, 195
Stickler syndrome, 200

Arrhythmia
  Carotid sinus syndrome, 28
  Glycogen storage disease type II, 276
  Hemochromatosis, 281
  Hyperthyroidism, 294
  Kearns-Sayre syndrome, 306
  LEOPARD syndrome, 113
  Stokes-Adams syndrome, 201
  Syndrome X, 205
  Tabatznik syndrome, 205
  Wolff-Parkinson-White syndrome, 229
Arterial calcification; *refer to* Calcification:
  arterial
Arterial dilatation
  Acromegaly, 235
  Contractural arachnodactyly, 44
  Cutis laxa, 49
  Ehlers-Danlos syndrome, 63
  Fragile X syndrome, 77
  Homocystinuria, 285
  Larsen syndrome, 112
  Marfan syndrome, 121
  Marfanoid hypermobility syndrome, 122
  Menkes disease, 319
  Neurofibromatosis I, 140
  Rendu-Osler-Weber syndrome, 176
  Turner syndrome, 214
Arterial dissection
  Ehlers-Danlos syndrome, 63
  Marfan syndrome, 121
  Marfanoid hypermobility syndrome, 122
  Noonan syndrome, 145
  Turner syndrome, 214
Arterial occlusion
  Behçet syndrome, 18
  Blue digit syndrome, 21
  Celiac axis compression syndrome, 31
  Chronic granulomatous disease of child-
    hood, 256
  Cogan syndrome, 43
  Degos syndrome, 51
  Ehlers-Danlos syndrome, 63
  Homocystinuria, 285
  Hypothenar hammer syndrome, 99
  Kawasaki syndrome, 106
  Leriche syndrome, 114
  Menkes disease, 319
  Mucopolysaccharidosis I-H, 327
  Neurofibromatosis I, 140
  Pachydermoperiostosis, 155
  Popliteal artery entrapment syndrome, 163

  Protein S deficiency, 354
  Quadrilateral space syndrome, 172
  Raynaud syndrome, 173
  Subclavian steal syndrome, 203
  Thoracic outlet syndrome, 208
  Tuberous sclerosis, 212
  Wallenberg syndrome, 222
  Williams syndrome, 227
Arterial rupture
  Ehlers-Danlos syndrome, 63
  Marfan syndrome, 121
  Neurofibromatosis I, 140
Arterial tortuosity/elongation
  Cutis laxa, 49
  Ehlers-Danlos syndrome, 63
  Menkes disease, 319
  Pachydermoperiostosis, 155
Arteriosclerosis/atherosclerosis
  Alkaptonuria, 243
  Arterial calcification of infancy, 12
  Blue digit syndrome, 21
  Cholesterol ester storage disease, 256
  Homocystinuria, 285
  Leriche syndrome, 114
  Mucolipidosis II, 323
  Mucopolysaccharidoses, 325
  Prader-Willi syndrome, 166
  Progeria, 168
  Werner syndrome, 224
Arteriovenous fistula
  Ehlers-Danlos syndrome, 63
  Rendu-Osler-Weber syndrome, 176
Arthropathy; arthritis
  Acromegaly, 235
  Agammaglobulinemia, X-linked, 5
  Alkaptonuria, 243
  Amyloidosis, 245
  Arthropathy-camptodactyly syndrome, 13
  Behçet syndrome, 18
  Calcium pyrophosphate dihydrate deposi-
    tion disease, 249
  Caplan syndrome, 26
  Dermo-chondro-corneal dystrophy of
    François, 54
  Diabetes mellitus, 262
  Farber disease, 268
  Felty syndrome, 70
  Fetal alcohol syndrome, 71
  Fluorosis, 269
  Glycogen storage disease type I, 275
  Gout, 280

Hemochromatosis, 281
Hemophilia, 282
Henoch-Schönlein syndrome, 91
Hydroxyapatite deposition disease, 286
Hyperlipoproteinemias, 287
Hyperparathyroidism (secondary), 290
Hypothyroidism, 300
Infantile multisystem inflammatory disease, 100
Jadassohn-Lewandowsky syndrome, 103
Lipoid dermatoarthritis, 115
Macrodystrophia lipomatosa, 119
Membranous lipodystrophy, 319
Mixed connective tissue disease, 131
Osteoarthropathy, familial idiopathic, 152
Osteolysis without nephropathy, 153
Osteoporosis-pseudoglioma syndrome, 154
Reiter syndrome, 174
Relapsing polychondritis, 175
Scleroderma, 186
Sickle cell anemia, 365
Sjögren syndrome, 192
Stagnant small-bowel syndrome, 198
Sterno-costo-clavicular hyperostosis, 199
Stickler syndrome, 200
Thevenard syndrome, 208
Weber-Christian syndrome, 223
Wilson disease, 383
Winchester syndrome, 384
Ascites
Alpha$_1$-antitrypsin deficiency, 243
Budd-Chiari syndrome, 25
Galactosialidosis, 271
Gaucher disease, 272
GM$_1$ gangliosidosis, 278
Hepatic fibrosis–renal cystic disease, 92
Hypothyroidism, 300
Meigs syndrome, 126
Ménétrier syndrome, 127
Nephrotic syndrome, 138
Ovarian hyperstimulation syndrome, 342
POEMS syndrome, 161
Turner syndrome, 214
Tyrosinemia type I, 378
Vitamin A intoxication, 380
Wilson disease, 383
Asymmetry
Bannayan-Riley-Ruvalcaba syndrome (localized overgrowth), 15
Beckwith-Wiedemann syndrome, 17
CHILD syndrome, 36

Coffin-Lowry syndrome, 42
Goltz syndrome, 83
Hemihypertrophy (idiopathic), 90
Hemophilia (sequela to bleeding), 282
Hereditary hemihypotrophy–hemiparesis–hemiathetosis syndrome
Hypomelanosis of Ito, 98
Incontinentia pigmenti, 100
Klippel-Feil syndrome (face), 109
Klippel-Trenaunay syndrome, 109
Macrodystrophia lipomatosa, 119
Maffucci syndrome, 119
Marfan syndrome (asymmetric form), 121
McCune-Albright syndrome, 125
MURCS association (face), 136
Neurofibromatosis I, 140
Noonan syndrome (head), 145
Oculo-auriculo-vertebral spectrum (face), 147
Opitz BBBG syndrome (head), 149
Oromandibular-limb hypogenesis (face), 152
Poland sequence (thoracic wall and upper limb), 162
Prader-Willi syndrome, 166
Proteus syndrome, 169
Romberg syndrome, 181
Saethre-Chotzen syndrome (face), 183
Scurvy (sequela), 362
Seckel syndrome, 188
Silver-Russell syndrome, 190
Sturge-Weber syndrome (head and face), 201
Tuberous sclerosis (digit), 212
Atlantoaxial instability
Aarskog syndrome, 2
Behçet syndrome, 18
Calcium pyrophosphate dihydrate deposition disease, 249
CREST syndrome, 46
Down syndrome, 57
Gout, 280
Grisel syndrome, 87
Hemophilia, 282
Klippel-Feil syndrome, 109
Marfan syndrome, 121
Mucolipidosis III, 324
Mucopolysaccharidoses, 325
Neurofibromatosis I, 140
Patterson syndrome, 347
Reiter syndrome, 174

Turner syndrome, 214
Winchester syndrome, 384

B

Basilar invagination
    Crouzon syndrome, 47
    Down syndrome, 57
    Hajdu-Cheney syndrome, 87
    Hyperparathyroidism, 290
    Hypoparathyroidism, 296
    Hypophosphatasia, 297
    Klippel-Feil syndrom, 109
    Mucopolysaccharidoses, 325
    Osteomalacia, 359
    Rickets, 359
Bladder: absent or small
    Cerebro-oculo-facio-skeletal syndrome, 33
    Polycystic kidney disease (infantile), 162
    Potter sequence, 166
    Sirenomelia, 192
Bladder: diverticula
    Cutis laxa, 49
    Diamond-Blackfan syndrome, 54
    Ehlers-Danlos syndrome, 63
    Fetal alcohol syndrome, 71
    Menkes disease, 319
    Prune-belly syndrome, 170
    Williams syndrome, 227
Bladder: dysfunction
    Berdon syndrome, 19
    Caudal dysplasia sequence, 31
    Cutis laxa, 49
    Diabetes mellitus, 262
    Ehlers-Danlos syndrome, 63
    Hinman syndrome, 93
    Hypothyroidism (adult), 300
    Neurofibromatosis I, 140
    Prune-belly syndrome, 170
    Shy-Drager syndrome, 190
    Tethered cord syndrome, 207
    Urofacial syndrome, 217
Bladder: large
    Bartter syndrome, 16
    Berdon syndrome, 19
    Diabetes insipidus, 261
    Diabetes mellitus, 262
    Hinman syndrome, 93
    Kaufman-McKusick syndrome, 106
    Megacystis-megaureter syndrome, 126
    Prune-belly syndrome, 170
Bleeding tendency

Afibrinogenemia (congenital), 241
Amyloidosis, 245
Bean syndrome, 17
Cogan syndrome, 43
Copper deficiency, 258
Cushing syndrome, 258
Ehlers-Danlos syndrome, 63
Hemophilia, 282
Hemorrhagic shock–encephalopathy syn-
    drome, 91
Hemosiderosis (idiopathic pulmonary),
    284
Henoch-Schönlein syndrome, 91
Hermansky-Pudlak syndrome, 284
Scurvy, 362
von Willebrand disease, 382
Wiskott-Aldrich syndrome, 228
Blepharophimosis
    Cerebro-oculo-facio-skeletal syndrome, 33
    CHARGE association, 34
    Dubowitz syndrome, 59
    Fetal alcohol syndrome, 71
    Freeman-Sheldon syndrome, 78
    Klein-Waardenburg syndrome, 108
    Marden-Walker syndrome, 121
    Michels syndrome, 127
    Opitz BBBG syndrome, 149
    Schwartz-Jampel syndrome, 185
    Smith-Lemli-Opitz syndrome type I, 370
Blue sclerae
    Aarskog syndrome, 2
    Chromosome 18 trisomy syndrome, 37
    Ehlers-Danlos syndrome, 63
    Hallermann-Streiff syndrome, 88
    Hyperphosphatasia, 297
    Incontinentia pigmenti, 100
    Iron deficiency anemia, 305
    Marfan syndrome, 121
    Marshall-Smith syndrome, 123
    Roberts syndrome, 179
    Silver-Russell syndrome, 190
    Turner syndrome, 214
Bone age: advanced
    Adrenal hyperplasia (congenital), 238
    Aldosteronism, primary, 241
    Beckwith-Wiedemann syndrome, 17
    Cockayne syndrome, 40
    Contractural arachnodactyly, 44
    Cushing syndrome, 258
    Gigantism, 236
    Homocystinuria, 285

Hyperthyroidism, 294
Lipodystrophies, 311
Marshall-Smith syndrome, 123
McCune-Albright syndrome, 125
Neurofibromatosis I, 140
Pseudohypoparathyroidism, 355
Sotos syndrome, 195
Tuberous sclerosis, 212
Weaver syndrome, 223
Bone age: advanced, newborn
Adrenal hyperplasia (congenital), 238
Beckwith-Wiedemann syndrome, 17
Greig cephalopolysyndactyly syndrome,
    86
Hyperthyroidism (maternal), 294
Larsen syndrome, 112
Marshall-Smith syndrome, 123
Simpson-Golabi-Behmel syndrome
    (carpal bones), 191
Weaver syndrome, 223
Bone age: delayed
Addison disease, 237
Aminopterin fetopathy, 8
Aspartylglucosaminuria, 247
Brachmann–de Lange syndrome, 22
Celiac disease, 254
Cephaloskeletal dysplasia, 32
Chromosomal abnormalities (Down syn-
    drome, Turner syndrome, etc.), 57,
    214
Coffin-Lowry syndrome, 42
Coffin-Siris syndrome, 42
Copper deficiency, 258
Cushing syndrome, 258
Cystinosis, 259
Deaf mutism–goiter–euthyroidism
Deprivation dwarfism, 260
de Morsier syndrome, 53
De Sanctis-Cacchione syndrome, 54
Diabetes mellitus, 262
Dubowitz syndrome, 59
Fanconi anemia, 69
Floating-Harbor syndrome, 75
Freeman-Sheldon syndrome, 78
Fucosidosis, 270
GAPO syndrome, 80
Glycogen storage disease type I, 275
Hypoparathyroidism, 296
Hypopituitarism (anterior lobe), 298
Hypothyroidism, 300
Incontinentia pigmenti, 100

Johanson-Blizzard syndrome, 103
KBG syndrome, 107
Kocher-Debré-Sémélaigne syndrome, 307
Laron syndrome, 309
Larsen syndrome, 112
Léri syndrome, 114
Lesch-Nyhan syndrome, 310
Lysinuric protein intolerance, 314
Marinesco-Sjögren syndrome, 122
Mauriac syndrome, 317
Mucolipidosis III, 324
Mucopolysaccharidoses, 325
Nephrotic syndrome, 138
Noonan syndrome, 145
Papillon-Lefèvre syndrome, 157
Patterson syndrome, 347
Phenylketonuria, 350
Prader-Willi syndrome, 166
Prasad syndrome, 354
Renal tubular acidosis, 358
Rickets, 359
Riley-Day syndrome, 178
Ritscher-Schinzel syndrome, 179
Rubinstein-Taybi syndrome, 182
Silver-Russell syndrome, 190
Thalassemia, 374
The 3-M syndrome, 208
Trichorrhexis nodosa syndrome, 212
Weill-Marchesani syndrome, 224
Wilson disease, 383
Zellweger syndrome, 386
Bone age: disharmony (carpal delay)
Chromosome 18 trisomy syndrome, 37
Homocystinuria, 285
Mucopolysaccharidosis IVA, 331
Sotos syndrome, 195
Brachydactyly
Aarskog syndrome, 2
Acrocallosal syndrome, 3
Acrorenal syndrome, 4
Chromosome 13 trisomy syndrome, 37
Chromosome 18 trisomy syndrome, 37
DOOR syndrome, 56
Down syndrome, 57
Du Pan syndrome, 60
Fanconi anemia, 69
Fetal alcohol syndrome, 71
Fibrodysplasia ossificans progressiva, 74
Fountain syndrome, 76
Goltz syndrome, 83
Goodman syndrome, 83

Hand-foot-genital syndrome, 89
Hanhart syndrome, 152
Holt-Oram syndrome, 94
Hyperthyroidism, 294
Hypoparathyroidism, 296
Hypophosphatasia, 297
Hypothyroidism, 300
Insensitivity to pain (congenital), 101
Juberg-Hayward syndrome, 104
Kabuki make-up syndrome, 104
KBG syndrome, 107
Keutel syndrome, 108
Larsen syndrome, 112
Lesch-Nyhan syndrome, 310
Möbius syndrome, 132
Mucolipidosis II, 323
Mucolipidosis III, 324
Mucopolysaccharidoses, 325
Neu-Laxova syndrome, 139
Noonan syndrome, 145
Oculo-dento-osseous dysplasia, 147
Opitz trigonocephaly syndrome, 149
Oro-facio-digital syndromes, 150
Oto-palato-digital syndrome type I, 154
Patterson syndrome, 347
Poland sequence, 162
Progeria, 168
Pseudohypoparathyroidism, 355
Pterygium syndromes, 171
Refsum disease, 357
Rothmund-Thomson syndrome, 181
Rubinstein-Taybi syndrome, 182
Rüdiger syndrome, 183
Silver-Russell syndrome, 190
Symphalangism-surdity syndrome, 205
TAR syndrome, 206
Weill-Marchesani syndrome, 224
Brain: atrophy
    Acrodermatitis enteropathica, 234
    Adrenoleukodystrophy, 239
    Alpers syndrome, 7
    Angelman syndrome, 10
    Aplasia cutis congenita, 12
    Ataxia-telangiectasia syndrome, 14
    Biotinidase deficiency, 248
    Börjeson-Forssman-Lehmann syndrome,
        22
    Canavan disease, 250
    Cardio-facio-cutaneous syndrome, 26
    Costello syndrome, 44
    Cushing syndrome, 258

Cystinosis, 259
Deprivation dwarfism, 260
De Sanctis-Cacchione syndrome, 54
Dyke-Davidoff-Masson syndrome, 60
Encephalo-cranio-cutaneous lipomatosis,
    66
Epidermal nevus syndrome, 66
Fucosidosis, 270
Galactosemia, 270
Glutaric aciduria type I, 274
GM_1 gangliosidosis, 278
Hallervorden-Spatz disease, 281
Hereditary hemihypotrophy– hemipare-
    sis–hemiathetosis syndrome
Hyperammonemic disorders, 286
Hypomelanosis of Ito, 98
Incontinentia pigmenti, 100
Krabbe disease, 307
Leigh disease, 309
Lesch-Nyhan syndrome, 310
Lissencephalies, 116
Maple syrup urine disease, 317
Membranous lipodystrophy, 319
Menkes disease, 319
Metachromatic leukodystrophies, 321
Mevalonic aciduria, 322
Neuroacanthocytosis, 335
Neuronal ceroid lipofuscinosis, 336
Ornithine transaminase deficiency
Proteus syndrome, 169
Pyruvate dehydrogenase complex defi-
    ciency, 356
Rett syndrome, 177
Reye syndrome, 177
Romberg syndrome, 181
Stiff-man syndrome, 200
Sturge-Weber syndrome, 201
Sulfite oxidase deficiency, 372
Usher syndrome, 218
Vitamin B_{12} deficiency, 381
West syndrome, 225
Zellweger syndrome, 386
Brain: dysgenesis
    Aicardi syndrome, 6
    Aminopterin fetopathy, 8
    Apert syndrome, 11
    Aplasia cutis congenita, 4
    Bobble-head doll syndrome, 21
    Cephaloskeletal dysplasia, 32
    Cerebro-reno-digital syndromes, 34
    Chromosomal abnormalities

Craniotelencephalic dysplasia, 46
Dandy-Walker syndrome, 50
de Morsier syndrome, 53
DiGeorge syndrome, 55
Encephalo-cranio-cutaneous lipomatosis,
    66
Epidermal nevus syndrome, 66
Eronen syndrome, 68
Fetal alcohol syndrome, 71
FG syndrome, 73
Foix-Chavany-Marie syndrome, 76
Frontonasal dysplasia, 78
Fryns syndrome, 79
Galloway-Mowat syndrome, 80
Gorlin syndrome, 85
Holoprosencephaly, 94
Hydrolethalus syndrome, 95
Hypomelanosis of Ito, 98
Incontinentia pigmenti, 100
Joubert syndrome, 103
Kallmann syndrome, 105
Kearns-Sayre syndrome, 306
Lhermitte-Duclos disease, 115
Lissencephalies, 116
Meckel syndrome, 125
Miller-Dieker syndrome, 130
Mulibrey nanism, 134
Muscle–eye–brain disease
Neu-Laxova syndrome, 139
Oculo-auriculo-vertebral spectrum, 147
Oro-facio-digital syndromes, 150
Pallister-Hall syndrome, 156
Pfeiffer syndrome, 160
Pseudotrisomy 13 syndrome, 170
Saethre-Chotzen syndrome, 183
Smith-Lemli-Opitz syndrome type I, 370
Smith-Lemli-Opitz syndrome type II, 371
Stoll-Charrow-Poznanski syndrome, 201
Walker-Warburg syndrome, 221
West syndrome, 225
Zellweger syndrome, 386
Brain dysgenesis and metabolic disorders
Glutaric acidemia
Methylmalonic acidemia, 322
Peroxisomal disorders, 349
Pyruvate dehydrogenase complex defi-
    ciency, 356
Sulfite oxidase deficiency, 372
3-Methylglutaconic aciduria
Branchial arch anomaly

Auriculo-osteodysplasia
Branchio-oculo-facial syndrome, 23
Branchio-oto-renal syndrome, 23
DiGeorge syndrome, 55
Hypertelorism–microtia–facial clefting
    syndrome, 98
Lacrimo-auriculo-dento-digital syndrome,
    111
Nager acrofacial dysostosis, 136
Oculo-auriculo-vertebral spectrum, 147
Postaxial acrofacial dysostosis,
Miller type, 164
Townes-Brocks syndrome, 210
Treacher Collins syndrome, 211
Breast abnormalities
Cowden syndrome, 44
Neurofibromatosis I, 140
Polycystic ovary syndrome, 351
Ulnar-mammary syndrome, 217
Bronchiectasis
Immotile cilia syndrome, 99
Kartagener syndrome, 105
Mounier-Kuhn syndrome, 133
Williams-Campbell syndrome, 228
Yellow nail syndrome, 230
Young syndrome, 230

C
Café au lait spots
Ataxia-telangiectasia syndrome, 14
Bannayan-Riley-Ruvalcaba syndrome, 15
Bloom syndrome, 20
Dubowitz syndrome, 59
Fanconi anemia, 69
Hemihypertrophy, 90
Jaffe-Campanacci syndrom, 103
LEOPARD syndrome, 113
Maffucci syndrome, 119
McCune-Albright syndrome, 125
Multiple endocrine neoplasia type IIB,
    135
Neurofibromatosis I, 140
Silver-Russell syndrome, 190
Tuberous sclerosis, 212
Calcaneus: multiple ossification centers; stip-
    pled calcification
Down syndrome, 57
GM_1 gangliosidosis, 278
Larsen syndrome, 112
Mucolipidosis II, 323

Calcification: adrenal glands
  Addison disease, 237
  Aldosteronism, 241
  Amyloidosis, 245
  Beckwith-Wiedemann syndrome, 17
  Cholesterol ester storage disease, 256
  Cushing syndrome, 258
  Nephrotic syndrome (congenital), 138
  Wolman disease, 385
Calcification: arterial
  Alkaptonuria, 243
  Aneurysm
  Arterial calcification of infancy, 12
  Atherosclerosis
  Burger disease
  Chondrodysplasia punctata (X-linked) and
      idiopathic infantile arterial calcifi-
      cation
  Congenital syphilis
  Cushing syndrome, 258
  Degos syndrome, 51
  Diabetes mellitus, 262
  Ductus arteriosus in infancy and child-
      hood, closed
  Ductus arteriosus, open
  Eisenmenger syndrome, 64
  Familial calcification of aorta and calcific
      aortic valve disease
  Glycogen storage disease type I, 275
  Gout, 280
  Homocystinuria, 285
  Hypercalcemia, idiopathic
  Hyperlipoproteinemia, 287
  Hyperparathyroidism, 290
  Hypoparathyroidism, 296
  Hypothyroidism, 300
  Iatrogenic (surgical conduits, etc.)
  Kawasaki syndrome, 106
  Leriche syndrome, 114
  Lipodystrophy (lipodystrophic diabetes),
      311
  Milk-alkali syndrome, 323
  Mycotic aneurysm
  Nephrotic syndrome, 138
  Osteogenesis imperfecta type II
  Oxalosis, 343
  Posttraumatic complications
  Progeria, 168
  Pseudoxanthoma elasticum
  Raynaud syndrome, 173
  Sarcoidosis

Singleton-Merten syndrome, 191
Syphilitic aortitis
Takayasu arteritis
Tumoral calcinosis, 377
Vitamin D intoxication, 382
Werner syndrome, 224
Calcification: basal ganglia
  Biotinidase deficiency, 248
  Carbonic anhydrase II deficiency, 252
  Cockayne syndrome, 40
  Down syndrome 57
  Fahr disease, 267
  Hallervorden-Spatz disease, 281
  Hemolytic uremic syndrome, 90
  Hyperparathyroidism, 290
  Hypoparathyroidism, 296
  Hypothyroidism, 300
  Lead intoxication
  Leigh disease, 309
  Lipoid proteinosis, 313
  Maple syrup urine disease, 317
  Nephrotic syndrome, 138
  Neurofibromatosis I, 140
  Phenylketonuria, 350
  Pseudohypoparathyroidism, 355
  Sturge-Weber syndrome, 201
  Tuberous sclerosis, 212
Calcification: bladder wall
  Hyperparathyroidism, 290
  Oxalosis, 343
  Prune-belly syndrome, 170
  Stevens-Johnson syndrome, 199
Calcification: cerebral gyriform
  Sturge-Weber syndrome, 201
  Tuberous sclerosis, 212
Calcification: chondral and/or periarticular
  Acromegaly, 235
  Alkaptonuria, 243
  Arterial calcification of infancy, 12
  Calcium pyrophosphate dihydrate deposi-
      tion disease, 249
  CREST syndrome, 46
  Fluorosis, 269
  GM_1 gangliosidosis, 278
  Gout, 280
  Hemochromatosis, 281
  Hyperparathyroidism, 290
  Hypoparathyroidism, 296
  Hypophosphatasia, 297
  Hypothyroidism, 300
  Keutel syndrome, 108

Milk-alkali syndrome, 323
Mixed connective tissue disease, 131
Multiple endocrine neoplasia type IIA, 135
Niemann-Pick disease, 336
Oxalosis, 343
Scleroderma, 186
Tietze syndrome, 209
Tumoral calcinosis, 377
Vitamin D intoxication, 382
Warfarin embryopathy, 222
Werner syndrome, 224
Wilson disease, 383
Zellweger syndrome, 386
Calcification: disc (intervertebral)
Aarskog syndrome, 2
Acromegaly, 235
Alkaptonuria, 243
Amyloidosis, 245
Calcium pyrophosphate dihydrate deposition disease, 249
Cockayne syndrome, 40
Gout, 280
Hemochromatosis, 281
Hypercalcemia
Hyperparathyroidism, 290
Hypophosphatasia, 297
Klippel-Feil syndrome, 109
Mucolipidosis II, 323
Sickle cell anemia, 365
Thalassemia (deferoxamine-treated), 374
Vitamin D intoxication, 382
Calcification: fingertip
CREST syndrome, 46
Epidermolysis bullosa, 67
Mixed connective tissue disease, 131
Raynaud syndrome, 173
Rothmund-Thomson syndrome, 181
Scleroderma, 186
Calcification: heart
Alkaptonuria, 243
Arterial calcification of infancy, 12
Hyperparathyroidism, 290
Marfan syndrome, 121
Mucopolysaccharidoses, 325
Singleton-Merten syndrome, 191
Calcification: intracranial
Arterial calcification of infancy, 12
Bannayan-Riley-Ruvalcaba syndrome, 15
Bean syndrome, 17
Biotinidase deficiency, 248
Carbonic anhydrase II deficiency, 252

Celiac disease, 254
Cerebro-oculo-facio-skeletal syndrome, 33
Cockayne syndrome, 40
Cystinosis, 259
Down syndrome, 57
Dyskeratosis congenita, 60
Encephalo-cranio-cutaneous lipomatosis, 66
Epidermal nevus syndrome, 66
Fahr disease, 267
Gorlin syndrome, 85
Hallermann-Streiff syndrome, 88
Homocystinuria, 285
Hyperlipoproteinemia, 287
Hyperparathyroidism, 290
Hypoparathyroidism, 296
Hypopituitarism (anterior lobe), 298
Hypothyroidism (adult), 300
Kallmann syndrome, 105
Kearns-Sayre syndrome, 306
Klippel-Trenaunay-Weber syndrome, 109
Lead intoxication
Lipodystrophies, 311
Lipoid proteinosis, 313
Maffucci syndrome, 119
Marinesco-Sjögren syndrome, 122
Marshall syndrome, 123
MELAS syndrome, 318
Membranous lipodystrophy, 319
Miller-Diecker syndrome, 130
Neu-Laxova syndrome, 139
Neurocutaneous melanosis sequence, 139
Neurofibromatosis I, 140
Neurofibromatosis II, 144
Oculo-auriculo-vertebral spectrum, 147
Oculo-dento-osseous dysplasia, 147
Papillon-Lefèvre syndrome, 157
Pelizaeus-Merzbacher disease, 348
Phenylketonuria, 350
Polyglandular autoimmune disease, 352
Porphyrias, 353
Pseudohypoparathyroidism, 355
Romberg syndrome, 181
Sturge-Weber syndrome, 201
Sulfite oxidase deficiency, 372
Tuberous sclerosis, 212
Vitamin D intoxication, 382
von Hippel–Lindau syndrome, 220
Weismann-Netter syndrome, 224
West syndrome, 225
Wilson disease, 383

Calcification: intraorbital
 Amyloidosis, 245
 Diabetes mellitus, 262
 Fraser syndrome, 77
 Hyperparathyroidism (primary), 290
 Milk-alkali syndrome, 323
 Oculo-dento-osseous dysplasia, 147
 Osteoporosis–pseudoglioma syndrome,
  154
 Sturge-Weber syndrome, 201
 Vitamin D intoxication, 382
 von Hippel–Lindau syndrome, 220
Calcification: larynx (premature, cartilage)
 Adrenal hyperplasia (congenital), 238
 Chondrodysplasia punctata
 Diastrophic dysplasia
 Hyperphosphatemia
 Idiopathic congenital laryngeal calcifica-
  tion
 Idiopathic infantile hypercalcemia
 Keutel syndrome, 108
 Vitamin D intoxication, 382
 Warfarin embryopathy, 222
Calcification: liver
 Amyloidosis, 245
 Chronic granulomatous disease of child-
  hood, 256
Calcification/ossification: external ear (pinna)
 Acromegaly, 235
 Addison disease, 237
 Alkaptonuria, 243
 Arterial calcification of infancy, 12
 Calcium pyrophosphate dihydrate deposi-
  tion disease, 249
 Cushing syndrome, 258
 Diabetes mellitus, 262
 Gout, 280
 Hyperparathyroidism, 290
 Hyperthyroidism, 294
 Hypoparathyroidism, 296
 Hypopituitarism (anterior lobe), 298
 Keutel syndrome, 108
 Relapsing polychondritis, 175
Calcification/ossification: soft tissue
 Alkaptonuria, 243
 Calcinosis universalis, 249
 Calcium pyrophosphate dihydrate deposi-
  tion disease, 249
 Chronic granulomatous diseaseof child-
  hood, 256
 Copper deficiency, 258

CREST syndrome, 46
Ehlers-Danlos syndrome, 63
Epidermal nevus syndrome, 66
Epidermolysis bullosa, 67
Fibrogenesis imperfecta ossium
Fluorosis, 269
Focal scleroderma, 75
Gorlin syndrome, 85
Gout, 280
Homocystinuria (vascular calcification),
 285
Hydroxyapatite deposition disease, 286
Hyperlipoproteinemia, 287
Hyperparathyroidism, 290
Hypoparathyroidism, 296
Hypophosphatasia, 297
Klippel-Trenaunay-Weber syndrome, 109
Madelung disease, 315
Maffucci syndrome, 119
Mandibuloacral dysplasia, 120
Milk-alkali syndrome, 323
Mixed connective tissue disease, 131
Multiple endocrine neoplasia type IIA, 135
Osteoma cutis, familial, 154
Oxalosis, 343
Pachydermoperiostosis, 155
Porphyrias, 353
Progeria (vascular calcification), 168
Pseudohypoparathyroidism, 355
Rothmund-Thomson syndrome, 181
Scleroderma, 186
Singleton-Merten syndrome, 191
Tietze syndrome, 209
Tumoral calcinosis, 377
Vitamin A intoxication, 380
Vitamin D intoxication, 382
Weber-Christian syndrome, 223
Werner syndrome, 224
Williams syndrome, 227
Wilson disease, 383
Zellweger syndrome, 386
Calcification: punctate osteoarticular (infants)
 Brachmann–de Lange syndrome, 22
 CHILD syndrome, 36
 Chromosome 18 trisomy syndrome, 37
 Cutis laxa (hips), 49
 Down syndrome, 57
 Fetal alcohol syndrome, 71
 Fetal hydantoin syndrome, 72
 GM_1 gangliosidosis (primarily tarsals),
  278

Hypopituitarism (anterior lobe), 298
Hypothyroidism (juvenile), 300
Keutel syndrome, 108
Metachromatic leukodystrophies, 321
Mucolipidosis II, 323
Mucopolysaccharidosis I-H, 327
Smith-Lemli-Opitz syndrome type I, 370
Warfarin embryopathy, 222
Zellweger syndrome, 386
Calcification: spleen
    Chronic granulomatous disease of child-
        hood, 256
    Sickle cell anemia, 365
Calculus: urinary tract
    Abetalipoproteinemia, 234
    Alkaptonuria, 243
    Calcinosis universalis, 249
    Cushing syndrome, 258
    Cystic renal disease
    Cystinosis, 259
    Cystinuria, 260
    Glycogen storage disease type I, 275
    Gout, 280
    Hemophilia, 282
    Hyperparathyroidism (primary), 290
    Hyperthyroidism, 294
    Lesch-Nyhan syndrome, 310
    Malabsorption syndrome, 119
    Milk-alkali syndrome, 323
    Osteomalacia, 360
    Oxalosis, oxaluria, 343
    Renal tubular acidosis (type I, carbonic
        anhydrase), 358
    Rickets (vitamin D, hypophosphatemic),
        359
    Short-bowel syndrome, 189
    Vitamin D intoxication, 382
    Williams syndrome, 227
    Wilson disease, 383
    Xanthine oxidase deficiency, 385
Camptodactyly
    Aarskog syndrome, 2
    Acro-fronto-facio-nasal dysostosis syn-
        drome
    Antley-Bixler syndrome, 11
    Arthropathy-camptodactyly syndrome, 13
    Cerebro-oculo-facio-skeletal syndrome, 33
    Christian syndrome, 36
    Chromosomal abnormalities (8, 13, 18,
        21)
    Contractural arachnodactyly, 44

Cranio-fronto-nasal dysplasia, 45
Fetal akinesia sequence, 71
Fetal alcohol syndrome, 71
Freeman-Sheldon syndrome, 78
Fryns syndrome, 79
Golden-Lakim syndrome, 82
Goltz syndrome, 83
Greig cephalopolysyndactyly syndrome,
    86
Holt-Oram syndrome, 94
Klein-Waardenburg syndrome, 108
Kuskokwim syndrome, 111
Lenz microphthalmia syndrome, 113
Marden-Walker syndrome, 121
Marfan syndrome, 121
Meckel syndrome, 125
Nail-patella syndrome, 137
Neu-Laxova syndrome, 139
Oculo-dento-osseous dysplasia, 147
Ophthalmo-mandibulo-melic dysplasia, 148
Oro-facio-digital syndrome I, 150
Poland sequence, 162
Pterygium syndrome, 171
Roberts syndrome, 179
Spondylocostal dysostosis (Jarcho-Levin
    syndrome), 197
Tel Hashomer camptodactyly syndrome,
    207
Trismus-pseudocamptodactyly syndrome,
    212
Weaver-Smith syndrome, 223
Williams syndrome, 227
Zellweger syndrome, 386
Cardiac valve thickening
    Alkaptonuria, 243
    Aspartylglucosaminuria, 247
    Geleophysic dysplasia
    Mannosidoses, 316
    Mucolipidoses (II, III), 323, 324
    Mucopolysaccharidoses, 325
    Osteodysplasty, precocious
Cardiomegaly
    Adrenal hyperplasia (congenital), 238
    Alpha$_1$-antitrypsin deficiency, 243
    Amyloidosis, 245
    Arterial calcification of infancy, 12
    Beckwith-Wiedemann syndrome, 17
    Carcinoid syndrome, 252
    Cardiomyopathies
    Cardiovocal syndrome, 27
    Carnitine deficiency syndromes, 253

Duchenne muscular dystrophy
Erdheim-Chester disease, 265
Fabry disease, 266
Friedreich ataxia
Gaucher disease, 272
Glycogen storage disease type II, 276
Hemochromatosis, 281
Hemolytic uremic syndrome, 90
Hypereosinophilic syndrome, 96
Hyperthyroidism, 294
Hypoparathyroidism, 296
Hypoplastic left heart syndrome
Hypoplastic right heart complex
Hypothyroidism, 300
Infants of the diabetic mother
Iron deficiency anemia, 305
Kasabach-Merritt syndrome, 106
Kawasaki syndrome, 106
Kugelberg-Welander syndrome, 110
Lutembacher syndrome, 118
Mitral valve prolapse syndrome
Mucolipidosis II, 323
Mucopolysaccharidosis I-H, 327
Mucopolysaccharidosis I-H/S, 328
Mucopolysaccharidosis I-S, 329
Myotubular myopathy
Pickwickian syndrome, 161
Polycythemia vera
Postcardiotomy syndrome, 164
Postmyocardial infarction syndrome, 166
Pseudoxanthoma elasticum
Pyruvate kinase deficiency anemia, 357
Relapsing polychondritis, 175
Rendu-Osler-Weber syndrome, 176
Sarcoidosis
Scleroderma, 186
Sialidosis, 364
Sickle cell anemia, 365
Singleton-Merten syndrome, 191
Takayasu arteritis
Thalassemia, 374
Twin-to-twin transfusion syndrome, 216
Vitamin B_1 deficiency, 381
Werner syndrome, 224
Cardiomyopathy
    Adrenal hyperplasia (congenital), 238
    Amyloidosis, 245
    Aspartylglucosaminuria, 247
    Carnitine deficiency syndrome, 253
    Degos syndrome, 51
    Duchenne muscular dystrophy

Emery-Dreifuss muscular dystrophy
Fabry disease, 266
Farber disease, 268
Fetal rubella syndrome
Friedreich ataxia
Fucosidosis type I, 270
Gaucher disease, 272
Geleophysic dysplasia
Glycogen storage disease type II, 276
Glycogen storage disease type III, 276
GM_1 gangliosidosis, 278
Hemochromatosis, 281
Hemolytic uremic syndrome, 90
Hyperphosphatasia, 293
Hyperthyroidism, 294
Hypothyroidism, 300
Kearns-Sayre syndrome, 306
Kugelberg-Welander syndrome, 110
Leigh disease, 309
LEOPARD syndrome, 113
Mannosidosis type I, 316
Mitochondrial diseases
Mucolipidosis II, 323
Mucolipidosis III, 324
Mucopolysaccharidoses, 325
Myotubular myopathy
Nemaline myopathy
Neuroacanthocytosis, 335
Niemann-Pick disease, 336
Noonan syndrome, 145
Pseudoxanthoma elasticum
Refsum disease, 357
Sarcoidosis
Scleroderma, 186
3-Hydroxy-3-methylglutaryl- coenzyme A
    lyase deficiency, 376
Toriello-Carey syndrome 210
Uremia
Vitamin B_1 deficiency, 381
Werdnig-Hoffmann disease
Carotid arteries, common origin
    Apert syndrome, 11
    Chromosomal abnormalities (trisomy 13,
        18, and 21 syndromes)
    DiGeorge syndrome, 55
Carpal fusion
    Acrocallosal syndrome, 3
    Acromegaly, 235
    Antley-Bixler syndrome, 11
    Apert syndrome, 11
    Baller-Gerold syndrome, 14

Carpenter syndrome, 29
EEC syndrome, 62
F syndrome, 68
Fetal alcohol syndrome, 71
Hand-foot-genital syndrome, 89
Holt-Oram syndrome, 94
Keratosis palmaris et plantaris familiaris
    (tylosis), 107
Klein-Waardenburg syndrome, 108
Kniest dysplasia
LEOPARD syndrome, 113
Multiple synostosis syndrome, 136
Occipital horn syndrome, 341
Oto-palato-digital syndrome type I, 154
Rothmund-Thomson syndrome, 181
Scleroderma, 186
Split-hand/split-foot deformities, 196
Spondylo-carpo-tarsal synostosis syn-
    drome, 197
Stickler syndrome, 200
Symphalangism-surdity syndrome, 205
Thalidomide embryopathy, 207
Townes-Brocks syndrome, 210
Turner syndrome, 214
Cataract
Alport syndrome, 8
Angelman syndrome, 10
Aniridia-Wilms tumor association, 10
Bardet-Biedl syndrome, 16
Branchio-oculo-facial syndrome, 23
Cerebro-oculo-facio-skeletal syndrome, 33
Cerebrotendinous xanthomatosis, 255
Clouston syndrome, 39
Cockayne syndrome, 40
Cutis verticis gyrata, 50
Diabetes mellitus, 262
Diaphyseal dysplasia, Engelmann type
Fronto-facio-nasal dysplasia, 78
Frontonasal dysplasia, 78
Galactokinase deficiency
Galactosemia, 270
Goltz syndrome, 83
Gorlin syndrome, 85
Hallermann–Streiff syndrome, 88
Homocystinuria, 285
Hypoparathyroidism, 296
Incontinentia pigmenti, 100
Jadassohn-Lewandowsky syndrome, 103
Klippel-Trenaunay-Weber syndrome, 109
Lactose intolerance, 308
Lowe syndrome, 314

Mannosidoses, 316
Marinesco-Sjögren syndrome, 122
Marshall syndrome, 123
Menkes disease, 319
Metachromatic leukodystrophies, 321
Mevalonic aciduria, 322
Microcephalic osteodysplastic primordial
    dwarfism, 127
Morning glory syndrome, 133
Multiple sulfatase deficiency, 334
Nail-patella syndrome, 137
Neu-Laxova syndrome, 139
Oculo-auriculo-vertebral spectrum, 147
Oculo-dento-osseous dysplasia, 147
Progeria, 168
Proteus syndrome, 169
Pseudohypoparathyroidism, 355
Rickets (vitamin D deficiency), 359
Roberts syndrome, 179
Rothmund-Thomson syndrome, 181
Rubinstein-Taybi syndrome, 182
Schwartz-Jampel syndrome, 185
Sialidosis, 364
Smith-Lemli-Opitz syndromes, 370, 371
Stickler syndrome, 200
Velo-cardio-facial syndrome, 219
Walker-Warburg syndrome, 221
Warfarin embryopathy, 222
Werner syndrome, 224
Wilson disease, 383
Zellweger syndrome, 386
Cerebellar dysgenesis/atrophy
Chédiak-Higashi syndrome, 35
Dandy-Walker syndrome, 50
Gerstmann-Sträussler-Scheinker syndrome
Joubert syndrome, 103
Lhermitte-Duclos disease, 115
Meckel syndrome, 125
Ritscher-Schinzel syndrome, 179
Romberg syndrome, 181
Stoll-Charrow-Poznanski syndrome, 201
Cherry-red spots
Farber disease, 268
Galactosialidosis, 271
GM$_1$ gangliosidosis, 278
GM$_2$ gangliosidosis: Sandhoff disease, 279
GM$_2$ gangliosidosis: Tay-Sachs disease, 279
Metachromatic leukodystrophies, 321
Multiple sulfatase deficiency, 334
Niemann-Pick disease, 336
Sialidosis, 364

Cherubic facies
  Neurofibromatosis I, 140
  Noonan syndrome, 145
  Ramon syndrome, 172
Choanal atresia/stenosis
  Amniotic band sequence, 9
  Antley-Bixler syndrome, 11
  Apert syndrome, 11
  Brachmann–de Lange syndrome, 22
  CHARGE association, 34
  Crouzon syndrome, 47
  DiGeorge syndrome, 55
  Marshall-Smith syndrome, 123
  Pfeiffer syndrome, 160
  Saethre-Chotzen syndrome, 183
  Schinzel-Giedion syndrome, 184
  Thalidomide embryopathy, 207
  Treacher Collins syndrome, 211
Chondrocalcinosis; *refer to* (1)
      Calcification: chondral and/or periar-
      ticular; (2) Calcification: punctate
      osteoarticular
Claudication
  Cauda equina syndrome, 30
  Leriche syndrome, 114
  Popliteal artery entrapment syndrome, 163
  Subclavian steal syndrome, 203
  Thoracic outlet syndrome, 208
Clavicle: aplasia/dysplasia
  CHILD syndrome, 36
  Fucosidosis, 270
  Goltz syndrome, 83
  Holt-Oram syndrome, 94
  Mandibuloacral dysplasia, 120
  Progeria, 168
  Restrictive dermatopathy, 176
Clavicle: broad or thickened
  Fucosidosis, 270
  GM_1 gangliosidosis, 278
  Holt-Oram syndrome, 94
  Mannosidoses, 316
  Menkes disease, 319
  Mucolipidoses, 323, 324, 325
  Mucopolysaccharidoses, 325
  Oculo-dento-osseous dysplasia, 147
  Sterno-costo-clavicular hyperostosis, 199
  Winchester syndrome, 384
Clavicle: defective ossification or destruction
      of the distal end
  Amyloidosis, 245
  Gout, 280

Hyperparathyroidism, 290
Lipoid dermatoarthritis, 115
Progeria, 168
Reiter syndrome, 174
Rickets, 359
Scleroderma, 186
Clavicle: lateral hook
  Brachmann–de Lange syndrome, 22
  Down syndrome, 57
  Holt-Oram syndrome, 94
  Meckel syndrome, 125
  Robin sequence, 180
  TAR syndrome, 206
Clavicle: slender
  Chromosome 13 trisomy syndrome, 37
  Chromosome 18 trisomy syndrome, 37
  Cockayne syndrome, 40
  Larsen syndrome, 112
  Progeria, 168
  Turner syndrome, 214
Cleft lip/palate
  Aarskog syndrome, 2
  Aase syndrome, 2
  Acrocallosal syndrome, 3
  Adams-Oliver syndrome, 4
  Aicardi syndrome, 6
  Aminopterin fetopathy, 8
  Amniotic band sequence, 9
  Apert syndrome, 11
  Bardet-Biedl syndrome, 16
  Brachmann–de Lange syndrome, 22
  Branchio-oculo-facial syndrome, 23
  Catel-Manzke syndrome, 30
  Caudal dysplasia sequence, 31
  CHARGE association, 34
  CHILD syndrome, 36
  Christian syndrome, 36
  Crouzon syndrome, 47
  Dubowitz syndrome, 59
  EEC syndrome, 62
  Femoral hypoplasia–unusual facies syn-
      drome, 70
  Fetal alcohol syndrome, 71
  Fetal hydantoin syndrome, 72
  Fetal valproate syndrome, 73
  Fronto-facio-nasal dysplasia, 78
  Frontonasal dysplasia, 78
  Gardner-Silengo-Wachtel syndrome, 81
  Goldberg-Shprintzen syndrome, 82
  Goltz syndrome, 83
  Gordon syndrome, 84

Gorlin syndrome, 85
Holoprosencephaly, 94
Hydrolethalus syndrome, 95
Hypertelorism–microtia–facial clefting
    syndrome, 98
Hypoglossia-hypodactylia syndrome, 98
Juberg-Hayward syndrome, 104
Larsen syndrome, 112
Marden-Walker syndrome, 121
Marfan syndrome, 121
Meckel syndrome, 125
Michels syndrome, 127
MURCS association, 136
Neu-Laxova syndrome, 139
Oculo-auriculo-vertebral spectrum, 147
Odonto-tricho-melic syndrome, 148
Opitz BBBG syndrome, 149
Oro-facio-digital syndrome I, 150
Oro-facio-digital syndrome II, 150
Oromandibular-limb hypogenesis, 152
Oto-palato-digital syndrome type I, 154
Pallister-Hall syndrome, 156
Postaxial acrofacial dysostosis,
    Miller type, 164
Pterygium syndromes, 171
Roberts syndrome, 179
Robin sequence, 180
Seckel syndrome, 188
Simpson-Golabi-Behmel syndrome, 191
Smith-Lemli-Opitz syndrome type I, 370
Smith-Lemli-Opitz syndrome type II, 371
Stickler syndrome, 200
Toriello-Carey syndrome, 210
Treacher Collins syndrome, 211
Clinodactyly
Aarskog syndrome, 2
Aminopterin fetopathy, 8
Bardet-Biedl syndrome, 16
Bloom syndrome, 20
Brachmann–de Lange syndrome, 22
Carpenter syndrome, 29
Cephaloskeletal dysplasia, 32
Cerebro-costo-mandibular syndrome, 33
Chromosomal abnormalities (13, 18, 21,
    etc.)
Cohen syndrome, 43
Cranio-fronto-nasal dysplasia, 45
DOOR syndrome, 56
Dubowitz syndrome, 59
EEC syndrome, 62
Ehlers-Danlos syndrome, 63

Fanconi anemia, 69
Fetal alcohol syndrome, 71
Fibrodysplasia ossificans progressiva, 74
Goltz syndrome, 83
Goodman syndrome, 83
Hand-foot-genital syndrome, 89
Holt-Oram syndrome, 94
Hypomelanosis of Ito, 98
Kabuki make-up syndrome, 104
Lenz microphthalmia syndrome, 113
Marfan syndrome, 121
Meckel syndrome, 125
Miller-Dieker syndrome, 130
Nail-patella syndrome, 137
Noonan syndrome, 145
Oculo-dento-osseous dysplasia, 147
Oro-facio-digital syndrome I, 150
Oro-facio-digital syndrome II, 150
Oto-palato-digital syndrome type I, 154
Poland sequence, 162
Prader-Willi syndrome, 166
Pterygium syndrome, 171
Roberts syndrome, 179
Rubinstein-Taybi syndrome, 182
Saethre-Chotzen syndrome, 183
Seckel syndrome, 188
Silver-Russell syndrome, 190
TAR syndrome, 206
Treacher Collins syndrome, 211
Weill-Marchesani syndrome, 224
Williams syndrome, 227
Zellweger syndrome, 386
Clitoromegaly
Adrenal hyperplasia (congenital), 238
Chromosome 18 trisomy syndrome, 37
Fraser syndrome, 77
Johanson-Blizzard syndrome, 103
Lipodystrophies, 311
Neurofibromatosis I, 140
Roberts syndrome, 179
Clubbing: digits
Acromegaly, 235
Cronkhite-Canada syndrome, 47
Hajdu-Cheney syndrome, 87
Hyperthyroidism; thyroid acropachy, 294
Hypothyroidism (myxedema), 300
Immotile cilia syndrome, 99
Larsen syndrome, 112
Osteoarthropathy, familial idiopathic, 152
Pachydermoperiostosis, 155
POEMS syndrome, 161

Rendu-Osler-Weber syndrome, 176
Seckel syndrome, 188
Clubfoot, metatarsus adductus
Aarskog syndrome, 2
Aminopterin fetopathy, 8
Amniotic band sequence, 9
Antley-Bixler syndrome, 11
Bloom syndrome, 20
Brachmann–de Lange syndrome, 22
Caudal dysplasia sequence, 31
Cephaloskeletal dysplasia, 32
Christian syndrome, 36
Chromosomal abnormalities
Dubowitz syndrome, 59
Ehlers-Danlos syndrome, 63
Femoral hypoplasia–unusual facies syndrome, 70
Fetal akinesia sequence, 71
Fetal valproate syndrome, 73
Freeman-Sheldon syndrome, 78
Gardner-Silengo-Wachtelsyndrome, 81
Homocystinuria, 285
Kuskokwim syndrome, 111
Larsen syndrome, 112
Marinesco-Sjögren syndrome, 122
Meckel syndrome, 125
Microcephalic osteodysplastic primordial dwarfism, 127
Mietens-Weber syndrome, 130
Möbius syndrome, 132
Mucopolysaccharidoses, 325
Nager acrofacial dsyostosis, 136
Nail-patella syndrome, 137
Noonan syndrome, 145
Potter sequence, 166
Pseudodiastrophic dysplasia
Pterygium syndromes, 171
Roberts syndrome, 179
Schinzel-Giedion syndrome, 184
Schwartz-Jampel syndrome, 185
Seckel syndrome, 188
Smith-Lemli-Opitz syndrome type I, 370
Trismus-pseudocamptodactyly syndrome, 212
Waardenburg anophthalmia syndrome, 220
Zellweger syndrome, 386
Coarctation of aorta
Cutis laxa, 49
Marfan syndrome, 121
Marfanoid hypermobility syndrome, 122

Neurofibromatosis I, 140
Sturge-Weber syndrome, 201
Tuberous sclerosis, 212
Turner syndrome, 214
Colitis
Behçet syndrome, 18
Chronic granulomatous disease of childhood, 256
Hemolytic uremic syndrome, 90
Hermansky-Pudlak syndrome, 284
Kawasaki syndrome, 106
Coloboma
Aniridia-Wilms tumor association, 10
Brachmann–de Lange syndrome, 22
Branchio-oculo-facial syndrome, 23
Cat-eye syndrome, 30
CHARGE association, 34
Cohen syndrome, 43
Contractural arachnodactyly, 44
Crouzon syndrome, 47
Delleman syndrome, 52
Epidermal nevus syndrome, 66
Fetal hydantoin syndrome, 72
Fronto-facio-nasal dysplasia, 78
Frontonasal dysplasia, 78
Goltz syndrome, 83
Gorlin syndrome, 85
Holoprosencephaly, 94
Joubert syndrome, 103
Marfan syndrome, 121
Meckel syndrome, 125
Morning glory syndrome, 133
Nager acrofacial dysostosis, 136
Nasopalpebral lipoma-coloboma syndrome, 137
Oculo-auriculo-vertebral spectrum, 147
Pallister-Hall syndrome, 156
Rubinstein-Taybi syndrome, 182
Sturge-Weber syndrome, 201
Treacher Collins syndrome, 211
Conjunctivitis
Acrodermatitis enteropathica, 234
Biotinidase deficiency, 248
Chronic granulomatous disease of childhood, 256
Cogan syndrome, 43
Kawasaki syndrome, 106
Reiter syndrome, 174
Relapsing polychondritis, 175
Sjögren syndrome, 192
Stevens-Johnson syndrome, 199

Corneal opacity, dystrophy, dysplasia
  Acrodermatitis enteropathica, 234
  Carpenter syndrome, 29
  Chédiak-Higashi syndrome, 35
  Cockayne syndrome, 40
  Cross syndrome, 47
  Cutis laxa, 49
  Dermo-chondro-corneal dystrophy of
      François, 54
  Fabry disease, 266
  Fanconi syndrome, 268
  Fryns syndrome, 79
  Galactosialidosis, 271
  Insensitivity to pain (congenital), 101
  Jadassohn-Lewandowsky syndrome, 103
  Kearns-Sayre syndrome, 306
  Lipodystrophies, 311
  Lowe syndrome, 314
  Mannosidoses, 316
  Mietens-Weber syndrome, 130
  Mucolipidosis III, 324
  Mucolipidosis IV, 325
  Mucopolysaccharidosis I-H, 327
  Mucopolysaccharidosis I-H/S, 328
  Mucopolysaccharidosis I-S, 329
  Mucopolysaccharidosis III, 330
  Mucopolysaccharidosis VII, 334
  Multiple sulfatase deficiency, 334
  Nasopalpebral lipoma-coloboma syn-
      drome, 137
  Neurofibromatosis II, 144
  Ophthalmo-mandibulo-melic dysplasia, 148
  Roberts syndrome, 179
  Warfarin embryopathy, 222
  Wilson disease, 383
  Winchester syndrome, 384
Coronary artery abnormalities
  Arterial calcification of infancy, 12
  Hyperlipoproteinemias, 287
  Hyperthyroidism, 294
  Kawasaki syndrome, 106
  Marfan syndrome, 121
  Werner syndrome, 224
Corpus callosum: agenesis/hypoplasia
  Acrocallosal syndrome, 3
  Aicardi syndrome, 6
  Andermann syndrome, 9
  Apert syndrome, 11
  Chromosome 18 trisomy syndrome, 37
  Cogan syndrome, 43
  Dandy-Walker syndrome, 50

Delleman syndrome, 52
de Morsier syndrome, 53
Fetal alcohol syndrome, 71
FG syndrome, 73
Frontonasal dysplasia, 78
Gorlin syndrome, 85
Joubert syndrome, 103
Lennox-Gastaut syndrome, 113
Mucolipidosis IV, 325
Neu-Laxova syndrome, 139
Oro-facio-digital syndrome I, 150
Oro-facio-digital syndrome II, 150
Rubinstein-Taybi syndrome, 182
Shapiro syndrome, 188
Toriello-Carey syndrome, 210
Coxa valga
  Carpenter syndrome, 29
  Caudal regression syndrome, 31
  Coffin-Lowry syndrome, 42
  Fucosidosis, 270
  Mannosidoses, 316
  Mucopolysaccharidoses, 325
  Occipital horn syndrome, 341
  Ophthalmo-mandibulo-melic dysplasia,
      148
  Oto-palato-digital syndrome type I, 154
  Prader-Willi syndrome, 166
  Progeria, 168
  Pseudohypoparathyroidism, 355
  Schwartz-Jampel syndrome, 185
  Stickler syndrome, 200
  Turner syndrome, 214
Coxa vara
  Arthropathy-camptodactyly syndrome, 13
  Femoral hypoplasia–unusual facies syn-
      drome, 70
  Hyperparathyroidism, 290
  Hyperphosphatasia, 293
  Hypophosphatasia, 297
  Hypothyroidism, 300
  Osteomalacia, 360
  Pseudohypoparathyroidism, 355
  Rickets, 359
  Schwartz-Jampel syndrome, 185
Cranial nerve: paresis/ paralysis; *refer to*
      Paralysis/paresis: cranial nerve
Craniosynostosis
  Aminopterin fetopathy, 8
  Antley-Bixler syndrome, 11
  Apert syndrome, 11
  Baller-Gerold syndrome, 14

Bardet-Biedl syndrome, 16
Carpenter syndrome, 29
Chromosomal syndromes
Cloverleaf skull deformity, 39
Cranio-fronto-nasal dysplasia, 45
Craniotelencephalic dysplasia, 46
Crouzon syndrome, 47
Fetal hydantoin syndrome, 72
FG syndrome, 73
Fucosidosis, 270
Hyperimmunoglobulinemia E syndrome, 96
Hyperthyroidism, 294
Hypophosphatasia, 297
Hypothyroidism (juvenile), 300
Jackson-Weiss syndrome, 102
Lowe syndrome, 314
Meckel syndrome, 125
Michels syndrome, 127
Mucolipidosis III, 324
Mucopolysaccharidosis I-H, 327
Mucopolysaccharidosis VI, 333
Opitz trigonocephaly syndrome, 149
Pfeiffer syndrome, 160
Rickets, 359
Saethre-Chotzen syndrome, 183
Seckel syndrome, 188
Shprintzen-Goldberg syndrome, 189
Sickle cell anemia, 365
Thalassemia, 374
Vitamin D intoxication, 382
Williams syndrome, 227
Cranium bifidum
Aminopterin fetopathy, 8
Aminopterin fetopathy-like syndrome, 9
Fronto-facio-nasal dysplasia, 78
Frontonasal dysplasia, 78
Cryptorchidism
Aarskog syndrome, 2
Adrenal insufficiency
Aniridia-Wilms tumor association, 10
Bardet-Biedl syndrome, 16
Beckwith-Wiedemann syndrome, 17
Brachmann–de Lange syndrome, 22
Carpenter syndrome, 29
Cerebro-oculo-facio-skeletal syndrome, 33
Cockayne syndrome, 40
Dubowitz syndrome, 59
Fanconi anemia, 69
Fetal akinesia sequence, 71
Fraser syndrome, 77
Gordon syndrome, 84

Gorlin syndrome, 85
Hallermann-Streiff syndrome, 88
Hypopituitarism (anterior lobe), 298
Kallmann syndrome, 105
Lenz microphthalmia syndrome, 113
LEOPARD syndrome, 113
Lowe syndrome, 314
Marfan syndrome, 121
Meckel syndrome, 125
Miller-Dieker syndrome, 130
Noonan syndrome, 145
Opitz BBBG syndrome, 149
Persistent müllerian duct syndrome, 159
Prader-Willi syndrom, 166
Prune-belly syndrome, 170
Pterygium syndromes, 171
Roberts syndrome, 179
Rothmund-Thomson syndrome, 181
Rubinstein-Taybi syndrome, 182
Saethre-Chotzen syndrome, 183
Seckel syndrome, 188
Smith-Lemli-Opitz syndrome type I, 370
Smith-Lemli-Opitz syndrome type II, 371
Splenogonadal fusion/limb deformity, 196
Testicular feminization, 373
Toriello-Carey syndrome, 210
Treacher Collins syndrome, 211
Urofacial syndrome, 217
Velo-cardio-facial syndrome, 219
Zellweger syndrome, 386
Cubitus valgus
Léri syndrome, 114
Turner syndrome, 214
Zellweger syndrome, 386
Cutis laxa
Cutis laxa, 49
Ehlers-Danlos syndrome, 63
Geroderma osteodysplastica, 81
Marfanoid hypermobility syndrome, 122
Occipital horn syndrome, 341
Opitz trigonocephaly syndrome, 149
Patterson syndrome, 347
Potter sequence, 166
Turner syndrome, 214
Weaver syndrome, 223

D
Diabetes mellitus
Cystinosis, 259
Femoral hypoplasia–unusual facies syndrome, 70

Glucagonoma syndrome, 274
Hemochromatosis, 281
Klinefelter syndrome, 108
Lipodystrophy (lipoid diabetes), 311
Mauriac syndrome, 317
McCune-Albright syndrome, 125
Patterson syndrome, 347
Polyglandular autoimmune disease, 352
Prader-Willi syndrome, 166
Renal–hepatic–pancreatic dysplasia, 176
SHORT syndrome, 265
Somatostatinoma syndrome, 371
Sotos syndrome, 195
Thalassemia, 374
Troell-Junet syndrome, 212
Turner syndrome, 214
Werner syndrome, 224
Diaphragmatic hernia
Brachmann–de Lange syndrome, 22
Cantrell syndrome, 25
Chromosome 13 trisomy syndrome, 37
Chromosome 18 trisomy syndrome, 37
DiGeorge syndrome, 55
Ehlers-Danlos syndrome, 63
Fetal hydantoin syndrome, 72
Fryns syndrome, 79
Marfan syndrome, 121
Digital defects: adactyly, oligodactyly, mon-
    odactyly
Acrorenal syndrome, 4
Amniotic band sequence, 9
Aplasia cutis congenita, 4
Baller-Gerold syndrome, 14
Brachmann–de Lange syndrome, 22
Charlie M syndrome, 152
CHILD syndrome, 36
Chorionic villus sampling–transverse limb
    deficiency
Chromosome 18 trisomy syndrome, 37
DOOR syndrome, 56
Down syndrome, 57
EEC syndrome, 62
Eronen syndrome, 68
Fetal hydantoin syndrome, 72
Fuhrmann syndrome, 79
Goltz syndrome, 83
Hand-foot-genital syndrome, 89
Hanhart syndrome, 152
Holt-Oram syndrome, 94
Hypoglossia-hypodactylia syndrome, 98

Keratosis palmaris et plantaris familiaris
    (tylosis), 107
Möbius syndrome, 132
Oculo-dento-osseous dysplasia, 147
Opitz trigonocephaly syndrome, 149
Oro-facio-digital syndrome I, 150
Oromandibular-limb hypogenesis, 152
Poland sequence, 162
Postaxial acrofacial dysostosis, Miller
    type, 164
Pterygium syndromes, 171
Roberts syndrome, 179
Splenogonadal fusion/limb deformity, 196
Thalidomide embryopathy, 207
Turner syndrome, 214
Ulnar-mammary syndrome, 217
Weyers oligodactyly syndrome, 226
Yunis-Varón syndrome
Zimmermann-Laband syndrome, 231
Disc calcification; *refer to* Calcification: disc
    (intervertebral)
Diverticulum: alimentary system
Cutis laxa, 49
Ehlers-Danlos syndrome, 63
Jadassohn-Lewandowsky syndrome, 103
Multiple endocrine neoplasia type IIA,
    135
Multiple endocrine neoplasia type IIB,
    135
Noonan syndrome, 145
Scleroderma, 186
Williams syndrome, 227
Dysostosis multiplex
Fucosidosis, 270
Galactosialidosi, 271
Mannosidoses, 316
Mucolipidosis II, 323
Mucolipidosis III, 324
Mucopolysaccharidosis I-H, 327
Mucopolysaccharidosis I-H/S, 328
Mucopolysaccharidosis II, 329
Mucopolysaccharidosis VII, 334
Sialidosis, 364

E
Ear, external: malformation
Aarskog syndrome, 2
Aminopterin fetopathy, 8
Aminopterin fetopathy-like syndrome, 9
Amniotic band sequence, 9

Aniridia-Wilms tumor association, 10
Antley-Bixler syndrome, 11
Baller-Gerold syndrome, 14
Beckwith-Wiedemann syndrome, 17
Bloom syndrome, 20
Börjeson-Forssman-Lehmann syndrome, 22
Branchio-oculo-facial syndrome, 23
Branchio-oto-renal syndrome, 23
Cat-eye syndrome, 30
Cerebro-costo-mandibular syndrome, 33
CHARGE association, 34
Chromosomal abnormalities (13, 18, 21, XO, etc.)
Coffin-Lowry syndrome, 42
Cohen syndrome, 43
Contractural arachnodactyly, 44
DiGeorge syndrome, 55
Dubowitz syndrome, 59
EEC syndrome, 62
Ehlers-Danlos syndrome, 63
Facio-auriculo-radial dysplasia, 69
Fanconi anemia, 69
Fetal akinesia sequence, 71
Fetal alcohol syndrome, 71
Fetal hydantoin syndrome, 72
FG syndrome, 73
Fibrochondrogenesis
Fraser syndrome, 77
Fryns syndrome, 79
GM_1 gangliosidosis, 278
Greig cephalopolysyndactyly syndrome, 86
Hydrolethalus syndrome, 95
Hyperphosphatasia, 293
Hypertelorism–microtia–facial clefting syndrome, 98
Klippel-Feil syndrome, 109
Lacrimo-auriculo-dento-digital syndrome, 111
Lenz microphthalmia syndrome, 113
LEOPARD syndrome, 113
Lissencephalies, 116
Marfan syndrome, 121
Meckel syndrome, 125
Möbius syndrome, 132
MURCS association, 136
Nager acrofacial dysostosis, 136
Neu-Laxova syndrome, 139
Noonan syndrome, 145
Oculo-auriculo-vertebral spectrum, 147

Opitz BBBG syndrome, 149
Oro-facio-digital syndrome II, 150
Oto-palato-digital syndrome type I, 154
Pallister-Hall syndrome, 156
Pallister-Killian syndrome, 156
Postaxial acrofacial dysostosis, Miller type, 164
Potter sequence, 166
Prader-Willi syndrome, 166
Relapsing polychondritis, 175
Renal-genital-ear anomalies, 175
Roberts syndrome, 179
Rubinstein-Taybi syndrome, 182
Saethre-Chotzen syndrome, 183
Schinzel-Giedion syndrome, 184
Seckel syndrome, 188
Shprintzen-Goldberg syndrome, 189
Smith-Lemli-Opitz syndrome type I, 370
Sturge-Weber syndrome, 201
Thalidomide embryopathy, 207
Townes-Brocks syndrome, 210
Treacher Collins syndrome, 211
VATER association, 218
Velo-cardio-facial syndrome, 219
Warfarin embryopathy, 222
Wildervanck syndrome, 226
Zellweger syndrome, 386
Zimmermann-Laband syndrome, 231
Ear, inner: anomaly
Apert syndrome, 11
Branchio-oto-renal syndrome, 23
Down syndrome, 57
Fetal rubella infection
Fountain syndrome, 76
Hypertelorism–microtia–facial clefting syndrome, 98
Klippel-Feil syndrome, 109
Multiple synostosis syndrome, 136
Neurofibromatosis, 140, 144
Oculo-auriculo-vertebral spectrum, 147
Pendred syndrome, 158
Treacher Collins syndrome, 211
Waardenburg syndrome, 221
Wildervanck syndrome, 226
Ear: low-set
Aminopterin fetopathy, 8
Brachmann–de Lange syndrome, 22
Carpenter syndrome, 29
Cat-eye syndrome, 30
Chromosomal abnormalities
DiGeorge syndrome, 55

Fetal akinesia sequence, 71
Fetal hydantoin syndrome, 72
Frontonasal dysplasia, 78
Gardner-Silengo-Wachtel syndrome, 81
Hajdu-Cheney syndrome, 87
Hallermann-Streiff syndrome, 88
Joubert syndrome, 103
Lissencephalies, 116
Noonan syndrome, 145
Oculo-auriculo-vertebral spectrum, 147
Oto-palato-digital syndrome type I, 154
Potter sequence, 166
Rubinstein-Taybi syndrome, 182
Schinzel-Giedion syndrome, 184
Schwartz-Jampel syndrome, 185
Seckel syndrome, 188
Shprintzen-Goldberg syndrome, 189
Smith-Lemli-Opitz syndrome type I, 370
Smith-Lemli-Opitz syndrome type II, 371
Treacher Collins syndrome, 211
Ear, middle: anomaly
    Apert syndrome, 11
    Branchio-oto-renal syndrome, 23
    Chromosome 13 trisomy syndrome, 37
    Chromosome 18 trisomy syndrome, 37
    DiGeorge syndrome, 55
    Duane syndrome, 59
    EEC syndrome, 62
    Fanconi anemia, 69
    Hypertelorism–microtia–facial clefting
        syndrome, 98
    Hypothyroidism, 300
    Klippel-Feil syndrome, 109
    Mucopolysaccharidoses, 325
    Multiple synostosis syndrome, 136
    Oro-facio-digital syndrome II, 150
    Oto-palato-digital syndrome type I, 154
    Renal-genital-ear anomalies, 175
    Robin sequence, 180
    Symphalangism-surdity syndrome, 205
    Treacher Collins syndrome, 211
    Turner syndrome, 214
    Wildervanck syndrome, 226
Ectodermal dysplasia
    Clouston syndrome, 39
    Ectodermal dysplasia (hypohidrotic), 61
    EEC syndrome, 62
    Marshall syndrome, 123
Ectrodactyly
    Acrorenal syndrome, 4
    Adams-Oliver syndrome, 4

Amniotic band sequence, 9
Brachmann–de Lange syndrome, 22
Chromosome 13 trisomy syndrome, 37
Chromosome 18 trisomy syndrome, 37
EEC syndrome, 62
Eronen syndrome, 68
Fuhrmann syndrome, 79
Goltz syndrome, 83
Hand-foot-genital syndrome, 89
Holt-Oram syndrome, 94
Hypoglossia-hypodactylia syndrome, 98
Möbius syndrome, 132
Poland sequence, 162
Roberts syndrome, 179
Split-hand/split-foot deformities, 196
Treacher Collins syndrome, 211
Zimmermann-Laband syndrome, 231
Eczema, eczematoid lesion
    Acrodermatitis enteropathica, 234
    Ataxia-telangiectasia syndrome, 14
    Chronic granulomatous disease of child-
        hood, 256
    Dubowitz syndrome, 59
    Ectodermal dysplasia (hypohidrotic), 61
    Hyperimmunoglobulinemia E syndrome, 96
    Hypoparathyroidism, 296
    Incontinentia pigmenti, 100
    Osteoarthropathy, familial idiopathic, 152
    Phenylketonuria, 350
    Shwachman syndrome, 363
    Wiskott-Aldrich syndrome, 228
Elbow: dislocation
    Aminopterin fetopathy, 8
    Brachmann–de Lange syndrome, 22
    Cerebro-costo-mandibular syndrome, 33
    Chromosome XXXXY syndrome
    Cloverleaf skull deformity, 39
    Coffin-Siris syndrome, 42
    Crouzon syndrome, 47
    Cutis laxa, 49
    Fanconi anemia, 69
    Larsen syndrome, 112
    Mietens-Weber syndrome, 130
    Multiple synostosis syndrome, 136
    Nail-patella syndrome, 137
    Neurofibromatosis I, 140
    Noonan syndrome, 145
    Occipital horn syndrome, 341
    Ophthalmo-mandibulo-melic dysplasia, 148
    Opitz trigonocephaly syndrome, 149
    Oto-palato-digital syndrome type I, 154

Pterygium (antecubital), 171
Seckel syndrome, 188
Encephalocele/meningocele
Amniotic band sequence, 9
Fraser syndrome, 77
Frontonasal dysplasia, 78
Meckel syndrome, 125
Walker-Warburg syndrome, 221
Warfarin embryopathy, 222
Epiphysis: cone-shaped/ball-in-socket defor-
mity
Apert syndrome, 11
Beckwith-Wiedemann syndrome, 17
Cockayne syndrome, 40
DOOR syndrome, 56
Hyperthyroidism, 294
Hypochondroplasia
Hypophosphatasia, 297
Oro-facio-digital syndrome I, 150
Oto-palato-digital syndrome type I, 154
Pseudohypoparathyroidism, 355
Scurvy, 362
Seckel syndrome, 188
Vitamin A intoxication, chronic, 380
Weill-Marchesani syndrome, 224
Epiphysis: large
Adrenal hyperplasia (congenital), 238
Beckwith-Wiedemann syndrome, 17
Hemophilia (hemarthrosis), 282
Hyperthyroidism, 294
Infantile multisystem inflammatory dis-
ease, 100
Sotos syndrome, 195
Epiphysis: punctate calcification; *refer to*
Calcification: punctate osteoarticular
(infants)
Erlenmeyer flask deformity
Gaucher disease, 272
Hypophosphatasia (adult), 297
Lead poisoning, sequela
Membranous lipodystrophy, 319
Niemann-Pick disease, 336
Oto-palato-digital syndrome type I, 154
Schwarz-Lélek syndrome, 185
Thalassemia, 374
Esophagus: dysfunction
Achalasia-adrenal-alacrima syndrome, 2
Amyloidosis, 245
Behçet syndrome, 18
Chronic granulomatous disease of child-
hood, 256

CREST syndrome, 46
Cutis laxa, 49
Diabetes mellitus, 262
Down syndrome, 57
Ehlers-Danlos syndrome, 63
Familial achalasia
Hyperthyroidism, 294
Hypothyroidism, 300
Kugelberg-Welander syndrome, 110
Mixed connective tissue disease, 131
Opitz BBBG syndrome, 149
Paraneoplastic syndrome, 344
Riley-Day syndrome, 178
Scleroderma, 186
Exophthalmos
Brachmann–de Lange syndrome, 22
Cardio-facio-cutaneous syndrome, 26
Cloverleaf skull deformity, 39
Craniosynostoses
Crouzon syndrome, 47
Erdheim-Chester disease, 265
Geroderma osteodysplastica, 81
Hyperthyroidism, 294
Infantile multisystem inflammatory dis-
ease, 100
Neu-Laxova syndrome, 139
Neurofibromatosis I, 140
Noonan syndrome, 145
Relapsing polychondritis, 175
Roberts syndrome, 179
Shprintzen-Goldberg syndrome, 189
Thalassemia, 374
Exostosis; spur; horn
Copper deficiency (metaphyseal spur), 258
Fetal alcohol syndrome (tibia), 71
Fibrodysplasia ossificans progressiva, 74
Hyperparathyroidism (metaphyseal spur),
290
Hypophosphatasia, 297
Iso-Kikuchi syndrome, 102
Menkes disease (metaphyseal spur), 319
Nail-patella syndrome (iliac horn), 137
Occipital horn syndrome, 341
Proteus syndrome (skull protuberances),
169
Scurvy (metaphyseal spur), 362
Tuberous sclerosis (exostoses), 212
Turner syndrome (exostosis of tibia), 214
Eyebrow abnormalities
Alopecia areata, totalis and universalis
(absent eyebrows)

Brachmann–de Lange syndrome (syn-
 ophrys), 22
Chromosome 3q1 (synophrys)
Chromosome 10q1 (fine, arched)
Chromosome 12p1 (lateral extension)
Chromosome 18 trisomy (discontinuous),
 37
Fucosidosis (heavy), 270
Hypertrichosis universalis congenita (dou-
 ble)
ICE syndrome: ichthyosis–cheek–eyebrow
 syndrome (absence of outer half)
KBG syndrome (redundant), 107
Klein-Waardenburg syndrome (heavy),
 108
Metaphyseal chondrodysplasia, McKusick
 type (sparse)
Monilethrix (sparse)
Mucopolysaccharidosis I-H (heavy), 327
Mucopolysaccharidosis VI (heavy), 333
Oto-palato-digital syndrome type I (lateral
 extension), 154
Progeria (absent), 168
Romberg syndrome (loss of median por-
 tion), 181
Rothmund-Thomson syndrome (sparse),
 181
Waardenburg syndrome (premature gray-
 ing), 221
Williams syndrome (medial flare), 227

F

Facial asymmetry
 Aminoperin fetopathy-like syndrome, 9
 Amniotic band sequence, 9
 Cardiofacial syndrome, 26
 Dyke-Davidoff-Masson syndrome, 60
 Epidermal nevus syndrome, 66
 Goltz syndrome, 83
 Klippel-Feil syndrome, 109
 Romberg syndrome, 181
 Saethre-Chotzen syndrome, 183
 Sturge-Weber syndrome, 201
 Velo-cardio-facial syndrome, 219
 Wildervanck syndrome, 226
Femoral head: flat and/or fragmented
 Adrenal hyperplasia (congenital), 238
 Avascular necrosis (various etiologies)
 Behçet syndrome, 18
 Chondroectodermal dysplasia

Congenital hip dysplasia/dislocation
Cushing syndrome, 258
Diabetes mellitus, 262
Gaucher disease, 272
Hemophilia, 282
Hyperparathyroidism (secondary), 290
Hypothyroidism, 300
Legg-Calvé-Perthes disease
Meyer dysplasia of femoral head
Mucopolysaccharidoses, 325
Multiple endocrine neoplasia type IIB,
 135
Osteochondritis dissecans
Rickets, 359
Sarcoidosis
Schwartz-Jampel syndrome, 185
Septic arthritis
Shwachman syndrome, 363
Sickle cell anemia, 365
Slipped capital femoral epiphysis (late
 phase)
Stickler syndrome, 200
Thalassemia, 374
Winchester syndrome, 384
Femoral head: slipped
 Cushing syndrome, 258
 Down syndrome, 57
 Gaucher disease, 272
 Gigantism (hyperpituitarism), 236
 Hemophilia, 282
 Hyperparathyroidism, 290
 Hypothyroidism, 300
 Idiopathic slipped capital femoral epiph-
  ysis
 Klinefelter syndrome, 108
 Pseudohypoparathyroidism, 355
 Renal osteodystrophy, 292
 Rickets, 359
 Satoyoshi syndrome, 184
 Scurvy, 362
 Shwachman syndrome, 363
 Turner syndrome, 214
 Zellweger syndrome, 386
Fibular ray defect (aplasia, hypoplasia, short)
 Acro-fronto-facio-nasal dysostosis syn-
  drome
 Du Pan syndrome, 60
 Facio-auriculo-radial dysplasia, 69
 Fuhrmann syndrome, 79
 Mietens-Weber syndrome, 130

Ophthalmo-mandibulo-melic dysplasia, 148
Weyers oligodactyly syndrome, 226
Fontanelle: delayed closure, large
  Aase syndrome, 2
  Aminopterin fetopathy, 8
  Aplasia cutis (scalp)
  Chromosome 13 trisomy syndrome, 37
  Chromosome 18 trisomy syndrome, 37
  Coffin-Lowry syndrome, 42
  Cranium bifidum
  Cutis laxa, 49
  Down syndrome, 57
  Fetal hydantoin syndrome, 72
  GAPO syndrome, 80
  Greig cephalopolysyndactyly syndrome, 86
  Hallermann-Streiff syndrome, 88
  Hypophosphatasia, 297
  Hypothyroidism, 300
  Infantile multisystem inflammatory disease, 100
  Oculo-auriculo-vertebral spectrum, 147
  Opitz BBBG syndrome, 149
  Oto-palato-digital syndrome type I, 154
  Pachydermoperiostosis, 155
  Progeria, 168
  Rubinstein-Taybi syndrome, 182
  Schinzel-Giedion syndrome, 184
  Silver-Russell syndrome, 190
  Wiedemann-Rautenstrauch syndrome, 226
  Winchester syndrome, 384
  Zellweger syndrome, 386
Fragile bones, pathologic fracture
  Aluminum intoxication, 245
  Antley-Bixler symdrome, 11
  Aspartylglucosaminuria, 247
  Copper deficiency, 258
  Cushing syndrome, 258
  Cutis laxa, 49
  Cystinosis, 259
  Dyskeratosis congenita, 60
  Fetal akinesia sequence, 71
  Gaucher disease, 272
  Geroderma osteodysplastica, 81
  Glycogen storage disease type I, 275
  GM_1 gangliosidosis type I, 278
  Homocystinuria, 285
  Hyperparathyroidism, 290
  Hyperphosphatasia, 293
  Hyperthyroidism, 294

Hypophosphatasia, 297
Insensitivity to pain (congenital), 101
Lowe syndrome, 314
Lysinuric protein intolerance, 314
Maffucci syndrome, 119
McCune-Albright syndrome, 125
Membranous lipodystrophy, 319
Menkes disease, 319
Mucolipidosis II, 323
Niemann-Pick disease, 336
Osteoporosis-pseudoglioma syndrome, 154
Oxalosis, 343
Progeria, 168
Renal tubular acidosis, 358
Rickets/osteomalacia, 359
Riley-Day syndrome, 178
Scurvy, 362
Stiff-man syndrome, 200
Thalassemia, 374
Thevenard syndrome, 208
Wilson disease, 383

G
Gallstone
  Caroli syndrome, 28
  Hemophilia, 282
  Hyperlipoproteinemias, 287
  Hyperparathyroidism (primary), 290
  Mirizzi syndrome, 131
  Pyruvate kinase deficiency anemia, 357
  Sickle cell anemia, 365
  Somatostatinoma syndrome, 371
  Spherocytosis, 372
  Thalassemia, 374
  Wilson disease, 383
Genital anomalies
  Aarskog syndrome, 2
  Adrenal hyperplasia (congenital), 238
  Amniotic band sequence, 9
  Bardet-Biedl syndrome, 16
  Chromosome 4p2 syndrome
  Chromosome 13 trisomy syndrome, 37
  Chromosome 18 trisomy syndrome, 37
  Chromosome XXXXY syndrome
  Denys-Drash syndrome, 53
  Down syndrome, 57
  Fetal alcohol syndrome, 71
  Fraser syndrome, 77
  Fryns syndrome, 79
  Gardner-Silengo-Wachtel syndrome, 81
  Hand-foot-genital syndrome, 89

Johanson-Blizzard syndrome, 103
Kaufman-McKusick syndrome, 106
Klinefelter syndrome, 108
LEOPARD syndrome, 113
Mayer-Rokitansky-Küster syndrome, 124
Nager acrofacial dysostosis, 136
Noonan syndrome, 145
Persistent müllerian duct syndrome, 159
Prune-belly syndrome, 170
Pterygium syndrome, popliteal, 171
Renal–genital–middle ear anomalies, 175
Roberts syndrome, 179
Robinow syndrome
Rüdiger syndrome, 183
Seckel syndrome, 188
Smith-Lemli-Opitz syndrome type I, 370
Smith-Lemli-Opitz syndrome type II, 371
Splenogonadal fusion/limb deformity, 196
Spondylocostal dysostosis (Jarcho-Levin
    syndrome), 197
Testicular feminization, 373
Turner syndrome, 214
Young syndrome, 230
Genu valgum (knock-knees)
Bardet-Biedl syndrome, 16
Cohen syndrome, 43
Hajdu-Cheney syndrome, 87
Hypophosphatasia, 297
Mucopolysaccharidoses, 325
Nail-patella syndrome, 137
Physiologic knock-knees
Rickets, 359
Genu varum (bowlegs)
Hyperparathyroidism, 290
Hyperphosphatasia, 293
Physiologic bowlegs
Rickets, 359
Turner syndrome, 214
Gigantism; macrosomia; overgrowth syn-
    dromes (generalized or regional)
Adrenal hyperplasia (congenital), 238
Beckwith-Wiedemann syndrome, 17
Fragile X syndrome, 77
Homocystinuria, 285
Hypersomatotropism (acromegaly, gigan-
    tism), 235
Infant of the diabetic mother
Klinefelter syndrome, 108
Lipodystrophy (lipoatrophic diabetes), 311
Marshall-Smith syndrome, 123
McCune-Albright syndrome, 125

Neurofibromatosis I, 140
Pallister-Killian syndrome, 156
Perlman syndrome, 159
Proteus syndrome, 169
Simpson-Golabi-Behmel syndrome, 191
Sotos syndrome, 195
Tuberous sclerosis, 212
Weaver syndrome, 223
Glaucoma
Aniridia-Wilms tumor association, 10
Ehlers-Danlos syndrome, 63
Gorlin syndrome, 85
Hallermann-Streiff syndrome, 88
Homocystinuria, 285
Klippel-Trenaunay-Weber syndrome, 109
Lowe syndrome, 314
Marfan syndrome, 121
Marshall syndrome, 123
Michels syndrome, 127
Mucopolysaccharidoses, 325
Neurofibromatosis I, 140
Oculo-auriculo-vertebral spectrum, 147
Oculo-dento-osseous dysplasia, 147
Stickler syndrome, 200
Sturge-Weber syndrome, 201
Treacher Collins syndrome, 211
von Hippel–Lindau syndrome, 220
Weill-Marchesani syndrome, 224
Zellweger syndrome, 386
Goiter
Cowden syndrome, 44
Hyperthyroidism, 294
McCune-Albright syndrome, 125
Multiple endocrine neoplasia type IIB, 135
Pendred syndrome, 158
Troell-Junet syndrome, 212
Weismann-Netter syndrome, 224
Gout
Glycogen storage disease type I, 275
Hyperlipoproteinemias, 287
Lesch-Nyhan syndrome, 310
Thalassemia, 374
Gynecomastia
Cowden syndrome, 44
Gorlin syndrome, 85
Hyperthyroidism, 294
Hypothyroidism (juvenile), 300
Infant of diabetic mother
Klinefelter syndrome, 108
McCune-Albright syndrome, 125
Paraneoplastic syndromes, 344

POEMS syndrome, 161
Reifenstein syndrome, 174

H

Hair: color abnormalities
Copper deficiency, 258
Cross syndrome, 47
Cystinosis, 259
Klein-Waardenburg syndrome, 108
Kwashiorkor, 308
Waardenburg syndrome, 221
Werner syndrome, 224
Hairline: low
Brachmann–de Lange syndrome, 22
Fetal hydantoin syndrome, 72
Fraser syndrome, 77
Klippel-Feil syndrome, 109
Noonan syndrome, 145
Oculo-auriculo-vertebral spectrum, 147
Turner syndrome, 214
Hamartomatoses, congenital
Bannayan-Riley-Ruvalcaba syndrome, 15
Cowden syndrome, 44
Delleman syndrome, 52
Encephalo-cranio-cutaneous lipomatosis,
66
Epiderma nevus syndrome, 66
Gorlin syndrome, 85
Hypomelanosis of Ito, 98
Incontinentia pigmenti, 100
Klippel-Trenaunay-Weber syndrome, 109
LEOPARD syndrome, 113
Maffucci syndrome, 119
Multiple endocrine neoplasia syndrome
type IIB, 135
Neurofibromatosis I, 140
Peutz-Jeghers syndrome, 159
Proteus syndrome, 169
Sturge-Weber syndrome, 201
Tuberous sclerosis, 212
von Hippel–Lindau syndrome, 220
Hand: contracture (claw hand)
Chromosome 13 trisomy syndrome, 37
Chromosome 18 trisomy syndrome, 37
Contractural arachnodactyly, 44
Diabetes mellitus, 262
Digitotalar dysmorphism, 56
Epidermolysis bullosa, 67
Fetal akinesia sequence, 71
Freeman-Sheldon syndrome, 78

Mucolipidoses, 323, 324, 325
Mucopolysaccharidoses
Hand and foot: short/stubby
Aarskog syndrome, 2
Acro-osteolysis, 152
Börjeson-Forssman-Lehmann syndrome,
22
Cephaloskeletal dysplasia, 32
Cockayne syndrome, 40
Cohen syndrome, 43
Down syndrome, 57
Fountain syndrome, 76
Fragile X syndrome, 77
Hypopituitarism (anterior lobe), 298
Kabuki make-up syndrome, 104
Léri syndrome, 114
Mucolipidoses, 323, 324, 325
Mucopolysaccharidoses, 325
Noonan syndrome, 145
Oro-facio-digital syndromes, 150
Prader-Willi syndrome, 166
Progeria, 168
Pseudohypoparathyroidism, 355
Smith-Magenis syndrome, 193
Weill-Marchesani syndrome, 224
Hemihypertrophy (localized or generalized)
Beckwith-Wiedemann syndrome, 17
Hemihypertrophy, 90
Klippel-Trenaunay syndrome, 109
Macrodystrophia lipomatosa, 119
Proteus syndrome, 169
Hernia, abdominal
Aarskog syndrome, 2
Amniotic band sequence, 9
Aniridia-Wilms tumor association, 10
Beckwith-Wiedemann syndrome, 17
Brachmann–de Lange syndrome, 22
Cantrell syndrome, 25
Carpenter syndrome, 29
CHARGE association, 34
Chromosomal abnormalities
Coffin-Lowry syndrome, 42
Coffin-Siris syndrome, 42
Cutis laxa, 49
Ehlers-Danlos syndrome, 63
Femoral hypoplasia–unusual facial syn-
drome, 70
Fetal alcohol syndrome, 71
Fetal hydantoin syndrome, 72
Fetal valproate syndrome, 73

Fibrodysplasia ossificans progressiva, 74
Freeman–Sheldon syndrome, 78
Geroderma osteodysplastica, 81
Goltz syndrome, 83
Hajdu-Cheney syndrome, 87
Homocystinuria, 285
Hypothyroidism, 300
Marshall-Smith syndrome, 123
Meckel syndrome, 125
Mucolipidosis II, 323
Mucopolysaccharidosis I-H, 327
Mucopolysaccharidosis II, 329
Mucopolysaccharidosis VI, 333
Opitz BBBG syndrome, 149
Pterygium syndromes, 171
Sandifer syndrome, 184
Shprintzen-Goldberg syndrome, 189
Splenogonadal fusion/limb deformity, 196
Testicular feminization, 373
Weaver syndrome, 223
Williams syndrome, 227
Hip: dislocation or subluxation
Aminopterin fetopathy, 8
Caudal dysplasia sequence, 31
Cerebro-costo-mandibular syndrome, 33
Cerebro-oculo-facio-skeletal syndrome, 33
Cloverleaf skull deformity, 39
Cutis laxa, 49
Down syndrome, 57
Ehlers-Danlos syndrome, 63
Fanconi anemia, 69
Farber disease, 268
Fibrodysplasia ossificans progressiva, 74
Geroderma osteodysplastica, 81
Habitual hip dislocation
Hallermann-Streiff syndrome, 88
Insensitivity to pain (congenital), 101
Larsen syndrome, 112
Marfan syndrome, 121
Möbius syndrome, 132
Mucolipidosis II, 323
Mucopolysaccharidosis I-H, 327
Nager acrofacial dysostosis,136
Opitz trigonocephaly syndrome, 149
Oto-palato-digital syndrometype I, 154
Poland sequence, 162
Prader-Willi syndrome, 166
Prune-belly syndrome, 170
Riley-Day syndrome, 178
Silver-Russell syndrome, 190
Stoll-Charrow-Poznanski syndrome, 201

Horn; *refer to* Exostosis
Hydrocephalus
Aase-Smith syndrome
Acrocallosal syndrome, 3
Aicardi syndrome, 6
Aminopterin fetopathy, 8
Aminopterin fetopathy-like syndrome, 9
Amniotic band sequence, 9
Apert syndrome, 11
Aplasia cutis congenita, 12
Bardet-Biedl syndrome, 16
Beemer lethal malformation
Bobble-head doll syndrome, 21
Caudal dysplasia sequence, 31
Cloverleaf skull deformity, 39
Cockayne syndrome, 40
Crouzon syndrome, 47
Cystinosis, 259
Dandy-Walker syndrome, 50
Diencephalic syndrome, 55
Epidermal nevus syndrome, 66
Farber disease, 268
Fetal alcohol syndrome, 71
Gorlin syndrome, 85
Hydrocephalus (familial)
Hydrolethalus syndrome, 95
Incontinentia pigmenti, 100
Infant of the diabetic mother
Kasabach-Merritt syndrome, 106
Klüver-Bucy syndrome, 110
Lissencephalies, 116
Mannosidoses, 316
Meckel syndrome, 125
Metachromatic leukodystrophies, 321
Miller-Dieker syndrome, 130
Mucolipidosis IV, 325
Mucopolysaccharidosis I-H, 327
Mucopolysaccharidosis VI, 333
Mulibrey nanism, 134
Neu-Laxova syndrome, 139
Neurocutaneous melanosis sequence, 139
Oro-facio-digital syndrome I, 150
Pfeiffer syndrome, 160
Pseudotrisomy 13 syndrome, 170
Riley-Day syndrome, 178
Ritscher-Schinzel syndrome, 179
Sjögren-Larsson syndrome, 369
Smith-Lemli-Opitz syndrome type I, 370
Smith-Lemli-Opitz syndrome type II, 371
Sotos syndrome, 195
Tuberous sclerosis, 212

VATER association, 218
Vitamin A intoxication, 380
Walker-Warburg syndrome, 221
Zellweger syndrome, 386
Hypercalcemia
Adrenal insufficiency
Aluminum intoxication, 245
Blue diaper syndrome, 249
Familial hypocalciuric hypercalcemia
Hyperparathyroidism, 290
Hyperthyroidism, 294
Hypophosphatasia, 297
Hypothyroidism, 300
Infantile hypercalcemia
Milk-alkali syndrome,
Multiple endocrine neoplasia type I, 134
Oxalosis, 343
Paraneoplastic syndromes, 344
Vitamin A intoxication, 380
Vitamin D intoxication, 382
Williams syndrome, 227
Hypercalciuria
Bartter syndrome, 16
Hyperparathyroidism, 290
Idiopathic hypercalciuria
Renal tubular acidosis, 358
Short-bowel syndrome, 189
Williams syndrome, 227
Hyperhidrosis
Chédiak-Higashi syndrome, 35
Dyskeratosis congenita, 60
Jadassohn-Lewandowsky syndrome, 103
Keratosis palmaris et plantaris familiaris
(tylosis), 107
Osteoarthropathy, familial idiopathic, 152
Pachydermoperiostosis, 155
POEMS syndrome, 161
Shapiro syndrome, 188
Silver-Russell syndrome, 190
TAR syndrome, 206
Hyperkeratosis
Cardio-facio-cutaneous syndrome, 26
Cowden syndrome, 44
Dyskeratosis congenita, 60
Jadassohn-Lewandowsky syndrome, 103
Keratosis palmaris et plantaris familiaris
(tylosis), 107
Papillon-Lefèvre syndrome, 157
Proteus syndrome, 169
Vohwinkel syndrome, 219

Hyperparathyroidism
Bartter syndrome, 16
Cystinosis, 259
McCune-Albright syndrome, 125
Multiple endocrine neoplasia type I, 134
Multiple endocrine neoplasia type IIA,
135
Neurofibromatosis I, 140
Oxalosis, 343
Hyperphosphatasemia
Hyperostosis–hyperphosphatemia syn-
drome, 97
Hyperphosphatasia, 293
Rickets, 359
Hyperphosphatemia
Acromegaly, 235
Hyperostosis–hyperphosphatemia syn-
drome, 97
Hyperparathyroidism (secondary), 290
Hypoparathyroidism, 296
Pseudohypoparathyroidism, 355
Transient hyperphosphatemia of infancy
Tumoral calcinosis, 377
Vitamin D intoxication, 382
Hyperpituitarism
Acromegaly, 235
Gigantism, 235
Hyperprolactinemia, 293
Hypertelorism (ocular, orbital)
Aarskog syndrome, 2
Acrocallosal syndrome, 3
Aminopterin fetopathy, 8
Aminopterin fetopathy-like syndrome, 9
Apert syndrome, 11
Beckwith-Wiedemann syndrome, 17
Brachmann–de Lange syndrome, 22
Branchio-genito-skeletal syndrome, 23
Branchio-oculo-facial syndrome, 23
Cardio-facio-cutaneous syndrome, 26
Cat-eye syndrome, 30
CHARGE association, 34
Chromosomal abnormalities
Cloverleaf skull deformity, 39
Coffin-Lowry syndrome, 42
Cranium bifidum
Crouzon syndrome, 47
Diamond-Blackfan syndrome, 54
DiGeorge syndrome, 55
Dubowitz syndrome, 59
Ehlers-Danlos syndrome, 63

Fetal akinesia sequence, 71
Fetal hydantoin syndrome, 72
FG syndrome, 73
Fraser syndrome, 77
Freeman-Sheldon syndrome, 78
Frontonasal dysplasia, 78
German syndrome
Gorlin syndrome, 85
Greig cephalopolysyndactyly syndrome, 86
Holt-Oram syndrome, 94
Hypertelorism–microtia–facial clefting
   syndrome, 98
Larsen syndrome, 112
LEOPARD syndrome, 113
Lissencephalies, 116
Marden-Walker syndrome, 121
Meckel syndrom 125
Mucopolysaccharidosis I-H, 327
Neu-Laxova syndrome, 139
Noonan syndrome, 145
Oculo-dento-osseous dysplasia, 147
Opitz BBBG syndrome, 149
Oro-facio-digital syndrome I, 150
Oromandibular-limb hypogenesis, 152
Oto-palato-digital syndrome type I, 154
Pallister-Killian syndrome, 156
Pfeiffer syndrome, 160
Potter sequence, 166
Pterygium syndromes, 171
Roberts syndrome, 179
Rubinstein-Taybi syndrome, 182
Saethre-Chotzen syndrome, 183
Schinzel-Giedion syndrome, 184
Seckel syndrome, 188
Simpson-Golabi-Behmel syndrome, 191
Sjögren-Larsson syndrome, 369
Sotos syndrome, 195
Teebi hypertelorism syndrome, 206
Thalassemia, 374
Treacher Collins syndrome, 211
Waardenburg syndrome, 221
Warfarin embryopathy, 222
Weaver syndrome, 223
Hypertension, systemic
Adrenal hyperplasia (congenital), 238
Aldosteronism (primary), 241
Alkaptonuria, 243
Alport syndrome, 8
Carcinoid syndrome, 252
Degos syndrome, 51
Fabry disease, 266

Hemolytic uremic syndrome, 90
Hyperphosphatasia, 293
Hyperthyroidism, 294
Mucopolysaccharidosis I-H, 327
Nephronophthisis, 138
Neurofibromatosis I, 140
Osteolysis with nephropathy, 153
Paraneoplastic syndromes, 344
Postcoarctectomy syndrome, 165
Progeria, 168
Riley-Day syndrome, 178
Sleep apnea syndrome, 193
Tuberous sclerosis, 212
Turner syndrome, 214
Williams syndrome, 227
Hypertrichosis
Bardet-Biedl syndrome, 16
Bloom syndrome, 20
Brachmann–de Lange syndrome, 22
Cerebro-oculo-facio-skeletal syndrome, 33
Chromosome 18 trisomy syndrome, 37
Coffin-Siris syndrome, 42
Epidermal nevus syndrome, 66
Fetal alcohol syndrome, 71
Fetal hydantoin syndrome, 72
Frontometaphyseal dysplasia
Hajdu-Cheney syndrome, 87
Hemihypertrophy, 90
Hypothyroidism (juvenile), 300
Leprechaunism, 310
Lipodystrophy (lipoatrophic diabetes), 311
Marshall-Smith syndrome, 123
Morgagni-Stewart-Morel syndrome, 132
Mucopolysaccharidoses, 325
Patterson syndrome, 347
POEMS syndrome, 161
Polycystic ovary syndrome, 351
Porphyrias, 353
Rubinstein-Taybi syndrome, 182
Schinzel-Giedion syndrome, 184
Thevenard syndrome, 208
Turner syndrome, 214
Winchester syndrome, 384
Hypocalcemia
DiGeorge syndrome, 55
Hyperparathyroidism (secondary), 290
Hypoparathyroidism, 296
Malabsorption syndrome, 119
Nephronophthisis, 138
Paraneoplastic syndromes, 344
Pseudohypoparathyroidism, 355

Renal tubular acidosis, 358
Rickets, 359
Hypogenitalism, hypogonadism
Bardet-Biedl syndrome, 16
Börjeson-Forssman-Lehmann syndrome, 22
Brachmann–de Lange syndrome, 22
Carpenter syndrome, 29
Chromosome XXXXY syndrome
Cockayne syndrome, 40
Cushing syndrome, 258
De Sanctis-Cacchione syndrome, 54
Down syndrome, 57
Ectodermal dysplasia (hypohidrotic), 61
Goltz syndrome, 83
Gorlin syndrome, 85
Hallermann-Streiff syndrome, 88
Hemochromatosis, 281
Hypopituitarism (anterior lobe), 298
Hypothyroidism, 300
Jaffe-Campanacci syndrome, 103
Kallmann syndrome, 105
Klinefelter syndrome, 108
Laron syndrome, 309
Laurence-Moon syndrome, 16
LEOPARD syndrome, 113
Marfan syndrome, 121
Mauriac syndrome, 317
Odonto-tricho-melic syndrome, 148
Prader-Willi syndrome, 166
Prasad syndrome, 354
Pseudohypoparathyroidism, 355
Reifenstein syndrome, 174
Rothmund-Thomson syndrome, 181
Seckel syndrome, 188
Thalassemia, 374
Turner syndrome, 214
Werner syndrome, 224
Hypoglycemia
Beckwith-Wiedemann syndrome, 17
Carnitine deficiency syndromes, 253
de Morsier syndrome, 53
Glycogen storage disease type I, 275
Glycogen storage disease type III, 276
Hyperinsulinism, 287
Hypopituitarism (anterior lobe), 298
Islet cell dysplasia
Laron syndrome, 309
Neurofibromatosis I, 140
Paraneoplastic syndromes, 344

Pseudohypoparathyroidism, 355
Silver-Russell syndrome, 190
Hypokalemia
Aldosteronism (primary), 241
Bartter syndrome, 16
Cystinosis, 259
Fanconi syndrome, 268
Kwashiorkor, 308
VIPoma syndrome, 379
Hypoparathyroidism
Hallermann-Streiff syndrome, 88
Paraneoplastic syndromes, 344
Polyglandular autoimmune disease, 352
Thalassemia, 374
Hypophosphatemia
Cystinosis, 259
Fanconi syndrome, 268
Hyperparathyroidism (neonatal), 290
Hyperparathyroidism (primary), 290
Malabsorption syndrome, 119
Paraneoplastic syndromes, 344
Rickets, vitamin D–resistant, 359
Vitamin D deficiency, 359
Hypopituitarism
Caudal dysplasia sequence, 31
de Morsier syndrome, 53
Deprivation dwarfism, 260
Diamond-Blackfan syndrome, 54
Diencephalic syndrome, 55
Fanconi anemia, 69
Pallister-Hall syndrome, 156
Shapiro syndrome, 188
Thalassemia, 374
Hypospadias
Aniridia-Wilms tumor association, 10
Branchio-genito-skeletal syndrome, 23
Chromosomal abnormalities
Dubowitz syndrome, 59
Fanconi anemia, 69
Fraser syndrome, 77
Gardner-Silengo-Wachtel syndrome, 81
Hand-foot-genital syndrome, 89
Lenz microphthalmia syndrome, 113
LEOPARD syndrome, 113
Male pseudohermaphroditism
Opitz BBBG syndrome, 149
Polycystic kidney disease (infantile), 162
Potter sequence, 166
Reifenstein syndrome, 174
Schinzel-Giedion syndrome, 184

Silver-Russell syndrome, 190
Smith-Lemli-Opitz syndrome type I, 370
Smith-Lemli-Opitz syndrome type II, 371
Splenogonadal fusion/limb deformity, 196
Toriello-Carey syndrome, 210
VATER association, 218
Zellweger syndrome, 386
Hypotelorism (ocular, orbital)
    Chromosome 13 trisomy syndrome, 37
    Craniosynostosis (metopic)
    Craniotelencephalic dysplasia, 46
    DiGeorge syndrome, 55
    Down syndrome, 57
    Fetal hydantoin syndrome, 72
    Holoprosencephaly, 94
    Meckel syndrome, 125
    Oculo-dento-osseous dysplasia, 147
    Opitz trigonocephaly syndrome, 149
    Phenylketonuria, 350
    Postaxial acrofacial dysostosis, Miller
        type, 164
    Williams syndrome, 227
Hypotension, systemic
    Addison disease, 237
    Carotid sinus syndrome, 28
    Hypopituitarism (anterior lobe), 298
    Neurofibromatosis I, 140
    Ovarian hyperstimulation syndrome, 342
    Riley-Day syndrome, 178
    Sheehan syndrome, 363
    Shy-Drager syndrome, 190
    Subclavian steal syndrome, 203

I

Ichthyosis, ichthyosiform lesion, thick skin
    Bloom syndrome, 20
    Cardio-facio-cutaneous syndrome, 26
    CHILD syndrome, 36
    Clouston syndrome, 39
    Epidermal nevus syndrome, 66
    Harlequin ichthyosis
    Hyperimmunoglobulinemia E syndrome,
        96
    Hypomelanosis of Ito, 98
    Jadassohn-Lewandowsky syndrome, 103
    Menkes disease, 319
    Metachromatic leukodystrophies, 321
    Mucolipidosis II, 323
    Mucopolysaccharidosis I-H/S, 328
    Multiple sulfatase deficiency, 334
    Neu-Laxova syndrome, 139

Pachydermoperiostosis, 155
PIBI(D)S syndrome, 160
Refsum disease, 357
Senter syndrome
Sjögren-Larsson syndrome, 369
Trichorrhexis nodosa syndrome, 212
Vohwinkel syndrome, 219
Werner syndrome, 224
Immune disorders
    Adenosine deaminase deficiency
    Agammaglobulinemia, X-linked, 5
    Alpha-chain disease, 244
    Ataxia-telangiectasia syndrome, 14
    Beckwith-Wiedemann syndrome, 17
    Bloom syndrome, 20
    Celiac disease, 254
    Cockayne syndrome, 40
    DiGeorge syndrome, 55
    Down syndrome, 57
    Dubowitz syndrome, 59
    Dyskeratosis congenita, 60
    Ehlers-Danlos syndrome, 63
    Fanconi anemia, 69
    Felty syndrome, 70
    Griscelli syndrome, 86
    Hallermann-Streiff syndrome, 88
    Henoch-Schönlein syndrome, 91
    Hyperimmunoglobulinemia E syndrome,
        96
    Hyperostosis-hyperphosphatemia syn-
        drome, 97
    Immotile cilia syndrome, 99
    Incontinentia pigmenti, 100
    Infantile multisystem inflammatory dis-
        ease, 100
    Mannosidoses, 316
    POEMS syndrome, 161
    Polyglandular autoimmune disease, 352
    Schwartz-Jampel syndrome, 185
    Shwachman syndrome, 363
    Sjögren syndrome, 192
    Turner syndrome, 214
    Wiskott-Aldrich syndrome, 228
    X-linked severe combined immunodefi-
        ciency
Intestinal pseudo-obstruction
    Amyloidosis, 245
    Celiac disease, 254
    Diabetes mellitus, 262
    Hypoparathyroidism, 296
    Hypothyroidism, 300

Intestinal pseudo-obstruction (idiopathic)
Kawasaki syndrome, 106
Porphyrias, 353
Scleroderma, 186
Sprue

J
Jaundice
Alagille syndrome, 6
Alpha$_1$-antitrypsin deficiency, 243
Bile plug syndrome, 19
Budd-Chiari syndrome, 25
Byler's disease
Dubin-Johnson syndrome, 265
Galactosemia, 270
Gilbert syndrome, 273
Hypopituitarism (anterior lobe), 298
Hypothyroidism, 300
Kawasaki syndrome, 106
Mirizzi syndrome, 131
Polysplenia (extrahepatic biliary atresia)
    syndrome, 163
Pyruvate kinase deficiency anemia, 357
Refsum disease (infantile), 357
Renal-hepatic-pancreatic dysplasia, 176
Rotor syndrome, 361
Sickle cell anemia, 365
Spherocytosis, 372
Thalassemia, 374
Tyrosinemia type 1, 378
Wilson disease, 383
Joint: degenerative changes
Acromegaly, 235
Diabetes mellitus, 262
Gaucher disease, 272
Insensitivity to pain (congenital), 101
Lipoid dermatoarthritis, 115
Macrodystrophia lipomatosa, 119
Relapsing polychondritis, 175
Riley-Day syndrome, 178
Scleroderma, 186
Thevenard syndrome, 208
Joint: dislocation/subluxation
Aminopterin fetopathy (hip, elbow), 8
Cat-eye syndrome, 30
Coffin-Siris syndrome, 42
Cutis laxa, 49
Dermo-chondro-corneal dystrophy of
    François, 54
Down syndrome, 57
Ehlers-Danlos syndrome, 63

Fanconi anemia (hip), 69
Farber disease (hip), 268
Fetal hydantoin syndrome, 72
Freeman-Sheldon syndrome, 78
Hajdu-Cheney syndrome, 87
Keratosis palmaris et plantaris familiaris
    (tylosis), 107
Larsen syndrome (multiple joints), 112
Lenz-Majewski dysplasia
Marfan syndrome, 121
Mucopolysaccharidoses, 325
Nager acrofacial dysostosis, 136
Nail-patella syndrome, 137
Neurofibromatosis I, 140
Noonan syndrome (radial head), 145
Oculo-dento-osseous dysplasia (hip), 147
Oto-palato-digital syndrome type I
    (elbow), 154
Pallister-Hall syndrome, 156
Pallister-Killian syndrome, 156
Potter sequence, 166
Pterygium syndromes, 171
Riley-Day syndrome (hip), 178
Schwartz-Jampel syndrome, 185
Seckel syndrome, 188
Silver-Russell syndrome (elbow, hip), 190
Smith-Lemli-Opitz syndrome type I, 370
Stickler syndrome, 200
TAR syndrome, 206
Thevenard syndrome, 208
Turner syndrome, 214
Joint laxity, hypermobility
Aarskog syndrome, 2
Achard syndrome
Bannayan-Riley-Ruvalcaba syndrome, 15
Börjeson-Forssman-Lehmann syndrome, 22
Chromosome XXXXY syndrome
Coffin-Lowry syndrome, 42
Coffin-Siris syndrome, 42
Cohen syndrome, 43
Cutis laxa, 49
Down syndrome, 57
Ehlers-Danlos syndrome, **63**
FG syndrome, 73
Goltz syndrome, 83
Hajdu-Cheney syndrome, 87
Hallermann-Streiff syndrome, 88
Hypermobility syndrome, 97
Johanson-Blizzard syndrome, 103
Larsen syndrome, 112
LEOPARD syndrome, 113

Lowe syndrome, 314
Marfan syndrome, 121
Marfanoid hypermobility syndrome, 122
Mucopolysaccharidosis IVA, 331
Multiple endocrine neoplasia type IIB, 135
Nail-patella syndrome, 137
Osteoporosis-pseudoglioma syndrome,
154
Pallister-Killian syndrome, 156
Rubinstein-Taybi syndrome, 182
Seckel syndrome, 188
Stickler syndrome, 200
The 3-M syndrome, 208
Velo-cardio-facial syndrome, 219
Wrinkly skin syndrome, 230
Zimmermann-Laband syndrome, 231
Joint: limited mobility
Aase-Smith syndrome
Addison disease, 237
Amyloidosis, 245
Antley-Bixler syndrome, 11
Apert syndrome, 11
Aplasia cutis congenita, 4
Brachmann–de Lange syndrome, 22
Cerebro-oculo-facio-skeletal syndrome, 33
Christian syndrome, 36
Chromosomal abnormalities (8, 13, 18,
XXXXY, etc.)
Cockayne syndrome, 40
Contractural arachnodactyly, 44
Dermo-chondro-corneal dystrophy of
François, 54
Diabetes mellitus, 262
Digitotalar dysmorphism, 56
Epidermolysis bullosa, 67
Fabry disease, 266
Farber disease, 268
Femoral hypoplasia–unusual facies syn-
drome, 70
Fetal akinesia sequence, 71
Fetal alcohol syndrome, 71
Fibrodysplasia ossificans progressiva, 74
Fluorosis, 269
Freeman-Sheldon syndrome, 78
German syndrome
GM$_1$ gangliosidosis, 278
Golden-Lakim syndrome, 82
Gordon syndrome, 84
Hemophilia, 282
Infantile multisystem inflammatory dis-
ease, 100

Klein-Waardenburg syndrome, 108
Kniest dysplasia
Kuskokwim syndrome, 111
Léri syndrome, 114
Macrodystrophia lipomatosa, 119
Mandibuloacral dysplasia, 120
Marden-Walker syndrome, 121
Mietens-Weber syndrome, 130
Mixed connective tissue disease, 131
Moore-Federman syndrome
Mucolipidoses, 323, 324, 325
Mucopolysaccharidoses, 325
Multiple synostosis syndrome, 136
Nail-patella syndrome, 137
Pachydermoperiostosis, 155
Progeria, 168
Pterygium syndromes, 171
Rigid spine syndrome, 178
Schwartz-Jampel syndrome, 185
Scleroderma, 186
Seckel syndrome, 188
Shprintzen-Goldberg-syndrome, 189
Sjögren-Larsson syndrome, 369
Stickler syndrome, 200
Symphalangism-surdity syndrome, 205
Trismus–pseudocamptodactyly syndrome,
212
Tumoral calcinosis, 377
Weill-Marchesani syndrome, 224
Winchester syndrome, 384
Zellweger syndrome, 386

K
Kidney: cyst
Apert syndrome, 11
Aplasia cutis congenita, 4
Asplenia syndrome, 13
Bardet-Biedl syndrome, 16
Beckwith-Wiedemann syndrome, 17
Branchio-oto-renal syndrome, 23
Cerebro-reno-digital syndromes, 34
Chromosomal abnormalities
DiGeorge syndrome, 55
Ehlers-Danlos syndrome, 63
Eronen syndrome, 68
Femoral hypoplasia–unusual facies syn-
drome, 70
Fetal alcohol syndrome, 71
Fetal hydantoin syndrome, 72
Fryns syndrome, 79
Glutaric aciduria type II, 274

Hemihypertrophy, 90
Hepatic fibrosis–renal cystic disease, 92
Joubert syndrome, 103
Kaufman-McKusick syndrome, 106
Lissencephalies, 116
Marden-Walker syndrome, 121
Meckel syndrome, 125
Nephronophthisis, 138
Oculo-auriculo-vertebral spectrum, 147
Opitz trigonocephaly syndrome, 149
Oro-facio-digital syndrome I, 150
Pallister-Hall syndrome, 156
Polycystic kidney disease; autosomal
    dominant, 162
Polycystic kidney disease; autosomal
    recessive, 162
Polysplenia syndrome, 163
Potter sequence, 166
Prune-belly syndrome, 170
Renal-hepatic-pancreatic dysplasia, 176
Roberts syndrome, 179
Smith-Lemli-Opitz syndrome type I, 370
Tuberous sclerosis, 212
VATER association, 218
von Hippel–Lindau syndrome, 220
Williams syndrome, 227
Zellweger syndrome, 386
Kidney: large
Acromegaly, 235
Amyloidosis, 245
Bartter syndrome, 16
Beckwith-Wiedemann syndrome, 17
Cystic kidney disease
Diabetes insipidus, 261
Diabetes mellitus, 262
Gaucher disease, 272
Glycogen storage disease type I, 275
Goodpasture syndrome, 84
Hemihypertrophy, 90
Hemolytic uremic syndrome, 90
Hemophilia (hemorrhage), 282
Henoch-Schönlein syndrome, 91
Hydronephrosis
Lipodystrophy (lipoatrophic diabetes), 311
Mucopolysaccharidoses, 325
Multilocular cystic nephroma
Nephrotic syndrome, 138
Niemann-Pick disease, 336
Oxalosis, 343
POEMS syndrome, 161
Sickle cell anemia, 365

Tuberous sclerosis, 212
Tyrosinemia type I, 378
Wolman disease, 385
Kidney: small
Alport syndrome, 8
Amyloidosis, 245
Bardet-Biedl syndrome, 16
Bartter syndrome, 16
Diabetes mellitus, 262
Gout, 280
Hyperparathyroidism, 290
Nephronophthisis, 138
Oxalosis, 343
Tuberous sclerosis, 212

L

Labia major: aplasia or hypoplasia
Brachmann–de Lange syndrome, 22
Chromosomal abnormalities
Femoral hypoplasia–unusual facies syn-
    drome, 70
Fetal alcohol syndrome, 71
Pterygium syndromes, 171
Robinow syndrome
Lacrimal system: abnormal
Achalasia-adrenal-alacrima syndrome, 2
Branchio-oculo-facial syndrome, 23
Branchio-oto-renal syndrome, 23
Ectodermal dysplasia, anhidrotic
EEC syndrome, 62
Epidermal nevus syndrome, 66
Fraser syndrome, 77
Hypomelanosis of Ito, 98
Johanson-Blizzard syndrome, 103
Lacrimo-auriculo-dento-digital syndrome,
    111
Mikulicz syndrome, 130
Nasopalpebral lipoma-coloboma syn-
    drome, 137
Riley-Day syndrome (alacrima), 178
Larynx: anomaly
Cardiovocal syndrome, 27
Cerebro-costo-mandibular syndrome, 33
Epidermolysis bullosa, 67
Fraser syndrome (atresia), 77
Jadassohn-Lewandowsky syndrome, 103
Larsen syndrome, 112
Lipoid proteinosis, 313
Marshall-Smith syndrome, 123
Multiple endocrine neoplasia type IIB, 135
Oculo-auriculo-vertebral spectrum, 147

Opitz BBBG syndrome, 149
Pallister-Hall syndrome, 156
Relapsing polychondritis, 175
Velo-cardio-facial syndrome (web), 219
Larynx: premature cartilage calcification;
    refer to Calcification: larynx
Lens: dislocation
    Ehlers-Danlos syndrome, 63
    Homocystinuria, 285
    Marfan syndrome, 121
    Spondyloepimetaphyseal dysplasia with
        joint laxity
    Stickler syndrome, 200
    Weill-Marchesani syndrome, 224
Lens: opacity
    Alport syndrome, 8
    Lowe syndrome, 314
    Osteoporosis-pseudoglioma syndrome,
        154
    Stickler syndrome, 200
Leukodystrophies, dysmyelination
    Adrenoleukodystrophies, 239
    Alexander disease, 242
    Canavan disease, 250
    Cockayne syndrome, 40
    Glutaric aciduria type I, 274
    Krabbe disease, 307
    Leigh disease, 309
    Metachromatic leukodystrophies, 321
    Mitochondrial encephalopathies and
        encephalomyopathies
    Mucopolysaccharidoses, 325
    Multiple sulfatase deficiency, 334
    Navajo neuropathy, 335
    Pelizaeus-Merzbacher disease, 348
    Phenylketonuria, 350
    Salla disease, 362
    3-Hydroxy-3-methylglutaryl-coenzyme A
        lyase deficiency, 376
    Zellweger syndrome, 386
Limb: anomaly (miscellaneous)
    Amniotic band sequence, 9
    Brachmann–de Lange syndrome, 22
    CHILD syndrome, 36
    Cloverleaf skull–limb anomalies, 39
    Cranioectodermal dysplasia, 45
    Duane syndrome, 59
    Du Pan syndrome, 60
    Epidermal nevus syndrome, 66
    Fetal hydantoin syndrome, 72
    Goltz syndrome, 83

Gorlin syndrome, 85
Hallermann-Streiff syndrome, 88
Holt-Oram syndrome, 94
Hypoglossia-hypodactylia syndrome, 98
Nager acrofacial dysostosis, 136
Odonto-tricho-melic hypohidrotic dyspla-
    sia
Ophthalmo-mandibulo-melic dysplasia,
    148
Opitz trigonocephaly syndrome, 149
Oromandibular-limb hypogenesis, 152
Potter sequence, 166
Prune-belly syndrome, 170
Pterygium syndromes, 171
Roberts syndrome, 179
Robin sequence, 180
Sirenomelia, 192
Splenogonadal fusion/limb deformity, 196
Tabatznik syndrome, 205
TAR syndrome, 206
Thalidomide embryopathy, 207
Treacher Collins syndrome, 211
VATER association, 218
Limb: overgrowth
    Hemangiomas
    Hemihypertrophy, 90
    Klippel-Trenaunay syndrome, 109
    Lymphangioma
    Macrodystrophia lipomatosa, 119
    Maffucci syndrome, 119
    Neurofibromatosis I, 140
    Proteus syndrome, 169
    Sturge-Weber syndrome, 201
    Tuberous sclerosis, 212
    von Hippel–Lindau syndrome, 220
Limb: reduction
    Adams-Oliver syndrome, 4
    Aminopterin fetopathy, 8
    Amniotic band sequence, 9
    Brachmann–de Lange syndrome, 22
    CHILD syndrome, 36
    Chorionic villus sampling
    EEC syndrome, 62
    Fetal alcohol syndrome, 71
    Goltz syndrome, 83
    Hypoglossia-hypodactylia syndrome, 98
    Möbius syndrome, 132
    Odonto-tricho-melic hypohidrotic dyspla-
        sia
    Oromandibular-limb hypogenesis, 152
    Poland sequence, 162

Postaxial acrofacial dysostosis, Miller type, 164
Prune-belly syndrome, 170
Pterygium syndrome (popliteal), 171
Roberts syndrome, 179
Sirenomelia, 192
TAR syndrome, 206
Lip defect: fistula, pit, etc.
   Branchio-oculo-facial syndrome, 23
   Hypoglossia-hypodactylia syndrome, 98
   Oro-facio-digital syndromes, 150
   Pterygium syndromes, 171
   Saethre-Chotzen syndrome, 183
Lipomatosis
   Encephalo-cranio-cutaneous lipomatosis, 66
   Macrodystrophia lipomatosa, 119
   Madelung disease, 315
   Nasopalpebral lipoma-coloboma syndrome, 137
   Opitz BBBG syndrome, 149
   Proteus syndrome, 169
Liver: cirrhosis
   Alpers syndrome, 7
   Alpha$_1$-antitrypsin deficiency, 243
   Caroli syndrome, 28
   CREST syndrome, 46
   Cruveilhier-Baumgarten syndrome, 48
   Galactosemia, 270
   Glycogen storage disease type III, 276
   Glycogen storage disease type IV, 277
   Hemochromatosis, 281
   Hemophilia, 282
   Hypothyroidism (adult), 300
   Lipodystrophy (lipodystrophic diabetes), 311
   Renal tubular acidosis, 358
   Sea-blue histiocyte syndrome, 188
   Thalassemia, 374
   Tyrosinemia type I, 378
   Weber-Christian syndrome, 223
   Wilson disease, 383
Liver: fatty infiltration
   Cushing syndrome, 258
   Cystic fibrosis
   Diabetes mellitus, 262
   Glycogen storage disease type I, 275
   Kwashiorkor, 308
   Lipodystrophies, 311
   Lipoproteinemia

Malabsorption syndrome, 119
Reye syndrome, 177
Lymphangiectasia, intestinal
   Aplasia cutis
   Cystic fibrosis
   DiGeorge syndrome, 55
   Hennekam syndrome
   Noonan syndrome, 145
   Turner syndrome, 214
Lymphatic abnormalities, lymphedema
   Klippel-Trenaunay syndrome, 109
   Meige-Nonne-Milroy disease, 126
   Neurofibromatosis I, 140
   Opitz BBBG syndrome, 149
   Yellow nail syndrome, 230

M

Macrocephaly; megalencephaly; macrocrania
   Alexander disease, 242
   Bannayan-Riley-Ruvalcaba syndrome, 15
   Beckwith-Wiedemann syndrome, 17
   Canavan disease, 250
   Cardio-facio-cutaneous syndrome, 26
   Cowden syndrome, 44
   Cranioectodermal dysplasia, 45
   Cronkhite-Canada syndrome, 47
   Dandy-Walker syndrome, 50
   Familial megalencephaly (autosomal dominant)
   FG syndrome, 73
   Fragile X syndrome, 77
   Glutaric aciduria type I, 274
   GM$_1$ gangliosidosis, 278
   GM$_2$ gangliosidosis: Tay-Sachs disease, 279
   Gorlin syndrome, 85
   Greig cephalopolysyndactyly syndrome, 86
   Growth hormone deficiency
   Hydrolethalus syndrome, 95
   Hyperphosphatasia, 293
   Hypomelanosis of Ito, 98
   Hypothyroidism, 300
   Infantile multisystem inflammatory disease, 100
   Klippel-Trenaunay-Weber syndrome, 109
   Laron syndrome, 309
   Lhermitte-Duclos disease, 115
   Maple syrup urine disease, 317
   Marfan syndrome, 121

Marshall-Smith syndrome, 123
Metachromatic leukodystrophies, 321
Methylmalonic acidemia, 322
Mucolipidoses, 323, 324, 325
Mucopolysaccharidoses, 325
Noonan syndrome, 145
Pituitary gigantism, 235
Porencephaly
Proteus syndrome, 169
Ritscher-Schinzel syndrome, 179
Schwarz-Lélek syndrome, 185
Silver-Russell syndrome, 190
Sotos syndrome, 195
3-Hydroxy-3-methylglutaryl-coenzyme A
    lyase deficiency, 376
Tuberous sclerosis, 212
Weaver syndrome, 223
Wiedemann-Rautenstrauch syndrome, 226
Zellweger syndrome, 386
Macrodactyly
Klippel-Trenaunay-Weber syndrome, 109
Lymphangioma
Macrodystrophia lipomatosa, 119
Maffucci syndrome, 119
Neurofibromatosis I, 140
Plexiform neuroma
Proteus syndrome, 169
Tuberous sclerosis, 212
Macroglossia
Acromegaly, 235
Amyloidosis, 245
Beckwith-Wiedemann syndrome, 17
Chromosome 4p trisomy syndrome
Down syndrome, 57
Familial macroglossia
Glycogen storage disease type II, 276
GM_1 gangliosidosis, 278
Hypothyroidism (cretinism), 300
Infant of diabetic mother
Kocher-Debré-Sémélaigne syndrome, 307
Mucopolysaccharidosis I-H, 327
Mucopolysaccharidosis, I-S, 329
Mucopolysaccharidosis, VI, 333
Neurofibromatosis I, 140
Macrophthalmia
Aniridia
Axial myopia
Ehlers-Danlos syndrome, 63
Glaucoma
Homocystinuria, 285
Lowe syndrome, 314

Marfan syndrome, 121
Neurofibromatosis I, 140
Proteus syndrome, 169
Sturge-Weber syndrome, 201
Weill-Marchesani syndrome, 224
Macrostomia
Angelman syndrome, 10
Barber-Say syndrome
Beckwith-Wiedemann syndrome, 17
Neu-Laxova syndrome, 139
Oculo-auriculo-vertebral spectrum, 147
Opitz trigonocephaly syndrome, 149
Pallister-Killian syndrome, 156
Simpson-Golabi-Behmel syndrome, 191
Treacher Collins syndrome, 211
Williams syndrome, 227
Malabsorption
Abetalipoproteinemia, 234
Acrodermatitis enteropathica, 234
Addison disease, 237
Agammaglobulinemia, X-linked, 5
Alpha-chain disease, 244
Amyloidosis, 245
Anderson syndrome
Anorexia nervosa
Blind loop syndrome, 20
Brown bowel syndrome
Carcinoid syndrome, 252
Celiac axis compression syndrome, 31
Celiac disease, 254
Chronic granulomatous disease of child-
    hood, 256
Cronkhite-Canada syndrome, 47
Cystic fibrosis
Dermatomyositis
Diabetes mellitus, 262
Diverticulosis of jejunum–macrocytic ane-
    mia–steatorrhea syndrome
Ehlers-Danlos syndrome, 63
Henoch-Schönlein syndrome, 91
Histiocytosis X
Hyperthyroidism, 294
Hypoparathyroidism, 296
Immune disorders and lymphoid hyperpla-
    sia
Johanson-Blizzard syndrome, 103
Kwashiorkor, 308
Lymphangiectasia
Malabsorption syndrome, 119
Menkes disease, 319
Multiple endocrine neoplasia type IIB, 135

Nephrotic syndrome, 138
Pancreatitis
POEMS syndrome, 161
Polyglandular autoimmune disease, 352
Postgastrectomy syndromes, 165
Protein-losing enteropathy
Scleroderma, 186
Short-bowel syndrome, 189
Shwachman syndrome, 363
Sprue
Stagnant small-bowel syndrome, 198
Steatorrhea, idiopathic
VIPoma syndrome, 379
Whipple disease
Wolman disease, 385
Zollinger-Ellison syndrome, 387
Malrotation, intestinal
Abdominal heterotaxy
Apple peel intestinal atresia
Asplenia syndrome, 13
Brachmann–de Lange syndrom, 22
Cantrell syndrome, 25
Cat-eye syndrome, 30
Chromosomal abnormalities (13, 18, 21, etc.)
Coffin-Siris syndrome, 42
Familial intestinal malrotation
FG syndrome, 73
Marfan syndrome, 121
Meckel syndrome, 125
Mobile cecum syndrome
Polysplenia syndrome, 163
Prune-belly syndrome, 170
Marfanoid appearance
Gorlin syndrome, 85
Homocystinuria, 285
Marfanoid hypermobility syndrome, 122
Multiple endocrine neoplasia type I, 134
Multiple endocrine neoplasia type IIB, 135
Mastoid: advance pneumatization
Acromegaly, 235
Dyke-Davidoff-Masson syndrome, 60
Lipodystrophy (lipoatrophic diabetes), 311
Mastoid: underdeveloped
Cockayne syndrome, 40
Hypothyroidism, 300
Mucopolysaccharidoses, 325
Oto-palato-digital syndrome type I, 154
Treacher Collins syndrome, 211

Mastoiditis
Chronic granulomatous disease of childhood, 256
Gradenigo syndrome, 85
Histiocytosis X
Immotile cilia syndrome, 99
Immune disorders
Wiskott-Aldrich syndrome, 228
Megacolon
Amyloidosis, 245
Celiac disease, 254
Cystic fibrosis
Dermatomyositis
Diabetes mellitus, 262
Fetal cytomegalovirus infection
Functional constipation
Hinman syndrome, 93
Hirschsprung disease, 93
Hypothyroidism, 300
Multiple endocrine neoplasia type IIB, 135
Muscular dystrophies
Neurofibromatosis I, 140
Neurogenic megacolon
Ogilvie syndrome, 148
Riley-Day syndrome, 178
Scleroderma, 186
Sotos syndrome, 195
Sprue
Metacarpals: short
Aplasia cutis congenita, 12
Beckwith-Wiedemann syndrome, 17
Brachmann–de Lange syndrome, 22
Cephaloskeletal dysplasia, 32
CHILD syndrome, 36
Chromosome 18 trisomy syndrome, 37
Cockayne syndrome, 40
Coffin-Siris syndrome, 42
Cohen syndrome, 43
Fanconi anemia, 69
Fetal alcohol syndrome, 71
Fibrodysplasia ossificans progressiva, 74
Gorlin syndrome, 85
Hand-foot-genital syndrome, 89
Holt-Oram syndrome, 94
Hypoparathyroidism, 296
Hypothyroidism, 300
Larsen syndrome, 112
Mucolipidoses, 323, 324, 325
Mucopolysaccharidoses, 325
Opitz trigonocephaly syndrome, 149

Oto-palato-digital syndrome type I, 154
Pallister-Hall syndrome, 156
Poland sequence, 162
Pseudohypoparathyroidism, 355
Refsum disease, 357
Rothmund-Thomson syndrome, 181
Saethre-Chotzen syndrome, 183
Silver-Russell syndrome, 190
Sjögren-Larsson syndrome, 369
Tabatznik syndrome, 205
Turner syndrome, 214
Weill-Marchesani syndrome, 224
Metaphyseal cupping
   Cephaloskeletal dysplasia, 32
   Copper deficiency, 258
   GM$_1$ gangliosidosis, 278
   Hypophosphatasia, 297
   Infantile multisystem inflammatory disease, 100
   Insensitivity to pain (congenital), 101
   Menkes disease, 319
   Phenylketonuria, 350
   Rickets, 359
   Scurvy (postfracture), 362
   Sickle cell anemia, 365
   Vitamin A intoxication, 380
Metaphyseal spur
   Adenosine deaminase deficiency
   Copper deficiency, 258
   Hyperparathyroidism, 290
   Hypophosphatasia, 297
   Menkes disease, 319
   Scurvy, 362
Microcardia
   Addison disease, 237
   Adrenal hyperplasia (congenital), 238
   Anorexia nervosa
   Asthenia
   Kwashiorkor, 308
Microcephaly
   Anencephaly
   Angelman syndrome, 10
   Aspartylglucosaminuria, 247
   Börjeson-Forssman-Lehman syndrome, 22
   Brachmann–de Lange syndrome, 22
   Cephaloskeletal dysplasia, 32
   Cerebro-oculo-facial skeletal syndrome, 33
   Christian syndrome, 36
   Chromosomal abnormalities (13, 18, 21, etc.)
   Cockayne syndrome, 40

   Coffin-Siris syndrome, 42
   Cohen syndrome, 43
   Craniosynostosis
   Cutis verticis gyrata, 50
   Deprivation dwarfism, 260
   De Sanctis-Cacchione syndrome, 54
   Dubowitz syndrome, 59
   Fanconi anemia, 69
   Fetal alcohol syndrome, 71
   Fetal brain disruption sequence, 72
   Fetal hydantoin syndrome, 72
   Fraser syndrome, 77
   Galloway-Mowat syndrome, 80
   Goldberg-Shprintzen syndrome, 82
   Goltz syndrome, 83
   Homocystinuria, 285
   Incontinentia pigmenti, 100
   Johanson-Blizzard syndrome, 103
   Juberg-Hayward syndrome, 104
   Kearns-Sayre syndrome, 306
   Krabbe disease, 307
   Lenz microphthalmia syndrome, 113
   Lesch-Nyhan syndrome, 310
   Lissencephalies, 116
   Marinesco-Sjögren syndrome, 122
   Meckel syndrome, 125
   Menkes disease, 319
   Microcephalic osteodysplastic primordial dwarfism, 127
   Noonan syndrome, 145
   Opitz trigonocephaly syndrome, 149
   PEHO syndrome, 158
   Prader-Willi syndrome, 166
   Pyruvate dehydrogenase complex deficiency, 356
   Riley-Day syndrome, 178
   Rubinstein-Taybi syndrome, 182
   Seckel syndrome, 188
   Smith-Lemli-Opitz syndrome type I, 370
   Smith-Lemli-Opitz syndrome type II, 371
   Stoll-Charrow-Poznanski syndrome, 201
   Tuberous sclerosis, 212
   Wrinkly skin syndrome, 230
Microcolon
   Apple peel intestinal atresia
   Hirschsprung disease, 93
   Inspissated milk syndrome
   Intestinal atresia, familial
   Meconium ileus
   Small left colon syndrome, 193

Microglossia
    Freeman-Sheldon syndrome, 78
    Hypoglossia-hypodactylia syndrome, 98
    Möbius syndrome, 132
    Oromandibular-limb hypogenesis, 152
    Pallister-Hall syndrome, 156
Micrognathia
    Acrogeria, 4
    Aminopterin fetopathy, 8
    Aminopterin fetopathy-like syndrome, 9
    Aniridia-Wilms tumor association, 10
    Bloom syndrome, 20
    Brachmann–de Lange syndrome, 22
    Catel-Manzke syndrome, 30
    Cat-eye syndrome, 30
    Cerebro-costo-mandibular syndrome, 33
    Cerebro-oculo-facio-skeletal syndrome, 33
    CHARGE association, 34
    Charlie M syndrome, 152
    Chromosome 13 trisomy syndrome, 37
    Chromosome 18 trisomy syndrome, 37
    Cockayne syndrome, 40
    Cohen syndrome, 43
    Contractural arachnodactyly, 44
    Cowden syndrome, 44
    DiGeorge syndrome, 55
    Dubowitz syndrome, 59
    Ehlers-Danlos syndrome, 63
    Femoral hypoplasia–unusual facies syndrome, 70
    Fetal akinesia sequence, 71
    Fetal alcohol syndrome, 71
    Fetal valproate syndrome, 73
    FG syndrome, 73
    Freeman-Sheldon syndrome, 78
    Fryns syndrome, 79
    GAPO syndrome, 80
    Gardener-Silengo-Wachtel syndrome, 81
    German syndrome
    Hajdu-Cheney syndrome, 87
    Hallermann-Streiff syndrome, 88
    Hydrolethalus syndrome, 95
    Hypoglossia–hypodactylia syndrome, 98
    Johanson-Blizzard syndrome, 103
    Klippel-Feil syndrome, 109
    Larsen syndrome, 112
    Mandibuloacral dysplasia, 120
    Marden-Walker syndrome, 121
    Marshall-Smith syndrome, 123
    Meckel syndrome, 125

    Miller-Dieker syndrome, 130
    Möbius syndrome, 132
    MURCS association, 136
    Nager acrofacial dysostosis, 136
    Neu-Laxova syndrome, 139
    Noonan syndrome, 145
    Oculo-auriculo-vertebral spectrum, 147
    Ophthalmo-mandibulo-melic dysplasia, 148
    Opitz trigonocephaly syndrome, 149
    Oro-facio-digital syndrome I, 150
    Oro-facio-digital syndrome II, 150
    Oromandibular-limb hypogenesis, 152
    Osteolysis with nephropathy, 153
    Pallister-Hall syndrome, 156
    Pallister-Killian syndrome, 156
    Postaxial acrofacial dysostosis, Miller type, 164
    Potter sequence, 166
    Progeria, 168
    Pterygium syndromes, 171
    Pycnodysostosis
    Roberts syndrome, 179
    Rubinstein-Taybi syndrome, 182
    Schwartz-Jampel syndrome, 185
    Seckel syndrome, 188
    Silver-Russell syndrome, 190
    Smith-Lemli-Opitz syndrome type I, 370
    Smith-Lemli-Opitz syndrome type II, 371
    Stickler syndrome, 200
    TAR syndrome, 206
    Treacher Collins syndrome, 211
    Turner syndrome, 214
    Velo-cardio-facial syndrome, 219
    Weaver syndrome, 223
    Williams syndrome, 227
    Zellweger syndrome, 386
Microphthalmia
    Adams-Oliver syndrome, 4
    Amniotic band sequence, 9
    Bardet-Biedl syndrome, 16
    Branchio-oculo-facial syndrome, 23
    Cat-eye syndrome, 30
    Cerebro-oculo-facio-skeletal syndrome, 33
    CHARGE association, 34
    Chromosomal abnormalities
    Cohen syndrome, 43
    Cross syndrome, 47
    Delleman syndrome, 52
    Fanconi anemia, 69
    Fetal alcohol syndrome, 71

Frontonasal dysplasia, 78
Goltz syndrome, 83
Hallermann-Streiff syndrome, 88
Holoprosencephaly, 94
Hydrolethalus syndrome, 95
Hypopituitarism (anterior lobe), 298
Incontinentia pigmenti, 100
Infant of diabetic mother
Lenz microphthalmia syndrome, 113
Meckel syndrome, 125
Neu-Laxova syndrome, 139
Oculo-auriculo-vertebral spectrum, 147
Oculo-dento-osseous dysplasia, 147
Osteoporosis–pseudoglioma
    syndrome, 154
Pallister-Hall syndrome, 156
Phenylketonuria, 350
Proteus syndrome, 169
Pseudohypoparathyroidism, 355
Roberts syndrome, 179
Thalidomide embryopathy, 207
Treacher Collins syndrome, 211
VATER association, 218
Warfarin embryopathy, 222
Microspherophakia
Alport syndrome, 8
Familial microspherophakia
Homocystinuria, 285
Hyperlysinemia
Klinefelter syndrome, 108
Lowe syndrome, 314
Mandibulofacial dysostosis, 211
Marfan syndrome, 121
Weill-Marchesani syndrome, 224
Microstomia
Bardet-Biedl syndrome, 16
Branchio-oculo-facial syndrome, 23
Cerebro-costo-mandibular syndrome, 33
Chromosome 18 trisomy syndrome, 37
Cowden syndrome, 44
Down syndrome, 57
Fetal akinesia sequence, 71
Freeman-Sheldon syndrome, 78
Hallermann-Streiff syndrome, 88
Hypertelorism–microtia–facial clefting
    syndrome, 98
Hypoglossia-hypodactylia syndrome, 98
Marden-Walker syndrome, 121
Oromandibular-limb hypogenesis, 152
Oto-palato-digital syndrome type I, 154
Schwartz-Jampel syndrome, 185

Trismus-pseudocamptodactyly syndrome,
    212
Microtia
CHARGE association, 34
DiGeorge syndrome, 55
Down syndrome, 57
FG syndrome, 73
Hypertelorism–microtia–facial cleft
    ing syndrome, 98
Kabuki make-up syndrome, 104
Lacrimo-auriculo-dento-digital syndrome,
    111
Nager acrofacial dysostosis, 136
Oculo-auriculo-vertebral spectrum, 147
Postaxial acrofacial dysostosis, Miller
    type, 164
Townes-Brocks syndrome, 210
Treacher Collins syndrome, 211
Wildervanck syndrome, 226
Mitochondrial disorders
Alpers syndrome, 7
Kearns-Sayre syndrome, 306
Leigh disease, 309
MELAS syndrome, 318
Menkes disease, 319
MERRF (myoclonus, epilepsy, and ragged
    red fibers)
Mitral valve disease
Alkaptonuria, 243
Contractural arachnodactyly, 44
Cutis laxa, 49
Ehlers-Danlos syndrome, 63
Floppy valve syndrome, 75
Fragile X syndrome, 77
Geleophysic dysplasia
Mannosidoses, 316
Marfan syndrome, 121
Marfanoid hypermobility syndrome, 122
Mitral valve prolapse syndromes
Mucolipidoses (II, III), 323, 324
Mucopolysaccharidoses (I-H, I-H/S, II,
    VII), 327, 328, 329, 334
Osteogenesis imperfecta (I, III, IV)
Pseudoxanthoma elasticum
Relapsing polychondritis, 175
Takayasu arteritis
Muscle: absent or deficient
Möbius syndrome, 132
Poland sequence, 162
Potter sequence, 166
Prune-belly syndrome, 170

Muscle: large
    Hoffmann syndrome (hypothyroidism,
        adult), 301
    Kocher-Debré-Sémélaigne syndrome, 307
    Lipodystrophy (lipoatrophic diabetes), 311
Muscular atrophy
    Arthrogryposis
    Charcot-Marie-Tooth disease, 34
    Duchenne muscular dystrophy
    Freeman-Sheldon syndrome, 78
    Glycogen storage disease type V, 277
    Kugelberg-Welander syndrome, 110
    Kuskokwim syndrome, 111
    Madelung disease, 315
    Multiple endocrine neoplasia type IIB,
        135
    Pancoast syndrome, 157
    Progeria, 168
    Rieger syndrome
    Schwartz-Jampel syndrome, 185
    Tethered cord syndrome, 207
    Werner syndrome, 224
Muscular hypertonicity
    Brachmann–de Lange syndrome, 22
    Canavan disease, 250
    Chromosome 13 trisomy syndrome, 37
    Chromosome 18 trisomy syndrome, 37
    Fahr disease, 267
    Freeman-Sheldon syndrome, 78
    Fucosidosis, 270
    Hypothyroidism (Hoffmann syndrome),
        300
    Krabbe disease, 307
    Machado-Joseph disease
    Melorheostosis
    Menkes disease, 319
    Satoyoshi syndrome, 184
    Schwartz-Jampel syndrome, 185
    Sjögren-Larsson syndrome, 369
    Stiff-man syndrome, 200
    Vitamin A intoxication, 380
    Weaver-Smith syndrome, 223
Muscular hypotonicity
    Aluminum intoxication, 245
    Börjeson-Forssman-Lehmann syndrome,
        22
    Canavan disease, 250
    Cerebro-oculo-facio-skeletal syndrome, 33
    Christian syndrome, 36
    Chromosome 5 partial short-arm deletion
    Chromosome 13 trisomy syndrome, 37

Chromosome XXXXY syndrome
Cohen syndrome, 43
Copper deficiency, 258
Cutis verticis gyrata, 50
Down syndrome, 57
Fetal alcohol syndrome, 71
FG syndrome, 73
Galactosemia, 270
Galloway-Mowat syndrome, 80
German syndrome
Geroderma osteodysplastica, 81
Glycogen storage disease type II, 276
GM_1 gangliosidosis, 278
GM_2 gangliosidosis: Tay-Sachs disease,
    279
Hyperparathyroidism (neonatal), 290
Hypomelanosis of Ito, 98
Hypothyroidism (infant), 300
Johanson-Blizzard syndrome, 103
Lissencephalies, 116
Lowe syndrome, 314
Lysinuric protein intolerance, 314
Mannosidoses, 316
Marfan syndrome, 121
Marinesco-Sjögren syndrome, 122
Methylmalonic acidemia, 322
Mulibrey nanism, 134
Multiple endocrine neoplasia type IIB, 135
Myasthenia syndromes
Myotonic dystrophy
Nemaline myopathy
Osteoporosis–pseudoglioma syndrome,
    154
Pallister-Killian syndrome type I, 370, 156
PEHO syndrome, 158
Prader-Willi syndrome, 166
Smith-Lemli-Opitz syndrome type I, 370
Werdnig-Hoffmann disease
Wrinkly skin syndrome, 230
Zellweger syndrome, 386
Myelopathy: acquired
    Adrenomyeloneuropathy, 239
    Calcium pyrophosphate dihydrate
        deposition disease, 249
    Central cord syndrome, 31
    Déjérine-Sottas syndrome, 52
    Fluorosis, 269
    Guillain-Barré syndrome, 87
    Kugelberg-Welander syndrome, 110
    Mucopolysaccharidosis I-H, 327
    Mucopolysaccharidosis I-H/S, 328

Mucopolysaccharidosis VI, 333
Paraneoplastic syndromes, 344
Schwartz-Jampel syndrome, 185
Myocardial infarction
    Alkaptonuria, 243
    Arterial calcification of infancy, 12
    Degos syndrome, 51
    Fabry disease, 266
    Homocystinuria, 285
    Kawasaki syndrome, 106
    Mucopolysaccharidoses (I-H, II, VI), 327,
        329, 333
    Pseudoxanthoma elasticum
    Takayasu arteritis
Myoclonus
    Gaucher disease, 272
    GM_2 gangliosidosis, 279
    Kearns-Sayre syndrome, 306
    Leigh disease, 309
    MELAS syndrome, 318
    Neuronal ceroid lipofuscinosis, 336
    Niemann-Pick disease, 336
    Opsoclonus-myoclonus syndrome, 150
    Progressive myoclonus epilepsy
    Reflex epilepsy
    Refsum disease, 357
    Sialidosis, 364
Myopathy
    Aluminum intoxication, 245
    Behçet syndrome, 18
    Carnitine deficiency syndromes, 253
    Christian syndrome: myopathic face, 36
    Cushing syndrome, 258
    Glycogen storage disease (types II, III, V),
        276, 277
    GM_1 gangliosidosis, 278
    Hypoparathyroidism, 296
    Hypothyroidism, 300
    Kawasaki syndrome, 106
    MELAS syndrome, 318
    Myasthenia gravis
    Myotubular myopathy
    Nemaline myopathy
    Paraneoplastic syndrome, 344
    Rigid spine syndrome, 178
    Xanthine oxidase deficiency, 385
Myopia
    Alagille syndrome, 6
    Alport syndrome, 8
    Aminopterin fetopathy, 8
    Brachmann–de Lange syndrome, 22

Branchio-oculo-facial syndrome, 23
Branchio-oto-renal syndrome, 23
Chromosomal abnormalities
Cohen syndrome, 43
Cranioectodermal dysplasia, 45
Ehlers-Danlos syndrome, 63
Fetal alcohol syndrome, 71
Hajdu-Cheney syndrome, 87
Homocystinuria, 285
Incontinentia pigmenti, 100
Marfan syndrome, 121
Marshall syndrome, 123
Marshall-Smith syndrome, 123
Mucopolysaccharidosis I-S, 329
Muscle–eye–brain disease
Noonan syndrome, 145
Proteus syndrome, 169
Rubinstein-Taybi syndrome, 182
Schwartz-Jampel syndrome, 185
Stickler syndrome, 200
Weill-Marchesani syndrome, 224

N
Nail: aplasia, hypoplasia, deformity, dystro-
        phy
    Acrogeria, 4
    Amniotic band sequence, 9
    Antley-Bixler syndrome, 11
    Aplasia cutis congenita (Adams-Oliver
        syndrome), 4
    CHILD syndrome, 36
    Chromosomal abnormalities (4, 8, 9, 13,
        18, XO, etc.)
    Clouston syndrome, 39
    Coffin-Siris syndrome, 42
    Cronkhite-Canada syndrome, 47
    DOOR syndrome, 56
    Dyskeratosis congenita, 60
    Ectodermal dysplasia, hereditary
    EEC syndrome, 62
    Epidermolysis bullosa, 67
    Eronen syndrome, 68
    Fetal alcohol syndrome, 71
    Fetal hydantoin syndrome, 72
    Fetal valproate syndrome, 73
    Fryns syndrome, 79
    Fuhrmann syndrome, 79
    Goltz syndrome, 83
    Hajdu-Cheney syndrome, 87
    Hallermann-Streiff syndrome, 88
    Hypothyroidism (infants), 300

Incontinentia pigmenti, 100
Iso-Kikuchi syndrome, 102
Jadassohn-Lewandowsky syndrome, 103
Larsen syndrome, 112
LEOPARD syndrome, 113
Mandibuloacral dysplasia, 120
Multiple synostosis syndrome, 136
Nail-patella syndrome, 137
Oto-palato-digital syndrome type I, 154
Pallister-Hall syndrome, 156
Polyglandular autoimmune disease, 352
Progeria, 168
Pterygium syndromes, 171
Roberts syndrome, 179
Rothmund-Thomson syndrome, 181
Rubinstein-Taybi syndrome, 182
Schinzel-Giedion syndrome, 184
Sotos syndrome, 195
Tricho-dento-osseous syndrome, 211
Trichorrhexis nodosa syndrome, 212
Warfarin embryopathy, 222
Weaver syndrome, 223
Williams syndrome, 227
Yellow nail syndrome, 230
Zimmermann-Laband syndrome, 231
Nail: discoloration
POEMS syndrome, 161
Wilson disease, 383
Yellow nail syndrome, 230
Nail: onycholysis
Hyperthyroidism, 294
Incontinentia pigmenti, 100
Iron deficiency anemia, 305
Porphyrias, 353
Stevens-Johnson syndrome, 199
Yellow nail syndrome, 230
Neck: cyst
Chromosomal abnormalities
Pterygium syndromes, 171
Roberts syndrome, 179
Neck: short
Aarskog syndrome, 2
CHARGE association, 34
Chromosome 18 trisomy syndrome, 37
Chromosome XXXXY syndrome
Contractural arachnodactyly, 44
Diamond-Blackfan syndrome, 54
Down syndrome, 57
Fetal alcohol syndrome, 71
Fetal hydantoin syndrome, 72
Freeman-Sheldon syndrome, 78

Fryns syndrome, 79
Hajdu-Cheney syndrome, 87
Hyperphosphatasia, 293
Joubert syndrome, 103
Klippel-Feil syndrome, 109
Kniest dysplasia
Meckel syndrome, 125
Neu-Laxova syndrome, 139
Noonan syndrome, 145
Pallister-Killian syndrome, 156
Schwartz-Jampel syndrome, 185
Smith-Lemli-Opitz syndrome type I, 370
Smith-Lemli-Opitz syndrome type II, 371
Spondylocostal dysostoses, 197
The 3-M syndrome, 208
Turner syndrome, 214
Warfarin embryopathy, 222
Neck: web, fold
Aase syndrome, 2
Bardet-Biedl syndrome, 16
Cerebro-costo-mandibular syndrome, 33
Chromosomal abnormalities: 13, 18, 21,
        XO, XXX, XXXX, XXXXY, etc.
Diamond-Blackfan syndrome, 54
DiGeorge syndrome, 55
Distichiasis-lymphedema syndrome, 56
Fetal alcohol syndrome, 71
Fetal hydantoin syndrome, 72
Freeman-Sheldon syndrome, 78
Golden-Lakim syndrome, 82
Hypothyroidism, congenital, 300
Klippel-Feil syndrome, 109
Lenz microphthalmia syndrome, 113
LEOPARD syndrome, 113
Meckel syndrome, 125
Noonan syndrome, 145
Pterygium syndromes, 171
Nephrocalcinosis
Alkaptonuria, 243
Alport syndrome, 8
Amelogenesis imperfecta– nephrocalci-
        nosis
Aminoaciduria
Amyloidosis, 245
Bartter syndrome, 16
Bicarbonate-induced nephrocalcinosis
Blue diaper syndrome, 249
Cushing syndrome; steroid therapy, 258
Ehlers-Danlos syndrome, 63
Glycogen storage disease type I, 275
Gout, 280

Hemolytic uremic syndrome, 90
Hepatic fibrosis–renal cystic disease, 92
Hypercalcemia
Hypercholesterolemia, 288
Hyperparathyroidism, 290
Hyperphosphatasia, 293
Hyperthyroidism, 294
Hypophosphatasia, 297
Hypothyroidism (juvenile), 300
McCune-Albright syndrome, 125
Milk-alkali syndrome, 323
Nail-patella syndrome, 137
Oxalosis, 343
Paraneoplastic syndromes, 344
Pseudohypoparathyroidism, 355
Renal tubular acidosis, 358
Rickets, vitamin D–resistant, 359
Shwachman syndrome, 363
Sickle cell anemia, 365
Sjögren syndrome, 192
Vitamin D intoxication, 382
Wilson disease, 383
Xanthine oxidase deficiency, 385
Zollinger-Ellison syndrome, 387
Nephropathy
Alagille syndrome, 6
Alkaptonuria, 243
Alport syndrome, 8
Amyloidosis, 245
Bardet-Biedl syndrome, 16
Bartter syndrome, 16
Behçet syndrome, 18
Carbonic anhydrase II deficiency, 252
Cockayne syndrome, 40
Cystinosis, 259
Cystinuria, 260
Denys-Drash syndrome, 53
Diabetes mellitus, 262
Fabry disease, 266
Fanconi syndrome, 268
Galloway-Mowat syndrome, 80
Gaucher disease, 272
Glycogen storage disease type I, 275
Glycogen storage disease type V, 277
Goodpasture syndrome, 84
Gout, 280
Hemolytic uremic syndrome, 90
Hemophilia, 282
Henoch-Schönlein syndrome, 91
Hepatic fibrosis–renal cystic disease, 92
Hyperparathyroidism, 290

Lesch-Nyhan syndrome, 310
Lowe syndrome, 314
Milk-alkali syndrome, 323
Nail-patella syndrome, 137
Nephronophthisis, 138
Nephrotic syndrome, 138
Osteolysis with nephropathy, 153
Oxalosis, 343
Paraneoplastic syndromes, 344
Pseudohypoaldosteronism type II, 84
Renal tubular acidosis, 358
Riley-Day syndrome, 178
Shwachman syndrome, 363
Sickle cell anemia, 365
Tyrosinemia type I, 378
Vitamin D intoxication, 382
Wilson disease, 383
Wiskott-Aldrich syndrome, 228
Zellweger syndrome, 386
Nerve and nerve root: enlargement
Acromegaly, 235
Charcot-Marie-Tooth disease, 34
Déjérine-Sottas syndrome, 52
Guillain-Barré syndrome, 87
Neurofibromatosis I, 140
Neurofibromatosis II, 144
Refsum disease, 357
Neurocutaneous syndromes
Ataxia-telangiectasia syndrome, 14
Cowden syndrome, 44
Encephalo-cranio-cutaneous lipomatosis, 66
Epidermal nevus syndrome, 66
Hypomelanosis of Ito, 98
Incontinentia pigmenti, 100
Klippel-Trenaunay-Weber syndrome, 109
Neurocutaneous melanosis sequence, 139
Neurofibromatosis I, 140
Rendu-Osler-Weber syndrome, 176
Sturge-Weber syndrome, 201
Tuberous sclerosis, 212
von Hippel–Lindau syndrome, 220
Neurodegenerative metabolic brain disorders
    in children
Aminoacid and organic acid metabolic
    disorders
Krabbe disease, 307
Leigh disease, 309
Lipoid proteinosis, 313
Lowe syndrome, 314
Lysosomal storage disease
Maple syrup urine disease, 317

Metachromatic leukodystrophies, 321
Mitochondrial dysfunction
 Peroxisomal disorders, 349
 Sulfite oxidase deficiency
 3-Hydroxy-3-methylglutaryl-coenzyme A
  lyase deficiency, 376
Neuropathy, peripheral
 Adrenoleukodystrophy and adreno-
  myeloneuropathy, 239
 Andermann syndrome, 9
 Cerebrotendinous xanthomatosis, 255
 Charcot-Marie-Tooth disease, 34
 Déjérine-Sottas syndrome, 52
 Fucosidosis, 270
 GM$_1$ gangliosidosis, 278
 Hajdu-Cheney syndrome, 87
 Hereditary sensory neuropathies
  Insensitivity to pain (congenital), 101
  Congenital sensory neuropathy
  Congenital sensory neuropathy with
   anhidrosis
  Familial dysautonomia
  Hereditary sensory radicular neuropa-
   thy
 Hyperthyroidism (thyrotoxic periodic
  paralysis), 294
 Krabbe disease, 307
 Lead intoxication
 Navajo neuropathy, 335
 POEMS syndrome, 161
 Porphyrias, 353
 Quadrilateral space syndrome, 172
 Refsum disease, 357
 Thevenard syndrome, 208
 Vitamin B$_1$ deficiency, 381
 Wernicke-Korsakoff syndrome, 225
Nipple: anomaly
 Adams-Oliver syndrome, 4
 Bannayan-Riley-Ruvalcaba syndrome, 15
 Brachmann–de Lange syndrome, 22
 Cerebro-oculo-facio-skeletal syndrome,
  33
 Chromosomal abnormalities
 Ectodermal dysplasia (hypohidrotic), 61
 EEC syndrome, 62
 Fetal hydantoin syndrome, 72
 Fraser syndrome, 77
 Johanson-Blizzard syndrome, 103
 Leprechaunism, 310
 Mucolipidosis II, 323
 Noonan syndrome, 145

Poland sequence, 162
Postaxial acrofacial dysostosis syndrome,
 Miller type, 164
Progeria, 168
Pterygium syndromes (Escobar syn-
 drome), 171
Schinzel-Giedion syndrome, 184
Ulnar-mammary syndrome, 217
Weaver syndrome, 223
Nose: bifid
 Cranio-fronto-nasal dysplasia, 45
 Fronto-facio-nasal dysplasia, 78
 Frontonasal dysplasia, 78
 Hypertelorism–microtia–facial clefting
  syndrome, 98
 Laurin-Sandrow syndrome, 113
 Oro-facio-digital syndrome II, 150
Nose: polyp
 Azoospermia–nasal polyposis
 Cystic fibrosis
 Immotile cilia syndrome, 99
 Kartagener syndrome, 105
 Peutz-Jeghers syndrome, 159
Nose: prominent/bulbous
 Alagille syndrome, 6
 Coffin-Lowry syndrome, 42
 Rubinstein-Taybi syndrome, 182
 Seckel syndrome, 188
 Smith-Lemli-Opitz syndrome
 Symphalangism-surdity syndrome, 205
 Velocardiofacial syndrome, 219
Nose: small
 Aarskog syndrome, 2
 Apert syndrome, 11
 Binder syndrome, 19
 Brachmann–de Lange syndrome, 22
 Chromosomal abnormalities (13, 18, 21,
  XXXXY, etc.)
 Femoral hypoplasia–unusual facies syn-
  drome, 70
 Fetal akinesia sequence, 71
 Fetal alcohol syndrome, 71
 Fetal hydantoin syndrome, 72
 Fetal valproate syndrome, 73
 Hallermann-Streiff syndrome, 88
 Marshall syndrome, 123
 Marshall-Smith syndrome, 123
 Miller-Dieker syndrome, 130
 Mucolipidosis II, 323
 Oculo-dento-osseous dysplasia, 147
 Opitz trigonocephaly syndrome, 149

Oto-palato-digital syndrome type I, 154
Pallister-Hall syndrome, 156
Pallister-Killian syndrome, 156
Pfeiffer syndrome, 160
Rothmund-Thomson syndrome, 181
Treacher Collins syndrome, 211
Waardenburg syndrome (thin nose), 221
Warfarin embryopathy, 222
Williams syndrome, 227
Nystagmus
Aniridia-Wilms tumor association, 10
Ataxia-telangiectasia syndrome, 14
Bardet-Biedl syndrome, 16
Börjeson-Forssman-Lehmann syndrome, 22
Cerebro-oculo-facio-skeletal syndrome, 33
Chédiak-Higashi syndrome, 35
Cockayne syndrome, 40
Cranioectodermal dysplasia, 45
de Morsier syndrome, 53
Epidermal nevus syndrome, 66
Fanconi anemia, 69
Fragile X syndrome, 77
Hajdu-Cheney syndrome, 87
Hallermann-Streiff syndrome, 88
Marinesco-Sjögren syndrome, 122
Mietens-Weber syndrome, 130
Noonan syndrome, 145
Parinaud syndrome, 158
Proteus syndrome, 169
Pseudohypoparathyroidism, 355
Stoll-Charrow-Poznanski syndrome, 201
Wallenberg syndrome, 222
Zellweger syndrome, 386

O
Obesity
Bardet-Biedl syndrome, 16
Börjeson-Forssman-Lehmann syndrome, 22
Carpenter syndrome, 29
Chromosomal abnormalities (4, 21, XO, XXY, XXXXY)
Cohen syndrome, 43
Cushing syndrome, 258
Morgagni-Stewart-Morel syndrome, 132
Pallister-Killian syndrome, 156
Pickwickian syndrome, 161
Polycystic ovary syndrome, 351
Prader-Willi syndrome, 166
Pseudohypoparathyroidism, 355

Sleep apnea syndrome, 193
Ulnar-mammary syndrome, 217
Omphalocele, gastroschisis
Beckwith-Wiedemann syndrome, 17
Cantrell syndrome, 25
Chromosomal abnormalities
Hypothyroidism, 300
Optic atrophy
Behr syndrome, 248
Bobble-head doll syndrome, 21
Brachmann–de Lange syndrome, 22
Cohen syndrome, 43
de Morsier syndrome, 53
Fetal alcohol syndrome, 71
Foster Kennedy syndrome, 76
GAPO syndrome, 80
GM_2 gangliosidosis: Tay-Sacks disease, 279
Hajdu-Cheney syndrome, 87
Hallervorden-Spatz disease, 281
Homocystinuria, 285
Hyperphosphatasia, 293
Incontinentia pigmenti, 100
Morning glory syndrome, 133
Multiple sulfatase deficiency, 334
Muscle–eye–brain disease
PEHO syndrome, 158
Refsum disease, 357
Vitamin B_1 deficiency, 381
Wolfram syndrome, 229, 264
Orbit: large
Craniosynostosis (coronal)
Glaucoma (congenital)
Hyperthyroidism, 294
Neurofibromatosis I, 140
Pseudotumor
Varix of orbital vein
Orbit: shallow
Apert syndrome, 11
Cloverleaf skull deformity, 39
Crouzon syndrome, 47
Larsen syndrome, 112
Marshall-Smith syndrome, 123
Mucopolysaccharidosis I-H, 327
Weill-Marchesani syndrome, 224
Orbit: small
Anophthalmos
Chromosome 13 trisomy syndrome, 37
Enucleation in childhood
Fibrous dysplasia
Hallermann-Streiff syndrome, 88

Oculo-dento-osseous dysplasia, 147
Osteoporosis-pseudoglioma syndrome,
    154
Paget disease
Ossification, soft tissue
    Ehlers-Danlos syndrome, 63
    Fibrodysplasia ossificans progressiva, 74
    Myositis ossificans progressiva, 74
    Osteoma cutis, 154
    Pachydermoperiostosis, 155
    Pseudohypoparathyroidism, 355
Osteolysis
    Ehlers-Danlos syndrome, 63
    Gorham syndrome, 84
    Hajdu-Cheney syndrome, 87
    Hyperparathyroidism, 290
    Keratosis palmaris et plantaris familiaris
        (tylosis), 107
    Kuskokwim syndrome, 111
    Mixed connective tissue disease, 131
    Osteolysis, familial expansile, 153
    Osteolysis with nephropathy, 153
    Osteolysis without nephropathy, 153
    Progeria, 168
    Rothmund-Thomson syndrome, 181
    Satoyoshi syndrome, 184
    Scleroderma, 186
    Singleton-Merten syndrome, 191
    Thevenard syndrome, 208
    Wegener granulomatosis
    Winchester syndrome, 384
Osteoporosis
    Acromegaly, 235
    Addison disease, 237
    Alkaptonuria, 243
    Aluminum intoxication, 245
    Anemias
    Aspartylglucosaminuria, 247
    Autosomal-recessive sparse hair
    Calcium hydroxyapatite crystal deposition
        disease, 286
    Celiac disease, 254
    Cerebro-oculo-facio-skeletal syndrome, 33
    Chromosomal abnormalities (13, 18, 21,
        XO, etc.)
    Cockayne syndrome, 40
    Contractural arachnodactyly, 44
    Copper deficiency, 258
    Cranioectodermal dysplasia, 45
    CREST syndrome, 46
    Cushing syndrome, 258

Deprivation dwarfism, 260
Diabetes mellitus, 262
Dyskeratosis congenita, 60
Ehlers-Danlos syndrome, 63
Epidermolysis bullosa, 67
Fanconi syndrome, 268
Farber disease, 268
Fibrodysplasia ossificans progressiva, 74
Focal scleroderma, 75
Gaucher disease, 272
Geroderma osteodysplastica, 81
Glycogen storage disease type I, 275
GM$_1$ gangliosidosis, 278
Goltz syndrome, 83
Gorham syndrome, 84
Gout, 280
Grant syndrome, 86
Hajdu-Cheney syndrome, 87
Hallermann-Streiff syndrome, 88
Hemochromatosis, 281
Hemophilia, 282
Homocystinuria, 285
Hypercalcemia, idiopathic
Hyperparathyroidism, 290
Hyperphosphatasia, 293
Hyperthyroidism, 294
Hypogonadism
Hypoparathyroidism, 296
Hypophosphatasia, 297
Hypopituitarism (anterior lobe), 298
Hypothyroidism, 300
Infantile multisystem inflammatory dis-
    ease, 100
Kawasaki syndrome, 106
Keratosis palmaris et plantaris familiaris
    (tylosis), 107
Laron syndrome, 309
Lowe syndrome, 314
Lysinuric protein intolerance, 314
Malabsorption syndrome, 119
Mannosidoses, 316
Mauriac syndrome, 317
Membranous lipodystrophy, 319
Menkes disease, 319
Metachromatic leukodystrophies, 321
Mixed connective tissue disease, 131
Mucolipidoses, 323, 324, 325
Mucopolysaccharidoses, 325
Muscular dystrophies
Niemann-Pick disease, 336
Osteolysis with nephropathy, 153

Osteoporosis-pseudoglioma syndrome, 154
Papillon-Lefèvre syndrome, 157
Phenylketonuria, 350
Prader-Willi syndrome, 166
Progeria, 168
Pseudohypoparathyroidism, 355
Pyruvate kinase deficiency anemia, 357
Refsum disease, 357
Renal tubular acidosis, 358
Rickets/osteomalacia, 359
Rothmund-Thomson syndrome, 181
Scleroderma, 186
Scurvy, 362
Sickle cell anemia, 365
Singleton-Merten syndrome, 191
Spherocytosis, 372
Thalassemia, 374
Thevenard syndrome, 208
Thoracic outlet syndrome, 208
Trichorrhexis nodosa syndrome (peripheral osteopenia), 212
Vitamin D intoxication, 382
Werner syndrome, 224
Wilson dusease, 383
Winchester syndrome, 384
Wolman disease, 385
Osteosclerosis: periosteal hyperostosis, endosteal hyperostosis
Calcium hydroxyapatite crystal deposition disease, 286
Epidermal nevus syndrome, 66
Erdheim-Chester disease, 265
Fibrogenesis imperfecta ossium
Fluorosis, 269
Fucosidosis, 270
Gardner syndrome, 80
Gaucher disease, 272
Hypercalcemia, idiopathic
Hyperostosis-hyperphosphatemia syndrome, 97
Hyperparathyroidism (treated), 290
Hyperthyroidism (thyroid acropathy), 294
Hypoparathyroidism, 296
Hypothyroidism (infants, juvenile), 300
Lead intoxication
Lipodystrophy (lipoatrophic diabetes), 311
Neurofibromatosis I, 140
Osteoarthropathy, familial idiopathic, 152
Osteomalacia, healing, 360
Oxalosis, 343
Pachydermoperiostosis, 155

Patterson syndrome, 347
POEMS syndrome, 161
Pseudohypoparathyroidism, 355
Renal osteodystrophy, 292
Rothmund-Thomson syndrome, 181
Schwarz-Lélek syndrome, 185
Sickle cell anemia, 365
Sterno-costo-clavicular hyperostosis, 199
Stoll-Charrow-Poznanski syndrome, 201
Trichorrhexis nodosa syndrome (axial osteosclerosis), 212
Tuberous sclerosis, 212
Vitamin A intoxication, 380
Vitamin D intoxication, 382
Weismann-Netter syndrome, 224
Williams syndrome, 227
Ovarian tumor or cyst
Gorlin syndrome, 85
Hypothyroidism (juvenile), 300
Lipodystrophy (lipoatrophic diabetes), 311
McCune-Albright syndrome, 125
Meigs syndrome, 126
Ovarian hyperstimulation syndrome, 342
Peutz-Jeghers syndrome, 159
Polycystic ovary syndrome, 351
Polysplenia syndrome, 163

P
Pancreas: dysplasia (cysts, fibrosis, etc.)
Meckel syndrome, 125
Polysplenia syndrome, 163
Renal-hepatic-pancreatic dysplasia, 176
Shwachman syndrome, 363
Zellweger syndrome, 386
Pancreas: exocrine insufficiency
Cystic fibrosis
Familial pancreatic enzyme insufficiency
Mucolipidosis II, 323
Paucity of interlobular bile ducts–exocrine pancreatic insufficiency
Pearson syndrome, 348
Renal-hepatic-pancreatic dysplasia, 176
Shwachman syndrome, 363
Pancreas: fat deposition
Cystic fibrosis
Johanson-Blizzard syndrome, 103
Obesity
Shwachman syndrome, 363
Pancreatitis in children
Cystic fibrosis
Glycogen storage disease type Ia, 275

Hereditary pancreatitis
Homocystinuria, 285
Hyperlipoproteinemia, 287
Hyperparathyroidism, 290
Idiopathic pancreatitis
Infection
Malnutrition
Maple syrup urine disease, 317
Methylmalonic acidemia, 322
Pearson syndrome, 348
3-Hydroxy-3-methylglutaryl-coenzyme A
　lyase deficiency, 376
Pancytopenia
Aase syndrome, 2
Diamond-Blackfan syndrome, 54
Dyskeratosis congenita, 60
Fanconi anemia, 69
Hypothyroidism (infants), 300
Paralysis/paresis
Adrenoleukodystrophy, 239
Brown-Séquard syndrome, 24
Carpal tunnel syndrome, 28
Central cord syndrome, 31
Charcot-Marie-Tooth disease, 34
Cross syndrome, 47
Cutis verticis gyrata, 50
Déjérine-Sottas syndrome, 52
Dyke-Davidoff-Masson syndrome, 60
Epidermal nevus syndrome, 66
Foix-Chavany-Marie syndrome, 76
Gorlin syndrome, 85
Guillain-Barré syndrome, 87
Hemophilia, 282
Hereditary hemihypotrophy–hemipare-
　sis–hemiathetosis syndrome
Kawasaki syndrome, 106
Kugelberg-Welander syndrome, 110
Lesch-Nyhan syndrome, 310
Locked-in syndrome, 117
Man-in-the barrel syndrome, 120
Mucopolysaccharidosis IVA, 331
Neuronal ceroid lipofuscinosis, 336
Oculo-auriculo-vertebral spectrum, 147
Pancoast syndrome, 157
Ramsay Hunt syndrome (facial nerve),
　173
Steele-Richardson-Olszewski syndrome,
　198
Sturge-Weber syndrome, 201
Tethered cord syndrome, 207

Paralysis/paresis: cranial nerve
Amyloidosis, 245
Behçet syndrome, 18
Cardiofacial syndrome, 26
Claude syndrome, 39
Craniodiaphyseal dysplasia
Craniometaphyseal dysplasia
Déjérine-Sottas syndrome, 52
Epidermal nevus syndrome, 66
Gorlin syndrome, 85
Gradenigo syndrome, 85
Hajdu-Cheney syndrome, 87
Henoch-Schönlein syndrome, 91
Horner syndrome, 95
Hyperthyroidism, 294
Jugular foramen syndrome, 104
Kawasaki syndrome, 106
Kearns-Sayre syndrome, 306
Möbius syndrome, 132
Neurocutaneous melanosis sequence, 139
Oromandibular-limb hypogenesis, 152
Paraneoplastic syndromes, 344
Parinaud syndrome, 158
Poland sequence, 162
Wallenberg syndrome, 222
Wildervanck syndrome, 226
Patella: aplasia, dysplasia, hypoplasia, dislo-
　cation
Kuskokwim syndrome (hypoplastic), 111
Nail-patella syndrome (absent or
　hypoplastic), 137
Neurofibromatosis I (absent), 140
Pterygium syndrome; popliteal type
　(absent or bipartite), 171
Stickler syndrome (dislocated), 200
Pectoral muscle deficiency
Holt-Oram syndrome, 94
Möbius syndrome, 132
Poland sequence, 162
Pectus carinatum
Coffin-Lowry syndrome, 42
Ehlers-Danlos syndrome, 63
Fetal alcohol syndrome, 71
Homocystinuria, 285
Hyperphosphatasia, 293
LEOPARD syndrome, 113
Marfan syndrome, 121
Mucopolysaccharidosis IVA and B, 331,
　332
Noonan syndrome, 145

Prune-belly syndrome, 170
Schwartz-Jampel syndrome, 185
The 3-M syndrome, 208
Pectus excavatum
    Aarskog syndrome, 2
    Coffin-Lowry syndrome, 42
    Cowden syndrome, 44
    Cutis laxa, 49
    Ehlers-Danlos syndrome, 63
    F syndrome, 68
    Fetal alcohol syndrome, 71
    Freeman-Sheldon syndrome, 78
    German syndrome
    Golden-Lakim syndrome, 82
    Homocystinuria, 285
    LEOPARD syndrome, 113
    Marfan syndrome, 121
    Noonan syndrome, 145
    The 3-M syndrome, 208
Pelvis: small, hypoplastic
    Caudal dysplasia sequence, 31
    Chromosome 13 trisomy syndrome, 37
    Chromosome 18 trisomy syndrome, 37
    Goltz syndrome, 83
    Molded baby syndrome, 132
    Sirenomelia, 192
    Weaver syndrome, 223
Penis: large
    Adrenal hyperplasia (congenital), 238
    Cerebro-oculo-facio-skeletal syndrome, 33
    Klippel-Trenaunay-Weber syndrome, 109
    Lipodystrophy, 311
    Megalourethra
    Neurofibromatosis I, 140
    Roberts syndrome, 179
Penis: small
    Aarskog syndrome, 2
    Aniridia-Wilms tumor association, 10
    Bardet-Biedl syndrome, 16
    CHARGE association, 34
    Chromosomal abnormalities
    Hypopituitarism (anterior lobe), 298
    Juberg-Marsidi syndrome
    Laron syndrome, 309
    Silver-Russell syndrome, 190
    Smith-Lemli-Opitz syndrome type I, 370
    Toriello-Carey syndrome, 210
Periauricular tags/pits
    Acrocallosal syndrome, 3
    Antley-Bixler syndrome, 11
    Beckwith-Wiedemann syndrome, 17

Branchio-oculo-facial syndrome, 23
Branchio-oto-renal syndrome, 23
Carpenter syndrome, 29
Cat-eye syndrome, 30
Chromosomal abnormalities
Coffin-Siris syndrome, 42
Delleman syndrome (postauricular tags),
    52
Frontonasal dysplasia, 78
Lenz microphthalmia syndrome, 113
Nager acrofacial dysostosis, 136
Oculo-auriculo-vertebral spectrum, 147
Townes-Brocks syndrome, 210
Treacher Collins syndrome, 211
Pericardial effusion
    Amyloidosis, 245
    Anemias
    Arthropathy-camptodactyly syndrome, 13
    Behçet syndrome, 18
    Degos syndrome, 51
    Erdheim-Chester disease, 265
    Gout, 280
    Hypothyroidism, 300
    Kawasaki syndrome, 106
    Mixed connective tissue disease, 131
    Nephrotic syndrome, 138
    Ovarian hyperstimulation syndrome, 342
    Postcardiotomy syndrome, 146
    Postmyocardial infarction syndrome, 166
    Reiter syndrome, 174
    Scleroderma, 186
    Stevens-Johnson syndrome, 199
    Superior vena cava syndrome
    Thalassemia, 374
    Turner syndrome, 214
    Vitamin B_1 deficiency, 381
    Wegener granulomatosis
    Yellow nail syndrome, 230
Periosteal cloaking
    GM_1 gangliosidosis, 278
    Goldbloom syndrome, 82
    Mucolipidosis II, 323
    Prostaglandin-induced hyperostosis
    Rickets, 359
    Scurvy, 362
Platyspondyly: nonskeletal dysplasia
    Aspartylglucosaminuria, 247
    Cushing syndrome, 258
    Ehlers-Danlos syndrome, 63
    Freeman-Sheldon syndrome, 78
    Fucosidosis, 270

Gaucher disease, 272
Geroderma osteodysplastica, 81
GM$_1$ gangliosidosis, 278
Hallermann-Streiff syndrome, 88
Homocystinuria, 285
Hyperphosphatasia, 293
Hypophosphatasia, 297
Hypopituitarism (anterior lobe), 298
Hypothyroidism, 300
Larsen syndrome, 112
Marshall syndrome, 123
Mucopolysaccharidosis IVA, 331
Osteoporosis-pseudoglioma syndrome,
    154
Patterson syndrome, 347
Rothmund-Thomson syndrome, 181
Schwartz-Jampel syndrome, 185
Severe combined immune deficiency
Sotos syndrome, 195
Thalassemia (deferoxamine-treated), 374
Polycythemia
    Asplenia syndrome, 13
    Beckwith-Wiedemann syndrome, 17
    Familial benign polycythemia
    Infant of diabetic mother
    Paraneoplastic syndromes, 344
    Pickwickian syndrome, 161
    Polycythemia vera
    Rendu-Osler-Weber syndrome, 176
    von Hippel–Lindau syndrome, 220
Polydactyly, postaxial
    Acrocallosal syndrome, 3
    Acro-fronto-facio-nasal dysostosis
    Acrorenal syndrome, 4
    Bardet-Biedl syndrome, 16
    Carpenter syndrome, 29
    Cerebro-reno-digital syndromes, 34
    Chromosome 13 trisomy syndrome, 37
    Fuhrmann syndrome, 79
    Goltz syndrome, 83
    Greig cephalopolysyndactyly syndrome, 86
    Kaufman-McKusick syndrome, 106
    Laurin-Sandrow syndrome, 113
    Meckel syndrome, 125
    Opitz trigonocephaly syndrome, 149
    Oro-facio-digital syndromes (II, III, IV),
        150
    Pallister-Hall syndrome, 156
    Pseudotrisomy 13 syndrome, 170
    Rubinstein-Taybi syndrome, 182
    Smith-Lemli-Opitz syndrome type I, 370

Smith-Lemli-Opitz syndrome type II, 371
    Weyers acrodental dysostosis, 226
Polydactyly, preaxial
    Bloom syndrome, 20
    Carpenter syndrome, 29
    Cerebro-reno-digital syndromes, 34
    Cranio-fronto-nasal dysplasia, 45
    Diamond-Blackfan syndrome, 54
    Down syndrome, 57
    Dubowitz syndrome, 59
    Fanconi anemia, 69
    Greig cephalopolysyndactyly syndrome, 86
    Holt-Oram syndrome, 94
    Lacrimo-auriculo-dento-digital syndrome,
        111
    Laurin-Sandrow syndrome, 113
    Nager acrofacial dysostosis, 136
    Poland sequence, 162
    Townes-Brocks syndrome, 210
    VATER association, 218
Polyps: alimentary tract
    Bannayan-Riley-Ruvalcaba syndrome, 15
    Behçet syndrome (inflammatory polyps),
        18
    Cowden syndrome, 44
    Cronkhite-Canada syndrome, 47
    Gardner syndrome, 80
    Menkes disease (gastric polyp), 319
    Peutz-Jeghers syndrome, 159
    Turcot syndrome, 214
Portal vein: hypertension
    Alagille syndrome, 6
    Alpha$_1$-antitrypsin deficiency, 243
    Banti syndrome, 15
    Budd-Chiari syndrome, 25
    Caroli syndrome, 28
    Cholesterol ester storage disease, 256
    Cruveilhier-Baumgarten syndrome, 48
    Cystic fibrosis
    Gaucher disease, 272
    Glycogen storage disease type III, 276
    Glycogen storage disease type IV, 277
    Hepatic fibrosis–renal cystic disease, 92
    Rendu-Osler-Weber syndrome, 176
    Wilson disease, 383
Postaxial deficiency syndromes
    Brachmann–de Lang syndrome, 22
    Postaxial acrofacial dysostosis, Miller
        type, 164
    Ulnar-mammary syndrome, 217
    Weyers oligodactyly syndrome, 226

Progeroid appearance, premature aging
  Acrogeria, 4
  Cockayne syndrome, 40
  Cutis laxa, 49
  Down syndrome, 57
  Geroderma osteodysplastica, 81
  Hajdu-Cheney syndrome, 87
  Hallermann-Streiff syndrome, 80
  Lipodystrophy (Bernardinelli-Seip syn-
      drome), 311
  Mandibuloacral dysplasia (Andy Gump
      appearance), 120
  Progeria, 168
  Rothmund-Thomson syndrome, 181
  Werner syndrome, 224
  Wiedemann-Rautenstrauch syndrome, 226
Prognathism
  Acromegaly, 235
  Angelman syndrome, 10
  Apert syndrome, 11
  Beckwith-Wiedemann syndrome, 17
  Binder syndrome, 19
  Cherubism
  Cloverleaf skull deformity, 39
  Cockayne syndrome, 40
  Crouzon syndrome, 47
  Down syndrome, 57
  Epidermolysis bullosa, 67
  Fetal alcohol syndrome, 71
  Fragile X syndrome, 77
  Geroderma osteodysplastica, 81
  Gorlin syndrome, 85
  Hajdu-Cheney syndrome, 87
  Hemihypertrophy (unilateral prog-
      nathism), 90
  Hypothyroidism (juvenile), 300
  LEOPARD syndrome, 113
  Mucolipidosis III, 324
  Mucopolysaccharidosis I-S, 329
  Multiple endocrine neoplasia type IIB, 135
  Myotonic dystrophy
  Oculo-dento-osseous dysplasia, 147
  Opitz BBBG syndrome, 149
  Sotos syndrome, 195
  Turner syndrome, 214
  Williams syndrome, 227
Protrusio acetabuli
  Alkaptonuria, 243
  Calcium pyrophosphate dihydrate deposi-
      tion disease, 249
  Cushing syndrome, 258
  Gout, 280
  Homocystinuria, 285
  Hyperparathyroidism, 290
  Hyperphosphatasia, 293
  Marfan syndrome, 121
  Osteolysis, multicentric
  Renal osteodystrophy, 292
  Rickets, 359
  Sickle cell anemia, 365
  Turner syndrome, 214
Pseudoarthrosis
  Amniotic band sequence, 9
  Kuskokwim syndrome, 111
  Neurofibromatosis I, 140
Pterygium
  Herrmann-Opitz syndrome
  Klippel-Feil syndrome, 109
  Nail-patella syndrome, 137
  Noonan syndrome, 145
  Pterygium syndromes, 171
  Turner syndrome, 214
Ptosis: eyelid
  Aarskog syndrome, 2
  Aniridia-Wilms tumor association, 10
  Carey-Fineman-Ziter syndrome, 180
  Cerebro-oculo-facio-skeletal syndrome,
      33
  CHARGE association, 34
  Chromosomal abnormalities
  Coffin-Siris syndrome, 42
  EEC syndrome, 62
  Fetal alcohol syndrome, 71
  Fetal hydantoin syndrome, 72
  Freeman-Sheldon syndrome, 78
  Horner syndrome, 95
  Mannosidoses, 316
  Myasthenia syndromes
  Myotonic dystrophy
  Nail-patella syndrome, 137
  Neurofibromatosis I, 140
  Noonan syndrome, 145
  Ocular fibrosis (congenital)
  Oculogastrointestinal muscular dystrophy
  Pachydermoperiostosis, 155
  Pallister-Killian syndrome, 156
  Parinaud syndrome, 158
  Proteus syndrome, 169
  Rubinstein-Taybi syndrome, 182
  Velo-cardio-facial syndrome, 219

Pubic bones: nonossification, delayed ossification
    Caudal dysplasia sequence, 31
    Cephaloskeletal dysplasia, 32
    Hypophosphatasia, 297
    Hypothyroidism, 300
    Larsen syndrome, 112
    Schinzel-Giedion syndrome, 184
    Sjögren-Larsson syndrome, 369
Pubic symphysis: wide
    Ehlers-Danlos syndrome (distraction during delivery), 63
    Fraser syndrome, 77
    Goltz syndrome, 83
    Prune-belly syndrome, 170
Pulmonary artery: aneurysm
    Behçet syndrome, 18
    Ehlers-Danlos syndrome, 63
    Hughes-Stovin syndrome, 95
    Marfan syndrome, 121
    Polyarteritis nodosa
    Takayasu arteritis
Pulmonary artery: rupture
    Cutis laxa, 49
    Ehlers-Danlos syndrome (IV, VI), 63
    Marfan syndrome, 121
Pulmonary artery: stenosis (valvular, peripheral)
    Alagille syndrome, 6
    Carcinoid syndrome, 252
    Cutis laxa, 49
    Keutel syndrome, 108
    LEOPARD syndrome, 113
    Noonan syndrome, 145
    Takayasu arteritis
    Turner syndrome, 214
    Williams syndrome, 227
Pulmonary hypertension, cor pulmonale
    Alpha$_1$-antitrypsin deficiency, 243
    Crouzon syndrome, 47
    Cutis laxa, 49
    Cystic fibrosis
    Ehlers-Danlos syndrome, 63
    Eisenmenger syndrome, 64
    Hemosiderosis (idiopathic pulmonary), 284
    Marfan syndrome, 121
    Mucopolysaccharidoses (I-H, I-H/S, II, VI), 327, 328, 329, 333
    Robin sequence, 180
    Scimitar syndrome, 186

Scleroderma, 186
Sickle cell anemia, 365
Sleep apnea syndrome, 193
Takayasu arteritis
Tuberous sclerosis, 212

R
Radius/radial ray: aplasia, hypoplasia
    Aase syndrome, 2
    Aminopterin fetopathy, 8
    Baller-Gerold syndrome, 14
    Brachmann–de Lange syndrome, 22
    Cat-eye syndrome, 30
    Chromosomal abnormalities (13, 18, etc.)
    Facio-auriculo-radial dysplasia, 69
    Fanconi anemia, 69
    Holt-Oram syndrome, 94
    Juberg-Hayward syndrome, 104
    Klippel-Feil syndrome, 109
    Lacrimo-auriculo-dento-digital syndrome, 111
    Laurin-Sandrow syndrome, 113
    Mietens-Weber syndrome, 130
    Nager acrofacial dysostosis, 136
    Oculo-auriculo-vertebral spectrum, 147
    Roberts syndrome, 179
    Rothmund-Thomson syndrome, 181
    Seckel syndrome, 188
    TAR syndrome, 206
    Thalidomide embryopathy, 207
    Treacher Collins syndrome, 211
    VATER association, 218
Raynaud phenomenon
    CREST syndrome, 46
    Mixed connective tissue disease, 131
    Raynaud syndrome, 173
    Scleroderma, 186
Retinopathy
    Aase syndrome, 2
    Aicardi syndrome, 6
    Alagille syndrome, 6
    Alport syndrome, 8
    Bardet-Biedl syndrome, 16
    Behçet syndrome, 18
    Cockayne syndrome, 40
    Cohen syndrome, 43
    Diabetes mellitus, 262
    Fetal alcohol syndrome, 71
    Gorlin syndrome, 85
    Holoprosencephaly, 94
    Hypomelanosis of Ito, 98

Incontinentia pigmenti, 100
Lipoid proteinosis, 313
Marshall syndrome, 123
Morning glory syndrome, 133
Muscle–eye–brain disease
Neurofibromatosis I, 140
Proteus syndrome, 169
Sotos syndrome, 195
Usher syndrome, 218
Velo-cardio-facial syndrome, 219
von Hippel–Lindau syndrome, 220
Waardenburg syndrome, 221
Walker-Warburg syndrome, 221
Wrinkly skin syndrome, 230
Retinopathy and errors of metabolism
Abetalipoproteinemia, 234
Hyperlipoproteinemia, 287
Kearns-Sayre syndrome, 306
Mucolipidosis IV, 325
Neuronal ceroid lipofuscinosis, 336
Ornithine aminotransferase deficiency
Peroxisomal disorders, 349
Refsum disease (classic type), 357
Sjögren-Larsson syndrome, 369
Rib: anomaly
Baller-Gerold syndrome, 14
Cerebro-costo-mandibular syndrome, 33
Chromosome XXY syndrome
Down syndrome, 57
Femoral hypoplasia–unusual facies syndrome, 70
Fetal hydantoin syndrome, 72
Goltz syndrome, 83
Gorlin syndrome, 85
Holt-Oram syndrome, 94
Incontinentia pigmenti, 100
Klippel-Feil syndrome, 109
Nager acrofacial dysostosis, 136
Noonan syndrome, 145
Oculo-auriculo-vertebral spectrum, 147
Opitz trigonocephaly syndrome, 149
Poland sequence, 162
Pterygium syndromes, 171
Spondylocostal dysostoses, 197
TAR syndrome, 206
Thoracic outlet syndrome, 208
VATER association, 218
Rib: 11 pairs or less
Chromosome 18 trisomy syndrome, 37
Down syndrome, 57

Femoral hypoplasia–unusual facies syndrome, 70
Ritscher-Schinzel syndrome, 179
Spondylocostal dysostosis, 197
Rib: flaring, anterior-end cupping
Adenosine deaminase deficiency with severe combined immunodeficiency and chondrodysplasia
Copper deficiency, 258
Farber disease, 268
GM$_1$ gangliosidosis, 278
Hypophosphatasia, 297
Menkes disease, 319
Rickets, 359
Scurvy, 362
Shwachman syndrome, 363
Thalassemia, 374
Rib: notching or erosion
Hyperparathyroidism, 290
Neurofibromatosis I, 140
Superior vena cava syndrome
Thalassemia, 374
Rib: slender, thin, or twisted
Aminopterin fetopathy, 8
Antley-Bixler syndrome, 11
Chromosome 8 trisomy syndrome
Chromosome 13 trisomy syndrome, 37
Chromosome 18 trisomy syndrome, 37
Cockayne syndrome, 40
Contractural arachnodactyly, 44
Down syndrome, 57
Gorlin syndrome, 85
Hallermann-Streiff syndrome, 88
Hyperparathyroidism, 290
Larsen syndrome, 112
Myotonic dystrophy
Myotubular myopathy
Neurofibromatosis I, 140
Progeria, 168
Scleroderma, 186
The 3-M syndrome, 208
Turner syndrome, 214
Werdnig-Hoffmann disease
Rib: wide or thickened, periosteal reaction
Acromegaly, 235
Adenosine deaminase deficiency with severe combined immunodeficiency and chondroosseous dysplasia
Chromosome 8 trisomy syndrome

Erdheim-Chester disease, 265
Fluorosis, 269
Fucosidosis, 270
Gaucher disease, 272
Gorlin syndrome, 85
Hyperphosphatasia, 293
Mannosidoses, 316
Mucolipidosis II, 323
Mucolipidosis III, 324
Mucopolysaccharidoses, 325
Niemann-Pick disease, 336
Oculo-dento-osseous dysplasia, 147
Pachydermoperiostosis, 155
Proteus syndrome, 169
Sickle cell anemia, 365
Sterno-costo-clavicular hyperostosis, 199
Thalassemia, 374
Tuberous sclerosis, 212
Weill-Marchesani syndrome, 224

S
Salivary duct: ectasia
  Mikulicz syndrome, 130
  Sarcoidosis
  Sjögren syndrome, 192
Salivary gland: abnormality
  Amyloidosis, 245
  Cystic fibrosis
  Hyperparathyroidism (primary), 290
  Hypoglossia-hypodactylia syndrome, 98
  Lacrimo-auriculo-dento-digital syndrome,
    111
  Mikulicz syndrome, 130
  Oculo-auriculo-vertebral spectrum, 147
  Treacher Collins syndrome, 211
Scrotum: bifid
  Aarskog syndrome, 2
  Bardet-Biedl syndrome, 16
  Chromosome 18 ring
  Chromosome XXXXY
  Pterygium syndrome (popliteal), 171
  Teebi hypertelorism syndrome, 206
  Triploidy
Self-mutilation
  Brachmann–de Lange syndrome, 22
  Congenital sensory neuropathy (with or
    without anhidrosis)
  Insensitivity to pain (congenital), 101
  Lesch-Nyhan syndrome, 310
  Mucolipidosis III, 324

Riley-Day syndrome, 178
Smith-Magenis syndrome, 193
Sella turcica: large
  Acromegaly and gigantism, 235
  Cushing syndrome, 258
  Empty sella syndrome, 65
  Hydrocephalus
  Hydrolethalus syndrome, 95
  Hypogonadism
  Hypopituitarism (empty sella), 298
  Hypothyroidism (juvenile), 300
  Mucolipidoses, 323, 324, 325
  Mucopolysaccharidoses, 325
  Nelson syndrome, 335
  Neoplasms
  Neurofibromatosis I, 140
  Oxycephaly
  Turner syndrome, 214
Sella turcica: small
  Cockayne syndrome, 40
  Deprivation dwarfism, 260
  Down syndrome, 57
  Growth hormone deficiency
  Hypopituitarism, 298
  Myotonic dystrophy
  Prader-Willi syndrome, 166
  Sheehan syndrome, 363
Shield-like thorax
  Chromosome 18 trisomy syndrome, 37
  Noonan syndrome, 145
  Turner syndrome, 214
Sinuses: advanced development
  Acromegaly, 235
  Dyke-Davidoff-Masson syndrome, 60
  Homocystinuria, 285
  Lipodystrophy (lipoatrophic diabetes), 311
  Marfan syndrome, 121
  Myotonic dystrophy
  Normal variant
  Turner syndrome, 214
Sinuses: underdeveloped or absent
  Binder syndrome, 19
  Cockayne syndrome, 40
  Down syndrome, 57
  Frontonasal dysplasia, 78
  Hypopituitarism, 298
  Hypothyroidism, 300
  Oto-palato-digital syndrome type I, 154
  Prader-Willi syndrome, 166
  Schwarz-Lélek syndrome, 185

Sickle cell anemia, 365
Thalassemia, 374
Treacher Collins syndrome, 211
Sinusitis
    Ataxia-telangiectasia syndrome, 14
    Cystic fibrosis
    Immotile cilia syndrome, 99
    Immune disorders
    Kartagener syndrome, 105
    Wiskott-Aldrich syndrome, 228
    Yellow nail syndrome, 230
    Young syndrome, 230
Skin: aplasia or hypoplasia
    Aplasia cutis congenita, 12
    Chromosome 4: del (4p) syndrome, 36
    Chromosome 13 trisomy syndrome, 37
    Delleman syndrome, 52
Skin: atrophy
    Acrogeria, 4
    Ataxia-telangiectasia syndrome, 14
    CREST syndrome, 46
    Focal scleroderma, 75
    Goltz syndrome, 83
    Hallermann-Streiff syndrome, 88
    Incontinentia pigmenti, 100
    Mandibuloacral dysplasia, 120
    Progeria, 168
    Rothmund-Thomson syndrome, 181
    Scleroderma, 186
    Weber-Christian syndrome, 223
Skin: dimple
    Antley-Bixler syndrome, 11
    Camptomelic dysplasia
    Caudal dysplasia sequence, 31
    Chromosome dup (9p) syndrome
    Chromosome del (18q) syndrome
    Fetal akinesia sequence, 71
    Freeman-Sheldon syndrome, 78
    Hypophosphatasia, 297
    Zellweger syndrome, 386
Skin: eruption, erythema, rash
    Acrodermatitis enteropathica, 234
    Biotinidase deficiency, 248
    Cowden syndrome, 44
    Darier disease
    Degos syndrome, 51
    Dermo-chondro-corneal dystrophy of
        François, 54
    De Sanctis-Cacchione syndrome, 54
    Dubowitz syndrome, 59
    Epidermal nevus syndrome, 66

Epidermolysis bullosa, 67
Fabry disease, 266
Farber disease, 268
Glucagonoma syndrome, 274
Hemolytic uremic syndrome, 90
Henoch-Schönlein syndrome, 91
Homocystinuria, 285
Horner syndrome, 95
Hyperlipoproteinemias, 287
Incontinentia pigmenti, 100
Infantile multisystem inflammatory dis-
    ease, 100
Juvenile xanthogranuloma
Kawasaki syndrome, 106
LEOPARD syndrome, 113
Lipoid dermatoarthritis, 115
Macrodystrophia lipomatosa, 119
Mixed connective tissue disease, 131
Osteoarthropathy, familial idiopathic,
    152
Phenylketonuria, 350
Pseudoxanthoma elasticum
Reiter syndrome, 174
Relapsing polychondritis, 175
Rothmund-Thomson syndrome, 181
Sea-blue histiocyte syndrome, 188
Sterno-costo-clavicular hyperostosis, 199
Stevens-Johnson syndrome, 199
Sweet syndrome, 204
Toxic shock syndrome, 210
Vitamin A intoxication, 380
Wiskott-Aldrich syndrome, 228
Skin: lesions in metabolic disorders
    Acrodermatitis enteropathica, 234
    Alkaptonuria, 243
    Argininosuccinic aciduria
    Biotinidase deficiency, 248
    Homocystinuria, 285
    Lipoid proteinosis, 313
    Phenylketonuria, 350
    Tyrosinemia II, 378
Skin: ossification
    Dermatomyositis
    Fibrodysplasia ossificans progressiva, 74
    Osteoma cutis, familial, 154
    Pseudohypoparathyroidism, 355
    Scleroderma, 186
Skin: photosensitivity
    Bloom syndrome, 20
    Cockayne syndrome, 40
    Pellagra

PIBI(D)S syndrome, 160
Porphyrias, 353
Skin: pigmentary abnormalities
  Acrodysostosis
  Acrogeria, 4
  Addison disease, 237
  Alkaptonuria, 243
  Ataxia-telangiectasia syndrome, 14
  Bannayan-Riley-Ruvalcaba syndrome, 15
  Bloom syndrome, 20
  Carbon baby
  Carney complex, 27
  Chédiak-Higashi syndrome, 35
  Clouston syndrome, 39
  Copper deficiency, 258
  Cronkhite-Canada syndrome, 47
  Cross syndrome, 47
  De Sanctis-Cacchione syndrome, 54
  Dyskeratosis congenita, 60
  Ectodermal dysplasia (hypohidrotic), 61
  EEC syndrome, 62
  Epidermal nevus syndrome, 66
  Fanconi anemia, 69
  Farber disease, 268
  Gaucher disease, 272
  Goltz syndrome, 83
  Gorlin syndrome, 85
  Hemihypertrophy, 90
  Hemochromatosis, 281
  Hermansky-Pudlak syndrome, 284
  Homocystinuria (malar flush), 285
  Hyperphosphatasia, 293
  Hypomelanosis of Ito, 98
  Incontinentia pigmenti, 100
  Jaffe-Campanacci syndrome, 103
  Klein-Waardenburg syndrome, 108
  Klippel-Trenaunay-Weber syndrome, 109
  Kuskokwim syndrome, 111
  LAMB syndrome, 27
  LEOPARD syndrome, 113
  Lipodystrophy, 311
  Maffucci syndrome, 119
  McCune-Albright syndrome, 125
  Melorheostosis
  Neurocutaneous melanosis sequence, 139
  Neurofibromatosis I, 140
  Noonan syndrome, 145
  Patterson syndrome, 347
  Peutz-Jeghers syndrome, 159
  POEMS syndrome, 161
  Polyglandular autoimmune disease, 352

  Porphyrias, 353
  Prader-Willi syndrome, 166
  Progeria, 168
  Proteus syndrome, 169
  Reflex sympathetic dystrophy syndrome
  Romberg syndrome, 181
  Rothmund-Thomson syndrome, 181
  Silver-Russell syndrome, 190
  Tuberous sclerosis, 212
  Turner syndrome, 214
  Vitamin A intoxication, 380
  Waardenburg syndrome, 221
  Weber-Christian syndrome, 223
  Wilson disease, 383
  Winchester syndrome, 384
Skin: tags
  Delleman syndrome, 52
  Frontonasal dysplasia (ear tag), 78
  Oculo-auriculo-vertebral spectrum, 147
  Tuberous sclerosis, 212
Skin: wrinkled, creased
  Acrogeria, 4
  Chromosome 2: del(2q) and wrinkly skin
  Costello syndrome: loose skin, 44
  Cutis laxa, 49
  Cutis verticis gyrata, 50
  Fetal brain disruption sequence, 72
  Michelin tire baby syndrome
  Pachydermoperiostosis, 155
  Prune-belly syndrome, 170
  Wrinkly skin syndrome, 230
Skull: asymmetry
  Dyke-Davidoff-Masson syndrome, 60
  Epidermal nevus syndrome, 66
  Hemimegalencephaly
  Opitz BBBG syndrome, 149
  Saethre-Chotzen syndrome, 183
  Sturge-Weber syndrome, 201
  Wildervanck syndrome, 226
Skull: defective ossification/congenital defect
  Aase syndrome, 2
  Acalvaria
  Adams-Oliver syndrome, 4
  Aminopterin fetopathy, 8
  Aminopterin fetopathy-like syndrome, 9
  Amniotic band sequence, 9
  Bardet-Biedl syndrome, 16
  Chromosomal abnormalities (13, 18,
    Down syndrome)
  Cranium bifidum
  Delleman syndrome, 52

Ehlers-Danlos syndrome, 63
Encephalocele
Epidermoid
Frontonasal dysplasia, 78
Hallermann-Streiff syndrome, 88
Hydrocephalus
Hyperparathyroidism, 290
Hypophosphatasia, 297
Hypothyroidism, 300
Lacunar skull
Menkes disease, 319
Neurofibromatosis I, 140
Noonan syndrome, 145
Occipital foramina
Oto-palato-digital syndrome type I, 154
Pachydermoperiostosis, 155
Parietal foramina
Progeria, 168
Restrictive dermatopathy, 176
Rickets, 359
Rubinstein-Taybi syndrome, 182
Zellweger syndrome, 386
Skull: "hair-on-end" appearance (generalized)
    Cyanotic congenital heart disease with
        polycythemia
    Iron deficiency anemia, 305
    Leukemia
    Lymphoma
    Multiple myeloma
    Polycythemia vera
    Pyruvate kinase deficiency anemia, 357
    Sickle cell anemia, 365
    Spherocytosis, 372
    Thalassemia, 374
Skull: thick
    Aase-Smith syndrome
    Acromegaly, 235
    Aspartylglucosaminuria, 247
    Cerebral atrophy
    Chromosome XXXXY syndrome
    Clouston syndrome, 39
    Cockayne syndrome, 40
    Coffin-Lowry syndrome, 42
    Cyanotic congenital heart disease
    Dyke-Davidoff-Masson syndrome, 60
    Fanconi anemia, 69
    Fibrous dysplasia (polyostotic)
    Fluorosis, 269
    Fountain syndrome, 76
    Fucosidosis, 270
    Homocystinuria, 285

Hyperphosphatasia, 293
Hypoparathyroidism, 296
Hypothyroidism, 300
Infantile multisystem inflammatory dis-
    ease, 100
Iron deficiency anemia, 305
Lipodystrophy (lipoatrophic diabetes), 311
Mannosidoses, 316
Marfan syndrome, 121
Marshall syndrome, 123
Microcephaly
Morgagni-Stewart-Morel syndrome, 132
Mucolipidosis II, 323
Mucopolysaccharidosis I-H, 327
Mucopolysaccharidosis II, 329
Mucopolysaccharidosis III, 330
Mucopolysaccharidosis VI, 333
Myotonic dystrophy
Neu-Laxova syndrome, 139
Oculo-dento-osseous dysplasia, 147
Osteopathia striata
Oto-palato-digital syndrome type I, 154
POEMS syndrome, 161
Polycythemia
Proteus syndrome, 169
Pseudohypoparathyroidism, 355
Pyruvate kinase deficiency anemia, 357
Renal osteodystrophy, 292
Rickets, treated, 359
Salla disease, 362
Schwarz-Lélek syndrome, 185
Sickle cell anemia, 365
Sjögren-Larsson syndrome, 369
Spherocytosis, 372
Thalassemia, 374
Tricho-dento-osseous syndrome, 211
Troell-Junet syndrome, 212
Tuberous sclerosis, 212
Vitamin D intoxication, 382
Weill-Marchesani syndrome, 224
Slender tubular bones; *refer to* Tubular bones:
    slender
Spinal canal: narrow
    Acromegaly, 235
    Alagille syndrome, 6
    Brachyolmia
    Calcium pyrophosphate dihydrate deposi-
        tion disease, 249
    Cauda equina syndrome, 30
    Gordon syndrome, 84
    Klippel-Feil syndrome, 109

Rickets (hypophosphatemic), 359
Sirenomelia, 192
Turner syndrome, 214
Weill-Marchesani syndrome, 224
Spinal canal: wide
    Arteriovenous malformation
    Diastematomyelia
    Idiopathic
    Intraspinal neoplasms
    Marfan syndrome, 121
    Meningomyelocele
    Neurofibromatosis I, 140
    Oto-palato-digital syndrome type 1, 154
    Tethered cord syndrome, 207
Split hand (lobster claw hand)
    Brachmann–de Lange syndrome, 22
    EEC syndrome, 62
    Goltz syndrome, 83
    Hypoglossia-hypodactylia syndrome, 98
    Möbius syndrome, 132
    Roberts syndrome, 179
    Treacher Collins syndrome, 211
Spur: bone; *refer to* Exostosis
Steatorrhea
    Abetalipoproteinemia, 234
    Celiac disease, 254
    Hypoparathyroidism, 296
    Immune disorder and lymphoid hyperplasia
    Intestinal pseudo-obstruction (idiopathic)
    Short-bowel syndrome, 189
    Somatostatinoma syndrome, 371
    Wolman disease, 385
Stomatitis
    Behçet syndrome, 18
    Chronic granulomatous disease of childhood, 256
    Degos syndrome, 51
    Glucagonoma syndrome, 274
    Iron deficiency anemia, 305
    Kawasaki syndrome, 106
    Polyglandular autoimmune disease, 352
    Stevens-Johnson syndrome, 199
Strabismus
    Aarskog syndrome, 2
    Adams-Oliver syndrome, 4
    Apert syndrome, 11
    Baller-Gerold syndrome, 14
    Bardet-Biedl syndrome, 16
    Brachmann–de Lange syndrome, 22
    Chromosomal abnormalities

Clouston syndrome, 39
Cohen syndrome, 43
Crouzon syndrome, 47
Duane syndrome, 59
Femoral hypoplasia–unusual facies syndrome, 70
Fetal alcohol syndrome, 71
Fetal hydantoin syndrome, 72
Freeman-Sheldon syndrome, 78
Goltz syndrome, 83
Gorlin syndrome, 85
Hallermann-Streiff syndrome, 88
Hypomelanosis of Ito, 98
Incontinentia pigmenti, 100
Johanson-Blizzard syndrome, 103
Marden-Walker syndrome, 121
Marinesco-Sjögren syndrome, 122
Marshall syndrome, 123
Mietens-Weber syndrome, 130
Möbius syndrome, 132
Mulibrey nanism, 134
Multiple synostosis syndrome, 136
Noonan syndrome, 145
Oculo-auriculo-vertebral spectrum, 147
Okihiro syndrome: Duane syndrome and radial dysplasia (DR syndrome)
Opitz BBBG syndrome, 149
Oro-facio-digital syndromes, 150
Oromandibular-limb hypogenesis, 152
Pallister-Killian syndrome, 156
Pfeiffer syndrome, 160
Prader-Willi syndrome, 166
Rubinstein-Taybi syndrome, 182
Saethre-Chotzen syndrome, 183
Seckel syndrome, 188
Smith-Lemli-Opitz syndrome type I, 370
Sotos syndrome, 195
Stoll-Charrow-Poznanski syndrome, 201
TAR syndrome, 206
Williams syndrome, 227
Stroke
    Afibrinogenemia (congenital), 241
    Alien hand syndrome, 7
    Amyloidosis, 245
    Antiphospholipid syndrome, 10
    Arterial calcification of infancy, 12
    Behçet syndrome, 18
    Cardiomyopathies
    Degos syndrome, 51
    Ehlers-Danlos syndrome, 63
    Fabry disease, 266

Foix-Chavany-Marie syndrome, 76
Hemophilia, 282
Homocystinuria, 285
Kearns-Sayre syndrome, 306
Leigh disease, 309
Man-in-the-barrel syndrome, 120
MELAS syndrome, 318
Mitral valve prolapse syndrome
Neurofibromatosis I, 140
Polycystic kidney disease, 162
Protein C deficiency
Protein S deficiency, 354
Pseudoxanthoma elasticum
Sickle cell anemia, 365
Sickle cell–hemoglobin C disease
Spherocytosis, 372
Sulfite oxidase deficiency, 372
Tuberous sclerosis, 212
Sutures: delayed closure and/or wide
  Acrogeria, 4
  Aminopterin fetopathy, 8
  Chromosomal abnormalities (13, 18, 21)
  Cranium bifidum
  Dandy-Walker syndrome, 50
  Deprivation dwarfism, 260
  Diencephalic syndrome, 55
  Growth hormone deficiency
  Hajdu-Cheney syndrome, 87
  Hallermann-Streiff syndrome, 88
  Hydrocephalus
  Hydrolethalus syndrome, 95
  Hyperparathyroidism, 290
  Hypoparathyroidism, 296
  Hypophosphatasia, 297
  Hypothyroidism, 300
  Laron syndrome, 309
  Lead intoxication
  Mandibuloacral dysplasia, 120
  Osteoarthropathy, familial idiopathic, 152
  Pachydermoperiostosis, 155
  Progeria, 168
  Pseudotumor cerebri
  Pycnodysostosis
  Rickets, 359
  Rubinstein-Taybi syndrome, 182
  Schinzel-Giedion syndrome, 184
  Silver-Russell syndrome, 190
  Vitamin A deficiency, 380
  Vitamin A intoxication, 380
  Wiedemann-Rautenstrauch syndrome, 226

Winchester syndrome, 384
Zellweger syndrome, 386
Symphalangism
  Apert syndrome, 11
  Möbius syndrome, 132
  Multiple synostosis syndrome, 136
  Poland sequence, 162
  Pterygium syndromes, 171
  Symphalangism-surdity syndrome, 205
Syndactyly
  Aarskog syndrome, 2
  Acrorenal syndrome, 4
  Aminopterin fetopathy, 8
  Amniotic band sequence, 9
  Apert syndrome, 11
  Aplasia cutis congenita, 12
  Bardet-Biedl syndrome, 16
  Bloom syndrome, 20
  Brachmann–de Lange syndrome, 22
  Carpenter syndrome, 29
  Chromosomal abnormalities (13, 18, 21,
    etc.)
  Cloverleaf skull deformity, 39
  Cohen syndrome, 43
  Cranio-fronto-nasal dysplasia, 45
  DOOR syndrome, 56
  Dubowitz syndrome (toes), 59
  EEC syndrome, 62
  Ehlers-Danlos syndrome, 63
  Epidermolysis bullosa, 67
  F syndrome, 68
  Fanconi anemia, 69
  Fetal hydantoin syndrome, 72
  FG syndrome, 73
  Fibrodysplasia ossificans progressiva, 74
  Fraser syndrome, 77
  Fuhrmann syndrome, 79
  Goltz syndrome, 83
  Gorlin syndrome, 85
  Greig cephalopolysyndactyly syndrome, 86
  Hallermann-Streiff syndrome, 88
  Hermann-Opitz syndrome
  Holt-Oram syndrome, 94
  Hypoglossia–hypodactylia syndrome, 98
  Hypomelanosis of Ito, 98
  Incontinentia pigmenti, 100
  Kaufman-McKusick syndrome, 106
  KBG syndrome, 107
  Lacrimo-auriculo-dentodigital syndrome,
    111

Laurin-Sandrow syndrome, 113
Lenz microphthalmia syndrome, 113
Meckel syndrome, 125
Möbius syndrome, 132
Multiple synostosis syndrome, 136
Nager acrofacial dysostosis, 136
Neu-Laxova syndrome, 139
Oculo-dento-osseous dysplasia, 147
Opitz trigonocephaly syndrome, 149
Oro-facio-digital syndrome I, 150
Oro-facio-digital syndrome II, 150
Oromandibular-limb hypogenesis, 152
Oto-palato-digital syndrome type I, 154
Pallister-Hall syndrome, 156
Pfeiffer syndrome, 160
Poland sequence, 162
Postaxial acrofacial dysostosis, Miller
    type, 164
Prader-Willi syndrome, 166
Pterygium syndromes, 171
Roberts syndrome, 179
Robin sequence, 180
Rothmund-Thomson syndrome, 181
Rubinstein-Taybi syndrome, 182
Saethre-Chotzen syndrome, 183
Silver-Russell syndrome, 190
Smith-Lemli-Opitz syndrome type I, 370
Spondylocostal dysostosis
    (Jarcho-Levin syndrome), 197
TAR syndrome, 206
Tel Hashomer camptodactyly syndrome,
    207
Triploidy
Waardenburg anophthalmia syndrome,
    220
Synophrys
    Aarskog syndrome, 2
    Brachmann–de Lange syndrome, 22
    Chromosomal abnormalities (13 trisomy;
        etc.), 37
    Gorlin syndrome, 85
    Hajdu-Cheney syndrome, 87
    Mucopolysaccharidosis III, 330
    Waardenburg syndrome, 221
Synostosis: humerus, radius, ulna
    Antley-Bixler syndrome, 11
    Cloverleaf skull deformity, 39
    Femoral hypoplasia–unusual facies syn-
        drome, 70
    Holt-Oram syndrome, 94
    Multiple synostosis syndrome, 136

Pfeiffer syndrome, 160
Symphalangism-surdity syndrome, 205
Synostosis: radioulnar
    Chromosome 18 trisomy syndrome, 37
    Chromosome XXXXX syndrome
    Chromosome XXXXY syndrome
    Chromosome XXXY syndrome
    Chromosome XXY syndrome
    Cloverleaf skull deformity, 39
    Ehlers-Danlos syndrome, 63
    Facio-auriculo-radial dysplasia, 69
    Femoral hypoplasia–unusual facies syn-
        drome, 70
    Fetal alcohol syndrome, 71
    Holt-Oram syndrome, 94
    Lacrimo-auriculo-dento-digital syndrome,
        111
    Multiple synostosis syndrome, 136
    Nager acrofacial dysostosis, 136
    Pfeiffer syndrome, 160
    Thalidomide embryopathy, 207

T
Tags/pits (periauricular); *refer to* Periauricular
    tags/pits
"Tail" (caudal appendage; sacral appendage)
    Crouzon syndrome, 47
    Goltz syndrome, 83
    Isolated anomaly
    Metatropic dysplasia
    Pallister-Killian syndrome, 156
Tarsal fusion
    Crouzon syndrome, 47
    F syndrome, 68
    Hand-foot-genital syndrome, 89
    Multiple synostosis syndrome, 136
    Spondylo-carpo-tarsal synostosis syn-
        drome, 197
    Tarsal coalition (an isolated abnormality)
    Turner syndrome, 214
Taurodontism
    Chromosome XXXXY
    Chromosome XXY
    Down syndrome, 57
    Tricho-dento-osseous syndrome, 211
Teeth: anodontia or hypodontia
    Aarskog syndrome, 2
    Acrofacial dysostosis, 3
    Bloom syndrome, 20
    Charlie M syndrome, 152
    Coffin-Lowry syndrome, 42

Crouzon syndrome, 47
Down syndrome, 57
Ectodermal dysplasia (hypohidriotic), 61
EEC syndrome, 62
Ehlers-Danlos syndrome, 63
Epidermal nevus syndrome, 66
GAPO syndrome (pseudoanodontia), 80
Goltz syndrome, 83
Hallermann-Streiff syndrome, 88
Hanhart syndrome, 152
Hypoglossia–hypodactylia syndrome, 98
Hypophosphatasia, 297
Incontinentia pigmenti, 100
Johanson-Blizzard syndrome, 103
Lacrimo-auriculo-dento-digital syndrome,
    111
Oculo-dento-osseous dysplasia, 147
Oro-facio-digital syndrome I, 150
Oro-facio-digital syndrome II, 150
Oto-palato-digital syndrome type I, 154
Pseudohypoparathyroidism, 355
Pycnodysostosis
Rothmund-Thomson syndrome, 181
Seckel syndrome, 188
Sjögren-Larsson syndrome, 369
Stoll-Charrow-Poznanski syndrome, 201
Weill-Marshesani syndrome, 224
Williams syndrome, 227
Teeth: delayed eruption/noneruption
Aarskog syndrome, 2
Acrodysostosis
Apert syndrome, 11
Brachmann–de Lang syndrome, 22
Branchio-genito-skeletal syndrome, 23
Charlie M syndrome, 152
Chondroectodermal dysplasia
Cleidocranial dysplasia
Down syndrome, 57
Dubowitz syndrome, 59
Fetal rubella infection
GAPO syndrome, 80
Gardner syndrome, 80
Goltz syndrome, 83
Hallermann-Streiff syndrome, 88
Hanhart syndrome, 152
Hypoparathyroidism, 296
Hypopituitarism (anterior lobe), 298
Hypothyroidism, 300
Incontinentia pigmenti, 100
Kocher-Debré-Sémélaigne syndrome, 307

Lacrimo-auriculo-dento-digital syndrome,
    111
Miller-Dieker syndrome, 130
Mucopolysaccharidoses, 325
Osteogenesis imperfecta
Osteoglophonic dysplasia
Osteopetrosis
Pallister-Killian syndrome, 156
Progeria, 168
Pseudohypoparathyroidism, 355
Pycnodysostosis
Rickets, 359
Robinow syndrome
Romberg syndrome, 181
SHORT syndrome, 265
Tricho-dento-osseous syndrome, 211
Tricho-rhino-pharyngeal dysplasia type I
Wiedemann-Rautenstrauch syndrome, 226
Williams syndrome, 227
Winchester syndrome, 384
Teeth: dental cyst
Branchio-genito-skeletal syndrome, 23
Gardner syndrome, 80
Gorlin syndrome, 85
Lowe syndrome, 314
Mucopolysaccharidosis I-H, 327
Mucopolysaccharidosis I-H/S, 328
Opitz BBBG syndrome, 149
Teeth: floating
Agranulocytosis and cyclic neutropenia
Desmoplastic fibroma
Fibrous dysplasia
Gaucher disease, 272
Gorlin cyst (calcifying odontogenic cyst)
Hemangioma
Histiocytosis X
Hyperparathyroidism (loss of lamina
    dura), 290
Lymphangioma
Neoplasms
Papillon-Lefèvre syndrome, 157
Periodontitis
Teeth: natal
Adrenal hyperplasia (congenital), 238
Chondroectodermal dysplasia
Fetal akinesia sequence, 71
Hallermann-Streiff syndrome, 88
Hypoglossia–hypodactylia syndrome, 98
Jadassohn-Lewandowsky syndrome, 103
Robin sequence, 180

Rubinstein-Taybi syndrome, 182
Short rib–polydactyly syndrome type IV
Sotos syndrome, 195
Wiedemann-Rautenstrauch syndrome, 226
Teeth: premature loss
Cleidocranial dysplasia
Groll-Hirschowitz syndrome
Hajdu-Cheney syndrome, 87
Hyperphosphatasia, 293
Hypophosphatasia, 297
Insensitivity to pain (congenital), 101
Jadassohn-Lewandowsky syndrome, 103
Mandibuloacral dysplasia, 120
Papillon-Lefèvre syndrome, 157
Pycnodysostosis
Tricho-dento-osseous syndrome, 211
Werner syndrome, 224
Teeth: single maxillary central incisor
Chromosomal abnormalities (XXX
    female; 18p2; 7q2)
Holoprosencephaly, 94
Hypomelanosis of Ito, 98
Hypopituitarism, 298
Telangiectasia
Ataxia-telangiectasia syndrome, 14
Bloom syndrome, 20
Carcinoid syndrome, 252
CREST syndrome, 46
De Sanctis-Cacchione syndrome, 54
Dyskeratosis congenita, 60
Fetal alcohol syndrome, 71
Fetal hydantoin syndrome, 72
Goltz syndrome, 83
Hemihypertrophy, 90
Klippel-Trenaunay syndrome, 109
Radiation-induced telangiectasia
Rendu-Osler-Weber syndrome, 176
Rothmund-Thomson syndrome, 181
Sternal malformation–angiodysplasia
    association, 198
Turner syndrome, 214
Wegener granulomatosis
Xeroderma pigmentosa
Testes: large
Adrenal rests
Fragile X syndrome, 77
Growth hormone treatment
Hemihypertrophy, 90
Hypothyroidism, juvenile, 300
Precocious puberty, idiopathic
Proteus syndrome, 169

Testicular microlithiasis
Tumors
X-linked mental retardation
Testes: small/dysplastic
Chromosome 18p2 syndrome
Chromosome XXXY syndrome
Chromosome XXYY syndrome
Chromosome XY gonadal dysgenesis
Denys-Drash syndrome, 53
De Sanctis-Cacchione syndrome, 54
Dyskeratosis congenita, 60
Klinefelter syndrome, 108
Myotonic dystrophy
Polyorchidism
Schwartz-Jampel syndrome, 185
Thorax: shield-like; *refer to* Shield-like tho-
    rax
Thrombocythemia
Henoch-Schönlein syndrome, 91
Kawasaki syndrome, 106
Paraneoplastic syndromes, 344
Thrombocytopenia
Banti syndrome, 15
Chédiak-Higashi syndrome, 35
Chromosome 13 trisomy syndrome, 37
Chromosome 18 trisomy syndrome, 37
Congenital thrombocytopenia
Dyskeratosis congenita, 60
Fanconi anemia, 69
HELLP syndrome, 89
Hemolytic uremic syndrome, 90
Hyperthyroidism, 294
Kasabach-Merritt syndrome, 106
Kawasaki syndrome, 106
Klippel-Trenaunay syndrome, 109
Mixed connective tissue disease, 131
Roberts syndrome, 179
Sea-blue histiocyte syndrome, 188
Shwachman syndrome, 363
TAR syndrome, 206
Wiskott-Aldrich syndrome, 228
Thumb: broad
Apert syndrome, 11
Carpenter syndrome, 29
Chromosome 13 trisomy syndrome, 37
Fibrodysplasia ossificans progressiva, 74
Greig cephalopolysyndactyly syndrome,
    86
Hand-foot-genital syndrome, 89
Larsen syndrome, 112
Léri syndrome, 114

Meckel syndrome, 125
Oto-palato-digital syndrome type I, 154
Pfeiffer syndrome, 160
Rubinstein-Taybi syndrome, 182
Weaver-Smith syndrome, 223
Thumb: large
    Klippel-Trenaunay-Weber syndrome, 109
    Macrodactyly (*refer to* p. 427)
    Macrodystrophia lipomatosa, 119
    Maffucci syndrome, 119
    Neurofibromatosis I, 140
    Proteus syndrome, 169
Thumb: short, hypoplastic, or absent
    Aminopterin fetopathy, 8
    Baller-Gerold syndrome, 14
    Brachmann–de Lange syndrome, 22
    Cephaloskeletal dysplasia, 32
    Chromosomal abnormalities (9, 18, etc.)
    Fanconi anemia, 69
    Fibrodysplasia ossificans progressiva, 74
    Hand-foot-genital syndrome, 89
    Holt-Oram syndrome, 94
    Juberg-Hayward syndrome, 104
    Oto-palato-digital syndrome type I, 154
    Pterygium syndrome, popliteal, 171
    Rubinstein-Taybi syndrome (short), 182
    Symphalangism-surdity syndrome, 205
    TAR syndrome, 206
    Thalidomide embryopathy, 207
    VATER association, 218
    Werner syndrome, 224
Thumb: triphalangeal (TPT)
    Aase syndrome, 2
    Chromosome 13 trisomy syndrome, 37
    Chromosome 22 trisomy syndrome, 30
    Diamond-Blackfan syndrome, 54
    DOOR syndrome, 56
    Duane syndrome, 59
    Fanconi anemia, 69
    Fetal hydantoin syndrome, 72
    Holt-Oram syndrome, 94
    Hypomelanosis of Ito, 98
    Isolated TPT
    Juberg-Hayward syndrome, 104
    Lacrimo-auriculo-dento-digital syndrome, 111
    Poland sequence, 162
    Thalidomide embryopathy, 207
    Townes-Brocks syndrome, 210
    VATER association, 218

Thyroid dysfunction
    Alagille syndrome, 6
    Cowden syndrome, 44
    Cystinosis, 259
    de Morsier syndrome, 53
    Deprivation dwarfism, 260
    DiGeorge syndrome, 55
    Down syndrome, 57
    Johanson-Blizzard syndrome, 103
    Kocher-Debré-Sémélaigne syndrome, 307
    McCune-Albright syndrome, 125
    Multiple endocrine neoplasiatype IIA, 135
    Multiple endocrine neoplasiatype IIB, 135
    Nephrotic syndrome, 138
    Paraneoplastic syndromes, 344
    Pendred syndrome, 158
    POEMS syndrome, 161
    Polyglandular autoimmune disease, 352
    Pseudohypoparathyroidism, 355
    Thalassemia, 374
    Troell-Junet syndrome, 212
    Tuberous sclerosis, 212
    Turner syndrome, 214
Toe: broad
    Chromosome XXXXY syndrome
    Greig cephalopolysyndactyly syndrome, 86
    Oto-palato-digital syndrome type I, 154
    Pfeiffer syndrome, 160
    Rubinstein-Taybi syndrome, 182
Tongue: abnormality
    Beckwith-Wiedemann syndrome (large), 17
    Cerebro-costo-mandibular syndrome (forked tip), 33
    Cleft tongue
    Down syndrome (fissured, protruding), 57
    Ehlers-Danlos syndrome (ability to touch the tip of the nose), 63
    Fissured tongue
    Glossopalatine ankylosis syndrome
    Hairy tongue (chromogenic bacteria, smokers, etc.)
    Hypoglossia-hypodactylia syndrome, 98
    Indifference to pain (ulcers)
    Isolated tongue hemiatrophy
    Kocher-Debré-Sémélaigne syndrome (large), 307
    Lesch-Nyhan syndrome (ulcers), 310
    Lingua cochlearis (spoon-shaped tongue) in multiple pterygium syndrome

Meckel syndrome (lobulated), 125
Mucopolysaccharidosis I-H (large, protruding), 327
Multiple endocrine neoplasia type IIB (thick, nodular), 135
Oculo-auriculo-vertebral spectrum (deformed), 147
Oro-facio-digital syndrome I (cleft, lobulated), 150
Oro-facio-digital syndrome II (lobulated), 150
Prominent tuberculum impar associated with maxillary arch duplication
Robinow syndrome (large)
Trachea: congenital stenosis/cartilage anomaly
Apert syndrome, 11
Asplenia syndrome, 13
Cloverleaf skull deformity, 39
Crouzon syndrome, 47
Down syndrome, 57
Hydrolethalus syndrome, 95
Pfeiffer syndrome, 160
Trachea/bronchi: premature cartilage calcification
Association with congenital heart disease
Chondrodysplasia punctata
Hyperphosphatemia
Hypervitaminosis D
Idiopathic infantile hypercalcemia
Idiopathic isolated congenital tracheobronchial calcification
Keutel syndrome, 108
Relapsing polychondritis, 175
Warfarin embryopathy, 222
Warfarin therapy in children and adults
Trachea: short
DiGeorge syndrome, 55
GM$_1$ gangliosidosis, 278
Möbius syndrome, 132
Nager acrofacial dysostosis, 136
Spondylocostal dysostosis (Jarcho-Levin syndrome), 197
Tracheoesophageal fistula
Apert syndrome, 11
Asymmetric crying facies
CHARGE association, 34
Chromosome 18 trisomy syndrome, 37
DiGeorge syndrome, 55
Oculo-auriculo-vertebral spectrum, 147
VATER association, 218

Tracheomalacia
Cerebro-costo-mandibular syndrome, 33
Hallermann-Streiff syndrome, 88
Larsen syndrome, 112
Tracheomegaly/tracheobronchomegaly
Cystic fibrosis
Ehlers-Danlos syndrome, 63
Immune disorders
Mounier-Kuhn syndrome, 133
Trigonocephaly
Chromosomal abnormalities
Familial trigonocephaly
Holoprosencephaly, 94
Opitz trigonocephaly syndrome, 149
Tubular bones: bowed
Antley-Bixler syndrome, 11
Brachmann–de Lange syndrome, 22
Cloverleaf skull deformity, 39
Contractural arachnodactyly, 44
Epidermal nevus syndrome, 66
Fuhrmann syndrome, 79
GM$_1$ gangliosidosis, 278
Hemihypertrophy, 90
Homocystinuria, 285
Hydrolethalus syndrome, 95
Hyperparathyroidism, 290
Hyperphosphatasia, 293
Hypophosphatasia, 297
Infantile multisystem inflammatory disease, 100
Klippel-Trenaunay syndrome, 109
Larsen syndrome, 112
Maffucci syndrome, 119
Mucolipidoses, 323, 324, 325
Mucopolysaccharidoses, 325
Neurofibromatosis I, 140
Occipital horn syndrome, 341
Ophthalmo-mandibulo-melicdysplasia, 148
Osteolysis with nephropathy, 153
Osteomalacia, 360
Oto-palato-digital syndrome type I, 154
Pseudohypoparathyroidism, 355
Rickets, 359
Schwarz-Lélek syndrome, 185
Weismann-Netter syndrome, 224
Tubular bones: broad
Gaucher disease, 272
GM$_1$ gangliosidosis, 278
Hyperphosphatasia, 293
Infantile multisystem inflammatory disease, 100

Iron deficiency anemia, 305
Léri syndrome, 114
Mucolipidoses, 323, 324, 325
Mucopolysaccharidoses, 325
Neu-Laxova syndrome, 139
Niemann-Pick disease, 336
Oculo-dento-osseous dysplasia, 147
Oto-palato-digital syndrome type I, 154
Schwarz-Lélek syndrome, 185
Singleton-Merten syndrome, 191
Thalassemia, 374
Tubular bones: cortical hyperostosis; thickening
Acromegaly, 235
Dubowitz syndrome, 59
Erdheim-Chester disease, 265
Gaucher disease, 272
Gigantism, 236
Hyperostosis-hyperphosphatemia syn-
drome, 97
Hyperparathyroidism, 290
Hyperphosphatasia, 293
Hypothyroidism, 300
Klippel-Trenaunay-Webersyndrome, 109
Lipodystrophies, 311
Mannosidoses, 316
McCune-Albright syndrome, 125
Neurofibromatosis I (hemorrhage), 140
Osteoarthropathy, familial idiopathic,
152
Pachydermoperiostosis, 155
Rickets, 359
Sickle cell anemia, 365
Tricho-dento-osseous syndrome, 211
Tuberous sclerosis, 212
Tumoral calcinosis, 377
Vitamin A intoxication, 380
Vitamin D intoxication, 382
Weismann-Netter syndrome, 224
Tubular bones: slender
Caudal dysplasia sequence, 31
Cockayne syndrome, 40
Contractural arachnodactyly, 44
Fetal akinesia sequence, 71
Hallermann-Streiff syndrome, 88
Hypopituitarism (anterior lobe), 298
Marshall-Smith syndrome, 123
Muscular disorders
Neurofibromatosis I, 140
Neurologic disorders
Osteogenesis imperfecta, type I, III, IV

Pterygium syndrome (lethal multiple
pterygium), 171
The 3-M syndrome, 208
Winchester syndrome, 384

U
Ulna/ulnar ray: aplasia, hypoplasia
Brachmann–de Lange syndrome, 22
Postaxial acrofacial dysostosis, Miller
type, 164
Roberts syndrome, 179
Ulnar-mammary syndrome, 217
Weyers oligodactyly syndrome, 226
Uterus: anomaly
Apert syndrome, 11
Beckwith-Wiedemann syndrome, 17
Chromosome 13 trisomy syndrome, 37
Chromosome 18 trisomy syndrome, 37
Fraser syndrome, 77
Hand-foot-genital syndrome, 89
Johanson-Blizzard syndrome, 103
Mayer-Rokitansky-Küster syndrome, 124
MURCS association, 136
Roberts syndrome, 179
Schinzel-Giedion syndrome, 184
Spondylocostal dysostoses (Jarcho-Levin
syndrome), 197

V
Vagina: atresia, occlusion
Antley-Bixler syndrome, 11
Dyskeratosis congenita, 60
EEC syndrome, 62
Fraser syndrome, 77
Mayer-Rokitansky-Küster syndrome, 124
MURCS association, 136
Renal-genital-ear anomalies, 175
Sirenomelia, 192
Varices, venous dilatation
Alpha$_1$-antitrypsin deficiency, 243
Banti syndrome, 15
Budd-Chiari syndrome, 25
Cruveilhier-Baumgarten syndrome, 48
Ehlers-Danlos syndrome, 63
Fabry disease, 266
Klippel-Trenaunay syndrome, 109
Maffucci syndrome, 119
Marfan syndrome, 121
Occipital horn syndrome, 341
Rendu-Osler-Weber syndrome, 176
Superior vena cava syndrome

Vasculopathy
Behçet syndrome, 18
Churg-Strauss syndrome, 38
Cogan syndrome, 43
Dermatomyositis
Familial polyarteritis nodosa
Giant-cell arteritis
Henoch-Schönlein syndrome, 91
Kawasaki syndrome, 106
Moyamoya
Reiter syndrome, 174
Relapsing polychondritis, 175
Sweet syndrome, 204
Takayasu arteritis
Wegener granulomatosis
Vasomotor symptoms
Carcinoid syndrome, 252
Dumping syndrome, 60
Horner syndrome, 95
Raynaud syndrome, 173
Reflex sympathetic dystrophy syndrome
Riley-Day syndrome, 178
Thevenard syndrome, 208
Veins: anomalies
Aplasia cutis congenita, 12
Asplenia syndrome, 13
Cruveilhier-Baumgarten syndrome, 48
Hepatic fibrosis–renal cysticdisease, 92
Polysplenia syndrome, 163
Scimitar syndrome, 186
Turner syndrome, 214
Wiedemann-Rautenstrauch syndrome, 226
Wrinkly skin syndrome, 230
Veins: occlusion (partial; complete)
Budd-Chiari syndrome, 25
Superior vena cava syndrome
Thoracic outlet syndrome, 208
Veins: thrombosis
Antiphospholipid syndrome, 10
Aplasia cutis congenita, 12
Behçet syndrome, 18
Budd-Chiari syndrome, 25
Carpal tunnel syndrome, 28
Congenital renal vein thrombosis
Glucagonoma syndrome, 274
Hereditary pancreatitis
Homocystinuria, 285
Hughes-Stovin syndrome, 95
Infants of diabetic mothers
Lemierre syndrome

Nephrotic syndrome, 138
Paget-Schroetter syndrome, 156
Polycythemia vera
Protein C deficiency
Protein S deficiency, 354
Superior vena cava syndrome
Tolosa-Hunt syndrome, 209
Vertebrae: anterior beaked body in children
Adenosine deaminase deficiency
Aspartylglucosaminuria, 247
Fucosidosis, 270
GM$_1$ gangliosidosis, 278
Hypothyroidism, 300
Mannosidoses, 316
Mucolipidoses, 323, 324, 325
Mucopolysaccharidoses, 325
Neuromuscular disorders
Niemann-Pick disease, 336
Normal variant, mild beaking (thora-columbar junction)
Phenylketonuria, 350
Thalassemia (deferoxamine-treated), 374
Vertebrae: malsegmentation, fusion, agenesis
Aicardi syndrome, 6
Alagille syndrome, 6
Apert syndrome, 11
Binder syndrome, 19
Caudal dysplasia sequence, 31
CHILD syndrome, 36
Crouzon syndrome, 47
Currarino triad, 49
Fanconi anemia, 69
Femoral hypoplasia–unusual facies syndrome, 70
Fetal alcohol syndrome, 71
Goltz syndrome, 83
Gorlin syndrome, 85
Holt-Oram syndrome, 94
Incontinentia pigmenti, 100
Infant of diabetic mother
Klippel-Feil syndrome, 109
Larsen syndrome, 112
LEOPARD syndrome, 113
MURCS association, 136
Noonan syndrome, 145
Oculo-auriculo-vertebral spectrum, 147
Pfeiffer syndrome, 160
Poland sequence, 162
Pterygium syndrome (multiple), 171
Robin sequence, 180

Robinow syndrome
Saethre-Chotzen syndrome, 183
Split notochord syndrome, 196
Spondylo-carpo-tarsal synostosis syndrome, 197
Spondylocostal dysostoses, 197
Tethered cord syndrome, 207
VATER association, 218
Wildervanck syndrome, 226
Vertebrae: tall
Antley-Bixler syndrome, 11
Chromosomal abnormalities
Freeman-Sheldon syndrome, 78
Hypotonia
Infantile multisystem inflammatory disease, 100
Proteus syndrome, 169
Spondylocostal dysostoses, 197
Voice abnormality
Brachmann–de Lange syndrome, 22
Cardiovocal syndrome, 27
Chromosome 5: del (5p) syndrome (cat-cry syndrome), 37
Cutis laxa, 49
Farber disease, 268
Hajdu-Cheney syndrome, 87
Hypopituitarism (anterior lobe), 298
Hypothyroidism, 300
Jadassohn-Lewandowsky syndrome, 103
Lipoid proteinosis, 313
Lowe syndrome, 314
Mucopolysaccharidosis I-H, 327
Opitz BBBG syndrome, 149

Progeria, 168
Relapsing polychondritis, 175
Rüdiger syndrome, 183
Schwartz-Jampel syndrome, 185
Smith-Lemli-Opitz syndrome type I, 370
Weaver syndrome, 223
Werner syndrome, 224

W
Wormian bones (sutural bones)
Acrogeria, 4
Aminopterin fetopathy, 8
Aplasia cutis congenita, 12
Copper deficiency, 258
Down syndrome, 57
Hajdu-Cheney syndrome, 87
Hallermann-Streiff syndrome, 88
Hydrocephalus
Hypophosphatasia, 297
Hypothyroidism (cretinism), 300
Infantile multisystem inflammatory disease, 100
Mandibuloacral dysplasia, 120
Menkes disease, 319
Normal variant
Osteoarthropathy, familial idiopathic, 152
Osteogenesis imperfecta (I, III, IV)
Pachydermoperiostosis, 155
Prader-Willi syndrome, 166
Progeria, 168
Schinzel-Giedion syndrome, 184
Zellweger syndrome, 386